Uppers, Downers, All Arounders

Physical and Mental Effects of Psychoactive Drugs

Fifth Edition

Darryl S. Inaba, Pharm.D.

Chief Executive Officer, Haight Ashbury Free Clinics
Associate Clinical Professor of Pharmacology,
University of California Medical Center, San Francisco

William E. Cohen

Communications and Education Consultant,
Haight Ashbury Detox Clinic
President, CNS Productions, Inc.™

CNS Publications, Inc.™
Ashland, Oregon

CNS Publications, Inc.™

Publisher: Paul J. Steinbroner
130 Third St.
P.O. Box 96
Ashland, OR 97520
Tel: (541) 488-2805   Fax: (541) 482-9252
Web Site: www.cnsproductions.com

Uppers, Downers, All Arounders, Fifth Edition
Second Printing
© 2004, William E. Cohen & Darryl S. Inaba
First Edition   © 1989
Second Edition   © 1993
Third Edition   © 1996
Fourth Edition   © 2000

Editor: **Carol A. Caruso**

Book Design: **Connie Wolfe/Data Management, Inc.**, Cedar Rapids, Iowa

Illustrations: **David Ruppe/Impact Publications**, Medford, Oregon

Cover Art: **Alexis Le Bars/Integrity Print Management**, Jacksonville, Oregon

Printing and Color Separations: **Cedar Graphics**, Cedar Rapids, Iowa

Student Study Guide & Peer Review: **Thomas G. Ten Eyck M.A., CADC II, CGAC,** Adjunct Professor of Addictions, Lewis & Clark Graduate School, Portland, Oregon, Mount Hood Community College, Gresham Oregon, and Chemeketa Community College, Salem, Oregon

Student Study Guide CD-ROM Design: **Sharp Design/Robert Sharp**, Medford, Oregon

Cowriter, Chapter 10: **Pablo Stewart, M.D.,** Chief of Psychiatry, Haight Ashbury Free Clinics, Associate Clinical Professor of Psychiatry, University of California, School of Medicine, San Francisco, California

Special thanks to:
Michael Aldrich, Ph.D., Curator, Fitz Hugh Ludlow Memorial Library, San Francisco, California
Daniel Amen, M.D., Psychiatrist and Founder of the Amen Clinic for Behavioral Medicine, Fairfield & Newport Beach, California
Rick Seymour, M.A., Editor, Journal of Psychoactive Drugs, Director of Training and Education, Haight Ashbury Free Clinics, San Francisco, California
David E. Smith, M.D., Founder, Haight Ashbury Free Clinics, San Francisco, California
Florence Sage, M.A., M.Ed., LPC, Social Sciences Faculty, Clatsop Community College, Astoria, Oregon

DISCLAIMER: Information in this book is in no way meant to replace professional medical advice or professional counseling and treatment.

Publisher's Cataloging-in-Publication
Inaba, Darryl.
   Uppers, downers, all arounders: physical and mental
effects of psychoactive drugs / Darryl S. Inaba, William
E. Cohen. — 5th ed.
   p. cm.
   Includes bibliographical references and index.
   LCCN: 00-105811
   ISBN 0-92654427-6
   1. Psychoactive drugs—Side effects. 2. Drug abuse—
Complications. I. Cohen, William E., 1941- II. Title

RM332.I43 2003   616.86
          QB103-200652

Printed in the United States of America

T his Fifth Edition of Uppers, Downers, All Arounders is lovingly dedicated to the memory of my father, Paul L. Steinbroner (1921–2001) who recently succumbed to the complications of Alzheimer's disease. Paul was a founding member of the company and served as its President for 10 years. His generosity and wisdom enabled us to establish CNS Productions 20 years ago. We are grateful for the opportunity he gave us.

Paul J. Steinbroner
Publisher

PREFACE

One of the major changes in the *Fifth Edition of Uppers, Downers, All Arounders* has been the technique of **highlighting key phrases** throughout each chapter to emphasize the most important idea in each paragraph or group of paragraphs to help the reader prioritize a large body of information.

The other major change has been the inclusion of a **Student Study Guide** on **CD-ROM** to further help the student learn the central themes and ideas presented. The Student Study Guide can be utilized in the computer or printed out and used independently of a computer. The Student Study Guide includes an introduction, a chapter outline, a guided review, key word/phrase identification, sample tests, a drug function test, and a complete glossary

In addition our **web site**, which can be accessed at *http://www.cnsproductions.com*, has been updated with articles and key links to enable the student to connect with additional information on substance abuse and treatment.

The information and quotations in this book are based on the experience and clinical expertise of the 130 staff members of the Haight Ashbury Detox Clinic in San Francisco, California, and on the experiences of more than 200,000 clients who have been treated at the Clinic over the past 37 years.

The Haight Ashbury Drug Detox Clinic's treatment program has one of the highest caseloads and best success rates in the country due in part to its success in drug education. The Clinic has found that objective nonjudgmental information about drugs and their effects is important in treatment and crucial in drug abuse prevention.

Note: In order to distinguish between trade (brand) names and chemical (generic) names of prescription and over-the-counter drugs, we have included the trademark symbol ® after all trade names.

CONTENTS

Psychoactive Drugs:
History & Classification

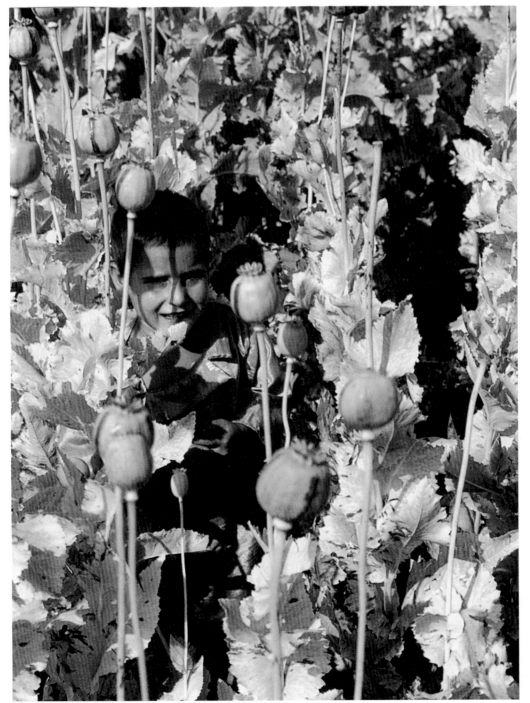

This poppy field in Afghanistan and others like it were used to produce 70% of the world's opium. Before the Taliban government fell it banned opium growing and for a brief period none was grown. It has since resumed. The vast profits from opium growing and heroin processing in Afghanistan and other countries, such as Myanmar (Burma), have funded wars, insurgencies, and terrorism activities throughout recent world history.
© 1990 Alain Labrousse.

INTRODUCTION

- **Five themes of drug use become apparent when studying history:**
  1. a basic need of human beings to cope with their environment and existence;
  2. the natural vulnerability of brain chemistry to psychoactive drugs;
  3. government and business involvement in selling and taxing drugs;
  4. technological advances in refining and synthesizing drugs;
  5. development of more efficient and faster methods of putting drugs in the body.

HISTORY OF PSYCHOACTIVE DRUGS

- **Prehistory & the Neolithic Period (8500–4000 B.C.):** The earliest human uses of psychoactive drugs involved plants and fruits whose mood-altering qualities were accidentally discovered and then deliberately cultivated.
- **Ancient Civilizations (4000 B.C.–A.D. 400):** Sumerian, Egyptian, Indian, Chinese, South American tribes, and other ancient cultures used opium, alcohol, *Cannabis* (marijuana), peyote, psychedelic mushrooms, and coca leaves.
- **Middle Ages (400–1400):** Psychoactive plants, such as belladonna and psilocybin mushrooms, were used by witches, shamans, and medicine men for healing and spiritual purposes.
- **Renaissance & the Age of Discovery (1400–1700):** Tobacco, coffee, tea, distilled alcohol, and opium smoking spread along the trade routes. Governments and merchants controlled much of the trade.
- **Age of Enlightenment & the Early Industrial Revolution (1700–1900):** New refinement techniques (e.g., morphine from opium), new delivery methods (e.g., hypodermic needle), and new manufacturing techniques (e.g., cigarette-rolling machines) increased use, abuse, and addiction liability. Temperance and prohibition movements also spread.
- **Twentieth Century:** Wider distribution channels, improved refinement technology, new synthetic drugs, and social/political changes increased legal and illegal use. Defining addiction as a disease and as a biochemical imbalance helped expand treatment options.
- **Today & Tomorrow:** The geopolitics of growing, refining, smuggling, and selling drugs affects the national security of dozens of countries. Alcohol, tobacco, marijuana, heroin, cocaine, and methamphetamines are still the drugs of choice but old and new rave club drugs are showing increased popularity, e.g., MDMA (ecstasy), GHB, ketamine, LSD, *Salvia divinorum,* and nitrous oxide. Finally federal and state drug policy is shifting from supply reduction to demand reduction.
- **Conclusions:** The history of man reflects the integral part psychoactive drugs have played in the social, economic, and emotional development of civilizations and while the current drug of choice often changes, the reasons for drug use remain the same. The "war on terrorism" and the so-called war on drugs both need long-term strategies that require imagination, resolve, patience, and intelligence.

CLASSIFICATION OF PSYCHOACTIVE DRUGS

- **What Is a Psychoactive Drug?** Psychoactive drugs can be identified by their street name, chemical name, or trade name. This book classifies most drugs by their general effects.
- **Major Drugs**
  - ◇ **Uppers:** Stimulants, such as cocaine, amphetamines, caffeine, and nicotine, force the release of energy chemicals. The strongest stimulants, cocaine and amphetamines, can produce an intense rush and ecstatic feelings.
  - ◇ **Downers:** Depressants include opioids (e.g., heroin), sedative-hypnotics, and alcohol. They depress circulatory, respiratory, and muscular systems; they control pain; they lower inhibitions; and they can induce euphoria.
  - ◇ **All Arounders:** Psychedelics, e.g., marijuana, LSD, MDMA (ecstasy), can cause some stimulation but mostly they alter sensory input and can cause illusions, delusions, and hallucinations.
- **Other Drugs & Addictions**
  - ◇ **Inhalants** include organic solvents, volatile nitrites, and nitrous oxide (laughing gas) and can induce the full range of upper, downer, or psychedelic effects depending on the specific substance and the amount used.
  - ◇ **Anabolic Steroids** and other sports drugs are used to enhance athletic performance by increasing endurance, muscle size, and/or aggression.
  - ◇ **Psychiatric Medications** include antidepressants, antipsychotics, and antianxiety drugs. They are prescribed to rebalance brain chemistry when there are mental problems.
  - ◇ **Compulsive Behaviors**, such as overeating, anorexia, bulimia, compulsive gambling, sexual compulsion, Internet addiction, compulsive shopping, and even codependency, affect many of the same areas of the brain influenced by psychoactive drugs.
- **Controlled Substances Act of 1970:** This act consolidated and updated most drug laws. Its aim was to reduce the availability, use, and abuse of psychoactive drugs.

HARDING'S PEN SPEEDS DRIVE AGAINST DRUGS

President Signs Congress Re-solution to Join with Other Nations in Limiting Supply

Negotiations to Open at Once with Land the Bases of Cocaine

COOLIDGE SIGNS BILL FOR DOPE-CURE FARMS

NEW U.S. LAW WILL HELP END NARCOTIC EVIL, SAVE ADDICTS

JANUARY, 20, 1929
All Drug Slave" Convicts Will

Los Angeles Times

HOOVER BACKS U.S. IN DOPE WAR

WASHINGTON, Jan 21 - President Hoover today sent a message to Congress rec-

Reagan, Congress Call for Drug War

Clinton to Announce New Drug Plan

volved in educating youths

's budget for the 1999 lls for spending $1.1 or drug-control mea- ll departments, rep- tly less than a 7 per-

and arti- ster- ma-

Washington

Bush plans hit on drug abuse

White House goal is to reduce 'crisis' by 25% in five years

INTRODUCTION

Athenian: *"Let us not then simply censure the gift of Dionysus as bad and unfit to be received into the State. For wine has many excellences.... Shall we begin by enacting that boys shall not taste wine at all until they are eighteen years of age; we will tell them that fire must not be poured upon fire, whether in the body or in the soul."*

Plato, 360 B.C., *The Laws*

Even 2,363 years ago societies had to grapple with the same positive and negative aspects of alcohol and other psychoactive drugs that the world struggles with in the twenty-first century. Whether it has been to alter states of consciousness, reduce pain, forget harsh surroundings, alter a mood, explore feelings, promote so-

cial interaction, escape boredom, medicate a mental illness, stimulate creativity, or enhance the senses, **throughout history some people have chosen to alter their perception of reality with substances**. Which drugs are used, how they are used, and how abuse is punished, treated, or prevented have varied from culture to culture and from century to century but certain themes transcend time and cultural makeup.

FIVE HISTORICAL THEMES OF DRUG USE

1. Human beings have a basic need to find ways to cope with their environment and existence.

Early man lived in a dangerous and mysterious environment that could inflict pain and death in an instant. Brutal weather, carnivorous animals, aggressive enemies, abusive relatives, and life-threatening diseases could wound, maim, or kill. Primitive and eventually civilized human beings have continually searched for ways to control these dangers. They drew cave pictures of animals 20,000 years ago in France to help in the hunt. They built the city of Jericho 10,000 years ago so they could grow and control their supply of food and protect themselves from their enemies. They worshipped hundreds of gods, praying for divine intervention that would let them survive. They fasted, danced incessantly, practiced self-hypnosis, chanted, inflicted pain on themselves, went without sleep, meditated, and used other nondrug methods so they could receive revelations from the gods (Furst, 1976; La Barre, 1979a). By chance and by experimentation **they found that ingesting certain plants could ease fear and anxiety, reduce pain, treat some illnesses, give pleasure, and let them talk to their gods** in order to control their environment. Our modern environment also has uncertainties, pains, illnesses, and fears (including fear of boredom) that can cause a person to experiment with and possibly abuse psychoactive drugs.

2. The human brain chemistry can be affected by psychoactive drugs to induce an altered state of consciousness or mood.

If psychoactive drugs did not affect human brain chemistry in a desirable manner, then they would not be used. All psychoactive drugs affect the primitive or old part of the brain that controls emotions, natural physiological functions (e.g., breathing, heart rate), emotional memories, sensory perception, physical and emotional pain, and instincts. They also affect the reasoning and memory centers of the new brain called the "neocortex." Parts of these survival mechanisms and neurochemicals in the brain evolved hundreds of millions of years ago in invertebrate creatures, such as insects and snails, and grew in complexity in vertebrate creatures, especially Homo sapiens (Nesse & Berridge, 1997).

3. Governments and businesses have been involved in cultivating, manufacturing, distributing, taxing, and prohibiting drugs.

The intensity of the demand for substances that could relieve pain and induce pleasure has matched the **struggles for control of the supplies**. The desire for control of the supplies has resulted in the

◇ use of opium by the medicine men of ancient Sumeria for their secret medicines;

◇ doling out of beer by the pharaohs of Egypt to keep their slaves building pyramids;

◇ **monopolization** of coca leaf growing by the Conquistadors in Peru to increase tax revenues for Spain;

◇ exportation of and **excise taxes** on whiskey, hemp, and tobacco to finance the American Revolution;

◇ sale of opium to China by Britain, France, Japan, and other imperial powers to **support their colonies**;

◇ growing and smuggling opium in Afghanistan to **support insurgency activities**;

◇ and **prohibition or restriction** of alcohol, tobacco, opium, and most every other psychoactive drug by virtually every country at one time or another to control excessive drug use.

4. Technological advances in refining and synthesizing drugs have increased the potency of these substances.

Over the centuries, various cultures have learned how to

◇ **distill** alcoholic beverages to higher potency (Arabia, tenth century);

◇ **refine** morphine from opium (Germany, 1803);

◇ refine cocaine from coca leaves (Germany, 1859);

◇ create alcohol sedation in pill form by synthesizing barbiturates (Germany, 1868 and 1908);

◇ **synthesize** the stimulant amphetamine to create a replacement for scarce cocaine (Germany, 1887 and 1932);

◇ **extract** LSD from the ergot fungus (Switzerland, 1938);

◇ **use the sinsemilla-growing technique** to increase the THC content of marijuana (United States, 1960–1980);

◇ **modify** the amphetamine molecules to produce designer drugs like MDA and MDMA (ecstasy) (United States, 1910–present).

These and other techniques have enabled drug users to put larger and more potent amounts of a substance in their bodies.

5. The development of more efficient and faster methods of putting drugs in the body has intensified the effects.

Technological and pragmatic discoveries have taught researchers and/or users to

◇ **mix** alcohol and opium for stronger effects (Sumeria, 4000 B.C.);

◇ **absorb** more juice from the chewed coca leaf by mixing it with charred oyster shells (Peru, 1450);

◇ **inhale** nitrous oxide to become giddy and high (England, 1800);

◇ **inject** morphine to put the drug directly into the bloodstream (England, 1855);

◇ **snort** cocaine to absorb the drug more quickly (Europe, 1900);

◇ dissolve LSD onto blotter paper so the drug can be absorbed on the tongue (United States, 1960s);

◇ **smoke** cocaine freebase and crack to intensify the high (United States, 1975–1985);

◇ **crush and inject time-release medications**, such as the opiate pain reliever OxyContin®, for a bigger rush (United States, 2003).

When the history of substance use is closely examined, the five themes identified above appear time and time again. By studying the recurrent nature of drug use and abuse, treatment and prevention solutions become clearer.

"Most of the crime in our city is caused by cocaine."
Police Chief of Atlanta, Georgia, 1911

HISTORY OF PSYCHOACTIVE DRUGS

PREHISTORY & THE NEOLITHIC PERIOD (8500–4000 B.C.)

Many of the drugs available today have antecedents in psychoactive plants that have been around for millions of years. It has been estimated that **4,000 plants yield psychoactive substances** although only about 150 have historically been used for that purpose. Approximately 60 of those plants are still used; opium, marijuana, coca, tea, betel, khat, coffee, tobacco, and plants that ferment into alcohol have been the most popular over the centuries (Austin, 1979).

Evidence exists that 50,000 years ago Neanderthals in Europe and Asia used medicinal and psychedelic plants such as the fly-agaric mushroom in shamanic religions as a way to deal with their environment. **The shaman, a combination priest/doctor, was the key figure in these religions and functioned as a conduit to the supernatural** using naturally induced (e.g., fasting and dancing) and drug-induced altered states of consciousness.

The use of psychoactive substances spread through tribal migration. One hypothesis maintains that the earliest Native Americans were Eurasians who migrated to the Americas about 10,000–15,000 years ago bringing their customs, religions, and drugs, like the hallucinogenic mescal bean and sophora seeds, with them (Furst, 1976; La Barre, 1979a).

Alcohol has been the most popular psychoactive substance over the millennia. This food/medicine/drug has been with us since Prehistoric times. Perhaps hunger, thirst, or curiosity made early humans eat or drink fruits that had begun to ferment (chemically change into alcohol due to airborne yeast). They also discovered that chewing starchy vegetation would provide the catalyst, found in saliva, to convert the more complex carbohydrates into alcohol. Liking the taste, the nutrition, and the psychoactive effects, particularly the drunken states that made them feel closer to their gods, they learned how to make fermented beverages themselves (O'Brien & Chafetz, 1991). They collected honey to ferment into mead, an alcoholic beverage; they cultivated grains to ferment starchy foods into beer; and finally they cultivated grapes and other fruits to make wine. These agricultural experiments are the earliest signs of organized efforts to guarantee a steady supply of a desirable psychoactive substance.

ANCIENT CIVILIZATIONS (4000 B.C.–A.D. 400)

Nomadic tribes had begun to settle into small agricultural communities 10,000–20,000 years ago and over the millennia gradually grew, accumulating power and influence. Great civilizations arose where the land was fertile, usually next to rivers such as the Tigris and Euphrates in the Middle East and the Nile in Egypt. **The earliest crops were wheat and barley, used to make bread and beer** (beer was much more nutritious than it is today) (Ganeri, Martell, & Williams, 1998). Asian civilizations used rice as a staple food and to make wine. **Some ancient cultures also cultivated the opium poppy and hemp plant (*Cannabis* or marijuana).**

ALCOHOL

Recently jars found in a neolithic kitchen in the Middle East, dating to 5000 B.C., contained a residue of wine (McGovern, Gluskee, Exner, & Voight, 1998). Wine was so prized that important citizens were buried with their own personal drinking cup (O'Brien, 1991). The **first written references to alcohol are Sumerian clay tablets from 4000 B.C.** found in ancient Mesopotamia (now Iraq and Iran). They contained recipes for using wine as a solvent for medications including opium.

Many ancient cultures considered alcohol, particularly wine, a gift from the gods. In legends Osiris gave alcohol to the Egyptians as did Dionysus to the Greeks and Bacchus to the Romans. In ancient Egypt a barley beer called *"hek"* was given as a reward to slaves building the great pyramids. The value of *hek* was such that bureaucrats were appointed to control its production. In a medical papyrus about 15% of the prescriptions contained beer or wine (Keller, 1984). In many cultures beer was the drink of the workers and wine of the pharaohs as evidenced by earthen jars in King Tut's tomb, which noted the year (vintage) of the wine and the location of the vineyard.

Rice wine was the drink of the masses in ancient China and later Japan but grape wine was more highly prized. In about 180 B.C. a gift of grape wine was sufficient to serve as a bribe to get a civil service job (Lee, 1987). The Jewish people have historically used wine as part of their religious and secular celebrations including circumcisions, weddings, and the Sabbath. Though the Hebrews had eight different wines for various rites and the highest percentage of drinkers, historically they had one of the lowest rates of alcoholism because drunkenness was frowned upon (Keller, 1984). Heredity probably was also part of the reason.

The reaction of the human brain and body to alcohol caused not only the desired effects but also side effects capable of causing social and health problems. As a result most **civilizations throughout history have placed religious, social, and legal controls on the use of alcohol and other drugs.** In fact there are 150 biblical references to alcohol, often warnings.

"Drunk at the right time and in the right amount, wine makes for a glad heart and a cheerful mind. Bitterness of soul comes of wine drunk to excess out of temper or bravado. Drunkenness excites the stupid to a fury to his own harm, it reduces his strength while leading to blows."

The <u>Bible</u>, Ecclesiasticus, 31, 27

One of the **earliest attempts at temperance (limiting drinking) occurred in China around 2200 B.C.** when the legendary Emperor Yu levied a tax on wine in order to curtail consumption. Centuries later, during the Chu dynasty (1122–249 B.C.), the penalties for drunkenness were extremely severe for the lower classes while the upper classes were given a chance at recovery (Cherrington, 1924).

"As to the ministers and officers who have been ... addicted to drink, it is not necessary to put them to death; let them be taught for a time.... If you disregard my lessons, then I ... will show you no pity."

Emperor Wu Wang, Founder of Chu dynasty, 1120 B.C.

Another early documented attempt to regulate alcohol use dates back to the Babylonian *Code of Hammurabi* in 1770 B.C. This code set forth standards of measurement for drink and outlined the responsibilities of tavern owners. (It also showed the status of women in ancient times.)

"If a 'sister of a god' open a tavern, or enter a tavern to drink, then shall this woman be burned to death."

<u>Code of Hammurabi</u>, Babylonia, 1770 B.C.

Heavy drinking was recognized as a problem by the Egyptians in 1500 B.C. when their hieroglyphics recommended the moderate consumption of beer. In ancient religious hymns (*Vedas*) **in India, alcohol was considered to cause falsity, misery, and darkness** while the favorable aspects of alcohol were dismissed. Greek soci-

ety appreciated the dangers of heavy drinking and recommended diluting wine with water. In spite of the fact that many ancient Greek poets, philosophers, and writers, including Plato, Homer, Anacreon, and Aeschilus, drank wine all day, every day, warnings abounded, reinforced with cautionary tales of battles lost due to drunkenness (O'Brien, 1991).

"Socrates took his place on the couch, and supped with the rest; and then libations were offered ... they were about to commence drinking, when Pausanias said, 'And now, my friends, how can we drink with least injury to ourselves? I can assure you that I feel severely the effect of yesterday's potations, and must have time to recover; and I suspect that most of you are in the same predicament, for you were of the party yesterday.'"

Plato, 360 B.C., <u>The Symposium</u>

Unfortunately the temperance of later Greek society embodied in **Dionysus (god of wine and ecstasy)** gave way to binge drinking in Roman society, encouraged by **Bacchus**, a more liberal version of Dionysus.

"The delights of wine and feasts were added to the religious elements of the bacchanals. When wine inflamed their minds, and night and promiscuity ... erased any feelings of modesty, all manner of corruptions began to be practiced."

<u>Ad Urbe Condita</u>, VIII, 5–8

Orgiastic drinking became such a problem in the Roman Empire that in A.D. 81 the Emperor Comitian destroyed half the nation's vineyards and prohibited the planting of new ones (Keller, 1984). The conflict between heavy consumption and temperance continued. By the fourth century A.D. heavy drinkers were led through town by a cord strung through their noses. Habitual offenders were tied with the nose cord and left for ridicule in the public square.

OPIUM

Remnants of ancient poppy plantations in Spain, Greece, northeast Africa, Egypt, and Mesopotamia (in the Mideast) give evidence of the early use of opium (Escohotado, 1999). For example, around 4000 B.C. the Sumerians in southern **Mesopotamia culti-**

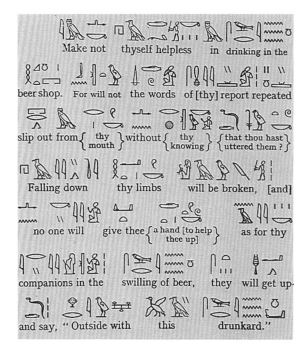

Make not thyself helpless in drinking in the beer shop. For will not the words of [thy] report repeated slip out from { thy mouth } without { thy knowing } { that thou hast uttered them? } Falling down thy limbs will be broken, [and] no one will give thee { a hand [to help] thee up } as for thy companions in the swilling of beer, they will get up and say, "Outside with this drunkard."

This Egyptian hieroglyphic from 1500 B.C. advised moderation in barley beer drinking as well as avoidance of other compulsive behaviors. Written Egyptian references to alcohol have been unearthed that date back to 3500 B.C.

Translation from *Precepts of Ani,* World Health Organization

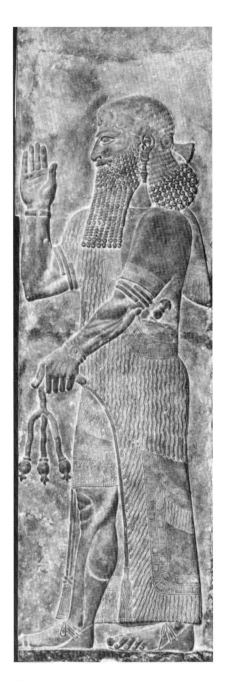

An Assyrian priest carries opium poppies as part of a ceremony to sacrifice a gazelle to the gods, circa eighth century B.C.
The Louvre Museum.

• •

vated the opium poppy in addition to barley and wheat, their basic agricultural crops. They named it *"Hul Gil,"* the plant of joy. The milky white fluid from the dried bulb was boiled to a sticky gum and chewed, burned and inhaled, or mixed with fermented liquids and drunk. It was **used for both its me-**dicinal properties of pain relief, cough suppression, and diarrhea control as well as its mental properties of sedation and euphoria (Hoffman, 1990). Because it was only ingested and not smoked as in later centuries, its bitter taste and the moderate concentration of active ingredients limited the abuse potential. Even the stalk of the poppy was used as fodder for the animals while the seeds were cooked in breads and other foods (Scarborough, 1995).

In ancient civilizations opium was used in many ways. Early Egyptian medical texts referred to it as a medicine and as a poison. In Egypt it was fed to crying babies to calm their discomfort and fears. In the *Odyssey* Homer spoke about an opium mixture, called *"nepenthe,"* given by Helen of Troy to Telemachus to banish unwanted feelings.

"Then Jove's daughter Helen bethought her of another matter. She drugged the wine with an herb that banishes all care, sorrow, and ill humour. Whoever drinks wine thus drugged cannot shed a single tear all the rest of the day, not even though his father and mother both of them drop down dead, or he sees a brother or a son hewn in pieces before his very eyes."
Homer, 700 B.C., Odyssey, IV, 221–226

Greek statues and paintings often show their gods and heroes, including Jason and Theseus, holding poppies, which they used to sedate their enemies (Hoffman, 1990). **Hippocrates, the Father of Medicine, recommended opium** as a painkiller and as a treatment for female hysteria. Centuries later in the Roman Empire Marcus Aurelius, writer, philosopher, and emperor (A.D. 161–181), would drink a potion of opium mixed with wine as a daily balm.

Even though opium was in short supply in Rome, the price was fixed by law. In A.D. 312 there were 793 stores that sold the substance and in fact the **excise tax on opium provided 15% of the city's revenue** (Escohotado, 1999). Because of its value drug fraud was common even 2,500 years ago. One of the duties of physicians was to detect counterfeit opium. The best opium was "thick and heavy and soporific to the smell, bitter to the taste, easily diluted in water, smooth, white, neither rough nor full of lumps" (Dioscorides, A.D. 70).

CANNABIS (marijuana)

Historically *Cannabis* was prized as **a source of fiber and oil, for its edible seeds, and as a medicine**. Archaeologists have found traces of hemp fibers in clothes, shoes, paper, and rope dating to 4000 B.C. in Taiwan, China although it was probably cultivated since Neolithic times around 9000 B.C. (Schultes & Hoffman, 1992; Stafford, 1982). According to legend, in 2737 B.C. the Chinese Emperor Shen-Nung studied, experimented on himself, and recorded his efforts to use *Cannabis* (*ma-fen*) as a medicine. In a medical herbal encyclopedia called the *"Pen-tsao,"* written in A.D. 100 but referring back to Shen-Nung's study of 364 drugs (including ephedra and ginseng), *Cannabis* is not only referred to as a medication but as **a substance with stupefying and hallucinogenic properties** (Schultes, 1992).

Medically, over the centuries, *Cannabis* has been recommended for constipation, rheumatism, absent-mindedness, female disorders, malaria, beriberi, and for the treatment of wasting diseases. The Chinese physician Hua T'o, in A.D. 200, recommended *Cannabis* as **an analgesic or painkiller for surgery** (Li, 1974).

India had an even more benevolent view of the psychoactive properties of *Cannabis*. Almost 1,500 years before the birth of Christ, the *Atharva-Veda* (sacred psalms) sang of *Cannabis* (bhang) as one of five sacred plants that gave freedom from distress, a long life, and visions (hallucinations). Other texts from India listed dozens of medicinal uses for the drug (Aldrich, 1977, 1997).

About 500 B.C. the Scythians, whose territory ranged from the Danube to the Volga River in Eastern Europe, threw *Cannabis* on hot stones

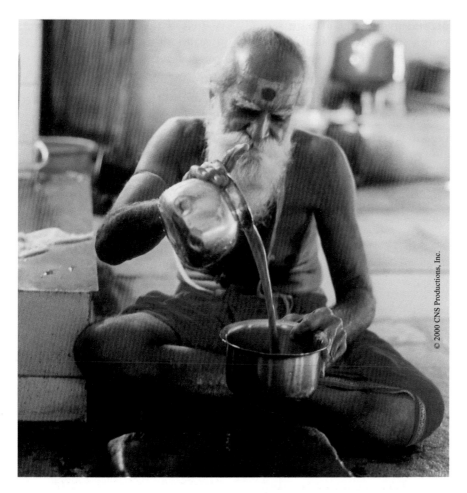

© 2000 CNS Productions, Inc.

This saddhu (Hindu ascetic) is making a beverage from Cannabis indica. *He grinds the leaves into a paste, filters out the remains of the plant by pouring water through cheesecloth, and then drinks the resulting infusion. He uses the drink as part of his religious belief system, for meditation, and concentration. He is a follower of the Hindu god Shiva. Shivites believe in the use of this intoxicant while many other Hindus do not believe in the use of* Cannabis. *The use of* Cannabis *for spiritual purposes in India goes back at least 3,500 years.*

brought with them were roasted and eaten during sacred rites, causing a sleepy delirium that lasted for days. Later on, cacti containing mescaline became another ceremonial hallucinogen of choice. Stone carvings and textiles depicting images of this plant **(San Pedro cactus)** were found at a Chavin temple in the Peruvian highlands and date back to 1300 B.C. Other South American cultures, including the Nazca and Chimu peoples, boiled the cacti for up to 7 hours and drank it to **produce hallucinations and communicate with the supernatural** (La Barre, 1979b). Evidence found in caves in what is now Texas implies ceremonial use of the *peyotl* or peyote cactus (which also contains mescaline) 3,000 years ago (Schultes, 1992). Ceremonial use of these plants was widespread but their foul taste and nauseating effects kept them from everyday use.

PSYCHEDELIC MUSHROOMS IN INDIA, SIBERIA, & MESOAMERICA

Archeology has suggested that the **sacramental use of mushrooms has been around since Paleolithic times**, about 7,000 years ago. Cave drawings from that era discovered in Algeria show shamanic figures enmeshed in mushrooms (possibly *Psilocybe mairei*) suggesting an early sacramental use (Stamets, 1996). In 1500 B.C. the *Vedas* of ancient India sang of a holy inebriant that proved to be an extract of the **Amanita muscaria mushroom**, also called the "fly agaric." The active ingredients are ibotenic acid and the alkaloid muscimole. In fact **Soma**, their name for the hallucinogen, was also the name of one of their most important gods. Over 100 holy hymns from the *Rig-Veda* are devoted to Soma.

placed in small tents and inhaled the vapors (Brunner, 1977).

"The Scythians then take the seed of this hemp and, crawling in under the mats, throw it on the red-hot stones, where it smoulders and sends forth such fumes that no Greek vapor bath could surpass it. The Scythians, transported with the vapor, shout for joy."
Herodotus, 460 B.C., *The Histories*, 4.75.1

Around A.D. 200 the **Greek physician Galen** wrote about hosts offering hemp to guests to stimulate enjoyment and promote hilarity. The hemp was

possibly mixed with wine to increase its potency. However for most ancient civilizations including Greece, Rome, and England, hemp's use as a fiber was predominant.

MESCAL BEAN, SAN PEDRO & PEYOTE CACTI (mescaline) IN MESOAMERICA

The **presence of dozens of hallucinatory plants in North and South America** gave rise to complex ceremonies overseen by shamans who came to positions of spiritual influence as did those in Neolithic times in Asia. The psychoactive mescal beans they

"It is drunk by the sick man as medicine at sunrise; partaking of it strengthens the limbs, preserves the legs from breaking, wards off all disease, and lengthens life. Then need and trouble vanish away."
Rig-Veda, 1500 B.C. (McKenna, 1992)

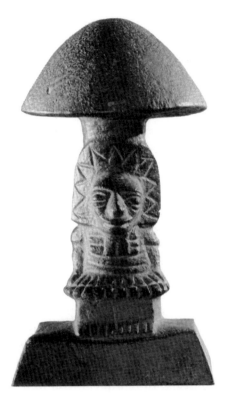

A Mayan stone god, sculpted in the shape of a mushroom (circa A.D. 5), is one of many sculptures of the psychedelic Psilocybe *mushroom. Some date back to A.D. 100.*

• •

The Soma cult had been brought to the Indus Valley of India by the Aryan (Indo-European) tribes to the north. The name "Soma" has been used to represent such diverse drugs as a mythical psychedelic in Aldous Huxley's novel *Brave New World* and a modern prescription muscle relaxant.

Though the *Amanita muscaria* also grows in North America, **it was the *Psilocybe* mushroom that was preferred by Aztec and Mayan cultures** in pre-Columbian Mexico (Schultes, 1992). Although there are more than 30,000 different identified species of mushroom, only 80 produce psilocybin and psilocin, the main active hallucinogenic ingredients. Of the many psychedelic mushrooms, *Psilocybe cubensis* is found growing in the widest areas (Stamets, 1996).

COCA LEAF & TOBACCO IN MESOAMERICA

The development of **plants containing stimulant alkaloids, e.g., to**bacco (nicotine) and coca leaves (cocaine)**, occurred 65–250 million years ago. The bitter alkaloids were the plants' way to keep dinosaurs, other herbivores, and insects away. It wasn't until approximately 5000 B.C. however that humans on a regular basis started drinking (in solution), chewing, snorting, and possibly smoking tobacco for religious ceremonies and for the stimulation. About the same time, they started chewing the coca leaf for stimulation, for nutrition, and to control their appetite when food was not available (Siegel, 1982). Burial sites unearthed on the north coast of Peru and dating back to 2500 B.C. contained bags that held coca leaves, flowers, and occasionally a chewed ball of coca leaves called *"cocada."* The coca was probably used to facilitate the deceased's journey through the afterlife. The word "coca" comes from the ancient South American Aymara Indian word *"khoka"* meaning "the tree" (Karch, 1996). Since the third century B.C. there have been hundreds of stone and wood sculptures of heads with cheeks enlarged due to a wad of coca leaves. Other mild stimulant **plants that have been popular in early times include the betel nut, the coffee bush, the khat shrub, and the ephedra bush**.

MIDDLE AGES (400–1400)

PSYCHEDELIC "HEXING HERBS"

Other psychedelics used over the centuries include **members of the nightshade family *Solanaceae* that contain the psychoactive chemicals atropine and scopolamine**. Members of this plant family include belladonna, henbane, mandrake root, and jimson weed or datura (thornapple). In the Middle Ages the various members of the nightshade family were sometimes used by medicine men and women who were later accused of witchcraft.

◇ **Datura** was often made into a salve and absorbed through the skin (McKenna, 1992).

◇ **Henbane** was referred to as early as 1500 B.C. in Egyptian medical texts. It was used as a painkiller and a poison. It was also used to mimic insanity, produce hallucinations, and generate prophecies.

◇ **Belladonna,** known as "witch's berry" and "devil's herb," dilates pupils, inebriates the user, and can cause hallucinations and delirium.

◇ **Mandrake** or mandragora, a root that often grows in the shape of a human body, was used in ancient Greece as well as in medieval times. Its properties, similar to those of belladonna and henbane, cause disorientation and delirium.

"... and then, after binding and stupefying the worthy shipmaster with mandragora or intoxication or otherwise, they take command of the ship, consume its stores and, drinking and feasting, make such a voyage."
Plato, 380 B.C., The Republic

Mandrake was considered an aphrodisiac in the 1400s in Italy and a century later Nicolo Machiavelli wrote a risqué comedy called the *"Madrigal"* about seduction and infidelity.

PSYCHEDELIC MOLD - ERGOT (St. Anthony's Fire)

Another psychedelic that has persisted through the ages is found in ergot, a brownish purple fungus, *Claviceps purpurea,* which **grows on infected rye/wheat plants. The psychedelic is lysergic acid diethylamide**, the natural form of the hallucinogen LSD. Ergot and its effects are referred to in ancient Greek and medieval European literature. It was recognized as a poison and a psychedelic as early as 600 B.C. Ergot in small doses was even used as a medication in the Middle Ages to induce childbirth.

Over the centuries there have been

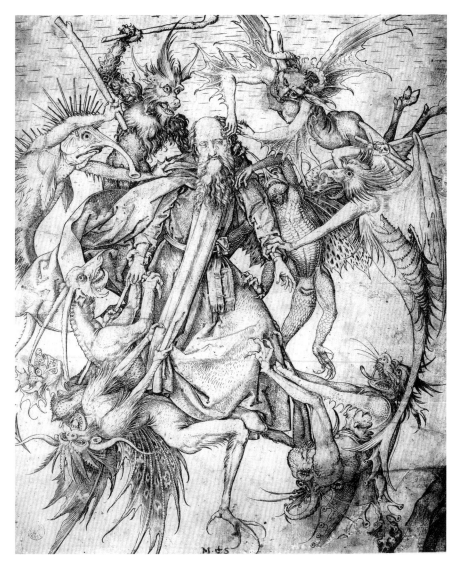

This fifteenth-century engraving by Martin Schongauer shows St. Anthony being assaulted by visions of sexual licentiousness and savage animals, visions similar to those caused by the ergot fungus found on spoiled rye or wheat cereal grasses. The chemical produced by the fungus is a natural source for lysergic acid, a naturally occurring form of LSD. St. Anthony's success in battling his demons and hallucinations associated him with ergotism and so St. Anthony's Fire became a synonym for the ergot-caused affliction. Ergotism was often fatal because it led to gangrene and extreme delirium. Museum of Fine Arts, Budapest, Hungary EMB Services for Publishers. Reprinted by permission. All rights reserved.

• •

numerous outbreaks of ergot poisoning when whole towns, particularly in rye-consuming areas of Eastern Europe, seemed to go mad, occasionally with great loss of life. In France in A.D. 944, 40,000 people are estimated to have died from an ergotism epidemic. There were outbreaks as recently as 1953 in France and Belgium. **Hallucinations, nervous convulsions, possibly permanent insanity, a burning sensation in the feet and hands,**

and gangrene that occasionally caused a loss of extremities—toes, feet, fingers, noses—were common. One of the outbreaks in A.D. 1039 gave the name "St. Anthony's Fire" to the affliction when a wealthy Frenchman and his son, who were afflicted with the disease, prayed to St. Anthony, a fourth-century saint who protects supplicants against fire, epilepsy, and infection. His and his son's recoveries inspired the father to build a hospital in Dauphiné, France

(where St. Anthony was buried) for the care of sufferers of ergotism.

FROM MEDICINE, TO PSYCHOACTIVE DRUG, TO POISON

Theophrastus, a Greek philosopher, emphasized that datura can be a **medicine at a low dose, a psychoactive drug at a moderate dose, and a deadly poison at a high dose**.

"One administers one drachma [of datura], if the patient must only be animated and made to think well of himself; double that, if he must enter delirium and see hallucinations; triple it, if he must become permanently deranged; give a quadruple dose if he is to die."

Theophrastus, 323 B.C., *Inquiry Into Plants*

Not only datura but ergot, opium, and most other psychoactive drugs can also follow this pattern. Opium sedates and suppresses pain at a low dose, causes euphoria at a higher dose, and depresses breathing to dangerous levels at a very high dose. Healers and shamans would experiment with various substances to find the correct dose to heal a patient or induce a trance state and probably lost a few patients in the process. Another example of dose-dependent effects is the coca leaf. Chewing a few coca leaves releases enough cocaine to keep a chewer awake and working. A large amount of chopped coca leaves, mixed with lime to increase absorption, will cause a mild high, keep the chewer chewing and awake for days while suppressing appetite. A very high dose of cocaine, refined from the coca leaf and injected, can freeze the heart and cause a fatal overdose.

Historically the ability to take higher doses of a drug to induce greater and more immediate psychoactive effects often leads users to flirt with addiction and the lethal end of the drug spectrum. Ironically one of the early uses of **opium was in a mixture called** *"theriaka"* (theriac) developed to counteract poisonings, a common fear of the wealthy. By the second century A.D. the amount of opium in theriac had increased to 40% of the total. Other poisons in low doses were administered on a regular basis to supposedly immunize users (build a tolerance) (Escohotado, 1999).

ALCOHOL & DISTILLATION

Alcohol consumption continued throughout the Middle Ages as **cultural attitudes bounced between abstention, temperance, and bingeing**. Christianity in its early days celebrated its faith with banquets of wine and bread but as the problems with alcohol increased, the ceremony (Eucharist) used less and less wine until it was only used symbolically. Inevitably **drinking became a moral cause**. St. Paul and others condemned the relaxed behavior caused by excessive drinking since it led users away from God. This change from paganism and the use of psychoactive substances to communicate with the supernatural gave way to a demand that faith alone be used to understand God.

Again the attitude towards alcohol wavered. In the later Middle Ages European monasteries and feudal lords used the *sirah* grape, imported during the Crusades, to cultivate their own vineyards and assure a supply of wine for their thirst, for their meals, for passing thirsty travelers, and for the Eucharist. Alcohol also killed bacteria and microorganisms that lived in water, so alcoholic drinks, along with boiled beverages, were often the only safe liquids to drink.

In spite of a Western attitude of distrust of science and knowledge, **technical advances in cultivation and purification (distillation) of alcohol made a difference in consumption**. Even though techniques for distillation of seawater and alcohol had been around for thousands of years (e.g., boiling the alcoholic beverage mead under a cloth that catches the evaporating alcohol and is wrung out), it wasn't until the eighth to fourteenth centuries

that knowledge of the techniques became widespread. This evaporation process was used to raise the alcohol content of beverages from 14% up to 40% (McKenna, 1992).

In one version of history an Arabian alchemist named Geber is credited with perfecting a wine distillation method in the eighth century A.D. In another version an Arabian physician, Rhazes, discovered distilled spirits. Whiskey distillation in Ireland was popular by the twelfth century, particularly because the cold damp climate was bad for grape cultivation (O'Brien, 1991). The word "whiskey" supposedly comes from the Gaelic *Usequebaugh*, which means "breath of life." In the thirteenth century two chemists in Switzerland, Arnaldus de Villanova and Raymone Lully, promoted distilled alcohol or *aqua vitae* (water of life) as a marvelous cure-all and longevity enhancer.

ISLAMIC SUBSTITUTES FOR ALCOHOL

In the *Koran*, **the holy book of Islam**, two minor references are made to wine but it is water that has relevance to the practice of the religion. Wine was not used as a sacrament in Islam and the **drinking of wine was frowned upon**. The prophet Mohammed did not mention wine, only that he chastised a drunkard for not performing his duties. Mohammed's brother-in-law, Ali, set the tone for alcohol in later Muslim societies.

"He who drinks gets drunk, he who is drunk, does nonsensical things, he who acts nonsensically says lies, and he who lies must be punished."
Ali (Escohotado, 1999)

So it was not alcohol per se that was shunned, it was what alcohol made a drinker do that was detested. However, through the centuries temperance gave way to prohibition, and objections to the debilitating effects of alcohol and other psychoactive drugs gave way to bans on any substance that could cause pleasure and make one for-

get their religious and moral duties. This attitude paralleled the attitude of Christianity during the Middle Ages.

The reasons that drew people to psychoactive substances remained, so some Muslims searched for alternatives. **Opium for the relief of pain**, both physical and mental, was seen as an acceptable substitute. It was used in Arab society as a general tonic much as it had been used by Roman nobility. Among other qualities it was supposed to ease the transition to old age. In later centuries **tobacco, hashish (concentrated *Cannabis*), and particularly coffee were employed as substitutes for alcohol** in order to provide stimulation, induce sedation, and alter consciousness. These substances were also used medicinally.

Khat, a stimulant that was permissible in Islamic cultures, was originally cultivated in the southern Arabian peninsula and the Horn of Africa. It was used during long prayer ceremonies to help the congregation stay awake. In A.D. 1238 the Arab physician Naguib Ad-Din distributed khat to soldiers to prevent hunger and fatigue while another Arab king, Sabr Ad-Din, gave it freely to subjects he had recently conquered to placate them and quell their revolutionary tendencies (Giannini, Burge, Shaheen, & Price, 1986).

COFFEE & TEA (caffeine)

Centuries after the **coffee plant *Coffea Arabica* was found growing wild in Ethiopia**, about A.D. 850, it was imported and intensely cultivated in Arabia (around the fourteenth century). Coffee was popularized by those who liked the stimulation but condemned by Orthodox Muslims because it was intoxicating although like khat it helped worshippers stay awake during long prayer ceremonies (Coste, 1984). The stimulating chemical caffeine made many ignore the mosque's condemnation. At first coffee was consumed by chewing the beans or by infusing them in water. Then during the later Middle Ages, coffee was **made even more potent once people learned how to roast and grind the**

beans, producing a tastier version. It was also used for medicinal purposes (e.g., diuretic, asthma treatment, and headache relief). It took 500 more years (1820) before caffeine, the active alkaloid in coffee and tea, was finally identified. Tea from the leaves of the **Thea sinensis** (*chinensis*) bush was supposedly used in China 4,700 years ago but the first written evidence of its use didn't appear until approximately A.D. 350. The fact that boiling water killed germs made it a popular drink. Cultivation of tea in Japan and development of tea ceremonies occurred about A.D. 800. Tea remains the heart of social and religious ceremonies to the present day (Harler, 1984). There are also approximately **60 other plants that contain caffeine, such as guarana, maté, yoco, kola nut, and cocoa.**

COCA IN THE NEW WORLD

Coca cultivation and ingestion of the stimulant coca leaf in Moche rituals in Peru occurred from A.D. 200–800. About A.D. 600 the early Incas also used coca, occasionally chewing it with tobacco. The Inca

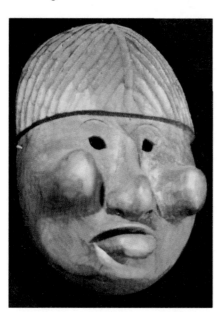

Colombian carving depicting a user's cheek stuffed with cocada, coca leaf mixed with powdered lime.
Courtesy of the Fitz Hugh Ludlow Memorial Library

Empire expanded and the coca leaf once again was involved in various shamanic rituals (Siegel, 1982). As with many substances that were used to contact the supernatural or achieve an altered state of consciousness, myths arose to explain the magical properties of the substance. Legend has it that almost 8 centuries ago in the Peruvian highlands the legendary Inca Emperor Manco Capac, worshipped as the divine son of the Sun god, brought the coca leaf to earth to satiate the hungry, strengthen the weak, and help them to forget their misfortunes (Scrivener, 1871). **All the nobility carried their precious supply of coca leaves in ornate bags** strapped to their wrists. A plentiful supply of the drug, which was considered divine, was buried with the nobility (White, 1989).

PSYCHEDELIC FUNGI & PLANTS IN THE AMERICAS

To the north of the Inca Empire, **about the time Columbus arrived in the Americas, the Aztec, Huichol, Cora, and Tarahumare Indians of Mexico were still digging up psychedelic plants**—peyote cactus (containing mescaline), "magic" psilocybin mushrooms, and the ololiuqui or morning-glory seed (containing hallucinogenic ergot alkaloids)—for their rituals. Later, missionaries wrote that the North American Indians used the drugs to communicate with the devil (Diaz, 1979). They were rarely used recreationally like alcoholic beverages, tobacco, or coca leaves.

RENAISSANCE & THE AGE OF DISCOVERY (1400–1700)

Two general trends continued the spread of psychoactive substances. Beginning with Portuguese, Spanish, British, French, and Dutch exploration, trade, and colonization, **Europeans encountered diverse cultures and unfa-**

miliar psychoactive plants. The most notable substances were coffee from Turkey and Arabia, tobacco and coca from the New World, tea from China, and the kola nut from Africa. Similarly, European explorers, soldiers, merchants, traders, and missionaries **carried their own culture's drug-using customs and drugs to the rest of the world.** Greater secularization of life (less control by churches), urbanization, spreading wealth, and growing personal freedom also increased use.

ALCOHOL

Laws limiting use of alcohol, particularly high-potency distilled beverages, were mostly based on the effects of overuse and the subsequent toxic effects as well as moral issues regarding lowered inhibitions that made the drinker forget his or her "duties." Switzerland and England passed closing-time laws in the thirteenth century. Even Scotland and Germany limited sales on religious days in the fifteenth century (O'Brien, 1991). But since the medicinal and recreational values of drinking were well established, laws were aimed more at temperance than prohibition, particularly since the increasing availability of **distilled beverages produced hefty tax revenues.**

COCA & THE CONQUISTADORS

One example of how the **economic and political needs of a country transformed the way a substance was used** is the interaction between the Spanish Conquistadors who colonized Peru in the 1500s and the native tribes' use of coca leaf. When the explorers/invaders arrived, coca leaf was used as a mild stimulant, as a reward, and as a way to suppress hunger and thirst.

"They carry them from some high mountains, to others, as merchandise to be sold, and they barter and change them for mantillas, and cattle, and salt, and other things."
Monardes, 1577

As the Incas cultivated a larger supply of the coca leaf some people chewed throughout the day, much as Americans drink coffee nowadays, but since the leaf was only 0.5% cocaine, it was not toxic. When the Conquistadors started to exploit the silver mines that they had discovered at extremely high altitudes in the Andes Mountains, they needed to find ways to keep the subjugated Indians working. The **Spanish started appropriating the Incan coca plantations** so they could keep the natives supplied with the stimulant. They planted so much that at times there was a glut on the market (Cleza de Leon, 1959). **Coca chewing increased dramatically as did revenue from the trade.** About 8% of the Spaniards living in Peru were involved in the coca trade and even had their own lobby back in Spain (Gagliano, 1994). Although the **tax revenues from the coca trade helped pay for the colony**, there were also many Spaniards who opposed the use of coca (Acosta, 1588). Even the church was torn between needing the revenue to pay for their missionary activities vs. revulsion at the way the Incas were exploited and doubt that someone chewing coca could be converted to Christianity. Native workers at the silver mining towns spent twice as much on coca leaves as they did for food (Karch, 1997).

TOBACCO CROSSES THE OCEANS

In 1492 after Christopher Columbus had crossed the Atlantic and landed in Hispaniola in the Caribbean, he noted the natives' use of tobacco. They **used it as a medicine for a wide variety of ailments** including headache, snakebite, stomach and heart pains, skin diseases, and toothaches. It was also widely used for rituals including planting, fertility, good fishing, consulting the spirits, and preparing magical cures. Shamans in South America **used the toxicity of tobacco to induce trance-like states** to awe their tribesmen (Benowitz & Fredericks, 1995). Columbus also noted that the Caribbean

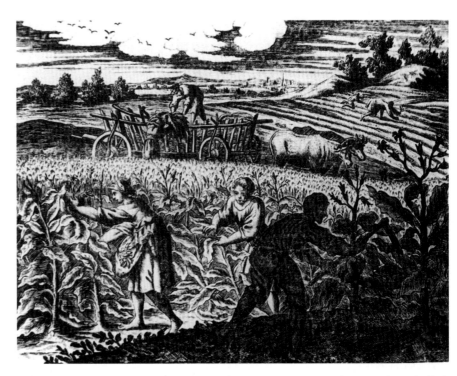

Starting about 1610 Virginia and Maryland produced tobacco crops that were planted, tilled, and picked by slave labor and which supported the Chesapeake Colonies for 2 centuries.
Courtesy of the National Library of Medicine, Bethesda, MD

natives snuffed *cohoba*, a potent hallucinogenic substance.

Soon the Spaniards and the British were exporting tobacco to Europe where it was received enthusiastically, originally as a medicine and later as a stimulant, mild relaxant, and mild euphoriant. **Sir Walter Raleigh brought "tobacco smoking for recreation" to the court of Queen Elizabeth** (Benowitz, 1995). In France tobacco was called "*nicotiana*" after Jean Nicot who described its medicinal properties. **Portuguese sailors introduced tobacco to Japan** where its cultivation began about 1605. The **Portuguese also introduced tobacco to China** where it was also highly regarded as a medicine. It was carried throughout China by soldiers, then banned, and then taxed. It was in vogue at the Emperor's court, then among the people, and then actively propagated throughout Asia. Despite sporadic attempts at prohibition by rulers, governments, and churches that thought tobacco use harmful to society, its use spread.

"The use of tobacco is growing greater and conquers men with a certain secret pleasure, so that those who have once become accustomed thereto can later hardly be restrained therefrom."
Sir Francis Bacon, 1620

Back in Europe the dangers of fire, the congregation of smokers in tobacco houses where radical ideas and politics were discussed, and the abuse of tobacco by the clergy led to **vigorous attacks by various authorities including King James I of England**.

"[Smoking is] a custome lothsome to the eye, hateful to the Nose, harmefull to the braine, dangerous to the Lungs, and the blacke stinking fume thereof, neerest resembling the horrible Stigian smoke of the pit that is bottomless."
James I, 1604

Pope Urban VIII forbade smoking under pain of excommunication. It was also forbidden in Turkey under pain of torture and death and banned by Czars Michael and Alexis in Russia under similar penalties (Benowitz, 1995). But smuggling and widespread covert use by clergy, by commoners, and by the nobility defeated all attempts at prohibition. Over the centuries the **craving for tobacco and the addictive qualities of nicotine have overwhelmed most calls for prohibition**.

From the beginning the economic power of trade in a substance that was both pleasurable and habit-forming was recognized. Eventually tobacco became a large source of revenue for many governments, especially for Spain and later for England and America.

COFFEE & TEA

Coffee drinking became widespread in Europe, first among wealthy classes, then, as quantities increased and prices declined, among the middle and lower classes. Coffee became a favorite drink as an alternative to alcohol. In cities such as Amsterdam, London, and later on Paris, New York, and Boston it was drunk in coffeehouses that became popular centers of intellectual, political, and literary discussion and news circulation. Coffee and tea were also popular in both Turkey and England where coffeehouses were closely watched by authorities as possible hotbeds of political dissent, sedition, and revolution.

Tea wasn't popular outside Asia until Dutch traders introduced it in Europe in 1610 and in America 40 years later. Then its popularity grew until it **became the center of social interaction and a ritualistic part of family life, e.g., afternoon tea**.

OPIUM RETURNS

During the Renaissance in the fifteenth and sixteenth centuries the use of opium in medicinal concoctions came back into favor when the works of the second-century **Greek physician Galen and the Moorish physi-**

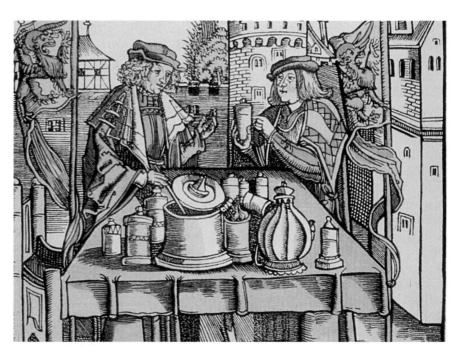

The preparation of theriac, the ancient cure-all, is depicted in this sixteenth-century woodcut. From H. Brunschwig, Das Neu Distiller Buch, *Strassburg, 1537.*
Courtesy of the National Library of Medicine, Bethesda, MD

cian Avicenna became widely taught in medical education (Acker, 1995). **Theriac, one of the opium preparations**, came into favor again. It was first described by Andromachus, physician to the Emperor Nero in A.D. 15. It originally contained more than 70 ingredients in addition to opium and Galen added over 30 more. It was prescribed for an incredible variety of illnesses including inflammation, diarrhea, madness, melancholy, headaches, anything involving pain, pestilence, and even nosebleeds. As usual many lookalike theriac preparations were being hawked in the marketplaces of Europe and the Middle East in later centuries. These bogus versions, called "treacle," were sold to the poor, letting them feel they could share in what George Bartisch called "a highly praiseworthy, imperial, royal, and princely medicine." Bartisch was a well-known physician/oculist in 1602 who recommended theriac for all the ailments of old age (Blanchard, 2000).

"This Theriac used daily serves old, cold, and enfeebled men. It awakens sexual appetite and intercourse. It strengthens and increases the manly nature and brings joy and desire."
Bartisch, 1602

In 1524 **Paracelsus** (Theophrastus von Hohenheim) returned from Constantinople to Western Europe with the **secret of laudanum**, a tincture of opium in alcohol (with henbane juice, crushed pearls, coral, amber, musk, and essential oils added). It was employed as a panacea or cure-all medication and, for many, a simple way to soothe a crying child. It was readily available, inexpensive, and soon was widely used (and abused) in all strata of society, unlike theriac that for centuries was reserved for the nobility and the wealthy. Laudanum was found in most home remedy chests. Parcelsus believed and widely promoted the idea that pain relief and sleep were part of the cure for any disease, so he medicated many of his patients with preparations containing opium (Karch, 1997). **A medicine that could kill pain and make one feel euphoric was highly prized in any society.**

AGE OF ENLIGHTENMENT & THE EARLY INDUSTRIAL REVOLUTION (1700–1900)

The development of refined forms of psychoactive drugs, new methods of use, and improved production techniques, along with governments' and merchants' economic motives, led not only to more users but also to more mental and physical problems including abuse and addiction.

DISTILLED LIQUORS & THE GIN EPIDEMIC

In addition to making one feel better, beer and wine had long been part of the European diet. Beer was much thicker than modern brews, contributing B vitamins and other nutrients to Europeans' daily intake. Wine used moderately was considered beneficial to health and had some food value. Distilled spirits (about 40% alcohol) had virtually no nutritional content and were most often used just to feel better and to get drunk.

Gin was first made in Holland during the 1600s from fermented mixtures of grains flavored with juniper berries. It became popular throughout Europe and when the **English Parliament encouraged production and consumption of gin**, urban alcoholism and the mortality rate skyrocketed. During the **London Gin Epidemic from 1710 to 1750**, the novelist Henry Fielding said that gin was the principal sustenance of more than 100,000 Londoners and he predicted that

"... should the drinking of this poison be continued at its present height, during the next 20 years, there will be by that time very few of the common people left to drink it."

Henry Fielding, 1740, Enquiry

It was estimated that one house in six in London was a gin house. Production went from 1.23 million gallons in 1700, to 6.4 million gallons in 1735, and 7 million gallons by 1751. The passage of the Tippling Act in 1751 prohibited distillers from selling gin. Prices rose and consumption declined back to about 2 million gallons. **It showed how unlimited availability of a desirable substance causes excess use. Only stiff taxes and the strict regulation of sales brought the epidemic under control.** One of the main objections to the availability of gin was that it hindered the production capabilities of the lower classes who were the producers of England's wealth (Abel, 2001). The upper class also felt that women who drank heavily gave birth to weak children, therefore threatening the supply of strong young men for the army and navy.

During the latter half of the eighteenth century, **rum was the chief medium of exchange in the slave trade and one of the mainstays of the economy of colonial America along with whiskey**. A farmer using a 25¢ bushel of corn could produce 2½ gallons of whiskey valued at $1.25 that could be shipped easily and not spoil (Skolnick, 1997). Around 1790 per capita consumption was three times what it is today. When the federal government enacted a tax on liquor, the farmers in western Pennsylvania led **the Whiskey Rebellion** that was broken up when George Washington sent troops. In 1801 Thomas Jefferson abolished the federal duty on liquor although later administrations reinstated this valuable source of revenue.

TOBACCO, HEMP, & THE AMERICAN REVOLUTION

Tobacco was introduced to the Jamestown colony in 1612. The first

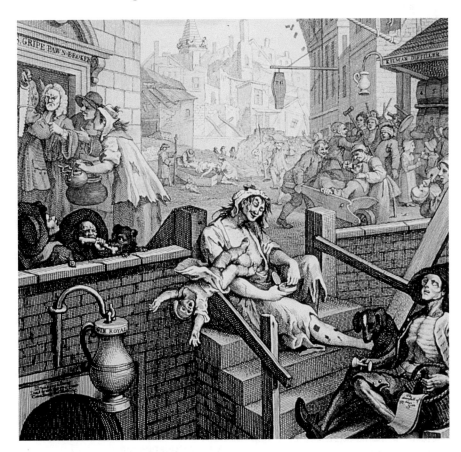

The Gin Epidemic devastated London from 1710 to 1750. Engraving by William Hogarth depicts "Gin Lane" c. 1751. A companion engraving "Beer Street" showed a happier group of drinkers and recommended beer as a way to drive gin out of vogue.

Courtesy of the National Library of Medicine, Bethesda, MD

shipment of *Nicotiana tabacum* (**Virginia leaf**) was sent to England by John Rolf, the husband of the Indian princess Pocahontas. **It became a financial mainstay for the southern colonies.** Virtually all of **it was chewed or smoked in cigars and pipes**. Tobacco was so important to America that sculptures of tobacco leaves and flowers were used to decorate the columns supporting the dome of the U.S. Capitol building, which was built in 1818 (Slade, 1989). Tobacco, along with rum (and continental currency or "continentals" that weren't worth much), helped finance much of the U.S. Revolutionary War. A lottery was also used to partially fund the Continental Army, making George Washington the first American to buy a government-sponsored lottery ticket.

Before the war **King George III of England sent a proclamation to America in 1764 to encourage the planting of hemp**, another important crop in the new American colonies, to send to England. "Hemp" is the word used to describe *Cannabis sativa* plants that are high in fiber content and generally low in psychoactive components. In later centuries "marijuana" came to be used to describe *Cannabis sativa* plants that are high in psychoactive ingredients. George III wanted to monopolize the hemp trade and required Americans to buy back hemp products from England made with their own hemp. George Washington directed colonists to comply but to retain much of their own hemp in America. His purpose was to **establish an American textile and rope industry** so the colonies could depend on a local supply. A single ship of that era used 1,000 yards of hemp rope to rig the sails and secure cargo. George Washington cultivated hemp at his Mount Vernon plantation and he too encouraged its production as a domestic source of rope and sails for the fledgling navy of the United States. There is no convincing evidence that *Cannabis* plants were used for their psychoactive effects in the American colonies. Until the Civil War hemp was the South's second largest crop behind cotton. But **because hemp was de**-pendent on slave labor, it was no longer profitable after the slaves were freed.

NITROUS OXIDE, OTHER ANESTHETICS, & OTHER INHALANTS

The **first anesthetic called "anodyne" (a liquid form of ether)** was discovered in 1730 by Frederick Hofmann, a German physician. It was used as a medicine, a drink, and an inhalant, often for intoxication because it was thought to be less harmful than alcohol.

Inhaling a gas (as opposed to smoking a drug) became more popular after Joseph Priestly discovered **nitrous oxide or "laughing gas"** in 1776. Its popularity was encouraged by Sir Humphry Davy in the early 1800s who suggested a nitrous oxide tavern as an alternative to saloons (Agnew, 1968).

"It is a clearly time-saving, exhilarating, angelizing ether; whereas spirituous liquors are besotting, brutalizing, devil-inspiring draughts which in the end clog the ideas whereas the etherial oxide sets them free."
Chemical Experimentalist, circa 1810 (Lynn, Walter, Harris, Dendy, & James, 1972)

Several other gases used for anesthesia were also developed, including **chloroform** in 1831. Both men and women participated in "gas frolics" in the 1830s. Later in the nineteenth century the refinement of various hydrocarbons (fossil fuels) into **volatile solvents** increased the range of substances that could be inhaled.

OPIUM TO MORPHINE TO HEROIN

For thousands of years opium had been used mostly as a medicine and tonic but as the Age of Enlightenment and the Industrial Revolution encouraged **technical developments and economic/political innovation**, the use of opiates often escalated into habituation, abuse, and addiction. The techni-

A GRAND EXHIBITION
OF THE EFFECTS PRODUCED BY INHALING NITROUS OXIDE, EXHILERATING, OR
LAUGHING GAS

WILL BE GIVEN AT *THE MASONIC HALL* *SATURDAY* EVENING, *5 PM.* 1845

30 GALLONS OF GAS will be prepared and administered to all in the audience who desire to inhale it.

MEN will be invited from the audience to protect those under the influence of the Gas from injuring themselves or others. This course is adopted that no apprehension of danger may be entertained. Probably no one will attempt to fight.

THE EFFECT OF THE GAS IS TO MAKE THOSE WHO INHALE IT, EITHER

LAUGH, SING, DANCE, SPEAK OR FIGHT, &c. &c.

according to the leading trait of their character. They seem to retain consciousness enough not to say or do that which they would have occasion to regret.

N.B. The Gas will be administered only to gentlemen of the first respectability. The object is to make The entertainment in every respect, a genteel affair.

* * * * * * * * * * * * * * * *

This simulation of an 1845 poster shows the excitement that accompanied a new mood-altering substance. For 25¢ a ticket a whiff of the gas was available. Inhalants and other substances were often looked at as substitutes for alcohol since that was the substance that caused the most problems.

cal developments were the spread of smoking as a means of using opium, the refinement of morphine from opium, the refinement of heroin from morphine, and the invention of the hypodermic needle to inject drugs directly into the body. The economic/political developments stemmed from recognition that **huge profits could be made from the opium drug trade**. That money could then finance other activities (e.g., excise taxes to finance exploration or wars of conquest). Under the British East India Company, the export of opium from their fields in India to the smokers in China increased from 13 tons in 1729 to 2,558 tons in 1839. The first Moghul Dynasty in India had developed poppy cultivation and ran the opium trade as a state monopoly around 1526 until the British took it over.

Opium Smoking

Opium smoking was first introduced to China about 1500 by Portuguese traders but didn't become popular for 200 more years. **Smoking put greater amounts of opium into the blood (via the lungs) more quickly and therefore into the brain sooner thus increasing the intensity of the effects.** Since the lungs had such a large surface area, large amounts could be absorbed rapidly. It also bypassed the distasteful flavor and resulted in a much more rapid onset of action. Dependence and repeated use were therefore more likely to develop through smoking thus causing a vast increase in opium use in China.

Morphine

The next development occurred in 1804 when a German pharmacist, Frederick W. Serturner, discovered how to refine *morphium* (morphine) from opium. Morphine is about **10 times more powerful than opium** and therefore a more effective pain reliever. Given the proliferation of wars the need for effective painkillers for wounded soldiers was high. Opium had been used in the American Revolutionary War in the eighteenth century but it was morphine that was used in the Crimean

War and most notably in the U.S. Civil War in the nineteenth century. Unfortunately the higher potency of the preparation caused greater changes in the human body leading to **more rapid development of tolerance** to the drug and therefore greater dependence. The increased use in wartime of morphine and the subsequent creation of dependent users generated the phrase "the soldier's disease." Some historians felt the scope of the problem was overstated. When opium was ingested (not smoked) and partly metabolized before reaching the brain, overdose was rarely a problem but the potency of morphine made overdose more common (Karch, 1996; Hoffman, 1990).

The other result of Serturner's refinement of morphine was the **discovery of active alkaloids in many other plants** (e.g., cocaine in the coca leaf) leading to more concentrated forms of a number of drugs.

Hypodermic Needle

Intravenous injection and infusion had been tried since the 1600s when several experimenters noticed that injecting an opium solution into a dog stupefied the animal quite quickly (Boyle, 1744). But it wasn't until 200 years later, around 1855, that the reusable hypodermic needle was invented. Some say that Charles Gabrial Pavras in France invented it but most credit the Scottish physician Alexander Wood with the revolutionary development. **Drugs could easily be put directly into the bloodstream causing more intense effects.** It also made it easier to overload the brain. Unfortunately Wood, through self-experimentation, managed to addict himself and his wife to morphine (Karch, 1998). The use of **the hypodermic needle also bypassed the natural barriers that protected the body from infection**, barriers such as skin, mucous membranes, lung tissue, stomach, and intestine walls. By the time of the Civil War morphine injection was common and by 1868 both opium and morphine had become cheaper than drinking alcohol and their use had spread even more.

Heroin

In 1874 **diacetyl morphine**, better known as "heroin," was refined from morphine at St. Mary's Hospital in London by C. R. Alder Wright but it wasn't until 1898 that the German Bayer Company began marketing Heroin® as a remedy for coughs, chest pains, and tuberculosis. At one time it was considered a possible cure for morphine addiction and alcoholism. Of course the greater intensity of the heroin high caused a **more rapid progression to abuse and addiction** but it wasn't until the twentieth century that heroin became a large problem on the world stage.

Opium Wars

Economic and political changes were the other factors that increased the use of drugs. For example, by the late 1700s China was known to be a potentially lucrative trading partner with many national riches like silk, jade, porcelains, and especially tea, all ripe for exploitation. **Colonial powers vied for the right to sell opium in China.** Because of the English addiction to tea, **the British government, through the East India Trading Company, grew opium in India to trade to China for silver in order to buy tea.** This complicated method of trade occurred because the Chinese government, which controlled the tea trade, would only accept silver as payment.

In the early 1800s China, now a land of 450 million people, had banned opium use and imports because of the terrible costs of crime, corruption, and addiction but the British, burdened by an unfavorable trade deficit due to the tea imports, insisted on their "right" of free trade. In 1839 Commissioner Lin Tse-hau, who had been appointed by the Manchu Emperor (Ch'ing Dynasty) to stop the opium trade, demanded that the traders surrender the tons of opium stored in their warehouses. "The Wars for Free Trade," as the British called them, or the "Opium Wars" (1839–42, 1856–60), as the rest of the world called them, were fought to enforce the British right to sell opium to Chinese traders. They, in turn, bribed government officials so they could sell the drug to all classes (Wallbank & Taylor, 1992; Hodgson, 1999). England and other countries that won both wars were **granted Hong Kong, greater trade concessions, and the unacknowledged right to sell opium**.

The resulting addiction of many Chinese, the indignities of China's defeat, and the unequal treaties imposed by Western countries after the Opium Wars continue to complicate China's relations with the West even today (Latimer & Goldberg, 1981).

FROM COCA TO COCAINE

One of the best examples of how refinement of a substance changes its use and addiction liability is the history of the coca leaf's transformation from a mild to a powerful stimulant. Until 1859 when Albert Nieman **isolated the alkaloid cocaine** from the coca leaf, the drug was chewed or chopped and kept on the gums, so the stimulatory effect was similar to several cups of espresso consumed over several hours. Once refined cocaine was available, the mild stimulation became an intense rush followed by ecstatic feelings and a powerful physical stimulation when injected, smoked, snorted, absorbed through the gums, or drunk. Various medical and commercial developments popularized the powerful stimulant, e.g.,

◇ the physician Karl Koller found that cocaine was a strong **topical anesthetic** that made eye surgery possible;

◇ a French chemist, Angelo Mariani, popularized his **cocaine wine** as a medicinal tonic (Vin Mariani);

◇ **Sigmund Freud published his treatise**, *Über Coca,* and suggested cocaine's use for a number of ailments.

"Here we would like to recapitulate the indications that Dr. Freud proposed for cocaine in July of last year; these are:
Coca as stimulant;
Coca in the treatment of gastric disorders;

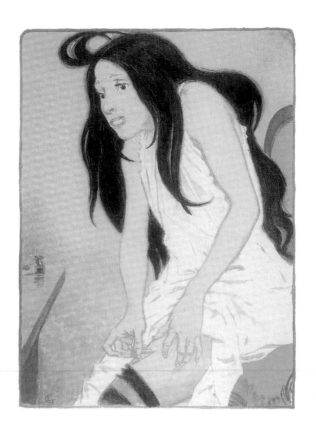

Morphinomanie. *Color lithograph by Eugene Samuel Grasset, 1897.* Philadelphia Museum of Art. Reprinted, by permission, SmithKline Beecham Corporation Fund for The Ars Medica Collection

Coca for the treatment of morphine and alcohol addicts;
Coca for the treatment of asthma; and
Coca as an aphrodisiac.
Guttmacher, 1885

Freud and others also used cocaine to feel better and relieve depression. There is evidence that the Father of Psychiatry became addicted for a while even though he denied that he had a problem. His writings in *Über Coca* about his craving for the drug and fear of being without it belied his denial.

"During the first hours of the coca effect one cannot sleep, but this sleeplessness is in no way distressing. I have tested this effect of coca, which wards off hunger, sleep, and fatigue and steels one to intellectual effort, some dozen times on myself."
Sigmund Freud, 1884

Though the manufacture and sale of coca wine and patent medicines spread rapidly, along with widespread

binge use and dependency, the **possibility of negative consequences was minimized**.

"As, at present, many authorities seem to harbor unjustified fears with regard to the internal use of cocaine. It is not out of place to stress that even subcutaneous injections—such as I have used with success in cases of long-standing sciatica [pinched sciatic nerve]—are quite harmless. For humans the toxic dose is very high, and there seems to be no lethal dose."
Sigmund Freud, 1884 (Byck, 1974)

It was only through the hindsight of a generation of abuse that the addictive nature of cocaine was seen and its widespread availability curtailed. Unfortunately the future generations often forget the lessons of the past.

TEMPERANCE & PROHIBITION MOVEMENTS

The widespread availability of distilled liquors, particularly rum in the

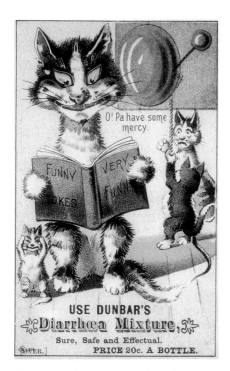

Opium was the usual active ingredient in diarrhea medications. It was also prescribed for almost every other illness because it could relieve pain. It was mostly used to treat symptoms rather than correct the disease state.
Courtesy of the National Library of Medicine, Bethesda, MD

• •

United States, led to increased bouts of drunkenness, violence, and public disruption. The **first temperance movement in the United States was started about 1785 by Dr. Benjamin Rush**, a noted physician and reformer who warned against overuse of alcohol but praised limited amounts for health reasons. The disease concept of alcohol was suggested by the early writings of Rush (Goodwin & Gabrielli, 1997).

"Strong liquor is more destructive than the sword. The destruction of war is periodic, whereas alcohol exerts its influence upon human life at all times and in all seasons."
Benjamin Rush, 1788

The first national temperance organization, **the American Temperance Society, was created in 1826** and it was supported by businessmen who

needed sober and industrious workers (Langton, 1995). The growth of these societies to more than 1,000 four years later did not stem the increased use of alcohol. Consumption peaked in 1830 in the United States with a yearly per capita consumption of 7.1 gallons of pure alcohol vs. 1.8 gallons today. In fact at Andrew Jackson's inauguration in 1833 the new President's staff stopped serving alcohol because they were afraid drunken revelers would destroy the White House.

It wasn't until 1851 that Maine passed the first prohibition law. Within 4 years one-third of the states had laws controlling the sale and use of alcohol and consumption fell to one-third of pre-Prohibition and Temperance levels. The Civil War stalled and in some cases reversed the Prohibition movement but after the war the **Women's Crusade, the Women's Christian Temperance Union, and the Anti-Saloon League (1893)** led the Temperance movement, which later became the Prohibition movement, into the twentieth century. The first facility that treated alcoholism opened in 1841 in Massachusetts.

OPIATES & COCAINE IN PATENT MEDICINES & PRESCRIPTION DRUGS

Over-the-counter medicines sold at the turn of the twentieth century had imaginative names, such as Mrs. Winslow's Soothing Syrup, Roger's Cocaine Pile Remedy, Lloyd's Cocaine Toothache Drops, and McMunn's Elixir

of Opium, all **loaded with opium, morphine, cocaine,** *Cannabis,* **and usually alcohol** (Armstrong & Armstrong, 1991). Needless to say, patent medicines were very popular in all strata of society and were used as a cure for any illness from lumbago to depression, much like nepenthe, theriac, and laudanum centuries before. The **manufacturers of these tonics did not need to list ingredients or back up their claims** regarding the medical usefulness of these products. Therefore many took tonics thinking they were more like medicine rather than potentially dangerous substances.

"It may strike you as strange that I who have had no pain—no acute suffering to keep down from its angles—should need opium in any shape. But I have had restlessness till it made me almost mad. . . . So the medical people gave me opium—a preparation of it, called morphine, and ether—and ever since I have been calling it my amreeta . . . my elixir."
Elizabeth Barrett Browning, 1837 (Aldrich, 1994)

One of the finest poets of the nineteenth century, Elizabeth Barrett Browning, became dependent on opium and morphine in much the same way that other middle- and upper-class European and American women of that era did, through their male **physicians**

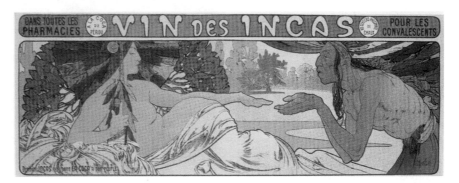

Ad for French tonic wine made with coca leaf extract. It promised to help the user's digestion and disposition (circa 1896 by Alphonse Mucha).
Courtesy of the estate of Timothy C. Plowman

• •

overprescribing psychoactive medications (iatrogenic addiction). In fact the **majority of addicts in the Victorian era were women** (Courtwright, 1982). Some of the more well-known female addicts were the writers Louisa May Alcott and Charlotte Bronte and the actress Sarah Bernhardt. Laudanum compounds and patent medicines were prescribed for anemia, angina, depression, menopause, and the vague complaint of neurasthenia or nervous weakness. Between 1860 and 1901 U.S. imports just of opium rose from 131,000 pounds to 628,000 pounds. In the mid-1880s there were an estimated 150,000–200,000 chronic opium users in the United States (Kandall, 1996).

Cocaine was almost as popular a patent medicine ingredient as opium. In 1887 the Hay Fever Association even declared cocaine to be its official remedy. It was offered for sale in drug stores, by mail order, and in catalogues. From its formulation in 1886 until 1903, **Coca-Cola® contained about 5 mg of cocaine** or one-third to one-half of a "line." Today the beverage contains caffeine and a coca-flavoring extract from which the cocaine has been removed (Karch, 1998). In fact Coca-Cola® continues to this day to be the largest single buyer of Trujillo coca leaf extract.

TWENTIETH CENTURY

FROM PIPES & SMOKELESS TOBACCO TO CIGARETTES

As governments and business companies exploited legal psychoactive substances, especially tea, coffee, alcohol, and tobacco, they became more readily available to the masses. Adding to this movement was the increased recreational use of these stimulants and depressants spurred by democratic governments that allowed greater personal freedom and the growth of a middle class (Matthee, 1995).

Tobacco use is an excellent example of this shift. Historically only small-to-moderate amounts of tobacco had been used—a pinch of snuff for the upper classes and some chopped leaf in

the cheek or in a pipe for the lower classes. At the beginning of the twentieth century, automation (particularly the **automatic cigarette-rolling machine** in 1884), a **milder strain of tobacco** that enabled smokers to inhale deeply, **advertising**, and a **more plentiful supply of the leaf** vastly expanded the market for cigarettes. Other factors that increased the mass use of cigarettes were public health campaigns against chewing tobacco and better cigarette paper (O'Brien, Cohen, Evans, & Fine, 1992).

The pioneer of the "mild" cigarette was the Camel® brand produced by R. J. Reynolds. During the 1920s this brand began to be actively **marketed to women, to young people, and to those who wanted to lose weight**. But even at the beginning of the twentieth century, smoking cigarettes, even with the milder strains of tobacco, was recognized as harmful. And as it had throughout history, the reaction to smoking was often distorted by passion.

"The cigarette has a violent action in the nerve centers, producing degeneration of the brain, which is quite rapid among boys. Unlike most narcotics, this degeneration is permanent and uncontrollable. I employ no person who smokes cigarettes."
Thomas A. Edison, 1914

Inspired by the success of Prohibition, antismoking efforts redoubled. State laws were passed prohibiting cigarettes but they were largely unenforceable and were repealed by the late 1920s. By the '30s **taxes on cigarettes provided a rich source of revenue** for federal and state governments, money that was sorely needed during the Depression and World War II. Cigarette packs were **distributed free to soldiers** during World War II and the Korean War. By the end of World War II demand for cigarettes sometimes exceeded supply and smoking was **considered socially acceptable**.

By mid-century smoking was entrenched in American society. It was a source of revenue for advertisers, retailers, tobacco farmers, the media, and government treasuries. Warnings of the health hazards of smoking were issued as early as 1945 by the Mayo Clinic and were echoed by the American Cancer

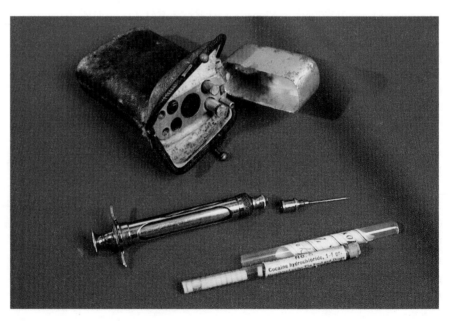

Drug kit on sale at Macys (circa 1908) included vials of cocaine, heroin, and a reusable syringe. Sears Roebuck also sold a drug kit.
Courtesy of the Fitz Hugh Ludlow Memorial Library

Society and various heart and physicians' organizations throughout the 1950s. The tobacco industry ridiculed health concerns and responded to health warnings with slogans, such as "Old Golds: for a treat instead of a treatment," and with the formation of The Tobacco Institute, the chief political lobbying group of the industry. In 1964 and 1967 the Surgeon General issued reports that concluded, "**Cigarette smoking is a health hazard.**" Smoking in the United States generally decreased through the '60s, then began rising during the '70s, and finally went into a long decline that continues into the present.

DRUG REGULATION

Though physicians understood the addictive and health liabilities of opiates and cocaine in the late 1800s, it took another 2 decades before regulation began in the United States. **The Pure Food and Drug Act (1906)** prohibited interstate commerce in misbranded and adulterated foods, drinks, and drugs and it required accurate labeling of the ingredients. **The Opium Exclusion Act (1909)** encouraged the gradual reduction in worldwide opium production and an eventual ban on smoking. Congress banned the importation of opium not intended for medical use the same year. **The Harrison Narcotic Act (1914)** controlled the sale of opium, opium derivatives, and cocaine in the United States by requiring all distributors to pay a tax on these drugs that could then be monitored by the federal government (Acker, 1995). These acts and others did, in fact, eliminate the over-the-counter availability of opiates and cocaine in the United States. Unfortunately the tight control of all supplies encouraged prescription drug diversion and the development of a huge illicit drug trade.

It wasn't only the growing importation of opiates and cocaine and the attendant health and social liabilities of the substances that spurred attempts at drug regulation. When cocaine and opiates made their way to minority and poor urban populations, they became a

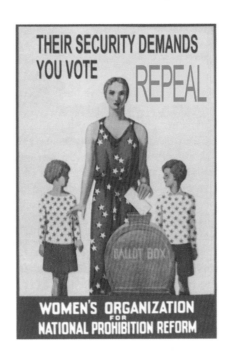

Unlike earlier posters urging protection of children from the evils of alcohol, this 1932 poster advocated protection from the evils of prohibition, namely crime, including corruption and murder.

Courtesy of the Strong Museum, Rochester, New York

●●●●●●●●●●●●●●●●●●●●●●●●●●●●●

matter of great political concern. Headlines about "drug-crazed Negroes," the "Yellow Peril" in regards to the Chinese immigrant use of opiates, along with warnings about sexual promiscuity and rape moved national and state legislatures to enact legislation (Kandall, 1996).

ALCOHOL PROHIBITION & TREATMENT

Between 1870 and 1915, one-half to two-thirds of the U.S. budget came from the tax on liquor. However, the new era in American politics, called the "Progressive Era," eliminated moderation or temperance as a viable choice. The anti-alcohol movement claimed that there could be no compromise with the "forces of evil." There was great debate over whether alcohol abuse was the result of or the cause of poverty with the majority calling it the cause.

It took 13 months to ratify the **Eighteenth Amendment (Prohibition) in 1920** prohibiting the manufacture

and sale of any beverage with an alcohol content greater than 0.5%. This was called "the noble experiment" but it wasn't only the United States that tried prohibition. Shorter noble experiments were tried in Iceland, Russia, parts of Canada, India, and Finland among others (Heath, 1995). It only took just 10 months to **repeal Prohibition 13 years later**. Americans hadn't changed their feelings about the benefits or liabilities of alcohol. They had simply found out that Prohibition created other serious problems for America in spite of the fact that **it did help control a number of serious health and social problems**. Cirrhosis of the liver and other alcohol-related diseases declined dramatically; domestic violence fell; violent crime dropped by two-thirds; and public drunkenness almost disappeared even though people still disregarded the law and drank in speakeasies or made bathtub gin and beer.

Unfortunately during tenure of the Eighteenth Amendment, along with the **Volstead Act that implemented it**, a new coalition of smugglers, strong-arm thieves, Mafia members, corrupt politicians, and crooked police had developed a lucrative trade in the distribution and sale of illicit alcohol. With the return of alcohol to legal status, this coalition turned to other illicit enterprises, including the expansion of their drug trade that handled heroin and cocaine. Whether this expansion of corruption would have gone on if Prohibition had continued is a matter for intense debate.

With the end of Prohibition alcoholism increased again, though it took 20 years for per capita drinking in the United States to reach pre-Prohibition levels. Higher levels of alcoholism were partly answered by the creation of an organization to help alcoholics recover. **Alcoholics Anonymous (AA), a spiritual program that teaches alcoholics 12 steps to recovery**, was founded in 1934 by two alcoholics, Bill Wilson and Doctor Bob Smith (Alcoholics Anonymous [AA], 1934). Over the years AA and its offshoots, such as Narcotics Anonymous, have proved themselves to be the most successful support/recovery programs in history (Trice, 1995). Other programs used the 12-step model to help narcotics addicts (NA), marijuana addicts (MA), overeaters (OA), gamblers (GA), adult children of alcoholics (ACoA), and even sexual addicts (SA).

The success of Alcoholics Anonymous and their cooperation with researchers, physicians, and organizations like the National Council on Alcoholism under Marty Mann was instrumental in convincing the public, hence the politicians, that alcoholism is a disease not a moral weakness.

MARIJUANA: FROM DITCHWEED TO SINSEMILLA

Though *Cannabis* (marijuana) had been widely used in patent medicines that were drunk, **marijuana smoking** wasn't really noticed in the United States until it was seen in Texas around 1910. Gradually it spread to the West and Southwest. To a certain extent alcohol prohibition spread the search for alternative highs. Another reason that marijuana was eventually listed as a narcotic and banned was an antimarijuana campaign by the Hearst newspapers in the 1930s. Publisher William Randolph Hearst had his papers popularize the Mexican word "marijuana" to make the drug sound more foreign and menacing. In addition when alcohol prohibition ended, there were a large number of federal drug-regulatory employees, particularly their boss **Harry Anslinger, who needed a new mission**. Marijuana seemed a likely target. Anslinger used the fear of rape and debauchery to support his opposition to marijuana. Due to the pressure to ban the drug, 46 states passed antimarijuana legislation.

The federal response to marijuana was the **1937 Marijuana Tax Act, which banned *Cannabis sativa*** (marijuana). The ban on growing and using marijuana occurred despite its use in numerous medicines for over 5,000 years though the discovery of newer medications lowered some of its medicinal value. Strangely enough, although marijuana was banned, its sterilized seeds could still be sold for birdseed under the new law. The growing of *Cannabis* in the United States for economic uses, e.g., hemp fiber for rope, paper, and oil, were also effectively prohibited except for a brief period during World War II when it was needed by the military.

During the 1950s, marijuana use was found mainly in a number of rural areas and in the inner cities while it was glamorized by jazz musicians and in the works of the beat generation poets and writers, chiefly Allen Ginsberg, Jack Kerouac, and Gregory Corso. By the 1960s a new generation began to defy prohibitions against marijuana, in part because they discovered it was not as demonic a drug as portrayed by the government and the media.

It was also a **symbol of youthful rebellion** against parents, against authority, and even against the war in Vietnam. Once it became popular, people started practicing different growing techniques. Bags of fertilizer, watering pipes and tubing, window garden boxes, and growing lights became hot items. The price of marijuana was low ($50 to $100 a pound) as was the concentration of THC, the active psychedelic ingredient, although stronger concentrations were grown but not readily available. It wasn't until the 1970s that the **sinsemilla-growing technique** (which increased the concentration of THC) was widespread and the price skyrocketed (*see Chapter 6*). Worldwide, in the 1960s, it was estimated that 250 million people were using marijuana (Fort, 1968).

AMPHETAMINES IN WAR & WEIGHT LOSS

Amphetamine was first synthesized in 1887 and methamphetamine in 1919 but it wasn't until the 1930s when they began to be used medically. Amphetamine was marketed in an inhaler as a **decongestant under the trade name Benzedrine®**. In other forms amphetamines were tried for the treatment of conditions such as low blood pressure, narcolepsy, epilepsy, schizophrenia, alcoholism, and barbiturate intoxication (Grinspoon & Hedblom, 1975). Its **appetite-suppressant qualities were soon recognized**, along with its calming and focusing effect on children diagnosed with what came to be known in later years as "attention-deficit/hyperactivity disorders" (ADHD).

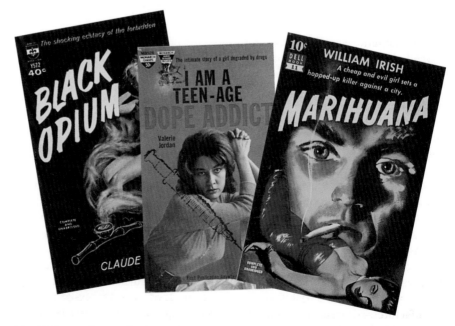

The 1950s saw dozens of pulp novels warning of the dangers of drugs. The "beat" poets and counterculture writers of the '60s reversed this trend.

From the beginning amphetamine's stimulating effects on the central nervous system were recognized and the drug was often used nonmedically (e.g., to stay awake or induce euphoria). These qualities were exploited during **World War II** when, in an attempt to improve the physical performance of soldiers, American, British, German, and Japanese army doctors routinely dispensed amphetamines (speed) to **fight fatigue, heighten endurance, and "elevate the fighting spirit"** (Marnell, 1997). Illicit amphetamine abuse also increased during the 1940s and 1950s among civilian truck drivers and workers engaged in monotonous factory jobs or college students who needed to cram for their exams. A popular song of the times was titled, "Who Put the Benzedrine® in Mrs. Murphy's Ovaltine®." Internationally, **excessive use in Japan after the war led to widespread abuse and thousand of cases of amphetamine psychosis** (Blum, 1984). Sweden also had a huge epidemic in the 1950s due to overuse for weight loss. Massive amounts of amphetamines were also dispensed during the Vietnam War—almost 225 million tablets of Dexedrine®. The publicity about marijuana and heroin use in Vietnam obscured the widespread use of amphetamines (Grinspoon, 1975).

The appetite-suppressant (anorexic) qualities led to the **massive use of amphetamines as diet drugs in the '50s and '60s**. In 1970 it is estimated that 6–8% of the American population were using 12 billion pills, tablets, and capsules containing legal amphetamines, mostly for weight loss.

Although they had been used to excess in the 1950s, amphetamines and methamphetamines were also the **fuel for the "hippie movement" and the "Summer of Love" in 1967**. As a reaction to the suddenly expanded use of these drugs, **The Controlled Substances Act of 1970 was passed**. Initially the legislation made it harder to manufacture and prescribe amphetamines in the United States but the street market expanded to fill the need. "Crosstops," smuggled in from Mexico, were the most popular but methamphetamine in powder or crystal form ("crank," "crystal") was also available.

SPORTS & DRUGS

Even in ancient Greece and Rome the rewards of success in sports were quite large. Plato noted that victory could bring large sums of money, homes, tax exemptions, and even deferment from serving in the army. With such rewards, the desire to excel led many athletes to try anything to improve performance, including extracts of mushrooms, donkey hooves, and plant seeds. These kinds of endeavors fell out of favor and it wasn't until the nineteenth and twentieth centuries that sports again became a rewarding endeavor. As the rewards increased, so did a win-at-any-cost attitude.

The **Cold War** inflamed athletic competition between the Free World and the Communist-bloc countries. This was very evident at the **Olympics** and other international sporting events during the 1950s and 1960s. The use of **anabolic androgenic steroids, stimulants, and other performance-enhancing drugs** became widespread.

"The athletes themselves came out and told that their coaches and scientists forced these drugs on them. And then they found the records that proved it. I've seen these [East] German girls; swimmers with their beards growing out. We used to dance with them after the meet. And their great strength— you didn't want to mess with any of them. They had muscles. They could knock you out."

Su Haa, Turkish Olympic Swim Team, 1972

By 1968 the **International Olympic Committee (IOC)** had defined performance-enhancing drug use, made a list of banned substances, and began drug testing (Australian Drug Foundation [ADF], 1999). The **National Collegiate Athletic Association (NCAA)** began drug testing 18 years later. By that time the proliferation of various steroids, the expansion of an underground steroid network in weightlifting gyms, the growing sophistication of street chemists, and the growth of over-the-counter nutritional supplements, including androstenedione, GHB, and creatine, had multiplied. Recent drug use incidents involving the 2000 Tour de France bicycling race, the 2000 Olympics in Australia, and the 2002 Winter Olympics in Utah emphasized that although testing and vigilance have increased, some athletes will still turn to illegal substances to give themselves an edge.

SEDATIVE-HYPNOTICS & PSYCHIATRIC MEDICATIONS

As the science of pharmacology took advantage of new technologies, drugs could be synthesized rather than having to rely on extracts from natural products. Sedatives, such as bromides, chloral hydrate, ether, and paraldehyde, gave way to barbiturates. The first one marketed was Veronal® (barbital) in 1903; phenobarbital came 10 years later and **eventually 50 barbiturates were used to induce sleep and calm anxiety**. Their use peaked in the 1930s and 1940s. Unfortunately the overprescribing of these drugs plus their addiction and overdose liability led to the development of Miltown® and other milder tranquilizers in the '50s and '60s (Hollister, 1983). **Benzodiazepines came to dominate the prescription downer market**, e.g., Librium®, Valium®, and later Xanax®, Klonopin®, and Halcion®. At one point in the 1980s, 100 million prescriptions were written each year for sedative-hypnotics.

The recognition of chemical brain imbalance as a cause of certain mental illnesses led to the development of **psychiatric medications** other than sedative and hypnotic drugs to treat mental illnesses. The development of **antipsychotics, lithium, antianxiety drugs, and antidepressants**, including tricyclics, MAO inhibitors, and later, SSRIs (selective serotonin reuptake inhibitors) such as Prozac®, led to a clearer understanding of both addictive

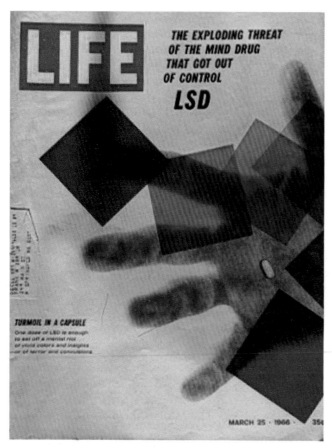

The hallucinogen LSD made a media splash in the 1960s as the public debated whether to accept it as a possible psychotherapeutic medication or to condemn it as a dangerous mind-altering drug.

processes and mental illnesses. The use of these medications to aid in detoxification, long-term abstinence, and relapse prevention became much more common since these psychiatric medications had a much lower addiction liability than standard sedative-hypnotics although they still had significant side effects.

LSD & THE NEW PSYCHEDELICS

Pharmacological developments led not only to synthetic depressants and psychiatric medications but also to new hallucinogenic drugs (psychedelics). For example, the active ingredient in **ergot fungus, called "LSD" (lysergic diethylamide), was isolated and extracted in 1938** in Switzerland by Albert Hoffman of Sandoz Pharmaceuticals although its hallucinogenic properties weren't discovered for five more years when he accidentally dosed himself with 250 micrograms, about 10 times a normal light dose.

"My visual field wavered and everything appeared deformed as in a faulty mirror. Space and time became more and more disorganized and I was overcome by a fear that I was going out of my mind. The worst part of it being that I was clearly aware of my condition."
Albert Hoffman, 1943

Due to his findings various groups, including the psychiatric community, started experimenting with LSD and other psychedelic drugs, seeing them as a potential treatment for mental illness, particularly schizophrenia, and as a way to examine and possibly gain insight into hidden memories and emotions. The army and the CIA experimented with them as mind-control drugs, as truth serums, and as a chemical weapon to disrupt the enemy's thought processes. Still others thought it would enhance human thought and emotions (Julien, 2001).

"Since my illumination of August, 1960, I have devoted most of my energies to try to understand the revelatory potentialities of the human nervous system and to make these insights available to others."
Timothy Leary, 1970

Dr. Timothy Leary encouraged the youth of the 1960s to "turn on, tune in, and drop out" to the apprehension and outrage of older generations and his bosses at Harvard University. The so-called guru of LSD advocated drug experimentation to alter the mind and to gain insight. Psychedelics such as LSD, marijuana, and psilocybin mushrooms were the most popular.

In the 1960s and in the years to come a flood of **synthetic psychedelic drugs, like MDA, DOB, DMT, PCP, 2CB, CBR (nexus), and particularly MDMA (ecstasy), were tried**. These drugs, combined with the new experimental attitude of the times and even newly rediscovered plant psychedelics like *Salvia divinorum*, made many believe in the slogan, "Better living through chemistry."

LEGAL & MEDICAL RESPONSES

The increase in drug use was met with attempts to address the problems of abuse, addiction, and crime brought on by the misuse of drugs. The methods tried were

◊ **supply reduction:** interdiction plus stricter laws concerning use;

◊ **demand reduction:** prevention coupled with treatment;

◊ **harm reduction:** medical or social techniques (e.g., methadone maintenance, free needle distribution, temperance) to reduce the physical and social damage of addiction.

As research findings were compiled, including the **discovery of brain chemicals, e.g., endorphins that acted like psychoactive drugs** (opiates), understanding of the process of addiction grew and treatment facilities expanded. Alcoholism and other addictions were slowly being defined and, to a certain extent, accepted as illnesses. **The treatment of addiction became a medical as well as a social science.** Some of the treatment protocols tried were therapeutic communities, treatment hospitals, free clinics, and 12-step fellowships.

METHADONE & HEROIN

Methadone, a long-acting opiate developed in Germany in the early 1940s, was the keystone of a program called "methadone maintenance." This program, designed to **substitute a legal opiate (methadone) for an illegal one (heroin)**, was developed during the 1960s in New York. Methadone isn't as intense as heroin and keeps the user on a more even keel, though it too is addictive. Methadone clinics spread throughout the United States to where there are now over 950 clinics that supply methadone to about 200,000 heroin addicts, 48,000 in New York City alone (American Methadone Treatment Association [AMTA], 2002). Methadone maintenance programs' original goals were to bring the illegal activities and addictive behavior of the heroin addict population under control. The idea was that if addicted people didn't have to steal for their drug, crime would go down, needle infections would be greatly reduced, and heroin addicts could bring some sanity to their lives. It was an early example of a **harm reduction goal that was targeted to benefit society** as well as the addict. Methadone maintenance continues today as the medical treatment model for opiate or opioid addiction; though there is still controversy and debate in the treatment community as to whether harm reduction should be a goal or a stepping stone on the way to total abstinence.

In the late '60s and '70s an unpopular war in Vietnam, along with a flood of opium from the Golden Triangle (Myanmar [Burma], Laos, and Thailand), encouraged the use of downers. A new group of heroin addicts was created during the years of America's involvement in the war; however, though half the soldiers in Vietnam had experimented with heroin and 20% of those had been addicted at one time, only 5% continued their heroin use after the war.

COCAINE & THE CRACK EPIDEMIC

After the two earlier eras of heavy cocaine use in 1880–1905 and 1920–1930, cocaine use became more limited. It was used primarily by some inner-city residents, underworld figures, jazz musicians, and high-society types. During the late '70s and early '80s, social amnesia about earlier problems with the stimulant, an excess of publicity, new ways of using, and more plentiful supplies promoted the drug. **Cocaine became a fashionable substance once again** (Siegel, 1982).

Snorting and injecting, the traditional methods for using cocaine, were supplemented by **smoking cocaine**. This new form of cocaine, developed in the 1970s, was **known originally as "freebase," and later as "crack" (cheap basing)**. Use went from after-hours clubs, to freebase parlors, to crack houses and individuals' apartments, and finally to street dealers (Hamid, 1992). The ensuing crack epidemic in the mid- and late 1980s was partly fueled by the media's heavy-handed news coverage but mostly by the effects of the drug itself. When smoked, cocaine reaches the brain in 7–10 seconds with a powerful rush. Unfortunately it only lasts a few minutes resulting in a crash that can be overcome by smoking again thus leading to an intense addiction. The other main reasons for crack's surge in use were the low cost of a "hit" and various socioeconomic forces in the inner city, including dissolution of family structures and lack of economic opportunities (Dunlop & Johnson, 1992). Experimentation and binge use were common in the suburbs but as the glamour of crack faded, it **moved to the inner city and heavy use became more prevalent among minorities**. Since the middle and upper classes began avoiding crack cocaine, newspaper coverage faded and all that was left were severe legal penalties for possession and use.

In the late 1980s, perhaps in response to the popularity of smoked cocaine, a slightly altered **smokable methamphetamine, called "ice,"** came onto the scene. Also called "L.A. glass" and "peanut butter," its mental effects were stronger and lasted longer than regular methamphetamines. The initial center of "ice" abuse was Hawaii. By the beginning of the 1990s and even into the 2000s, its use hadn't spread as rapidly as had been feared. However, most of the methamphetamine confiscated recently has been this slightly different form of the drug, the difference being that most of it is for snorting and injecting.

TODAY & TOMORROW

Overall, illicit drug use has declined since its peak in 1979 and 1980; however, the **age of first use of almost all psychoactive drugs has gone down**. Younger and younger people are using drugs experimentally and socially and are getting into habituation, abuse, and addiction. In fact one of the most reliable predictors of developing drug problems and addiction is early-onset drug use. There has been a slight increase in illicit drug use since 1990 but an even greater increase in severe drug abuse over the past 2 decades. The problems with current drug use often have less to do with the actual drug effects and more to do with social ramifications. The most obvious examples are political consequences and health care system overload not just in the United States but throughout the world.

THE GEOPOLITICS OF DRUGS

Heroin

Heroin use has continued its increased popularity into the twenty-first century in the United States, particularly **Mexican black tar and brown heroin** and the relatively new **Colombian white heroin**. New poppy fields

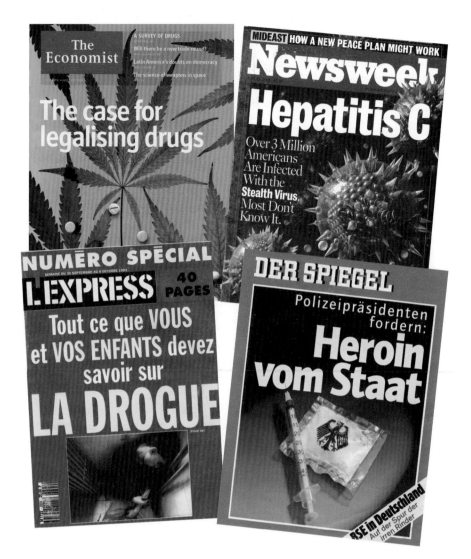

The Economist *from Great Britain,* Der Spiegel *from Germany,* L'Express *from France, and* Newsweek *from the United States are a testament to the variety of social consequences of drug use.*

are popping up not only in Colombia but also in Brazil, Chile, Bolivia, and Venezuela. About one-half of all heroin seizures in the United States in 2000 were from South America. According to congressional testimony by the Drug Enforcement Administration (DEA), much of the heroin is smuggled across the U.S./Mexican border with most of the traffic being controlled by Mexican crime organizations. Even Southeast Asian-based traffickers find it easier to smuggle their **China white heroin** through that route (DEA, 2001a). Because of the increased sources, the purity of heroin has gone up from 5% to 24% while the price has dropped in half

(Office of National Drug Control Policy [ONDCP], 2001).

Internationally the biggest change has been with **Afghan opium and heroin**, particularly in light of the "war on terrorism" in response to the attacks of September 11, 2001, at the World Trade Center in New York, in rural Pennsylvania, and in Washington, D.C. Afghanistan had been the largest grower of opium for many years; providing 4,000 tons or about 75% of the world's supply in 2000. Various groups including the **Taliban and members of the Northern Alliance used the profits to fund insurgencies and/or terrorist activities**, starting with the war

against the former Soviet Union. In November of 2000 Mullah Mohammed Omar, the Taliban's leader, banned poppy growing and heroin refining. The government destroyed fields, set fire to heroin laboratories, and jailed farmers to enforce the ban. In a United Nations field survey in January of 2001 most of the poppy fields were gone although large stores of crops from previous years were warehoused and many farmers saved seeds to replant when the Taliban fell (Associated Press [AP], 2001). **Reports in 2002 showed that it was back to business as usual and most of the poppy fields in Afghanistan have been replanted.** The new Afghan government pledges to eradicate opium but as the country recovers from decades of strife, opium is still the most lucrative crop.

Changes in Southeast Asia, particularly in Myanmar (Burma) the largest producer in the Golden Triangle, have cut production to half the levels of the 1990s. Unfortunately others are always willing to take up the slack as long as there is a market. Thus production has started to rise. The money involved in heroin trafficking is in the billions of dollars, particularly if sold overseas. For example, in 2001 the current price for a standard 700-gram (about 1½ pounds) weight of pure China white heroin was

◇ $2,500 to $3,200 in Myanmar (Burma),
◇ $7,400 to $9,200 in the city of Bangkok, Thailand,
◇ $13,440 to $15,876 in Hong Kong,
◇ $60,000 to $70,000 in the United States.

It takes 10–12 kilograms (kg) of raw opium to make 1 kg of heroin (DEA, 2001b).

Though there is a growing internal market for heroin in the countries that grow and smuggle heroin (about one-fourth of the total crop), the profits still lie in selling it to users in wealthy countries.

The huge profits can buy a lot of guns, bombs, ground-to-air missiles, and bribes and can also finance insurgencies that can't be supported by legitimate means. For example, after World War II the Kuomintang, under **Chiang Kai Shek**, fled from mainland China to Taiwan and Burma. They had been involved with the Green Gang, the leading criminal group in Shanghai that handled heroin among their other illegal activities. **The United States turned a blind eye when they continued growing opium along the Thailand/ Burmese border with China, thus acting as a buffer between Southeast Asia and the Chinese Communists.** The drug gangs had extensive armies made mostly of Kuomintang army members. Taiwan protected members of the Hong Kong triads that handled a lot of the trade, including kingpins such as godfather White Powder Ma. Recently the democratization of Taiwan has prompted a crackdown on some of the criminal activities.

During the Vietnam War the United States again turned a blind eye to drug growing and trafficking by the hill tribesmen (Hmong) so that they would support the effort against the North Vietnamese and Viet Cong. Now that the Cold War is a thing of the past the United States is applying pressure to Thailand and other former "frontline" buffers to Communism to control their drug trafficking (Observatoire Geopolitique des Drogues, 1996).

Cocaine

Geopolitics is also important in cocaine production and smuggling. **Virtually all cocaine is grown in South America**, specifically Colombia, Peru, and Bolivia, and the traffickers continue to infiltrate the economic, political, law enforcement, and military institutions of these countries. Colombia has been in a state of civil war and unrest for more than half a century, originally because of insurgency movements but in the last 20 years cocaine has been the catalyst. In addition countries that are transit routes for smuggling, especially Mexico but also Jamaica, Haiti, the Dominican Republic, the Bahamas, and Puerto Rico, are necessarily vulnerable to corruption

and bribery. About **65% of cocaine smuggled into the United States comes through the U.S./Mexican border**. In 1999 the government had to reassess its estimates of the level of cocaine importation when some highly publicized drug busts yielded very high tonnage—it was estimated that a single Colombian cocaine network was responsible for 30 metric tons a month (ONDCP, 1999). The *U.S. Household Survey* documented that at least 1.2 million Americans used cocaine on a regular basis during 2001 (Substance Abuse and Mental Health Services Administration [SAMHSA], 2002).

HIV, AIDS, & HEPATITIS C

Although **sexually transmitted diseases (STDs)** have been around for millennia, the spread of the **HIV virus** and **AIDS** since the 1980s has been unique and has had a profound impact on society. Worldwide, at the beginning of the new millennium, 21.8 million people have died while over 36.1 million are living with HIV or AIDS; 95% of those are in developing countries. In the United States 448,000 have died and 774,467 are living with HIV or AIDS (Centers for Disease Control [CDC], 2002).

Initially in the United States the HIV virus was spread by unsafe sex, mostly in the gay community but as more people became infected, transmission by **contaminated needles caused an explosion of infections** in the IV drug-using population. Overseas, AIDS is spread primarily by heterosexual sex and secondarily by contaminated needles. In one survey an average of 19% of injection drug users (IDUs) entering treatment tested positive for the HIV virus, a drop from the 50% infection rate at the beginning of the 1990s.

Unfortunately HIV/AIDS hasn't been the only major infection. The prevalence rate among IDUs for hepatitis C (HVC), a liver infection that can be fatal, is up around 85% to 90%. Drug use can also **spread HIV and HVC through high-risk sexual practices** that often occur when inhibitions

are lowered by the drug's effects or by the need to trade sex for drugs (CDC, 2002).

METHAMPHETAMINES

The mid-1990s saw street chemists developing **newer, somewhat safer, and more effective ways of manufacturing illicit methamphetamines** sold as "crank," "crystal," "meth," and "speed." Some of the drugs are produced on small stovetop operations but most of the manufacture and wholesaling is done by Mexican trafficking organizations or by independent gangs in Mexico and the United States. They either manufacture the drugs in Mexico and smuggle them into the United States or they supply raw materials and personnel to set up labs in the United States, mostly in California. Since there are fewer restrictions in Mexico on **precursor chemicals like ephedrine and pseudoephedrine, drugs needed to manufacture speed**, the Mexican nationals have an advantage over the biker gangs and independents that used to manufacture most of the methamphetamine. International efforts to limit the availability of precursor chemicals has lowered the purity of street meth by half (DEA, 2001a). There has also been a large increase in the use of methamphetamines in the midwestern and southern United States. From 1993 to 1999, admissions to drug treatment facilities for amphetamines, mainly methamphetamines, went from 13.8 per 100,000 up to 31.8 per 100,000 (Treatment Episode Data Sets [TEDS], 2001). In addition **methamphetamine abuse is spreading to a number of other countries including the Philippines and Thailand where small methamphetamine pills called "ya ba" have become extremely popular**, particularly among young people and students (TEDS, 2001; Leinwand, 2002).

MODAFINIL (Provigil®)

A stimulant that has recently come on the market, modafinil (Provigil®) does not act on the same parts of the brain as amphetamines or methamphetamines but causes many of the same

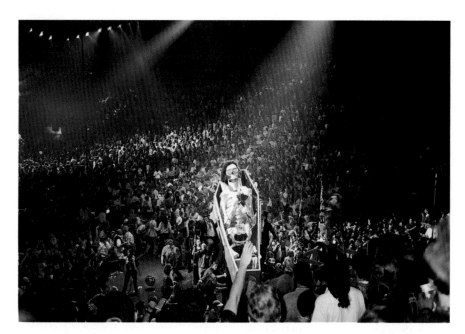

In the 1960s and 1970s it was psychedelic happenings, concerts with light shows, rock music, and LSD and marijuana while in the 2000s it has become rave parties with laser light shows, techno music, and ecstasy, GHB, and marijuana. One of the constants has been the Grateful Dead concerts, such as this Mardi Gras extravaganza, that continue to this day even with the death of Jerry Garcia.

Courtesy of Haight Ashbury Rock Medicine © 1991

effects: wakefulness, some euphoria, increased locomotor activity, and alterations in mood, perception, thinking, and feelings. It is reinforcing when administered in experiments. It was originally approved just for narcolepsy but from the beginning more prescriptions were written than were justified by cases of narcolepsy. Many of the original reports on the drug in the *Physicians' Desk Reference* sound similar to the original reports on other stimulants, including amphetamines. Time will tell as to any extended adverse reactions that may arise from use of the drug.

CLUB DRUGS

One of the biggest changes in the last few years has been a **reemergence of the psychedelic clubs and rock music parties of the '60s and '70s** only now they are called "rave clubs," "rave parties," or just "music parties." The comparisons are inevitable.

◊ In the 1960s there were oil lamp light shows, rock concerts, and drugs. Now it's laser light shows, technorave recorded music, and drugs.

◊ Then it was MDA. Now it's MDMA (ecstasy); they are both called "love drugs."

◊ Then it was STP, PCP, and Quaaludes®. Now it's nexus, ketamine (special K), Rohypnol®, and GHB.

◊ Then it was high-dose LSD (windowpanes and microdots). Now it's low-dose LSD (mostly blotter acid).

◊ Then it was no-name beer and wine. Now it's name brand whiskeys like Cuervo Gold® and Stolichnaya Vodka®, fruit or light beers, and wine coolers.

◊ Then the THC content of pot, "herb," and weed averaged 1–3 %. Now "chronic" and "bud" average 8–14%.

◊ Then cocaine was "blow" and "toot" in powdered form. Now it includes smokable crack cocaine.

◊ Then amphetamines included "crank," "crosstops," "beans," and "cartwheels." Now ya ba and smokable methamphetamine ("ice," "glass") have been added.

◊ Then partygoers inhaled glue, metallic paint, poppers, and nitrous oxide in large tanks (blue nuns). Now embalming fluid, gasoline additives, and nitrous oxide in small whipping cream propellant canisters are popular.

◊ Then a speedball was heroin and cocaine, now it's ecstasy and OxyContin® or ecstasy and hydrocodone (Vicodin®).

◊ Then you "huffed" amyl nitrite (poppers or "snappers"). Now it's isobutyl or isoamyl nitrite (sold as tape head cleaner or sneaker whitener).

◊ Then you could catch herpes, "clap," hepatitis B and syphilis. Now it's also chlamydia, venereal warts, hepatitis C, and HIV/AIDS.

The most common drug used at these rave parties, **MDMA (ecstasy, "X," "E," "Adam," and rave), is a psycho-stimulant**. One dose can cost $20 to $30. MDMA users claim that it promotes closeness and empathy, along with a loss of inhibitions that can trigger a strong urge to socialize, dance, and keep active. Dilution and adulteration are common with MDMA; PMA (paramethoxyamphetamine) and other stimulants are often found in bogus MDMA.

Another drug that has seen more abuse in recent years is **GHB (gammahydroxybutyrate), a sedative**. This drug was originally developed as an anaesthetic-induction medication and is occasionally used in Europe to treat narcolepsy and alcohol or opiate dependence. It was banned in the United States because youths were using it as a sedative, to induce euphoria, and for its anabolic or muscle-building effects. It has also been used by sexual predators to induce amnesia in their victims. Nausea, vomiting, myoclonic seizures, short comas, and a number of deaths from respiratory depression, particularly when used in combination with alcohol, have been reported. Emergency room mentions for GHB and MDMA quadrupled from 1998–2000 (Drug Abuse Warning Network [DAWN], 2002). Dextromethorphan (DXM), which acts as a depressant, is also used.

MARIJUANA (*Cannabis*) & HEALTH

At the start of the twenty-first century, marijuana is the most widely used illicit drug in the United States and in many countries such as Canada, Mexico, Costa Rica, El Salvador, Panama, Australia, and South Africa (National Institute on Drug Abuse [NIDA], 1998). **High-potency marijuana continues to be widely available** (up to 14 times as strong as varieties available in the 1970s). High-potency marijuana was always available but it was just not very plentiful. Just as the refinement of coca leaves into cocaine and opium into morphine and heroin led to greater abuse with those drugs, so have better sinsemilla-cultivation techniques increased the compulsive liability of marijuana. As with cocaine and heroin, the higher-potency marijuana commands a much steeper price, a 10- to 30-fold increase since the early 1970s.

The biggest story continues to be **attempts to legalize medical marijuana**. In 2001 the Supreme Court of the United States ruled that federal law prohibits dispensing the drug to seriously ill patients to relieve their pain and nausea even if the individual state allows it. The ruling applies to California, Alaska, Arizona, Colorado, Hawaii, Maine, Nevada, Oregon, and Washington, states that allow the use of medical marijuana by prescription. Recently several quasi legal *Cannabis* **clubs that dispense medical marijuana** were raided by the federal government to support the decision. By contrast Canada just passed a law to allow seriously ill patients to grow and smoke marijuana. The 300 Canadians that were already exempted from Canadian drug laws will be joined by thousands more.

The **drive to legalize or at least decriminalize marijuana continues**. A 2001 *USA TODAY*/CNN/Gallup Poll survey found that 34% of Americans favor full legalization of marijuana while other polls show that 70% support medical marijuana. The National Organization for the Reform of Marijuana Laws (NORML) and other groups have been pressing for legalization of marijuana for over 25 years with only limited success. Opponents of medical marijuana contend that legalization is a cover for use of marijuana as a euphoriant, that there is not enough sound medical evidence of the drug's usefulness in medical treatment, and that other drugs are medically more effective. The controversy and legal battles are likely to continue well into the future.

TOBACCO, HEALTH, & THE LAW

After a rise in smoking among American junior high and high school students in the 1990s, smoking has started to decline again in the 2000s. It has continued its decline among the 18-and-above age groups since the peak smoking year of 1962. **Between 1962 and 2001 per capita tobacco use declined by more than 30%** (SAMHSA, 2002). This decline originally resulted from the U.S. Surgeon General's Report on the dangers of smoking in 1964. Since then continuing research on dangerous health effects from smoking, antismoking campaigns, warnings printed on packaging, legislation prohibiting smoking on aircraft and in public places, lawsuits against tobacco companies, and restrictions placed on tobacco advertising have had their effect.

When the heads of the major tobacco companies appeared before Congress in the 1990s, they testified that cigarettes were not addictive or dangerous. The public soon began to realize that, indeed, the **tobacco industry did know about the addictive nature and health dangers of tobacco**. In fact in 2001 Philip Morris' international arm, in a memo to the Czech Republic, tried to convince them not to enact antismoking policies by showing how the thousands of premature deaths from smoking could save them health care, pension, and housing payments. Fortunately about 3,500 cigarette smokers do quit each day. Unfortunately 1,178 die prematurely each day in the United States from the effects of smoking. Increased smoking among women worldwide **increased lung cancer deaths past those from breast cancer** (Konietzko, 2001).

The tobacco companies have tried to keep their revenues up by **developing foreign markets**. They also have tried to sustain the U.S. market by marketing generic brands, cutting prices, as well as targeting females, minorities, and younger smokers.

In 1998 in the biggest class-action lawsuit settlement ever, the **major tobacco companies agreed to pay $246 billion over a period of 25 years** to the various states aimed toward programs to prevent teenagers from smoking and to help defray the medical costs associated with diseases caused by smoking or chewing tobacco. Unfortunately many of the states used the largest percentage of the money to defray the costs of other programs rather than for the stated purposes. In addition the change in the presidency in 2000 from Democratic to Republican reduced the aggressiveness of the U.S. Attorney General's office in pursuing legal action against the tobacco companies through reduced funding for existing lawsuits and declined to pursue new ones. However, on an individual and even state level, the lawsuits continue. Ironically, despite the heavy negative publicity and multiple court losses, tobacco companies' stocks dramatically increased in value during the 1990s and early 2000s despite a recession.

OXYCONTIN® (oxycodone) & VICODIN® (hydrocodone)

The onset of OxyContin® abuse shows how a technological change can increase problems with an existing drug. OxyContin® was developed in the late 1990s as a **time-release version of oxycodone** an opiate originally sold as Percodan®. Opiate addicts discovered that when crushed the drug loses its time-release capabilities and when swallowed or injected it gives a powerful almost **heroin-like high**. A rash of pharmacy robberies, forged prescriptions, and overdoses caused the DEA to send out warnings. In response the manufacturer, Purdue Pharma, is developing a new formulation that releases Narcan®, a drug that counteracts the effects of oxycodone, from capsules if the medication is crushed, thus counteracting the rush and high of the OxyContin®.

Hydrocodone (Vicodin®) is the most widely abused prescription opiate, a title that used to belong to codeine-based prescriptions. Hydrocodone caused less nausea but still has the same addictive potential as codeine. The number of people who take painkillers like hydrocodone for nonmedical reasons has risen from 500,000 in 1990 up to 1.2 million in 2001. Recently a number of cases of rapid-onset hearing loss caused by heavy abuse of Vicodin® have been reported.

ALCOHOL HANGS ON

The drug that has never been out of favor is alcohol. It is still widely used by every age group and in every country (except Muslim nations). As in the past, used separately or in combination with other psychoactive drugs, **alcohol still kills over 130,000 persons a year** in the United States compared to only 8,000 killed by all other illicit psychoactive drugs combined. In 2001 there were an estimated **13 million alcoholic Americans** and though that figure is just 5.6% of the population, alcoholics make up 10% to 15% of those in hospitals and 10% to 20% of those in nursing homes (SAMHSA, 2002).

Research into the causes and treatment of alcoholism and addiction in general has intensified over the last 10 years. The areas of focus include **genetic components of susceptibility, neurobiology of satiation, pharmacological interventions to reduce cravings, and refinement of treatment techniques** such as brief intervention and getting the primary physician more involved in diagnosing at-risk patients.

BEHAVIORAL ADDICTIONS (e.g., eating disorders, compulsive gambling)

"If I won all the money in the world, I'd have to move to a different world. If I won all the money in the world, there'd be no action, there'd be no game because there'd be no other players."
45-year-old compulsive gambler

A study of MRI brain scans of gamblers showed that the areas of the brain activated by winning or losing are the same as those activated by cocaine. In addition the blood flow increases, the heart rate goes up, and sweating increases. This and other research strongly suggests that **compulsive behaviors have many of the same signs and symptoms as drug addiction**. These include compulsive gambling, compulsive overeating, bulimia, anorexia, sexual addiction, Internet addiction, and even compulsive shopping. This and other research strongly suggests that some compulsive behaviors have many of the same symptoms and similar brain activity as drug addiction (Blum et al., 2000). Besides genetic components the environmental components such as fast-food restaurants with high-fat/high-sugar foods, the growth of the Internet, shopping networks, easily accessible pornography, and the explosion of gambling establishments have greatly increased the chances to practice these addictions.

COURT-REFERRED TREATMENT

Drug policy has shifted in the past 20 years from a heavy emphasis on supply reduction (stopping drugs at the borders, raiding laboratories, legislation, etc.) to an **equal emphasis on demand reduction** (treatment on demand, drug courts, prevention, etc.). In 2000, 61% of Californian voters passed Proposition 36, which requires a treatment option for nonviolent drug users on their first and second offense; about 37,000 offenders will be eligible. The budget is around $120 million a year but the state estimates that $250 million will be saved by keeping thousands out of jail if the treatment option works as planned.

About 40 states already use drug courts where a first-time offender can be **diverted from jail time to treatment**. From the first one started in 1989 in Dade County, Florida, the number has grown to more than **700 drug courts nationwide** (Drug Policy Research Center [DPRC], 2000). There is controversy over a number of aspects of drug courts but most agree that if they are successful, the savings to society financially and socially are quite large. This direction in treatment is known as "coerced treatment" since many addicts would not have voluntarily entered treatment had it not been legally mandated. Coerced treatment has demonstrated better outcomes than voluntary treatment according to David Deitch, Director of the Pacific Southwest Addiction Technology Transfer Center at the University of San Diego.

CONCLUSIONS

Some historians have suggested that the drive to alter states of consciousness is as essential to human nature as the drive to survive and procreate (Siegal, 1982). This concept is tenable if one understands that the use of psychoactive substances can create a drive or compulsion to continue using that supersedes many survival instincts. Botanical, pharmacological, and technological advances have increased the concentration and delivery methods of these drugs such that they overwhelm the brain's ability to rebalance itself more quickly than with the original substances. If one then couples the drive to overuse these substances with economic, political, and spiritual motives, then the influence of drugs on our development as human beings can be better understood.

The basic reasons for wanting to change one's perception of reality and consciousness will probably stay the same in succeeding generations and psychoactive drugs or other compulsive behaviors are ways that people will choose to try to bring about that change. It is, therefore, crucial to understand psychoactive drugs because they will affect us directly (physically and mentally) or indirectly (economically and socially) for the rest of our lives.

With the traumatic events of September 11, 2001, and the subsequent "war on terrorism", and invasions of Afghanistan and Iraq, the so-called war on drugs seems less pressing. Although violence and terrorism have been with us as long as the use and abuse of mind-altering substances, there are no easy answers. Any resolutions of the problems will only be temporary because the environment that escalates political or religious resolve into violence and drug use into abuse and addiction will always be with us. Continued research is needed to understand the roots of both problems but unfortunately **geopolitical considerations often get in the way of sensible and logical solutions**. Possible solutions to both situations need imagination, patience, intelligence, and resolve.

CLASSIFICATION OF PSYCHOACTIVE DRUGS

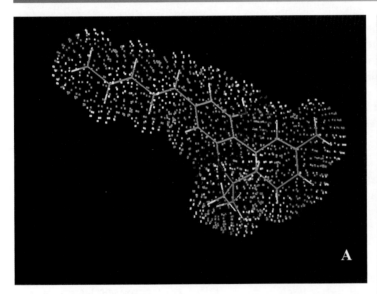

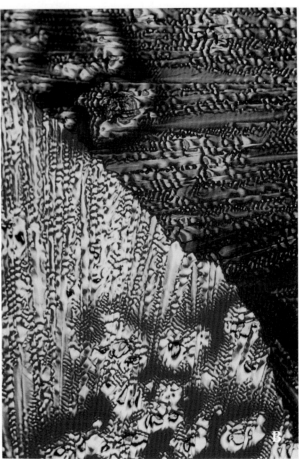

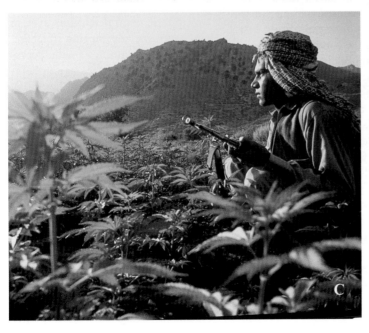

A drug such as marijuana can be examined theoretically as a molecule (A), microscopically as a crystal (B), or sociologically as a source of financing for insurgencies (C).

Molecular graphics image produced using the MidasPlus® package from the Computer Graphics Laboratory, University of California, San Francisco (supported by NIH P41 RR-01081). Crystalline photomicrograph courtesy of Michael W. Davidson, © 1999, Institute of Molecular Biophysics, Florida State University, Tallahassee, FL. Uzbekistan marijuana field photograph reprinted, by permission, Alain Labrousse.

WHAT IS A PSYCHOACTIVE DRUG?

◊ In ancient Egypt the Pharaoh Ramses might have defined a psychoactive drug as the beer he gave his pyramid workers to keep them happy.

◊ In second century B.C. Greece the physician Galen would have defined it as theriac, an opium-based cure-all he prescribed for his patients.

◊ A poisoned Frenchman in the Middle Ages could have defined it as the infected rye grain (ergot) he accidentally ate.

◊ About A.D. 1550 Spanish Conquistadors in Peru would have defined it as the coca leaves they gave to the native laborers to keep them working in the silver mines.

◊ A wounded soldier in the U.S. Civil War might say it was the injection of morphine that relieved his pain and caused euphoria.

◊ A pilot in World War II would have defined it as the amphetamine the medic gave him to stay awake on a night bombing run.

◊ In the 1990s an AIDS patient might define a psychoactive drug as a joint of marijuana that controls nausea.

◊ A law enforcement officer might define a psychoactive drug by its legal classification as a Schedule I, II, III, or IV substance whose illegal use and sale carry legal penalties.

◊ A member of Gamblers Anonymous might define a psychoactive drug as a video poker machine available at the local tavern.

"A psychoactive drug is any substance that when injected into a rat gives rise to a scientific paper."
Darryl Inaba, Pharm.D., CEO, Haight Ashbury Free Clinics

Each culture, each generation, each profession, and particularly each user has a definition of what constitutes a psychoactive drug. To complicate matters, most people who take psychoactive drugs on a regular basis use more than one substance.

DEFINITION

Our definition of **a psychoactive drug is any substance that directly alters the normal functioning of the central nervous system**. Today there are more psychoactive drugs to choose from than at any time in history. Modern transportation, a more open society, the ability to purchase drugs over the Internet, greater financial incentives for drug dealing, easy access to legal psychoactive drugs like tobacco, alcohol, caffeine, and prescription medications, and new refinement and synthesis techniques have all come together to increase availability of these chemicals to all strata of society.

CHEMICAL, TRADE, & STREET NAMES

The difficulty categorizing psychoactive drugs is that they have chemical names, trade names, and street names. For example, **street names** like "blunts," "chronic," and "bammer" for marijuana; "boulya," "24–7," and "beamers" for crack cocaine; ecstasy, and "E," for MDMA; and "chiva," "H," and "shit," for heroin evolve almost daily among drug users. Each commonly used and abused substance may have 20 or more informal names. Just as confusing is the continued synthesis of newer psychoactive drugs with **chemical names** such as methylenedioxymethamphetamine (MDMA) and 4-bromo 2,5 dimethoxy phenethylamine (2CB). **Trade names** such as Zoloft® instead of its chemical name sertraline, or OxyContin® instead of oxycodone further confuse the issue of how to classify psychoactive drugs.

Lawmakers have to be careful when outlawing a drug since they must describe its exact chemical formula. Customs officials have to examine imported herbal medicines carefully because some of them contain natural forms of restricted psychoactive substances.

CLASSIFICATION BY EFFECTS

A more practical way of classifying these substances is by their overall effects. Thus the terms **"uppers" for stimulants, "downers" for depressants, and "all arounders" for psychedelics** have been chosen to describe the most commonly abused psychoactive drugs. Then there are other drugs that don't fit neatly into one of these categories but that can be defined by their purpose, such as performance-enhancing **sports drugs, inhalants, and psychiatric medications** (e.g., antidepressants).

Caution: *Since drug effects depend on amount, frequency, and duration of use as well as the makeup of the user and the setting in which the drug is used, reactions to psychoactive substances can vary radically from person to person and even from dose to dose. Our information about the action of drugs on the body should be used as a general guideline and not as an absolute guide to the effects. It should not, in any way, be construed as medical advice.*

MAJOR DRUGS

UPPERS (stimulants)

Uppers, central nervous system stimulants, include **cocaine** (freebase, crack), **amphetamines** (meth, "crystal," speed, "crank," "ice"), **amphetamine congeners** (Ritalin®, diet pills), **plant stimulants** (khat, betel nuts, ephedra, yohimbe), **lookalike stimulants, caffeine, nicotine**, and newer synthetic substances like Modafinil®.

Physical Effects

The usual effect of a small-to-moderate dose is excessive **stimulation of the nervous system** creating energized muscles, increased heart rate, increased blood pressure, insomnia, and decreased appetite. Frequent use of the stronger stimulants (cocaine and amphetamines) over a period of a few days will deplete the body's energy chemicals and exhaust the user. If large amounts are used or if the user is extrasensitive, heart, blood vessel, and seizure problems can occur. Although tobacco is a comparatively weak stimulant, its long-term health effects can be dangerous, e.g., cancer, emphysema, and heart disease.

Mental/Emotional Effects

A small-to-moderate dose of the stronger stimulants can make someone **feel more confident**, outgoing, eager to perform, and excited. It can also **cause a certain rush** or ecstatic feeling depending on the physiology of the user and the specific drug. Larger doses can cause jitteriness, **anxiety**, anger, rapid speech, and **aggressiveness**. Prolonged use of the stronger stimulants can cause extreme anxiety, **paranoia**, anhedonia (inability to experience pleasure), and mental confusion. Overuse of strong stimulants can even mimic a **psychosis**.

DOWNERS (depressants)

Downers, central nervous system depressants, are divided into four main categories:

◇ **Opiates & Opioids:** opium, morphine, codeine, heroin, oxycodone (OxyContin®, Percodan®), hydrocodone; (Vicodin®), methadone, hydromorphone (Dilaudid®), meperidine (Demerol®), propoxyphene (Darvon®);

◇ **Sedative-Hypnotics:** benzodiazepines, e.g., alprazolam (Xanax®), diazepam (Valium®), clonazepam (Klonipin®), flunitrazepam (Rohypnol®); barbiturates, e.g. butalbital, zolpidem (Ambien®), meprobamate (Miltown®);

◇ **Alcohol:** beer, wine, and hard liquors;

◇ **Others:** antihistamines, skeletal muscle relaxants, lookalike sedatives, and bromides.

Physical Effects

Small doses of downers **depress the central nervous system**, which slows heart rate and respiration, relaxes muscles, decreases coordination, induces sleep, dulls the senses, and most importantly, especially with opiates and opioids, diminishes pain. Opiates and opioids can also cause constipation, nausea, and pinpoint pupils, which is why they're used to control diarrhea and headaches. Excessive drinking or sedative-hypnotic use can slur speech and cause digestive problems. Sedative-hypnotics and alcohol in large doses or in combination with other depressants can cause dangerous respiratory depression and coma. Large-dose use or prolonged use of any depressant can cause sexual dysfunction and tissue dependence.

Mental/Emotional Effects

Initially, small doses (particularly with alcohol) seem to act like stimulants because **they lower inhibitions thus inducing freer behavior**. But as more of the drug is taken the overall depressant effect begins to dominate, relaxing and dulling the mind, diminishing anxiety, and controlling some neuroses. Certain downers can also **induce euphoria** or a sense of well-being. Long-term use of any depressant can **cause physical and psychic dependence**.

ALL AROUNDERS (psychedelics)

All arounders (hallucinogens or psychedelics) are substances that can distort perceptions and induce illusions, delusions, or hallucinations. There are five classifications for psychedelics:

◇ Ergots/Indoles: **LSD, psilocybin mushrooms**, ayahuasca, and DMT;

◇ Phenylalkylamines: peyote (mescaline), **MDMA (ecstasy)**, MDA, 2CB, & ibogaine;

◇ Anticholinergics: belladonna, datura, jimson weed;

◇ Cannabinoids: **marijuana,** hashish;

◇ Others: **ketamine, PCP**, nutmeg, *Amanita* mushrooms.

Physical Effects

Most hallucinogenic plants, particularly cacti and some mushrooms, **cause nausea and dizziness**. Marijuana increases appetite and makes the eyes bloodshot. LSD raises the blood pressure and causes sweating. **MDMA and even LSD act like stimulants**. Generally, except for PCP and ketamine that act as anesthetics, the physical effects are not as dominant as the mental effects.

Mental/Emotional Effects

Most often psychedelics **distort sensory messages** to and from the brain stem, the sensory switchboard for the mind, so that many external stimuli, particularly visual, touch, and auditory ones, are intensified or altered (**illusions**). Imaginary sensory messages (**hallucinations**) can also be created by the brain, along with distorted thinking (**delusions**).

OTHER DRUGS & ADDICTIONS

There are three other groups of drugs that can stimulate, depress, or confuse the user: inhalants, anabolic steroids and other sports drugs, and psychiatric medications.

INHALANTS (deliriants)

Inhalants are gaseous or liquid substances that are inhaled and absorbed through the lungs. They include **organic solvents**, such as glue, gasoline, metallic paints, gasoline additives (STP®) and household sprays; **volatile nitrites**, such as amyl, butyl, or cyclohexyl nitrite (also called "poppers"); and **anesthetics**, especially nitrous oxide (laughing gas).

Physical Effects

Most often there is **central nervous system depression**. Dizziness, slurred speech, unsteady gait, and drowsiness are seen early on. Some inhalants **lower blood pressure** causing the user to faint or lose balance. Since they are depressants they cause drowsiness, stupor, coma, and asphyxiation.

The organic solvents can be quite **toxic to cells** in the lung, brain, liver, kidney tissues, and even the blood.

Mental/Emotional Effects

With small amounts, **impulsiveness, excitement, mental confusion, and irritability** are common. Some inhalants cause a rush through a variety of mechanisms. Larger amounts can cause **delirium and some hallucinations**.

ANABOLIC STEROIDS & OTHER SPORTS DRUGS

Anabolic-androgenic steroids are the most common **performance-enhancing drugs**. Others include stimulants (e.g., amphetamines, ephedrine, caffeine), human growth hormone (HGH), HCG, herbal/nutritional supplements (e.g., creatine, androstenedione), and some therapeutic drugs (e.g., painkillers, beta-blockers, diuretics).

Physical Effects

Anabolic steroids **increase muscle mass and strength**. Prolonged use can cause acne, high blood pressure, shrunken testes, and masculinization in women.

Mental/Emotional Effects

Anabolic steroids often cause a **stimulant-like high, increased confidence, and increased aggression**. Prolonged large-dose use can be accompanied by outbursts of anger known as "rhoid rage."

PSYCHIATRIC MEDICATIONS

These medications are used by psychiatrists and others in an expanding field known as "psychopharmacology" to try to **rebalance irregular brain chemistry** that has caused mental problems, drug addiction, and other compulsive disorders. The most common are **antidepressants** (e.g., Tofranil®, Prozac®, Zoloft®), **antipsychotics** (e.g., Resperidol®, Zyprexa®), and **antianxiety** drugs (e.g., Xanax®, BuSpar®) including panic disorder drugs (e.g., Inderal®). These drugs are being prescribed more and more frequently de-

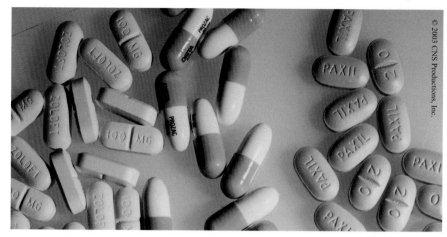

In the last few years, the number of available psychiatric drugs has increased. The most popular have been the new selective serotonin reuptake inhibitors (SSRIs) (e.g., Zoloft®, Prozac®, and Paxil®).

spite the fact that the national incidence of the disorders has remained fairly constant over the past 30 years.

Physical Effects

Psychiatric medications are accompanied by a **wide variety of physical side effects**, particularly on the heart, blood, and skeletal-muscle systems, but their mental and emotional effects are the most important. Side effects, adverse reactions, and toxic effects are especially severe with antipsychotic drugs (also called "neuroleptic drugs").

Mental/Emotional Effects

Antidepressants counteract depression by manipulating brain chemicals, such as serotonin, that **elevate mood**. Antipsychotics manipulate dopamine to **control schizophrenic mood swings and hallucinations**. Antianxiety drugs also manipulate brain chemicals, such as GABA, to **inhibit anxiety-producing thoughts**.

COMPULSIVE BEHAVIORS

Behaviors such as **eating disorders** (compulsive overeating, anorexia, bulimia), **compulsive gambling, sexual compulsion, Internet addiction, compulsive shopping, and even codependency** affect many of the same areas of the brain impacted by compulsive use of psychoactive drugs.

Physical Effects

The major physical effects of compulsive behaviors are generally confined to **neurological and chemical changes in the brain's reward pathway** except with eating disorders when excessive or extremely limited food intake can lead to cardiovascular problems, diabetes, nutritional diseases, and obesity.

Mental/Emotional Effects

The development of tolerance, psychological dependence, and even withdrawal symptoms exist with compulsive behaviors as do abuse and addiction. The compulsion to gamble or overeat is every bit **as strong as drug-seeking behavior**.

CONTROLLED SUBSTANCES ACT OF 1970

The Comprehensive Drug Abuse Prevention and Control Act of 1970, better known as the Controlled Substances Act was enacted to **reduce the burgeoning availability and use of psychoactive drugs** that occurred in the 1960s in the United States. The act consolidated and updated most drug laws that had been passed in the twentieth century. The **Drug Enforcement Administration** was made responsible for enforcing the provisions of the act.

The key provisions were to classify all psychoactive drugs, to control their manufacture, sale, and use, to limit imports and exports, and to define criminal penalties. Five levels or schedules of drugs were defined based on abuse liability, its value as a medication, its history of use and abuse, the risk to public health, and in a few cases, political considerations.

◇ Schedule I includes heroin, LSD, marijuana, peyote, psilocybin, mescaline, and MDMA. These drugs have a high abuse potential and supposedly no accepted medical use.

◇ Schedule II substances have a high abuse potential with severe psychic or physical dependence liability even though there are medical uses for the drugs. They include cocaine, methamphetamine, opium, morphine, hydromorphone, codeine, meperidine, oxycodone, and methylphenidate (Ritalin®).

◇ Schedule III substances have less abuse potential and include Schedule II drugs when used in compounds with other drugs. Schedule III drugs include Tylenol® with codeine, some barbiturate compounds, and paregoric.

◇ Schedule IV drugs have even less abuse potential and include chloral hydrate, meprobamate, fenfluramine, diazepam (Valium®) and the other benzodiazepines, and phenobarbital.

◇ Schedule V substances have very low abuse potential because they contain very limited quantities of narcotic and stimulant drugs. Examples of Schedule V are Robitussin AC® (DXM), and Lomotil®. Some of these drugs are sold over the counter.

CHAPTER SUMMARY

INTRODUCTION

1. Psychoactive drugs and drug-seeking behaviors have always been extremely influential in all aspects of human endeavors. Historically five themes have affected the use and abuse of these substances:

◇ a basic need of human beings to cope with their environment;

◇ a brain chemistry that can be affected by certain substances to induce an altered state of consciousness;

◇ government and business involvement in growing, manufacturing, distributing, taxing, and prohibiting drugs;

◇ technological advances in refining and synthesizing drugs;

◇ development of more efficient and faster methods for putting drugs into the body.

HISTORY OF PSYCHOACTIVE DRUGS

Prehistory & the Neolithic Period (8500–4000 B.C.)

2. More than 4,000 plants yield psychoactive substances. Their use dates back 50,000 years or more.

3. Psychoactive drugs have been used throughout history as a shortcut to an altered consciousness, to relieve pain, and for spiritual rituals.

Ancient Civilizations (4000 B.C.–A.D. 400)

4. Drugs and methods of use gradually spread as contact among different cultures increased.

5. Alcohol (beer and wine), opium, *Cannabis*, peyote cacti, psychedelic mushrooms, coca, and tobacco were the earliest psychoactive drugs employed by ancient civilizations.

6. Alcohol was considered a gift from the gods and it was used as a food, a reward, a medicine, and for sacred or shamanic rituals. It is often mentioned in the *Bible* with warnings about overindulgence.

7. Opium has been used to stop pain, control diarrhea, stop coughs, lessen anxiety, promote sleep, and induce euphoria.

8. *Cannabis* was used in China and India as a medicine, a food, a fiber, and a euphoriant.

9. *Amanita* mushrooms were used in Asia and Mesoamerica for visions and sacred ceremonies.

10. The peyote and San Pedro cacti (mescaline), the coca leaf (cocaine), the *Psilocybe* mushroom (psilocybin), and tobacco (nicotine) were used in Mesoamerica before the birth of Christ and that use continues to this day. Other stimulant alkaloids from plants include betel nut, coffee, khat, and ephedra.

Middle Ages (400–1400)

11. Psychedelic plants from the nightshade family (e.g., datura, belladonna, henbane, mandrake) were employed in religious, magic, or social ceremonies throughout history and especially in the Middle Ages. Their active ingredients include scopolamine and atropine.

12. Psychedelic mold on infected rye plants (which produced LSD-like symptoms) caused ergot poisonings in the Middle Ages and beyond.

13. A psychoactive substance can be a medicine, a drug, and a poison depending on the dose. Sometimes it can be a food or drink.

14. During the Middle Ages distillation was discovered. It increased the alcoholic content of beverages through evaporation and condensation. Before distillation about 14% alcohol was the strongest alcohol available.

15. In many Islamic countries, tobacco, hashish, and especially cof-

fee were employed as substitutes for alcohol that was forbidden by the holy book of the Islamic religion, the *Koran*.

16. The use of coffee and tea spread to Europe and became extremely popular. Sixty other plants contain caffeine.

17. The coca leaf, peyote cactus, *Psilocybe* mushroom, and ololiuqui were used in the Americas in pre-Columbian times, mostly by the ruling classes.

Renaissance & the Age of Discovery (1400–1700)

18. Exploration, trade, and colonization by European explorers brought back various drugs to Europe and carried European drugs, principally alcohol and the newly discovered tobacco, to other peoples.

19. Laws limiting alcohol use, along with taxes for use, were tried in most countries but the medicinal and recreational uses, along with high tax revenues, were so widespread that the laws often failed.

20. In South America Spanish Conquistadors defeated the Incas and took control of coca leaf production. They grew it for profit, to pay workers, and to stimulate the peasants to work longer in the silver mines.

21. Tobacco, which was used in the Americas as a medicine, for rituals, and to induce trance-like states, was introduced to Europe and back to the colonized Americas in the 1500s. Tobacco and hemp helped support many colonies.

22. Coffee houses and afternoon tea helped spread the popularity of coffee and tea drinking.

23. Opium was used as a cure-all throughout history. Scientists and physicians such as Galen in the second century, Avicenna in the eleventh century, and Parcelsus in the sixteenth century introduced theriac and laudanum to succeeding generations.

Age of Enlightenment & the Early Industrial Revolution (1700–1900)

24. During this period new refinement techniques and new methods of using were developed.

25. Consumption of distilled liquors like rum, gin, and whiskey increased alcohol abuse, sometimes to epidemic proportions as in the Gin Epidemic in London (1710–1750). Consumption had been encouraged then discouraged by the British Parliament.

26. The American Revolution was supported by the export of and taxes on tobacco (Virginia leaf mostly), hemp (textile/ rope industry), and rum.

27. In the nineteenth century nitrous oxide (laughing gas), an anesthetic, was used at inhalant parties as an intoxicant. Other anesthetics that came into use were chloroform and ether. Later hydrocarbon distillates were also inhaled.

28. The refinement of morphine from opium (1804) and heroin from morphine (1874), along with the invention of the hypodermic needle (1855) and the widespread use of morphine in wartime to control pain, expanded the addictive use of opiates.

29. The Opium Wars between England and China in the early to mid-1800s were fought for the right of the British (East India Trading Company) to sell opium to China (under the Manchus) in order to improve the British balance of trade. Other European powers also took part.

30. In the second half of the nineteenth century the refinement of cocaine from coca, its use as a topical anesthetic, the popularization of cocaine by Freud, and the manufacture of stimulant wines, such as Vin Mariani, led to the first cocaine epidemic.

31. The Temperance movement, begun in the eighteenth century by Dr. Benjamin Rush and others in the United States, led to state prohibition laws and temperance societies.

32. Patent medicines at the turn of the twentieth century frequently contained opium, cocaine, and alcohol as their active ingredients. Overprescribing by physicians, usually to women, often led to abuse (iatrogenic addiction).

Twentieth Century

33. Cigarettes gradually replaced cigars and chewing tobacco as the most popular method of nicotine consumption due to automatic cigarette-rolling machines, advertising, a milder strain of tobacco, and plentiful supplies. Women, young people, soldiers, and dieters were often targeted. Use (and taxes) increased through the first half of the century and then began to decline following public health campaigns and legal restrictions.

34. The Pure Food and Drug Act (1906), the Opium Exclusion Act (1909), and the Harrison Narcotic Act (1914) were passed to control opiates and cocaine. Racial biases often influenced legislation.

35. The Eighteenth Amendment (alcohol prohibition) and the supporting Volstead Act lasted from 1920 to 1933. They helped create the multi-billion dollar illegal drug business. The widespread abuse of alcohol encouraged the creation of Alcoholics Anonymous (AA) in 1934, the most successful drug treatment program in history.

36. Marijuana smoking was banned in 1937 by the Marijuana Tax Act. Marijuana became a symbol of the beat generation in the 1950s and the hippie generation in the 1960s. The sinsemilla-growing technique increased the psychoactive properties of marijuana starting in the '70s.

37. Amphetamines, first popularized in the 1930s as a decongestant, were used by soldiers on both sides in World War II to fight fatigue.

They were used and abused as diet drugs in the '50s and '60s. Methamphetamines such as "crank," "crystal," and "ice" became the drugs of choice.

38. Anabolic steroids and other performance-enhancing drugs (e.g., stimulants) became widely used in the Olympics and other sports competitions due to the Cold War and the large amounts of money involved in winning. Drug testing by the IOC and NCAA curbed many of the abuses.

39. Sedative-hypnotics and tranquilizers started with bromides and barbiturates and switched to Miltown® and benzodiazepines, such as Valium® and Xanax®, in the '50s and '60s. Psychiatric medications, including antipsychotics, antianxiety drugs, lithium, and antidepressants, also became accepted starting in the '50s and vastly expanding in the '90s.

40. LSD and other hallucinogenic drugs, especially designer psychedelics including MDA, DMT, and MDMA, were developed starting in the '40s and exploding in the '60s.

41. Supply reduction and demand reduction were tried in order to limit the growth of illegal drug use.

42. Methadone maintenance was developed as a harm-reduction technique to control heroin use. The Vietnam War expanded heroin use although not as much as experts thought it would.

43. Regular cocaine use and smokable cocaine (freebase, crack) use became popular in the late '70s and '80s.

44. Sexually transmitted diseases and contaminated needle diseases, especially HIV (AIDS) and hepatitis C, became endemic in the drug-using community. Besides dirty needles, drug-induced high-risk sexual practices encouraged the spread.

Today & Tomorrow

45. Overall drug use has declined since 1979 and 1980 although the age of first use has gotten younger and hard-core users have increased.

46. The geopolitics of drugs has seen countries corrupted and revolutions supported by the sale of heroin and cocaine. Mexican tar, Colombian white, China white, and Afghan heroin among others have flooded the world market. With the defeat of the Taliban, Afghanistan will again be the number one opium grower in the world. The Cold War made countries look away from drug trafficking as a way to finance revolutions and civil wars. The amount of cocaine and heroin entering the United States has gone up thus forcing the price down.

47. Street chemists have figured easier ways to synthesis methamphetamines by using precursor chemicals that aren't as tightly controlled.

48. The rave clubs are the 1990s and 2000s version of the psychedelic clubs of the '60s and '70s. LSD, methamphetamine, nitrous oxide, and marijuana are still around but MDA is now MDMA, Quaaludes® are Rohypnol® or GHB, and live acid rock bands are technorave recorded CDs.

49. Marijuana use has remained fairly constant although the potency of commonly available "pot" has greatly increased due to sinsemilla-cultivation techniques. The big battles are over the legalization of medical marijuana sold through *Cannabis* clubs.

50. Tobacco remains the target of class-action lawsuits while smoking in the United States has declined although marketing pushes by tobacco companies has increased smoking throughout the world. Lung cancer deaths among women have increased due to increased smoking.

51. OxyContin®, a time-release opioid, has been abused since its release when addicts learned to crush the capsules for a heroin-like high. Hydrocodone (Vicodin®) is the most widely abused prescription opioid.

52. Alcohol remains the number one drug problem in most of the world. There are over 13 million Americans with a drinking problem.

53. There is growing recognition that behavioral addictions, such as eating disorders and compulsive gambling, are very similar to drug addictions in the way they affect the brain.

54. Drug policy has shifted from supply reduction to demand reduction. Drug courts and laws like California's Proposition 36, which mandates the availability of treatment to nonviolent drug offenders, has the support of the public and the drug-treatment community.

Conclusions

55. The "war on terrorism" and the so-called war on drugs will be with us for a long long time and any solutions will take imagination, resolve, and intelligence.

CLASSIFICATION OF PSYCHOACTIVE DRUGS

What Is a Psychoactive Drug?

56. Though people define psychoactive substances in a variety of ways, our definition is "a psychoactive drug is any substance that directly alters the normal functioning of the central nervous system."

57. A psychoactive drug can be called by its chemical name, trade name, or street name.

58. Drugs can be classified by their effects: uppers (stimulants), downers (depressants), and all arounders (psychedelics). The other psychoactive drug groups are inhalants, sports drugs, and psychiatric medications.

Major Drugs

59. Uppers include cocaine, amphetamines, diet pills, and the plant stimulants (e.g., khat, betel nuts,

caffeine, tobacco). Major effects are increased energy, feelings of confidence, raised heart rate and blood pressure, and euphoria with stronger stimulants. Overuse can cause jitteriness, anger, depletion of energy, anhedonia (lack of ability to feel pleasure), and paranoia, along with damage to the heart, lungs, and blood vessels.

60. Downers include opiates (e.g., heroin, codeine), sedative-hypnotics (e.g., benzodiazepines, barbiturates), and alcohol (beer, wine, and distilled liquor). These drugs depress circulatory, respiratory, and muscular systems. The stronger opiates and sedative-hypnotics can initially cause euphoria. Prolonged use can cause health problems and dependence.

61. All arounders include marijuana, LSD, MDMA (ecstasy), PCP, psilocybin mushrooms, and pey-

ote. Major mental effects are illusions, hallucinations, and confused sensations. Physically many psychedelics cause stimulation but marijuana usually causes relaxation.

Other Drugs & Addictions

62. Other psychoactive drugs include

◇ inhalants, which are depressants but also cause dizziness and delirium accompanied by confusion;

◇ steroids and other sports drugs, which are used to enhance performance through muscle growth or relief from pain;

◇ and psychiatric drugs, which help rebalance brain chemistry disrupted by mental illness (e.g., antidepressants, antipsychotics, antianxiety drugs).

63. Certain addictive behaviors, including gambling, compulsive eat-

ing, anorexia, bulimia, sexual compulsivity, compulsive shopping, and even Internet addiction, cause neurological and chemical changes much the same way as drug addictions.

Controlled Substances Act of 1970

64. The Controlled Substances Act of 1970 was enacted to limit the availability, use, and abuse of psychoactive substances. Through the Drug Enforcement Administration (DEA), the act categorized dangerous substances into five schedules. Schedules I and II include the major psychoactive drugs, e.g., heroin, cocaine, marijuana, and methamphetamine (drugs with a high-abuse potential) and define criminal penalties for possession, intent to sell, and use.

REFERENCES

Alcoholics Anonymous. (1934, 1976). *Alcoholics Anonymous*. New York: Alcoholics Anonymous World Services, Inc.

Abel, E. L. (2001). The Gin Epidemic: Much ado about what? *Alcohol & Alcoholism, 36*(5), 401–405.

Acker, C. J. (1995). Opioids and opioid control: History. In J. H. Jaffe (Ed.), *Encyclopedia of Drugs and Alcohol* (Vol. II, pp. 763–769). New York: Simon & Shuster Macmillan.

Acosta, J. (1588). *Historia Natural y Moral de las Indias*. English translation by C. R. Markham. London: Hakluyt Society, 1880.

Agnew, L. R. (1968). On blowing one's mind (19th century style). *Journal of the American Medical Association (JAMA)*, pp. 61–62.

Aldrich, M. R. (1977). Tantric cannabis use in India. *Journal of Psychoactive Drugs, 9*(3), 227–233.

Aldrich, M. R. (1994). Historical notes on women addicts. *Journal of Psychoactive Drugs, 26*(1), 61–64.

Aldrich, M. R. (1997). History of therapeutic cannabis. In M. L. Mathre (Ed.), *Cannabis in Medical Practice*. Jefferson, NC: McFarland & Company, Inc.

American Methadone Treatment Association. (2002). 217 Broadway, New York, NY, 10007.

Associated Press. (2001, January 15). Taliban virtually wipes out Afghanistan's opium crop. Nando Media, Associated Press [Online]. Available: *http://www.nandotimes.com*

Armstrong, D., & Armstrong, E. M. (1991). *The Great American Medicine Show*. New York: Prentice Hall.

Austin, G. A. (1979). *Perspectives on the History of Psychoactive Substance Use*. DHEW Publication No. (ADM) 79–81.

Australian Drug Foundation. (1999). The history of drug use in sport. *http://www.adf.org.au/archive/asda/history.html*

Benowitz, N., & Fredericks, A. (1995). History of tobacco use. In J. H. Jaffe (Ed.), *Encyclopedia of Drugs and Alcohol* (Vol. III, pp. 1032–1036). New York: Simon & Schuster Macmillan.

Bible. (1990). Ecclesiasticus, 31, 27. *The New Jerusalem Bible Translation*. New York: Doubleday.

Blanchard, D. (2000). *Theriac: George Bartisch*. Portland, OR: Blanchard's Books.

Blum, K. (1984). *Handbook of Abusable Drugs*. New York: Gardner Press, Inc.

Blum, K., Braverman, E. R., Cull, J. G., Holder, J. M., Luck, R., Lubar, J., Miller, D., & Comings, D. E. (2000). Reward deficiency syndrome (RDS): A biogenetic model for the diagnosis and treatment of impulsive, addictive, and compulsive behaviors. *Journal of Psychoactive Drugs, 32*(1).

Boyle, R. (1744). *The Works: Of the Usefulness of Natural Philosophy*. London (out of print).

Brunner, T.F. (1977). Marijuana in ancient Greece and Rome? The literary evidence. *Journal of Psychoactive Drugs, 9*(3).

Centers for Disease Control. (2002). AIDS statistics from the Centers for Disease Control [Online]. *http://www.cdc.gov*

Cherrington, E. H. (Ed.). (1924). *Standard Encyclopedia of the Alcohol Problem* (Vol. II). Westerville, OH: American Issue Publishing.

Cleza de Leon. (1959). The Incas. Translated by Harriet de Onis. *The Civilization of the American Indian Series* (Vol. 53). Tulsa, OK: University of Oklahoma Press.

Coste, R. (1984). Coffee production. In *Encyclopaedia Britannica* (Vol. 4, pp.

818–820). Chicago: Encyclopaedia Britannica.

Courtwright, D. (1982). *Dark Paradise: Opiate Addiction in America Before 1940.* Cambridge, MA: Harvard University Press.

Diaz, J. L. (1979). Ethnopharmacology and taxonomy of Mexican psychodysleptic plants. *Journal of Psychoactive Drugs, 11*(1–2), 71–101.

Dioscorides. (A.D. 70). In M. Wellman (Ed.) (1906–1914, reprinted in 1958), *Pedanii Dioscuridis Anazarbei De materia medica* (3 volumes).

Drug Abuse Warning Network. (2002). *Year End 2001 Emergency Department Data.* Rockville, MD: Substance Abuse and Mental Health Services Administration.

Drug Enforcement Administration. (2001a). Congressional testimony by Errol J. Chavez, Special Agent in Charge, DEA. April 13, 2001 [Online]. Available: *http://www.usdoj.gov/dea/pubs/cngrtest/ct041301.htm*

Drug Enforcement Administration. (2001b). The price dynamics of Southeast Asian heroin. Drug Intelligence Brief [Online]. Available: *http://www.usdoj.gov/dea*

Drug Policy Research Center. (2000). What makes drug courts succeed or fail. *Drug Policy Research Center Newsletter*: Rand Corporation, June, 2000.

Dunlop, E., & Johnson, B. D. (1992). The setting for the crack era: Macro forces, micro consequences (1960–1992). *Journal of Psychoactive Drugs, 24*(4), 307–322.

Escohotado, A. (1999). *A Brief History of Drugs.* Rochester, VT: Park Street Press.

Fort, J. (1968). A world view of marijuana. *Journal of Psychoactive Drugs, 2*(1), 1–14.

Freud, S. (1884). *Uber Coca.* In R. Byck (Ed.) (1974), *The Cocaine Papers of Sigmund Freud.* New York: Stonehill.

Furst, P. T. (1976). *Hallucinogens and Culture.* San Francisco: Chandler & Sharp Publishers, Inc.

Gagliano, J. (1994). *Coca Production in Peru, The Historical Debates.* Tucson, AZ & London: University of Arizona Press.

Ganeri, A., Martell, H. M., & Williams, B. (1998). Beer. *World History Encyclopedia.* New York: Barnes & Noble.

Giannini, A. J., Burge, H., Shaheen, J. M., & Price, W. A. (1986). Khat: Another drug of abuse. *Journal of Psychoactive Drugs, 18*(2), 155–158.

Goodwin, D. W., & Gabrielli, W. F. (1997). Alcohol: Clinical aspects. In J. H.

Lowinson, P. Ruiz, R. B. Millman, & J. G. Langrod (Eds.), *Substance Abuse: A Comprehensive Textbook* (3rd ed., pp.142–147). Baltimore: Williams & Wilkins.

Grinspoon, L., & Hedblom, P. (1975). *The Speed Culture: Amphetamine Use and Abuse in America.* Cambridge, MA: Harvard University Press.

Guttmacher, H. (1885). New medications and therapeutic techniques concerning the different cocaine preparations and their effects. In R. Byck (Ed.) (1974), *The Cocaine Papers of Sigmund Freud.* New York: Stonehill.

Hamid, A. (1992). The developmental cycle of a drug epidemic: The cocaine-smoking epidemic of 1981–1991. *Journal of Psychoactive Drugs, 24*(4), 337–348.

Harler, C. R. (1984). Tea production. In *Encyclopaedia Britannica* (Vol. 18, pp. 16–19). Chicago: Encyclopaedia Britannica.

Heath, D. B. (1995). Alcohol: History. In J. H. Jaffe (Ed.), *Encyclopedia of Drugs and Alcohol* (Vol. I, pp. 70–78). New York: Simon & Schuster Macmillan.

Herodotus. (460 B.C.). *The Histories. 1.202,* 4.75.1.

Hodgson, B. (1999). *Opium: A Portrait of the Heavenly Demon.* San Francisco: Chronicle Books.

Hoffman, J. P. (1990). The historical shift in the perception of opiates: From medicine to social medicine. *Journal of Psychoactive Drugs, 22*(1), 53–62.

Hollister, L. E. (1983). The pre-benzodiazepine era. *Journal of Psychoactive Drugs, 15*(1–2), 9–13.

James I. (1604). *A Counter-Blaste to Tobacco.* Reprinted in 1954. London: The Rodale Press.

Julien, R. M. (2001). *A Primer of Drug Action.* New York: W. H. Freeman and Company.

Kandall, S. R. (1996). *Substance and Shadow: Women and Addiction in the United States.* Cambridge, MA: Harvard University Press.

Karch, S. B. (1996). *The Pathology of Drug Abuse.* Boca Raton, FL: CRC Press.

Karch, S. B. (1997). *A Brief History of Cocaine.* Boca Raton, FL: CRC Press.

Karch, S. B. (1998). *Drug Abuse Handbook.* Boca Raton, FL: CRC Press.

Keller, M. (1984). Alcohol consumption. In *Encyclopaedia Britannica* (Vol. 1, pp. 437–450). Chicago: Encyclopaedia Britannica.

Konietzko, N. (2001, September 24). Report at 11th Annual Congress of the European Respiratory Society.

La Barre, W. (1979a). Shamanic origins of religion and medicine. *Journal of Psychoactive Drugs, 11*(1–2), 7–11.

La Barre, W. (1979b). *Peyotl* and mescaline. *Journal of Psychoactive Drugs, 11*(1–2), 33–39.

Langton, P. A. (1995). Temperance movement. In J. H. Jaffe (Ed.), *Encyclopedia of Drugs and Alcohol* (Vol. III, pp. 1019–1023). New York: Simon & Schuster Macmillan.

Latimer, D., & Goldberg, J. (1981). *Flowers in the Blood: The Story of Opium.* New York: Franklin Watts.

Leary, T. (1970). The religious experience: Its production and interpretation. *Journal of Psychoactive Drugs, 3*(1), 76–86.

Lee, J. A. (1987). Chinese, alcohol and flushing: Sociohistorical and biobehavioral considerations. *Journal of Psychoactive Drugs, 19*(4), 319–327.

Leinwand, D. (2002, August 21). 10 held in smuggling of "Nazi Speed." *USA Today.*

Li, H. L. (1974). An archeological and historical account of *Cannabis* in China. *Economic Botany, 28,* 437–438.

Lynn, E. J., Walter, R. G., Harris, L. A., Dendy, R., & James, M. (1972). Nitrous oxide: It's a gas. *Journal of Psychoactive Drugs, 5*(1), 1–7.

Marnell, T. (Ed.). (1997). *Drug Identification Bible.* Denver: Drug Identification Bible.

Matthee, R. (1995). Exotic substances: The introduction and global spread of tobacco, coffee, cocoa, tea, and distilled liquor, sixteenth to eighteenth centuries. In R. Porter & M. Teich (Eds.), *Drugs and Narcotics in History.* Cambridge, England: Cambridge University Press.

McGovern, P., Gluskee, D. L., Exner, L. J., & Voight, M. M. (1998). Archeology: Neolithic resinated wine. *Nature: 381,* 480–481.

McKenna, T. (1992). *Food of the Gods.* New York: Bantam Books.

Monardes, N. (1577). *Joyfull Newes Out of the Newe Founde Worlde.* Translated by J. Frampton. (Reprinted in 1967). New York: AMS Press, Inc.

Nesse, R. A., & Berridge, K. C. (1997). Psychoactive drug use in evolutionary perspective. *Science, 278,* 63–65.

National Institute on Drug Abuse. (1998). Current trends in drug use worldwide. *NIDA Notes, 13*(2).

O'Brien, R., & Chafetz, M. (1991). *The Encyclopedia of Alcoholism* (2nd ed.). New York: Facts On File.

O'Brien, R., Cohen, S., Evans, G., & Fine, J. (1992). *The Encyclopedia of Drug*

Abuse (2nd ed.). New York: Facts On File.

Observatoire Geopolitique des Drogues. (1996). *The Geopolitics of Drugs*. Boston: Northeastern University Press.

Office of National Drug Control Policy. (1999). *National Drug Control Strategy, 1999*. Rockville, MD: National Drug Clearinghouse.

Office of National Drug Control Policy. (2001). *National Drug Control Strategy, 2001*. Rockville, MD: National Drug Clearinghouse.

Plato. (360 B.C.) The Symposium, The Republic, The Laws. In L. R. Loomis (Ed.), *Plato, Five Great Dialogues*. New York: Gramercy Books.

Scarborough, J. (1995). The opium poppy in Hellenistic and Roman medicine. In R. Porter & M. Teich (Eds.), *Drugs and Narcotics in History*. Cambridge, England: Cambridge University Press.

Schultes, R.E., & Hofmann, A. (1992). *Plants of the Gods*. Rochester, VT: Healing Arts Press.

Scrivener (1871). On the coca leaf and its use in diet and medicine. *Medical Times and Gazette*. In R. Byck (Ed.) (1974), *The Cocaine Papers of Sigmund Freud*. New York: Stonehill.

Siegel, R. K. (1982). History of cocaine smoking. *Journal of Psychoactive Drugs, 14*(4).

Skolnik, A. A. (1997). Lessons from US history of drug use. *Journal of the American Medical Association (JAMA), 277*(24), 1919–1921.

Slade, J. (1989). The tobacco epidemic: Lessons from history. *Journal of Psychoactive Drugs, 21*(3), 281–291.

Stafford, P. (1982). *Psychedelics Encyclopedia* (Vol. 1, p. 157). Berkeley, CA: Ronin Publishing.

Stamets, P. (1996). *Psilocybin Mushrooms of the World*. Berkeley, CA: Ten Speed Press.

Substance Abuse and Mental Health Services Administration. (2002). *National Household Survey on Drug Abuse: Population Estimates 2001*.

Rockville, MD: SAMHSA, Office of Applied Studies.

Treatment Episode Data Sets. (2001). Treatment Episode Data Sets [Online]. Available: *http://www.DrugAbuse Statistics.SAMHSA.gov*

Trice, H. M. (1995). Alcoholics Anonymous. In J. H. Jaffe (Ed.), *Encyclopedia of Drugs and Alcohol* (Vol. I, pp. 85–92). New York: Simon & Schuster Macmillan.

Wallbank, T. W., & Taylor, A. M. (1992). A short history of the Opium Wars. *Civilizations Past and Present: Chapter 29*. New York: Addison-Wesley Publishing Co.

White, P. T. (1989). Cocaine's deadly reach. *National Geographic, 175*(1).

Heredity, Environment, Psychoactive Drugs

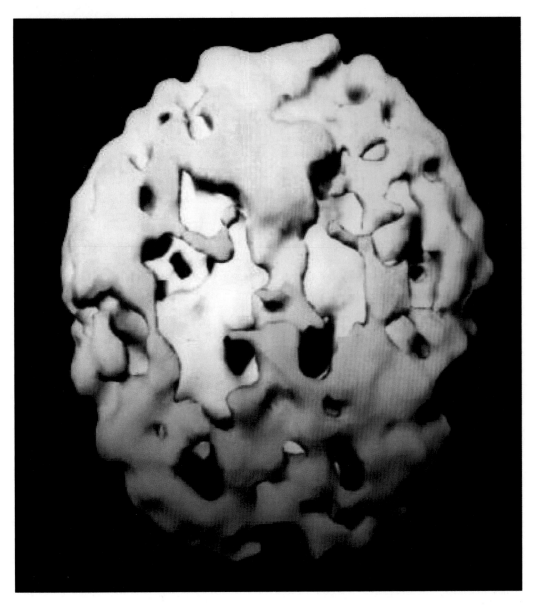

*T*his single photon emission computerized tomography (SPECT) scan of the brain of a long-time heroin addict shows an overall decrease in cerebral activity. The areas with a moth-eaten look are actually areas of the brain that have been suppressed or inactivated by the drug. Normally the brain has a more even appearance.

Courtesy of the Amen Clinic for Behavioral Medicine

HOW PSYCHOACTIVE DRUGS AFFECT US

- **How Drugs Get to the Brain:** A psychoactive drug is absorbed into body tissue and distributed in the bloodstream via the circulatory system.
  - ◊ **Routes of Administration & Drug Absorption:** Drugs can be absorbed through inhaling, injecting, mucous membrane absorption, oral ingestion, or contact absorption.
  - ◊ **Drug Distribution:** Psychoactive drugs travel through the bloodstream and finally cross the blood-brain barrier to the central nervous system. The drugs will either cause an effect, be ignored, be absorbed, or be transformed.
- **The Nervous System:** The two main parts of the nervous system are the peripheral nervous system (autonomic and somatic systems) and the central nervous system (brain and spinal cord).
  - ◊ **Peripheral Nervous System:** This two-part system controls involuntary body functions, relays sensory information, and sends instructions to muscles and organs.
  - ◊ **Central Nervous System:** The brain and spinal cord receive information from the peripheral nervous system, analyze it, and then send appropriate action messages to the involved organs and muscles.
  - ◊ **Old Brain-New Brain:** Craving for psychoactive drugs resides mostly in the old brain.
  - ◊ **The Reward/Reinforcement Center:** This area of the old brain gives a surge of satisfaction when a bodily or environmental need is met. Psychoactive drugs affect this center directly.
  - ◊ **On/Off Switches:** While craving resides in the reward/reinforcement center, current research is focusing on the areas of the brain that stop craving.
  - ◊ **Morality & the Reward/Reinforcement Center:** The conflict between the cravings of the old brain and the societal restraints of the new brain are as old as civilization.
  - ◊ **Neuroanatomy:** Psychoactive drugs affect the nerve cells of the brain and spinal cord and alter the way messages are transmitted.
  - ◊ **Neurotransmitters & Receptors:** Neurochemicals called "neurotransmitters" transmit messages across the tiny gap (synaptic cleft or gap) between nerve cells. When psychoactive drugs modify or mimic the way these neurotransmitters function, they cause physical, mental, and emotional effects.
- **Physiological Responses to Drugs:** In addition to direct effects, phenomena such as tolerance, tissue dependence, psychological dependence, and withdrawal determine a user's reaction to psychoactive drugs.
- **Basic Pharmacology:** Drug metabolism and elimination, along with a drug's molecular size, solubility, half-life and dose-response relationships, help determine the effects a drug will have on a user.

FROM EXPERIMENTATION TO ADDICTION

- **Desired Effects vs. Side Effects:** People use psychoactive drugs to change their mood, to get high, to self-medicate, to be social, and for a number of other reasons. Drugs also cause undesired effects (side effects, adverse reactions, and toxic effects) particularly with prolonged or high-dose use.
- **Levels of Use:** The amount, frequency, and duration of drug use help indicate levels of use: abstinence, experimentation, social/recreational use, habituation, abuse, and addiction.
- **Theories of Addiction:** Theories of addiction emphasize genetic factors, environmental influences, psychoactive drugs themselves, compulsive behaviors, or a combination of those factors as the basis for addiction.
- **Heredity, Environment, Psychoactive Drugs, & Compulsive Behaviors:** These factors determine at what level a person might use psychoactive drugs.
  - ◊ **Heredity:** Family history can indicate a genetic susceptibility to compulsive drug use.
  - ◊ **Environment:** The pressures and stress of growing up, particularly if there is abuse, can make people more susceptible to addiction especially if there is a strong hereditary component. Availability of the drug and peer pressure are also strong environmental factors.
  - ◊ **Psychoactive Drugs:** Drugs can activate a genetic/environmental susceptibility to drug abuse and addiction. They cause alterations in brain chemistry, structure, activity, and function, which can intensify drug-using behavior.
  - ◊ **Compulsive Behaviors:** Compulsive gambling, eating, shopping, sexuality, and other uncontrolled behaviors can cause changes in brain function and neurochemistry, particularly to the reward/reinforcement center, similar to those caused by psychoactive drugs.
- **Alcoholic Mice & Sober Mice:** Classic experiments with mice strongly suggest an interrelationship between heredity, environment, psychoactive drugs, and levels of use.
- **Compulsion Curves:** The way heredity, environment, and regular drug use combine to increase susceptibility to addiction can be visualized with compulsion graphs.
- **Conclusions:** Any examination of drug or behavioral addiction should focus on the totality of one's life not just on the specific drug or behavioral problem.

8D · THURSDAY, MARCH 19, 1998 · USA TODAY

HEALTH AND EDUCATION

Strain of stress can be drain on brain

By Karen S. Peterson
USA TODAY

Dealing with stress effectively not only protects one's general health: It can help keep memory and mental abilities strong as we age, ers are learning.

Stress actually can dam hippocampus, an area of th governing learning and m says neurologist Richard Re *The Longevity Strategy: H Live to 100 Using the Brai Connection* (Wiley, $22.95).

"It is no longer just common to avoid stress, to reframe str situations and see them in tern challenges" to reduce the feelin pressure, he says. Paying attentio stress is a necessity. "Stress cau brain damage."

Research reported this week the *Proceedings of the Nation Academy of Sciences* reinforces h analysis. A Princeton-Rockefelle University team finds the production of new cells in the hippocampus of monkeys is diminished under stress.

The fact that new cells are produced in their brains at all may amaze some scientists.

"There has been enormous skepticism for several decades that this was possible," Princeton researcher beth Gould says. "Up to this point, there been a lot of resistance to the idea, but I t people are going to change their attitude

Earlier research established the growth new cells in the olfactory bulbs of rats, area used in the sense of smell, she says. "I ours is the first to demonstrate growth in t primate brain."

In her study, male monkeys that had a ways lived alone were placed in small cage

Study Tracks Cocaine's Impact On Brain Function

Effects reported to be long-lasting

BALTIMORE SUN

Heavy use of cocaine impairs memory, manual dexterity and decision-making for at least a month after the drug was last taken, accord ing to a new study of drug users researchers at the National Instit on Drug Abuse.

The study, led by neurologi ren I. Bolla of the Johns H University, adds to the evider the powerful high experie cocaine users is accomp long-lasting harm to brain ing.

NIDA said the study documents be- ˟anges that appear to cor- ˟es found in brain

NIDA said the study documents behavio
respo
sca

Twins study shows smarts mostly in the genes

By Lisa M. Krieger
EXAMINER MEDICAL WRITER

New research

A focus on functions

Abuse sets kids up for big problems

Researcher: Urge to bet rewires brain

The Associated Press

LAS VEGAS — The excitement and risk taking of betting can change the brain's chemistry and create compulsive gamblers, a Harvard professor told casino executives at their annual meeting this week.

"Addi...

y Kim Painter
SA TODAY

˟avior
history of sexual or phys orted by up s and is linke n pregnancy ting disorder studies find. /s, though le similar cons rvey suggests tes are simila n previous stu statewide su national surve to claims th nany other ser

---

HOW PSYCHOACTIVE DRUGS AFFECT US

"We have centers in the brain that reinforce pleasurable and rewarding experiences, so much so that in experimental animals, the animal will continue to stimulate it, even to the point of not eating or drinking . . . and dying . . . so that the power of this pleasure or reward is an intense, driving experience. We believe that addicting drugs have the potential to take over, or subvert, or hijack some of those reward mechanisms."

Dr. Ivan Diamond, Director, Gallo Research Institute

At the beginning of the twenty-first century psychoactive drug research continues to examine the neurochemistry and genetics of craving. However,

there has been a subtle **shift of focus from "Why do we crave a drug?" to "Why can't we stop craving a drug?"** Research continues on the reward pathway in the brain that encourages use and abuse but interest has grown about the mechanisms that are supposed to signal satiation and shut off the craving (Koob & Le Moal, 2001; Nestler, Barrot, & Self, 2001). Other research is focusing on different genetic factors, such as those that signal a low level of response to drug use as a risk factor for addiction (Schuckit & Smith, 2001). In addition the role of other brain chemicals besides dopamine in the craving and addiction process is being studied. However, before studying the neurochemistry of craving and satiation, this chapter will examine how drugs get to the brain in the first place.

HOW DRUGS GET TO THE BRAIN

Psychoactive drugs are substances that directly affect the central nervous system and cause physical and mental changes. Factors that determine their effects and abuse potential include the drug's

◇ **route of administration,**

◇ **speed of transit to the brain,**

◇ **affinity for nerve cells and neurotransmitters.**

ROUTES OF ADMINISTRATION & DRUG ABSORPTION

There are five common ways that drugs enter the body: **(1) inhaling,**

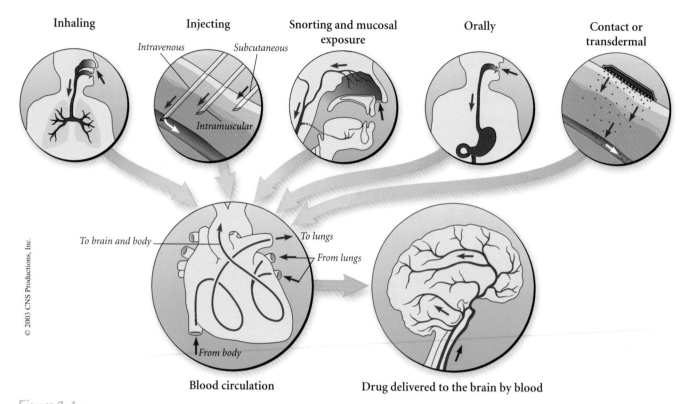

Inhaling Injecting Snorting and mucosal exposure Orally Contact or transdermal

Intravenous *Subcutaneous*

Intramuscular

© 2003 CNS Productions, Inc.

To brain and body *To lungs*

From lungs

From body

Blood circulation Drug delivered to the brain by blood

Figure 2-1 •

Whether inhaled (and absorbed in the lungs), injected (in a vein, muscle, or under the skin), snorted (through the nasal mucosa), drunk (and absorbed by the small intestine), or absorbed by contact (with the skin), the drug enters the bloodstream and eventually makes its way to the brain.

(2) injecting, (3) mucous membrane absorption, (4) oral ingestion, and (5) contact absorption (Fig. 2-1). The methods are arranged in the order of the speed with which they will reach the brain and spinal cord and begin to have an effect.

Inhaling

When a person smokes a marijuana joint or freebase cocaine or inhales ("huffs") nitrous oxide, the vaporized drug enters the lungs and is **rapidly absorbed through capillaries lining the air sacs (alveoli) of the bronchi**. From the capillaries (tiny blood vessels) the drug-laden blood travels back to the veins and then to the heart where it is pumped directly to the brain and other organs and tissues of the body. Inhaling acts more quickly than any other method of use (**7–10 seconds before the drug reaches the brain** and begins to cause changes).

Since the effects are felt so quickly and only a small amount of the drug is absorbed with each puff or breath, users can regulate the amount of drug they are receiving (titration). For example, cigarette smokers titrate the amount of nicotine they put in their bloodstream by controlling how often they smoke and how deeply they inhale. Currently Roxanne Laboratories, the only maker of synthetic THC (Marinol®) the most psychoactive ingredient in marijuana, is developing a deep lung aerosol spray and a nasal spray as delivery systems for medical marijuana that would avoid the hazards of smoking (Institute of Medicine, 1999).

Injecting

Substances such as heroin, cocaine, and methamphetamine (meth) can be injected directly into the body with a hypodermic syringe by three methods:

◊ **intravenous** (IV or "slamming"): directly into the bloodstream by way of a vein;

◊ **intramuscular** (IM or "muscling"): into a muscle mass;

◊ **subcutaneous** ("skin popping"): under the skin.

Injection is a quick and potent way to absorb a drug (**15–30 seconds intravenously or 3–5 minutes in a muscle or under the skin**). Because a large amount of the drug enters the blood at one time, injecting a strong psychoactive drug intravenously is **most likely to produce an intense rush** or flash of euphoria similar to a sexual orgasm. The slower routes of administration will produce euphoria but will not cause a rush. The drug will build up more slowly (Jaffe, Knapp, & Ciraulo, 1997). This rush is the main reason that some users prefer IV use of heroin, cocaine, and methamphetamine. In addition none of the drug is wasted as occurs with sidestream smoke, poor nasal absorption, or destruction by other body fluids and metabolism when taken orally.

The large bolus (amount) of drugs from injecting can cause exaggerated reactions and even an overdose since the illicit user is often not sure of the purity or identity of the drug. Once injected there is no turning back since the drugs are in an enclosed system and the effects will inevitably take their course. **Injecting is the most dangerous method of use** because it bypasses most of the body's natural defenses, thereby exposing the user to many health problems, such as hepatitis B and C, abscesses, HIV infection, and undissolved particles or additives that can cause embolisms, infections, or other illnesses.

Mucous Membrane Absorption

Certain drugs in powdered form, especially cocaine, heroin, and methamphetamine, can be **snorted into the nose (insufflation)** and absorbed by the capillaries enmeshed in the mucous membranes lining the nasal passages. The effects are usually more intense and occur more quickly than with the oral route because the drug initially bypasses digestive acids, enzymes, and the liver. A nasal spray containing a tranquilizer has been used in Sweden to calm cancer-stricken children undergoing chemotherapy (Ljungman et al., 2000). A similar mucosal absorption method involves placing a drug, such as crushed coca leaves (mixed with ash or soda lime) or tobacco, on the **mucous membranes under the tongue (sublingually) or between the gums and cheek (buccally) (3–5 minutes for effects to begin** for the above two methods). Trials with a marijuana nasal gel or sublingual preparation for mucosal absorption are under review. In hospices for terminally ill patients too weak for an oral dose of a painkiller, they use **morphine suppositories (10–15 minutes for effects to begin)**. The drug is absorbed through mucosal tissues lining the rectum. Vaginal absorption of drugs is also occasionally employed. Some users employ these last two methods for recreational/abusive/addictive drug use.

Oral Ingestion

When someone swallows an ecstasy tablet or drinks a beer, **the drug passes through the esophagus and stomach to the small intestine where it is absorbed into the capillaries enmeshed in the intestinal walls**. The capillaries feed the drug into the veins that carry it to the liver where it is partly metabolized (first-pass metabolism). It is then pumped back to the heart and subsequently to the rest of the body. **The effects of drugs taken by this method are delayed (20–30 minutes)**. About 10–20% of alcohol is me-

tabolized by the stomach in men who have more gastric metabolizing enzymes, so women will generally have higher blood alcohol levels for the same amount consumed.

Drugs enter the capillaries lining the walls of the small intestine through passive transport (absorption). This occurs because many drugs move from an area of high concentration of that drug to areas of low concentration of that same drug. Fat-soluble drugs, which include most psychoactive drugs, move readily across most biological barriers (membranes). Alcohol is both water- and fat-soluble (Wilkinson, 2001).

Contact Absorption

Drugs can be applied to the skin through **saturated adhesive patches** that allow measured quantities of the drug to be passively absorbed over a

long period of time (up to 7 days). It sometimes takes 1 to 2 days for therapeutic effects to begin. This noninvasive **transdermal absorption** method is used in nicotine patches to help smokers quit, fentanyl patches to control pain, clonidine patches to reduce drug withdrawal symptoms or reduce blood pressure, and heart medication patches to control angina (heart pain). **Skin creams and ointments** are absorbed through the skin, as is DMSO, a penetrating solvent that enhances the absorption of many drugs through the skin. LSD in liquid form is rapidly absorbed by ocular capillaries when it is placed on the eye.

DRUG DISTRIBUTION

No matter how a drug enters the circulatory system it is eventually distributed by the bloodstream to the rest

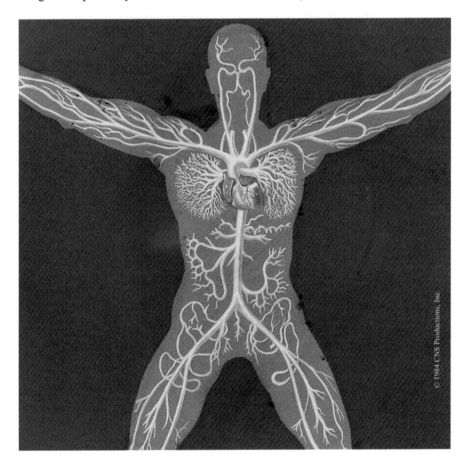

Figure 2-2 •

This drawing shows a small fraction of the veins and arteries of the circulatory system that, in an adult, carry an average of 5 liters (about 6 quarts) of blood to every part of the body. Miles of tiny capillaries then deliver the drug-laden blood to tissues, especially the nerve cells of the central nervous system. The circulatory system also carries the drug and its metabolites away from the brain and other tissues by running 500 gallons of blood a day through the kidneys.

of the body. The drug may be carried inside the blood cells, in the plasma outside the cells, or it might hitch a ride on protein molecules. Drug molecules then circulate and travel to and through every organ, fluid, and tissue in the body where they will either (1) **cause a direct effect,** (2) **be ignored,** (3) **be stored** (usually in fat cells), (4) **or be biotransformed** into metabolites or chemical variations of the original drug, some of which can also cause psychoactive effects.

The distribution of a drug within the body depends not only on the characteristics of the drug but on blood volume as well. The lighter the person, the less blood volume there is, so a child of 12 might only have 3 to 4 quarts of blood to dilute the drug instead of the **6 to 8 quarts of blood in a large adult circulatory system**. The effect of a drug on a specific organ or tissue is also dependent on the number of blood vessels reaching that site. For example, veins and arteries saturate the heart muscles and since all drugs pass through these vessels, a drug such as

cocaine can have a direct effect on heart function. Bones and muscles have fewer blood vessels, so most drugs will have less effect at these sites.

Most important, within only 10–15 seconds after entering the bloodstream, the drug will reach the gateway to the central nervous system, the protective blood-brain barrier. On the other side of the barrier the drug will have its greatest effects on the brain and spinal cord.

The Blood-Brain Barrier

The drug-laden blood flows through the internal carotid arteries in the neck toward the central nervous system, also called the "CNS." The walls of the capillaries enmeshed in the nerve cells and glial cells of the CNS consist of **tightly sealed epithelial cells that allow only certain substances to penetrate**. Normally substances such as toxins, viruses, and bacteria can't cross this barrier. One class of drugs that can infiltrate this blood-brain barrier is psychoactive

drugs (stimulants, depressants, psychedelics, inhalants). Psychotropic drugs, such as antipsychotics or antidepressants, also cross this barrier as do most steroids and some muscle relaxants.

The blood-brain barrier is not completely formed in humans at birth and does not become fully functional until a child is 1 to 2 years old. So ingesting toxic chemicals can be especially dangerous to the fetus during pregnancy.

A key reason why many psychoactive drugs, including nicotine, alcohol, and marijuana, cross this barrier is that they are fat-soluble (lipophilic) and **since the brain is essentially fatty, it readily absorbs fat-soluble substances**. This method of drug transfer is called "passive transport." For example, morphine is partly fat-soluble so it takes somewhat longer to cross the barrier than the more fat-soluble heroin. Cocaine hydrochloride and other drugs that are water-soluble, hitchhike across the blood-brain barrier by attaching onto protein molecules going across the barrier. This method is known as **"active transport"** (Wilkinson, 2001). Most substances that are **water-soluble** (hydrophilic), such as antibiotics, are prevented from entering the brain. As mentioned, alcohol is both lipophilic and hydrophilic.

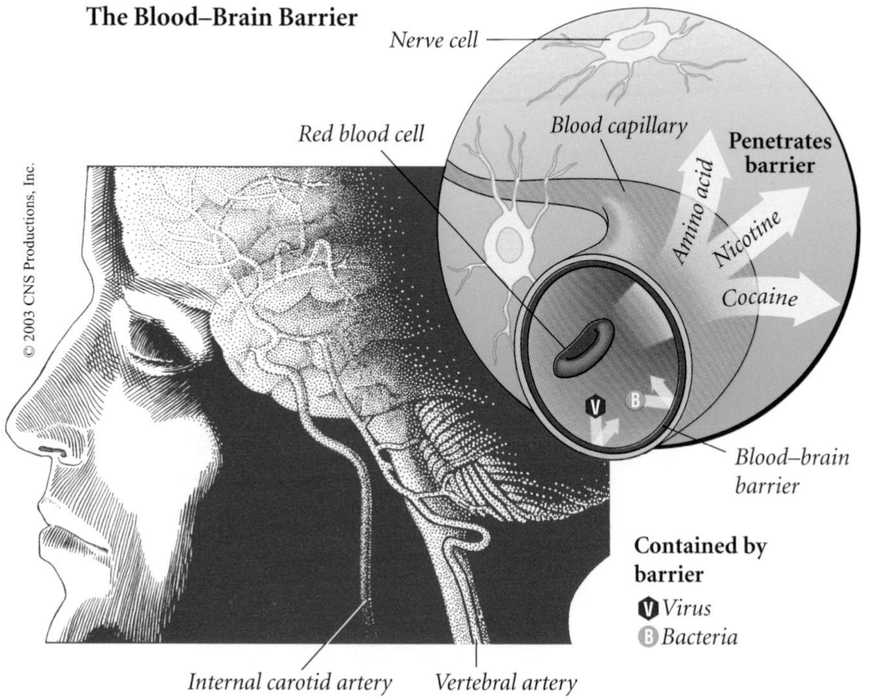

THE NERVOUS SYSTEM

Since the principal target of psychoactive drugs is the central nervous system, it is important to understand how this network of **100 billion nerve cells and 100 trillion connections** works.

◇ The **central nervous system (CNS)** is half of the complete nervous system. It contains the brain and spinal cord. It is better protected (the skull and spine) than most of the peripheral nervous system.

◇ The **peripheral nervous system (PNS)** is the other half of the nervous system. It connects the central nervous system with its internal

The Blood–Brain Barrier

Nerve cell

Red blood cell

Blood capillary

Penetrates barrier

Amino acid

Nicotine

Cocaine

Blood–brain barrier

Contained by barrier
Ⓥ *Virus*
Ⓑ *Bacteria*

© 2003 CNS Productions, Inc.

Internal carotid artery   Vertebral artery

Figure 2-3 •
The inset shows the wall of a capillary in the brain whose tightly sealed cells (astrocytes), with no clefts, pores, or gaps, act as a barrier to most substances. Psychoactive substances, which are fat-soluble, cross this barrier.

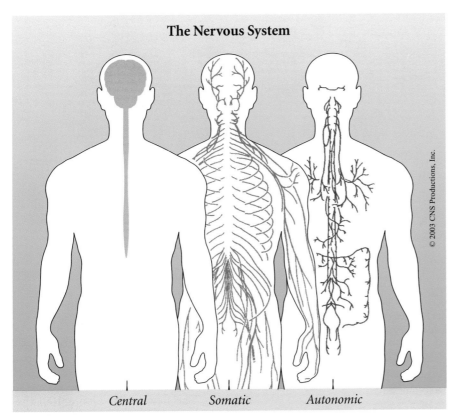

The Nervous System

Central   Somatic   Autonomic

© 2003 CNS Productions, Inc.

Figure 2-4 •

The three parts of the complete nervous system function together to transmit, interpret, store, and respond to information from the environment and from other parts of the body.

and external environments. The peripheral nervous system is further divided into the autonomic and the somatic systems.

PERIPHERAL NERVOUS SYSTEM

The **autonomic nervous system controls involuntary internal functions** such as circulation, digestion, respiration, glandular output, and genital reactions. It consists of the

◇ **sympathetic division**, which helps the body respond to stress;

◇ **parasympathetic division**, which conserves the body's resources and restores homeostasis (physiological balance);

◇ **enteric division**, which controls smooth muscles in the gut.

The autonomic system automatically helps us breathe, sweat, pump blood, release adrenaline, and so forth, to preserve a stable internal environment. For example, sympathetic nerves speed up the heart in response to stress while parasympathetic nerves slow it down when the threat passes.

Though many cell bodies of the autonomic nervous system are located in the brain (hypothalamus) and spinal cord, they reach out to the affected organs and muscles. This means that since psychoactive drugs cross the blood-brain barrier, they can also speed up, slow down, or disrupt these involuntary functions in addition to triggering emotional and mental effects. This is why cocaine can raise the heart rate, constrict blood vessels, and cause heightened sexual sensations.

The **somatic nervous system transmits sensory information** through sensory neurons that reach the skin, muscles, and joints. It tells the central nervous system (CNS) about the environment and about limb and muscle position. It then transmits any instructions from the CNS back to skeletal muscles, allowing the body to respond.

CENTRAL NERVOUS SYSTEM

The central nervous system, especially the brain, acts as a combination switchboard and computer, **receiving messages from the peripheral nervous system, analyzing those messages, and then sending responses** to the appropriate systems of the body: nervous, muscular, skeletal, circulatory, respiratory, digestive, excretory, endocrine, and/or reproductive. The CNS also enables us to reason and make judgments about our environment.

Psychoactive drugs can alter information sent to our brain from our environment, they can disrupt messages sent back to the various parts of the body, and they can disrupt thinking. Psychoactive drugs not only affect the nervous system, they can affect the other systems of the body as well. They can affect them directly while passing through the organ or tissue and they can affect them indirectly by manipulating nerve cell chemistry in the brain that then sends messages back to that organ. For example, alcohol can irritate the lining of the stomach and it can alter liver cells directly. It can also slow respiration and muscular reflexes indirectly through the CNS.

OLD BRAIN-NEW BRAIN

The brain can be described several ways.

◇ It can be anatomically divided into its component parts (spinal cord, brain stem [medulla, pons, cerebellum], midbrain, diencephalon, and the two cerebral hemispheres).

◇ It can be described by function (e.g., vision center, motor cortex, somatosensory cortex, hearing centers).

◇ It can be divided by location (hindbrain, midbrain, forebrain).

For the purposes of understanding how psychoactive drugs work and what causes addiction, we have found it valuable to look at the brain in an evolutionary sense. **The evolutionary perspective looks at physiological changes in the brain as survival adaptations**

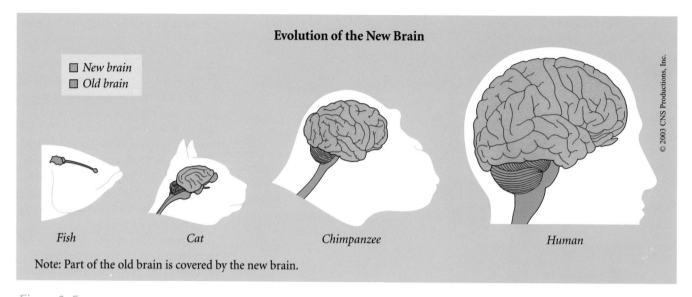

Evolution of the New Brain

☐ *New brain*
☐ *Old brain*

Fish   *Cat*   *Chimpanzee*   *Human*

Note: Part of the old brain is covered by the new brain.

© 2003 CNS Productions, Inc.

Figure 2-5 •

On the evolutionary scale, from a fish, to a cat, to a chimpanzee, and finally to a human being, the new brain has grown in proportion to the old brain. Though the new brain is much larger, the old brain tends to override it, particularly in times of stress.

(Nesse & Berridge, 1997; Nesse, 1994). For example, the evolutionary development of a desire for sweet-tasting substances helped survival by identifying food that could supply quick energy for fight/flight reactions. The instinctual desire for sex assured offspring that could guarantee survival of the species.

The evolutionary perspective also theorizes that **psychoactive drugs have an affinity for natural survival mechanisms** and initially cause desirable effects. The problem is that since refined and potent psychoactive drugs are so new in the evolutionary time scale and are more powerful than naturally occurring substances, the body and brain have not had time to adapt to their effects. The net effect is that they can end up being antisurvival. Using the evolutionary perspective, the two major parts of the brain are defined as the "old brain" and the "new brain."

Old Brain

The old brain, also called the "primal brain," consists of the **brain stem, cerebellum, and mesocortex or midbrain, which contains the limbic system** (the emotional center). The spinal cord can be considered part of this old-brain system. The old brain exists in all animals from a fish to a human being

(Fig. 2-5). The three main functions of the old brain are

◇ **regulating physiological functions** of the body (e.g., respiration, heartbeat, body temperature, hormone release, muscle movement);

◇ **experiencing basic emotions and cravings** (e.g., anger, fear, hunger, thirst, lust, pleasure);

◇ **imprinting survival memories** (e.g., that green plant tastes good, this bad smell signifies danger).

The old brain responds to internal changes and memories or external influences from the environment. For example, if a person has not had enough liquid, the old brain recognizes the body's thirst and triggers a craving for water. If a deer hears a twig snap in the woods, its old brain registers fear and triggers a desire to escape from that danger. If a man and a woman are in a sensual situation, they might desire sex.

When anyone uses psychoactive drugs, most often it is the old brain that is involved in craving and addiction. **It is the old brain that retains addiction memories**, memories of the experience of drug use and memories of how it felt; memories that can be triggered again and again, encouraging drug use (Boening, 2001; Nestler, 2001).

New Brain

The new brain, also called the **"neocortex" (cerebrum and cerebral cortex)**, processes information that comes in from the old brain, from different areas of the new brain, or from the senses via the peripheral nervous system. If a human being is thirsty and craves water, the new brain can help locate the nearest source of water. If there is danger, the new brain might figure out a smarter way of avoiding that danger instead of just running away. **The new brain allows us to speak, reason, create, and remember.** Over millions of years, but particularly the last 200,000 years, the new brain in humans has grown over the old brain until it has folded in on itself to make room for all the billions of new cells (Suzuki, 1994). The further along the evolutionary scale, the larger and more complex the new brain (Fig. 2-5).

However, the old brain is the senior partner; the new brain is the latecomer. Whenever the two brains are challenged by a crisis, such as fear or anger, there's an automatic tendency to revert to old-brain function. And since the **craving to use a psychoactive drug almost always resides in the old brain**, the desire for the pleasure, pain relief, and excitement that drugs promise can be very powerful. That **craving can override the new brain's rational arguments** that say, "Too expensive," or "Bad side effects," or "There's a midterm exam in the morning, so no partying tonight."

"The impact of that drug, the impact of that sensation and how it immobilized me and made me incapable of dealing with the simplest realities of walking to the bus, of going into my office, of getting on the phone, and of picking up my children was so frightening to me that I did not want to repeat it. I was however very compelled to repeat the use of methamphetamine, which I did for years."

Recovering meth abuser

If a person is to live a balanced life, there has to be good communication between the old brain and new brain. This communication is disrupted by psychoactive drugs.

THE REWARD/ REINFORCEMENT CENTER

The specific area of the old brain that **encourages a human being to remember and repeat an action that promotes survival** is called the "reward/reinforcement center." **It is also the part of the brain that is most affected by psychoactive drugs.** Technically it is referred to as the **"mesolimbic dopaminergic reward pathway"** (Fig. 2-6). This network gives animals and human beings a feeling of satisfaction when they fulfill a craving or even anticipate fulfilling a craving that has been triggered by an instinct, a physical imbalance, or an emotional memory (Bassareo & Di Chiara, 1999). And, just as important, it gives a sense of relief similar to the euphoria of reward when pain is moderated or eliminated (Goldstein, 2001). When this center is activated, **it tells the person, "Do it again, do it again, do it again," until that craving is satisfied.**

Nucleus Accumbens

The most important part of the reward pathway is a small group of nerve cells called the "medial forebrain bundle" that contains the nucleus accumbens septi (aka nucleus accumbens). This area of the brain was first pinpointed in 1954 by Canadian biologist Dr. James Olds (Olds & Milner, 1954). What Dr. Olds and others have hypothesized, and to a large extent proven, is that **the nucleus accumbens is a powerful motivator (reinforcer)**. Experimentally a rat had an electrode attached to its nucleus accumbens and then connected to an electrical switch. When the rat began pressing the switch activating that part of its brain, it wouldn't stop. In fact it was so powerful a reinforcer that the rat would press the switch 5,000 times an hour. It wouldn't eat, it wouldn't sleep, it would just keep pushing the switch. The experiment was tried on human beings. An electrode was implanted in the nucleus accumbens and they were given a switch that stimulated that part of the brain. Similar to the rats they pushed it again and again and again.

Dr. Olds, Dr. Robert Heath, and other researchers found that **many psychoactive drugs also stimulate this same reward/reinforcement center** (Olds, 1956). For example, when they had the rat push a lever that gave it a shot of cocaine, the rat would push that lever in much the same way it pushed the switch for the electrical stimulation of the nucleus accumbens. In fact the rats would keep pushing the lever to the exclusion of everything else. They would push it until they died of thirst or starvation.

The actions of the rats were similar to those of human beings who use certain psychoactive drugs. People also respond to the message to do it again, do it again, do it again. **The longer they use, the stronger the "do it again" message becomes.**

The other major parts of the mesolimbic reward pathway are the **ventral tegmental area (VTA), the lateral hypothalamus, and the prefrontal cortex.** The reward pathway can be activated by psychoactive drugs at any of these locations and through

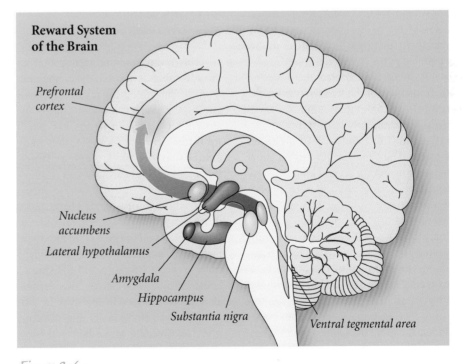

Reward System of the Brain

Prefrontal cortex

Nucleus accumbens

Lateral hypothalamus

Amygdala

Hippocampus

Substantia nigra

Ventral tegmental area

Figure 2-6 •

The reward/reinforcement center or pathway is really a combination of several structures in the old brain that are activated when the person fulfills some emotion or feeling that has arisen, such as hunger, thirst, or sexual desire. The principle parts are the ventral tegmental area, nucleus accumbens, lateral hypothalamus, and a small area of the prefrontal cortex.

Courtesy of Kenneth Blum, John Cull, Eric Braverman, & David Comings

different mechanisms, depending on the substance used. Alcohol might activate the nucleus accumbens via the globus pallidus, heroin through the VTA, and cocaine directly through the nucleus accumbens (Stahl, 2000).

The intense experience from the drug also changes the orbitofrontal cortex, the area of the brain that selects the more pleasurable activity. This alteration of neurochemistry causes normal activities to become even less pleasurable, leading the user to depend on the substance for intense experiences (Volkow, 2001).

Satiation Centers

Normally when repetition of the survival action finally satisfies the hunger, thirst, sex drive, or other desire, the craving is turned off until the need arises again. This **satiation center is crucial in keeping craving and satiation in balance**. In actuality there are several areas that make up each satiation center although there seem to be fewer areas than are involved in craving. For example, thirst seems to involve 22 areas of the brain whereas satiation of that thirst involves just 3 areas in the cingulate gyrus (Denton et al., 1999).

Animals can't control the drives of their instincts or the messages from the reward/reinforcement center on their own. They can only keep trying to satisfy them until the satiation center kicks in. The complete reward/satiation network involving several kinds of neurotransmitters (brain chemicals) was developed over millions of years in all animals as a way to reinforce survival instincts. Recent research has suggested that when this system is activated, **the memory of the action that caused the reward is more strongly imprinted**. The more intense the reward, the more ingrained the memory, and so the more likely the action will be repeated (Wicklegren, 1998).

When the reward/reinforcement center is activated by refined psychoactive drugs, the impact is so strong that they can **imprint the emotional memory of euphoria or pain relief more deeply than most natural survival**

memories. When these deeply imprinted memories are then activated by an experience or memory, they can induce a stronger craving and disrupt communication with the new brain. In recent experiments a number of cocaine users watched a video about using cocaine. Magnetic resonance imaging (MRI) scans of their brains showed activation of craving in the brain as did their subjective reports of their feelings. When shown nature videos, the craving and activation of the brain did not appear. Conversely a control group of nonaddicts showed no such activation or craving when shown any of the visual drug cues (Childress, 1999).

"When I started drinking, everything went blank in my mind as far as thinking, feelings, emotions. So I like kind of started getting used to it. I said, 'Well that numbed me the first time.' I didn't think of how I was abused or the sexual molestation, so I just continued on, every day, and then I got used to the alcohol."
42-year-old recovering polydrug abuser

The reward/reinforcement center in the old brain is intimately connected with the physiological regulatory centers of the body (autonomic nervous system). Thus **when drugs are used for intoxication or pleasure, they necessarily affect physiological functions**, especially heart rate and respiration; stimulants speed up these functions while depressants slow them down. Psychedelics seem to have a greater effect on the new brain although they will also affect physiological functions in the old brain (e.g., LSD stimulates, marijuana sedates). Most drugs also affect memory in one way or another because emotionally tinged memories involve the amygdala and hippocampus in the old brain.

What makes human beings unique is that starting around the age of 3 or 4 years old, the neocortex (new brain) becomes more complex and capable. Its strength comes from survival lessons and problem-solving skills taught from

birth by parents, relatives, schoolteachers, neighbors, and friends.

In most cases, as people continue to grow up they learn how to **integrate the drives of the old brain and the common sense of the new brain**. Unfortunately some people lose full use of this ability (usually due to genetic abnormalities, a chaotic or abusive childhood, and/or psychoactive drugs) often leading to mental illness or addiction. These people come to rely on one part of the brain. For example, someone with a mood disorder, such as major depression or bipolar disease, is buffeted by the emotional memories of their old brain. Another person with an obsessive-compulsive disorder could be stuck in an area of their new brain where an obsessive idea is repeated constantly in the prefrontal cortex (C. Pepper, personal communication, 1991). **Psychoactive drugs hijack the survival mechanism, thus disrupting this integration** (Hyman, 1998).

"You keep thinking your best thinking got you into this. So then you start to question your own thinking and then you think, 'Well, I think I'm pretty smart. My best thinking got me to do this.' So that's pretty scary for you right there."
38-year-old compulsive gambler

ON/OFF SWITCHES

A good deal of current research has changed its focus from why do we crave drugs to **why can't we stop craving drugs**. What happens at the other end of the reward system after craving has been activated? Are the changes to the on/off switches that govern craving and satiation permanent or reversible?

"There are switches that allow there to be changes in the way genes work, that they can be turned on or turned off. One of the things that alcohol does is it turns on and turns off some genes. And as it does this it changes the proteins in those cells and the enzymes that those proteins function as, and

that changes the communication between the cells, ultimately leading to a change in the network of the cells and you get a different kind of behavior."
Dr. Ivan Diamond, Director, Gallo Research Institute

There are a number of theories or ideas about how psychoactive drugs disrupt the on/off switches of the reward/reinforcement center and the satiation centers.

◇ One concept is that since the feeling of reward did not originate from an essential need of the body, **there is no satiation point** and so the on/off switches do not come into play.

◇ Another concept is that the **on/off switches become stuck**. The mechanism that normally informs the brain that a craving has been satisfied becomes damaged by the use of refined powerful substances. It becomes stuck in the "on" position, so the person never reacts to the fact that the task has been completed. The use of the drug then continues until the drug runs out or the user hits bottom (Koob & Le Moal, 1997).

"Crack tastes like more, that's all I can say. You take one hit, it's not enough, and a thousand is not enough. You just want to keep going on and on because it's like a 10-second head rush right after you let the smoke out and you don't get that effect again unless you take another hit."
32-year-old recovering crack addict

◇ Another theory postulates that the **on/off switches are ignored or overridden** because the user wants to continue the euphoria or pain-relief experiences from the psychoactive drug's effect on the reward/reinforcement center.

◇ A fourth idea is that **psychoactive substances disrupt communication between the two brains** directly (Hyman, 1996). They incapacitate areas of the new brain (thinking and insight) and disconnect its con-

trol of the instinctive or automatic old brain.

"I don't like being stuck on stupid, like tweaking all the time. When I'm doing speed, I'm just in this whole little world (can't get me out of it), finding something, nothing, and everything in the dirt."
24-year-old polydrug addict

◇ Finally, certain behaviors, such as compulsive sex, gambling, and risk-taking, also originate in the primal brain and so are subject to addictive behavioral patterns (Hyman, 1998). This **disruption of the on/off switches due to a behavioral addiction** can feed into a drug addiction.

The longer the drug is used or the behavior is practiced, the more the brain changes and the harder it becomes to restore it to healthy functioning.

MORALITY & THE REWARD/ REINFORCEMENT CENTER

"It was like I was two people. My inner self would try to communicate to me that, 'This is not you,' you know what I mean? My outer self would communicate to me, 'This is who you have to be.' So I was caught in between two entities, you know, the entities of what is good to you or what is good for you."
44-year-old recovering heroin addict

The Trappist Monk Thomas Merton wrote about the conflict between desire and common sense in more poetic terms than old brain vs. new brain.

"As long as pleasure is our end, we will be dishonest with ourselves and with those we love. We will not seek their good but only our own pleasure. Authentic love requires times of self-sacrifice. It requires that people monitor the sensations and feelings and moods of others, not just those of themselves."
Thomas Merton (Merton, 1955)

"Get addicts together and everyone's like, 'Me first.' Even me. You know, we fight about who's going to go first. It's always about me, me, me, you know. It's just about the selfishness of it and wanting to feel good."
19-year-old polydrug abuser

Since the reward/reinforcement center and the rest of the primal brain react more quickly and intensely than the neocortex, **it takes a powerful conscious effort to override cravings and desires from the old brain even when reason tells us those feelings are anti-survival**. The Greek philosopher Plato wrote almost 2,400 years ago that

"Passions, and desires, and fears make it impossible for us to think."
Plato, 400 B.C.

Christian, Buddhist, Islamic, and **almost all theologies (and even atheistic ethical structures) teach that one must resist most primal cravings (including psychoactive drugs) in order to live a moral or fulfilling life**. Freud, in the 1880s, wrote about how the superego tries to rein in the primal urges of the id (Freud, 1884/1995). Throughout human history primal urges, intense emotional memories, and desires have been pitted against reason, common sense, and morality. But if these primal urges are activated by abnormal biology caused by drug use or behavioral addictions rather than normal desires, is it fair to cast addicts as merely being morally weak? And how should the law deal with addicts who commit crimes?

NEUROANATOMY

Nerve Cells

Understanding the precise way messages are transmitted by the nervous system is crucial to understanding how psychoactive drugs affect a user's physical, emotional, and mental functioning. For example, if a dentist drills into a lower left molar, the damaged sensory fibers of the mandibular nerve

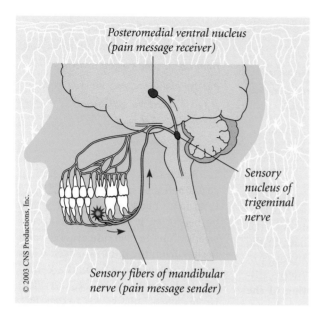

Figure 2-7 •

View of the nerves that would transmit a message of pain from a drilled left molar through the trigeminal nerve to the thalamus.

Posteromedial ventral nucleus (pain message receiver)

Sensory nucleus of trigeminal nerve

Sensory fibers of mandibular nerve (pain message sender)

of the peripheral nervous system (Fig. 2-7) send tiny electrical pain signals via the trigeminal nerve to the sensory nucleus in the spinal cord. **A rapid signal is immediately relayed to the primal brain** and cerebellum in the central nervous system where a reflex action might jerk the head away from the drill. **A slower signal continues to the thalamus at the top of the brainstem,** which identifies the signals as painful and then forwards them to the sensory cortex where the intensity and location of the pain is identified. The signal is also forwarded to the frontal cortex where the cause of the pain is identified and a possible course of action decided. The brain might tell the patient's neck muscles to continue to move the head away from the drill, it might instruct the jaw to bite the dentist's finger, or it might tell the vocal muscles to ask the dentist to prescribe a painkiller. **Nerve impulses might fire up to 1,000 pulses a second** at speeds approaching 270 miles per hour, depending on the size of the nerve (Diagram Group, 1991).

The building blocks of the nervous system, the nerve cells, are called **"neurons"** (Fig. 2-8). Each neuron has four essential parts: (1) **dendrites,** which receive signals from other nerve cells and relay them through the cell body; (2) **the cell body** (soma), which nourishes the cell and keeps it alive; (3) **the axon,** which carries the message from the cell body to (4) **terminals,** which then relay the message to the dendrites, cell body, or even terminals of the next nerve cell. A single cell might have anywhere from a few contacts up to 150,000 contacts with other cells' dendrites. For example, a spinal motor cell might receive 8,000 contacts on its dendrites and 2,000 on its cell body. A Purkinje cell in the cerebellum might have as many as 150,000 contacts available (Fig. 2-9). It is estimated that there are 100 trillion connections among nerve cells. Of course only a fraction of the synapses will fire at any given time (Purves et al., 1997; Kandel, Schwartz, & Jessell, 1991).

The length of a neuron is determined by the length of the cell body, dendrites, terminals, and particularly

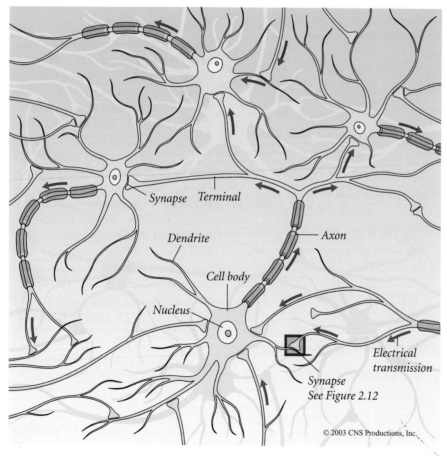

Synapse   Terminal

Dendrite

Axon

Cell body

Nucleus

Electrical transmission

Synapse See Figure 2.12

Figure 2-8 •

Stylized depiction of how nerve cells connect with each other. The dendrites, cell bodies, and even terminals receive signals from the terminals of other nerve cells. The transmitted signal then travels through the axon to the next set of terminals and the message is retransmitted. The process continues until the appropriate part of the nervous system is reached.

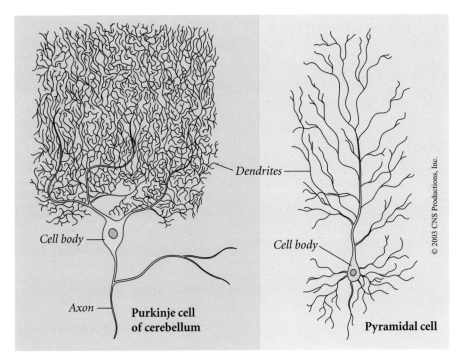

© 2003 CNS Productions, Inc.

Figure 2-9 •

A two-dimensional tracing of a Purkinje cell shows just a fraction of the dendrites that receive signals from other cells. A three-dimensional view of the cell would show tens of thousands of contacts.

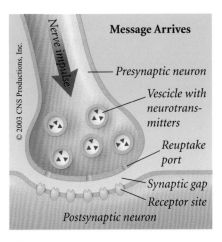

© 2003 CNS Productions, Inc.

Figure 2-10 •

This is a simplified version of the synapse between nerve cells. The electrical message (nerve impulse) arrives at the junction of two nerve cells, the synaptic gap or cleft.

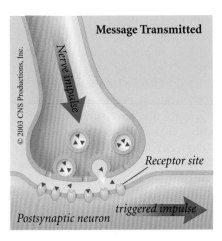

© 2003 CNS Productions, Inc.

Figure 2-11 •

The electrical message is retriggered in the postsynaptic neuron by neurotransmitters slotting into specialized receptors.

the axon, which varies from a fraction of a millimeter between brain cells, a foot between the tooth and brain, to several feet between the spinal cord and toe. Terminals of one nerve cell do not touch the adjoining nerve cell because a microscopic gap, called a **"synaptic gap" or "synaptic cleft,"** exists between them. This gap is 15–50 nm wide. A nanometer (nm) is one billionth of a meter. A million synaptic gap widths added together barely total 1 inch.

The message is transmitted electrically within the neuron but when it arrives at the synaptic cleft it almost always jumps this gap from the presynaptic terminal to the postsynaptic receptor, not as an electrical signal but as **microscopic bits of messenger chemicals called "neurotransmitters"** (Fig. 2-11). These bits of chemicals have been **synthesized within the neuron and stored in tiny sacs called "vesicles."** This chemical signal is then converted back to an electrical signal and travels to the next synapse where it's again converted to a chemical signal. This complete transmission proc-

ess across the gap between nerve cells is called a "synapse." **Electrical and chemical signals alternate until the message reaches the appropriate section of the brain or body.** Some synaptic gaps are one-tenth the width of normal synapses. At these junctures the signal is transmitted electrically. Our focus is on the synapses that need neurotransmitters to jump the gap.

NEUROTRANSMITTERS & RECEPTORS

Although the first neurotransmitters were discovered in the 1920s (acetylcholine) and 1930s (norepinephrine), it was the discovery in the mid-1970s of endorphins and enkephalins, which produce the same effects as opioid drugs, that finally **gave an understanding of how psychoactive drugs work in the brain and body.** For the first time, reaction and addiction to psychoactive drugs could be described in terms of specific naturally occurring chemical and biological processes.

◇ **Endorphins and enkephalins are called "endogenous opioids."** En-

dogenous means "originating or produced within the body or organism."

◇ **Morphine, heroin, and other opium derivatives or synthetics are called "exogenous opioids."** Exogenous means "originating or produced outside the organism."

Once the existence of endorphins and enkephalins was confirmed, the search for other natural neurochemicals that mimic psychoactive drugs began in earnest. Over the next 20–30 years researchers were able to identify and then correlate dozens of psychoactive drugs

TABLE 2–1   PSYCHOACTIVE DRUG/NEUROTRANSMITTER RELATIONSHIPS

Drug	Neurotransmitters Directly Affected
Alcohol	GABA (gamma-aminobutyric acid), met-enkephalin, serotonin
Benzodiazepines	GABA, glycine
Marijuana	Anandamide, acetylcholine
Heroin	Endorphin, enkephalin, dopamine
LSD	Acetylcholine, dopamine, serotonin
Nicotine	Epinephrine, endorphin, acetylcholine
Cocaine & amphetamines	Epinephrine, norepinephrine, serotonin, dopamine, acetylcholine
MDA, MDMA	Serotonin, dopamine, epinephrine, norepinephrine
PCP	Dopamine, acetylcholine, alpha-endopsychosin

with the neurotransmitters they affect (Table 2-1).

One implication of the research implies that virtually any psychoactive drug works because it mimics or disrupts naturally occurring chemicals in the body that have specific receptor sites. It means that **psychoactive drugs cannot create sensations or feelings that don't have a natural counterpart in the body**. It also implies that human beings can naturally create virtually all of the sensations and feelings they try to get through drugs although many of them are not as intense as those received through highly concentrated drugs. Here are some examples.

◇ A genuine scare will force the release of adrenaline that will mimic part of an amphetamine rush.

◇ Prolonged running produces a runner's high through the release of endorphins and enkephalins, similar to a modified heroin rush.

◇ Sleep or sensory deprivation can produce true hallucinations through the same neurotransmitters and mechanisms affected by peyote.

◇ Relaxation and stress-reduction exercises can calm restlessness through glycine and GABA modulation, similar to the effects of benzodiazepines.

One big difference between natural sensations and drug-induced sensations is that drugs have side effects, particularly if used to excess, while the natural methods of producing the desired effects usually have no side effects. In addition the more a drug is used, the weaker the effects become (due to tolerance) and the harder it becomes to reproduce the desired sensations. Increased doses to achieve the same desired effect increase the toxicity of side effects. With natural sensations the opposite is usually true. The desired effects become easier to reproduce with practice. Another key difference is that natural biochemical responses return to a normal state after the response is completed while drugs continue to affect the user's biochemistry until they have been metabolized.

Neurotransmitter research seems to indicate that **some people are drawn to certain drugs because they have an imbalance in one or more neurotransmitters** and have discovered through experimentation and self-medication that a specific drug or **drugs would help correct that imbalance temporarily**. For example, people who are born with low endorphin/enkephalin levels or who have damaged their ability to make these chemicals might have a propensity for opioid and alcohol use. Similarly those with low

epinephrine and norepinephrine (natural stimulants) may be predisposed to amphetamine or cocaine use. This is because those drugs mimic the deficient neurotransmitters and make the user feel normal, satisfied, and in control.

"After I got PMA [para methoxy amphetamine] like down, I never went back to ecstasy again because PMA was like such like a better feeling like it was like, it's the derivative of MDMA [ecstasy], that's the feeling that releases all your serotonin, that's what I wanted."
17-year-old recovering meth addict

Major Neurotransmitters

Amines (e.g., catecholamines)

◇ **Acetylcholine (ACh)** is the first known neurotransmitter. It is mostly active at nerve-muscle junctions (e.g., cardiac inhibition, vasodilation) and it also helps control mental acuity, memory, and learning. Acetylcholine imbalance has been implicated in Alzheimer's disease.

◇ **Norepinephrine (NE) and epinephrine (E)** are the second two neurotransmitters to be discovered. They are classified as catecholamines and function as stimulants when activated by a demand from the body for energy. Besides stimulating the autonomic nervous system, they also affect motivation, hunger, attention span, confidence, and alertness. The neurotransmitters are also known as "adrenaline" and "noradrenaline."

◇ **Dopamine (DA)** was discovered in 1958. This catecholamine helps regulate fine motor muscular activity, emotional stability, satiation, and the reward/reinforcement center. Dopamine is intimately involved in drug use and abuse. Parkinson's disease destroys dopamine-producing areas of the brain, thereby inducing erratic and limited motor movements. Excess dopamine causes many of the effects of schizophrenia.

◇ **Histamine** controls inflammation of tissues and allergic response. It also helps regulate emotional behavior and sleep.

◇ **Serotonin** helps control mood stability including depression and anxiety, appetite, sleep, and sexual activity. MDMA (ecstasy) forces the release of these neurotransmitters. Many antidepressant drugs, including Prozac® and Paxil®, are aimed at increasing the amount of serotonin in the synaptic gaps by blocking their reabsorption, thus elevating mood.

Opioid Peptides

◇ **Enkephalins, endorphins, and dynorphins** were discovered in 1973. A number of these opioid peptides are involved in the regulation of pain, the mitigation of stress (emotional and physical), the immune response, stomach activity, and a number of other physiological functions.

Amino Acids

◇ **GABA (gamma-aminobutyric acid)** is the brain's main inhibitory neurotransmitter and is involved in 25% to 40% of all synapses in the brain. It controls impulses, muscle relaxation, and arousal and generally slows the brain down.

◇ **Glycine,** an inhibitory neurotransmitter, is found mostly in the spinal cord and brain stem. It is also prominent in protein synthesis and slows the brain down.

◇ **Glutamic acid (glutamate, glutamine),** an important excitatory neurotransmitter, is one of the major amino acids and plays a major role in cognition, motor function, and sensory function. Strangely it is also a precursor for GABA, an inhibitory neurotransmitter.

Tachykinin

◇ **Substance "P," a peptide** found in sensory neurons, conveys pain impulses from the peripheral nervous system to the central nervous system. Enkephalins block release of substance "P."

Lipid Neurotransmitter

◇ **Anandamide,** discovered in 1995, has an affinity for receptor sites, discovered 3 years earlier, that accommodate THC, the main active ingredient in marijuana. It is found in the limbic system and the areas responsible for integration of sensory experiences with emotions as well as those controlling learning, motor coordination, and memory. It also can act as an analgesic or pain reliever. There are many more cannabinoid receptors in the brain than there are opioid receptors, so even though THC is not as efficient as anandamide in activating these receptors, their sheer number will cause wide-ranging effects.

Pituitary Peptide

◇ **Corticotropin (ACTH, cortisone)** aids the immune system, healing, and stress control.

Gas

◇ **Nitric oxide** is involved in message transmission to the intestines and other organs including the penis (erectile function). It also plays a part in regulation of emotions. When mice are bred without nitric oxide, they exhibit aggression, along with bizarre and excessive sexual behavior (Snyder, 1996). Nitric oxide (NO) is often confused with the anesthetic nitrous oxide (NO$_2$).

Hormones

◇ **Adenosine** functions as an autoregulatory local hormone. Most cells contain adenosine receptors that when activated inhibit some cell functions.

Besides the 16 listed above at least 100 more neurotransmitters have been discovered. Researchers have also discovered hundreds of receptor types, each one with a different molecular composition of proteins. A **receptor is designed to receive a compatible neurotransmitter**. There are often multiple receptors on a dendrite or cell body that can accommodate a single type of neurotransmitter. The neurotransmitter

serotonin has at least seven types of serotonin receptor sites (e.g., 5-HT1A, 5-HT4) in the brain, each one causing a slightly different effect.

Each nerve cell produces and sends only one type of neurotransmitter, one exception being some epinephrine nerve cells that also produce norepinephrine. Conversely **a single nerve cell can have receptors for several different types of neurotransmitters**. A serotonin receptor will not accommodate dopamine but a single nerve cell can contain dopamine and serotonin receptors. In addition the release of one neurotransmitter usually has a cascade effect. For example, the release of serotonin from one neuron will trigger the release of enkephalin in another neuron that then triggers dopamine from a third neuron in the brain's emotional center, which will result in a feeling of well-being.

Advanced Neurochemistry

Message transmission (Fig. 2-12) occurs when the incoming electrical signal (1) forces the release of neurotransmitters (2) from the vesicles (3) and sends them across the synaptic gap (4). On the other side of the gap the neurotransmitters will slot into precise and complex receptor sites (5). These receptor sites are structural protein molecules that when activated by a neurotransmitter cause an ion molecular gate (6) to open, allowing sodium (7), potassium, or chloride ionic electrical charges in or out.

◇ **Excitatory neurotransmitters increase cell firings** by opening the gate and allowing positive sodium ions in.

◇ **Inhibitory neurotransmitters reduce cell firings** by allowing negative chloride ions in and pushing positive potassium ions out.

When enough excitatory neurotransmitters cause sufficient movement of the positively charged sodium ions and the **total voltage reaches a certain action potential** (about 40–60 mv or millivolts), it fires the signal (8). It is the electrical-charge sum of all the acti-

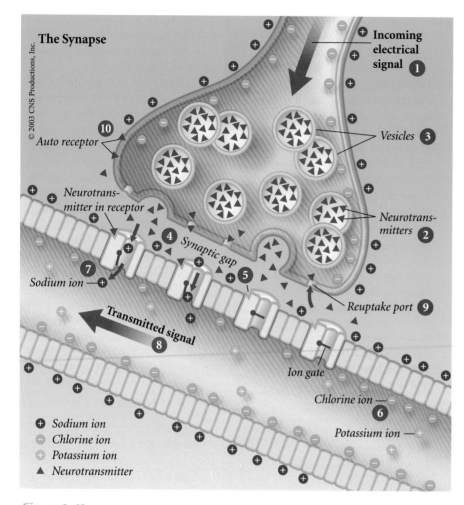

The Synapse

© 2003 CNS Productions, Inc.

Incoming electrical signal **1**

10 *Auto receptor*

Neurotransmitter in receptor

Vesicles **3**

Neurotransmitters **2**

4

Synaptic gap

7

5

Sodium ion

Transmitted signal **8**

Reuptake port **9**

Ion gate

Chlorine ion **6**

Potassium ion

⊕ *Sodium ion*
⊖ *Chlorine ion*
⊕ *Potassium ion*
▲ *Neurotransmitter*

Figure 2-12 •

This is a more complex illustration of what occurs neurochemically and electrically at the synaptic gap. To truly depict the complexity of what happens at the synaptic gap would require dozens of illustrations.

vated receptor sites that can cause the cell to reach its action potential and fire off the signal. If enough inhibitory neurotransmitters keep the voltage below the action potential, the cell is inhibited from firing.

◊ The process where the neurotransmitter directly affects electrical transmission in the receiving neuron is called the "**first messenger system.**"

◊ If the received neurotransmitters cause other biological and chemical changes that then affect the electrical transmission, it is called a "**second messenger system.**" The same neurotransmitter can be a first messenger in one part of the nervous system and a second messenger in another. Second messengers use G-

protein-coupled receptors to synthesize neurotransmitters.

(Stahl, 2000; Hoffman & Taylor, 2001)

As neurotransmitters complete their job in the receptors they are released back into the synaptic gap and are reabsorbed by the sending nerve cell membrane (reuptake ports [9]) and returned to the vesicles, ready to fire again. The reuptake ports use special molecules (transport carriers) as part of **active transport pumps** to move the neurotransmitters through these membranes. Some of the neurotransmitters don't make it back to the reuptake ports of the sending neurons and are metabolized by enzymes surrounding the nerve cells.

The amount of neurotransmitters available for message transmission is

constantly monitored by autoreceptors (10) on the sending neuron. If there are too many neurotransmitters, the cell slows their synthesis and release. If there are too few, it speeds up the process. In addition the number of receptor sites is altered to compensate for variations in the number of neurotransmitters.

◊ If the cell senses there are too many neurotransmitters, it will decrease the number of receptor sites to slow message transmission (**down regulation**).

◊ If there are too few neurotransmitters available to trigger the message, the receiving neuron will increase the number of receptor sites so the few neurotransmitters remaining can be more active (**up regulation**).

This information will be crucial later in this section to understand how tolerance, dependence, withdrawal, and addiction occur due to psychoactive drug use.

This description of the normal process of neural transmission is still greatly simplified but it is possible to see that it would be easy to induce significant changes in human functioning by making small changes at this molecular level.

Agonist & Antagonist

Psychoactive drugs are used because they alter the process of message transmission. The two most common ways drugs act are as agonists and as antagonists. Drugs that bind to receptors and

◊ **mimic or facilitate the effects of neurotransmitters are called "agonists";**

◊ **block neurotransmitters are called "antagonists";**

◊ **partly mimic the effects of neurotransmitters are called "partial agonists";**

◊ **stabilize the receptor so it doesn't react are called "inverse agonists."**

(Ross & Kenakin, 2001)

A drug will sometimes disrupt communication in more than one of the above ways, e.g., acting as an agonist at low doses and an antagonist at high doses. Drugs act in a number of other ways. They can

◇ **block the release of neurotransmitters** from the vesicles; heroin works this way on substance "P";

◇ **force the release of neurotransmitters** by entering the presynaptic neurons, thus causing an exaggerated effect. Cocaine works this way on norepinephrine and dopamine; ecstasy works this way on serotonin;

◇ **prevent neurotransmitters from being reabsorbed** into the sending neuron, thereby causing them to remain in the synapse to slot into receptors again to induce more intense effects (e.g., SSRI antidepressants, such as Prozac®, prevent the reuptake of serotonin, thus elevating mood);

◇ **inhibit an enzyme that helps synthesize neurotransmitters** to slow the nerve cell's production of neurotransmitters (e.g., heart medications that lower blood pressure by blocking production of norepinephrine, which can raise blood pressure);

◇ **inhibit enzymes that metabolize neurotransmitters** in the synaptic gap, thus increasing the number of active neurotransmitters. Methamphetamine inhibits monoamine oxidase and catechol-O-methyltransferase enzymes that metabolize norepinephrine and epinephrine;

◇ **interfere with the storage of neurotransmitters** allowing them to seep out of vesicles and become degraded, thus causing a shortage of those neurotransmitters;

◇ do a combination of these interactions (Snyder, 1996).

Sometimes the disruption of neurotransmitters is useful (blocking pain messages), sometimes desirable (releasing stimulatory chemicals), and sometimes it is extremely dangerous (blocking inhibitory neurotransmitters that control violent behavior). For example, a stimulant, such as **cocaine, will force the release of norepinephrine** (a stimulatory chemical) **and dopamine** (a pleasure-inducing chemical) from the vesicles and then prevent them from being reabsorbed. The net result is more of both those neurotransmitters available to exaggerate existing messages and stimulate new ones (Fig. 2-13). The user will stay up past normal exhaustion and feel alert until the neurotransmitters are depleted.

A depressant, such as heroin, will act like a second messenger by mimicking enkephalins and slot into opioid (enkephalin) receptors, thus **inhibiting the release of substance "P,"** a pain-transmitting neurotransmitter (Fig. 2-14). This is the reason that heroin and opioids lessen pain. Heroin also slots into substance "P" receptor sites on the receiving neurons without causing pain and acts like an antagonist, further blocking pain transmission. Finally it attaches itself to certain receptor sites in the reward/reinforcement center inducing a euphoric sensation. This too is a desired effect. Unfortunately it also attaches itself to the breathing center, thereby depressing respiration. This is a dangerous effect (O'Brien, 2001; Schuckit, 2000b).

An all arounder (psychedelic or hallucinogen), such as LSD, will release some stimulatory neurotransmitters but mostly it will **alter messages from the external environment**; sounds may become visual distortions and visual images may become distorted sounds. This intermixing of senses is known as "synesthesia." Other psychedelics create hallucinations by blocking the action of acetylcholine.

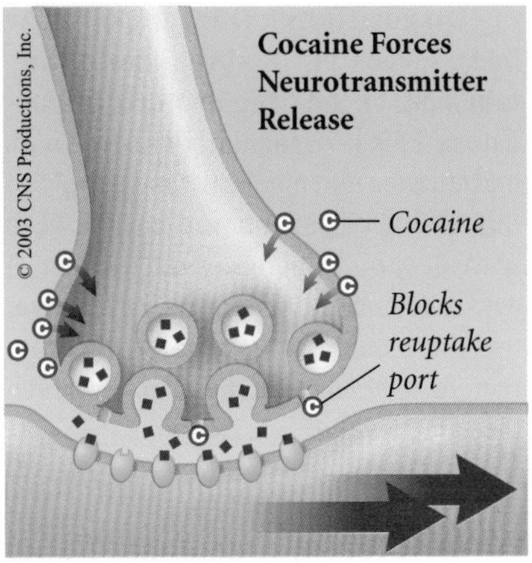

PHYSIOLOGICAL RESPONSES TO DRUGS

It is the way in which psychoactive drugs interact with neurotransmitters, nerve cells, and other tissues that helps determine how drugs affect people and why it is difficult to control their levels of use. Factors such as **tolerance, tissue dependence, psychological dependence, withdrawal, and drug metabolism** can moderate or intensify these effects.

TOLERANCE

The body regards any drug it takes as a toxin. Various organs, especially the liver and kidneys, try to eliminate the chemical before it does too much damage. But if the use continues over a long period of time, **the body is forced**

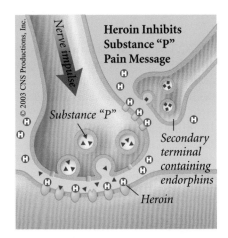

Figure 2-13 •

Cocaine forces the release of extra neurotransmitters and blocks their reabsorption, thus increasing the frequency and therefore the intensity of the electrical signal in the postsynaptic neuron.

Figure 2-14 •

Heroin inhibits the release of substance "P" and helps block most of the neurotransmitters that do get through, so the electrical signal is greatly weakened each time it crosses a substance "P" synapse.

to change and adapt to develop tolerance to the continued input of foreign substances. The net result is that **the user has to take larger and larger amounts to achieve the same effect**.

"It got to the point where it wasn't working anymore. You know, I'd drink and I'd still be sad, and I'd drink more, and I had, it got to the point where I had to drink so much more to not feel anything. You know, it was like I was drunk all day long."

17-year-old recovering alcoholic

The body adapts to an upper, such as methamphetamine, in order to minimize the stimulant's effect on the heart and other systems, so the drug appears to weaken with each succeeding dose if it's used frequently. One dose of methamphetamine on the first day of use will energize a user and trigger a euphoria that can only be matched by 20 doses on the 100th day of use.

"When I first started, I remember having a huge reaction to a small amount of speed. Inside of a year I could shoot a spoon of it easily, which is a pretty fair amount, and it finally got to a point where I couldn't even sleep unless I'd done some."

Recovering 34-year-old meth user

Although **some tolerance develops with the use of any drug**, a user needs to cross a certain level of use for the development of tolerance to accelerate. For example, if a user takes 5 or 10 milligrams (mg) of diazepam, a sedative, every few days, the development of tolerance is minimal. But if they start taking it two or three times a day, they will need to increase dosage up to 100 or more milligrams a day to achieve the same effect. Cases of 1,000 mg a day, 100–200 times the standard dose, have been recorded (O'Brien, 2001).

In experiments with rats 1 hour of access to self-administered cocaine per session did not increase intake or tolerance. However, 6 hours of access esca-

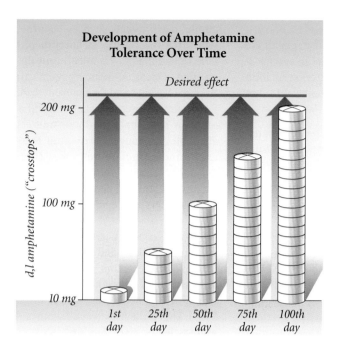

Development of Amphetamine Tolerance Over Time

Desired effect

d,l amphetamine ("crosstops")

200 mg

100 mg

10 mg

1st day | 25th day | 50th day | 75th day | 100th day

Figure 2-15 •
This graph shows the gradually increasing amounts of amphetamine needed to produce stimulation or euphoria over time.

lated tolerance and **increased the hedonic set point that is defined as "an individual's preferred level of pharmacological effects from a drug"** (Ahmed & Koob, 1998). The development of tolerance varies widely, depending mostly on the qualities of the drug itself. But it also depends on the amount, frequency, and duration of use, the chemistry of the user, and the psychological state of mind of the user. There are several different kinds of tolerance.

Kinds of Tolerance

Dispositional Tolerance. The body speeds up the breakdown (metabolism) of the drug in order to eliminate it. This is particularly the case with barbiturates and alcohol. An example of this biological adaptation can be seen with alcohol. It increases the amount of cytocells and mitochondria in the liver that are available to neutralize the drug; therefore more has to be drunk to reach the same level of intoxication.

Pharmacodynamic Tolerance. Nerve cells become less sensitive to the effects of the drug and even produce an antidote or antagonist to the drug. With opioids the brain will generate more opioid receptor sites, down regulate them, and produce its own antagonist, cholecystokinin.

Behavioral Tolerance. The brain learns to compensate for the effects of the drug by using parts of the brain not affected. A drunk person can make himself appear sober when confronted by police but might be staggering again a few minutes later.

Reverse Tolerance. Initially one becomes less sensitive to the drug but as it destroys certain tissues and/or as one grows older, the trend is suddenly reversed and **the user becomes more sensitive and therefore less able to handle even moderate amounts**. This is particularly true in alcoholics when, as the liver is destroyed, it loses the ability to metabolize the drug. An alcoholic with cirrhosis of the liver can stay drunk all day long on a pint of wine because the raw alcohol is passing through the body repeatedly, unchanged.

"At first I could drink a lot, for about 8 or 9 years. They'd say I finished 10 or more highballs in the bar but I'd never get falling-down drunk. I'd be pretty high but never passed out. Now, especially since my liver is only slightly smaller than a Volkswagen and not doing its job, if I drink over about 4 drinks, I can't walk one of those

white lines a cop makes you walk if he thinks you're DUI."

43-year-old alcohol user

Acute Tolerance (tachyphylaxis). In these cases **the brain and body begin to adapt almost instantly** to the toxic effects of the drug. With tobacco, for example, tolerance and adaptation begin to develop with the first puff. Someone who tries suicide with barbiturates can develop an acute tolerance and survive the attempt. They could be awake and alert even with twice the lethal dose in their systems, even if they've never taken barbiturates before.

Select Tolerance. The body develops tolerance to mental and physical effects at different rates. With opiates and depressants the dose needed to achieve an emotional high comes closer and closer to the lethal physical dose of that drug (Fig. 2-16). For example, a barbiturate induces sleep and causes a slight euphoria on the first day it is taken. Within a week it still induces sleep but no longer causes euphoria, so the user needs five pills to feel good. Unfortunately the user has not developed tolerance to the respiratory depression effects of the barbiturate, so

that effect is more severe and can be potentially lethal.

"As many pills as I had, I would take. I didn't really care about overdose, which I did many times."

Former barbiturate user

Inverse Tolerance (kindling). The person becomes more sensitive to the effects of the drug as the brain chemistry changes. A marijuana or cocaine user after months of getting a minimal effect from the drug will all of a sudden get an intense reaction. A cocaine or methamphetamine addict becomes more sensitive to the toxic effects after continued use, thus developing a greater risk of heart attack or stroke.

TISSUE DEPENDENCE

Tissue dependence is the **biological adaptation of the body** due to prolonged use of drugs. It is often quite extensive particularly with downers. In fact with certain drugs the body can change so much that the **tissues and organs come to depend on the drug just to stay functional**. For example, since the number of cytocells and mitochondria in the liver of an alcohol user increase with repeated use to keep the

drug from poisoning the drinker, when alcohol is discontinued their numbers return to normal levels if the liver hasn't been damaged. But once tissue dependence has set in, abrupt cessation of the drug can trigger dramatic and dangerous withdrawal reactions.

"I would start to feel very abnormal after 2 or 3 hours and it was like trying to maintain until I could begin to feel normal. And that was the only kind of normal that I knew, Darvon®-induced normality."

Recovering Darvon® user

PSYCHOLOGICAL DEPENDENCE & THE REWARD-REINFORCING ACTION OF DRUGS

In the past a drug was called addicting only if clear-cut tissue dependence developed, as evidenced by objective physical signs of withdrawal, but with breakthroughs in modern neurochemical research more subtle changes in body chemistry can be measured. In addition **psychological dependence has been recognized in recent years as an important factor in the development of addictive behavior.** Researchers, such as Dr. Anna Rose Childress at Veterans Hospital in Philadelphia, have shown that psychological dependence actually produces many physical effects, meaning that defining drug dependence as strictly physical or strictly mental is not accurate (Childress, McElgin, Mozley, Reivich, & O'Brien, 1996).

Drugs cause an altered state of consciousness and distorted perceptions pleasurable to the user. These reinforce continued use of the drug. Psychological dependence can therefore result from the continued misuse of drugs to avoid life's problems and boredom or from their continued use to compensate for inherited deficiencies in brain-reward neurotransmitters.

Drugs also have the innate ability to guide and **virtually hypnotize the user into continual use (called the "positive reward-reinforcing action of drugs").** In the animal experiments

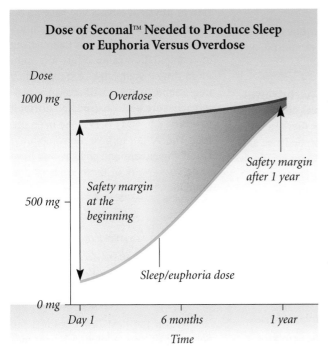

Dose of Seconal™ Needed to Produce Sleep or Euphoria Versus Overdose

Dose

1000 mg — Overdose

500 mg — Safety margin at the beginning

Safety margin after 1 year

Sleep/euphoria dose

0 mg

Day 1   6 months   1 year

Time

Figure 2-16 •

With many drugs, tolerance to mental effects develops at a different rate than tolerance to physical effects. If a user increases the amount of barbiturate they take in order to continue their high, tolerance to the respiratory depressant effects don't increase as quickly as tolerance to the mental effects, so an overdose (potentially fatal physical effects) becomes more likely.

in which rats were trained to press a lever that would feed them heroin or other drugs intravenously, they would continue to press the lever even before physical dependence had developed, showing that a psychoactive drug in and of itself can reinforce the desire to continue use.

"I have a choice about the first snort of cocaine I take. I have no choice about the second."
Recovering cocaine user

WITHDRAWAL

When the user stops taking a drug that has created tolerance and tissue dependence, the body is left with an altered chemistry. There might be an overabundance of enzymes, receptor sites, or neurotransmitters. Without the drug to support this altered chemistry, the body all of a sudden tries to return to normal. Withdrawal is defined as the **"body's attempt to rebalance itself after cessation of prolonged use of a psychoactive drug."** All the things the body was kept from doing while taking the drug, it does to excess while in withdrawal. For example, consider how the desired effects of heroin are quickly replaced by unpleasant withdrawal symptoms once a long-time user stops taking the drug (Table 2-2).

In fact with many compulsive users the **fear of withdrawal is one reason they keep using.** They dread the aches, pains, insomnia, vomiting, cramps, and occasional convulsions that accompany withdrawal.

"I have at times wished I was dead. That's how severe it would be. I've seen people in jail try to hang themselves. I've seen people in jail shoot their own urine to try and get the heroin out of the urine that's left in there. That's a terrible terrible feeling. One of the worst feelings is to be sick from withdrawal."
72-year-old recovering heroin user

Because the withdrawal as well as the fear of withdrawal can be so severe,

TABLE 2–2 OPIOID EFFECTS VS. WITHDRAWAL SYMPTOMS

(Withdrawal effects are often the opposite of the drug's direct effects.)

Effects	Withdrawal Symptoms
Numbness	becomes pain
Euphoria	becomes anxiety, depression, or craving
Dryness of mouth	becomes sweating, runny nose, tearing, and increased salivation
Constipation	becomes diarrhea
Slow pulse	becomes rapid pulse
Low blood pressure	becomes high blood pressure
Shallow breathing and suppressed cough	become coughing
Pinpoint pupils	become dilated pupils
Sluggishness	becomes severe hyper-reflexes and muscle cramps

many treatment programs use mild drugs to temper these symptoms. Withdrawal from opiates, alcohol, many sedatives, and even nicotine seems to be triggered by an area of the brainstem known as the "locus ceruleus." Drugs like Catapres®, Vasopressin®, and Baclofen®, which act to quiet down this part of the brain, partially block out the withdrawal symptoms of these drugs.

Kinds of Withdrawal

There are three distinct types of withdrawal symptoms: nonpurposive, purposive, and protracted.

Nonpurposive Withdrawal. Nonpurposive withdrawal consists of **objective physical signs** that are a direct result of the tissue dependence and are directly observable upon cessation of drug use by an addict. These include seizures, sweating, goose bumps, vomiting, diarrhea, and tremors.

"When I ran out, it was severe. I mean body convulsions, long memory lapses, cramps that were just enough to— you couldn't stand them. And it lasted for about 5 days—the actual convulsions, the cramps, and the pain and

stuff. And then it took another couple of weeks before I ever felt anywhere near normal."
Recovering 18-year-old heroin user

Purposive Withdrawal. Purposive withdrawal results from either **addict manipulation** (hence "purposive" or "with purpose") or from a psychic conversion reaction from the expectation of the withdrawal process. Psychic conversion is an **emotional expectation of physical effects** that have no biological explanation. Since a common behavior of most addicts is malingering or manipulation in an effort to secure more drugs, sympathy, or money, they may claim to have withdrawal symptoms that are very obscure and difficult to verify, e.g., "My nerves are in an uproar. You've got to give me something, Doc!" Physicians and pharmacists have to be very aware of these kinds of manipulations.

"It takes a doctor 30 minutes to say no but it only takes him 5 minutes to say yes. We used to share doctors that we could scam. We called them 'croakers.'"
Recovering 33-year-old heroin user

Within the past few decades, the portrayal of drug addiction by the media, books, movies, and television has resulted in another kind of purposive withdrawal. When they run out of drugs, younger addiction-naive drug users expect to suffer withdrawal symptoms similar to those portrayed in the media. They experience a wide range of reactions even though tissue dependence has not truly developed. Treatment personnel need to avoid overreacting to these symptoms. Further, as previously mentioned, Dr. Childress has demonstrated that psychological dependence can cause many physical symptoms not directly attributable to biological changes in the body.

Protracted Withdrawal (environmental triggers & cues). A major danger to maintaining recovery and preventing a drug overdose during relapse is protracted withdrawal (also called "post acute withdrawal syndrome" or "PAWS"). This is a **flashback or recurrence of the addiction withdrawal symptoms** and triggering of a heavy craving for the drug long after an addict has been detoxified. The cause of this reaction (similar to a posttraumatic stress phenomenon) often happens when some sensory input (odor, sight, noise) stimulates the memories experienced during drug use or withdrawal that evokes a desire for the drug by the addict. For instance, the odor of burnt matches or burning metal (smells that occur when cooking heroin) several months after detoxification may cause a heroin addict to suffer some withdrawal symptoms. Any white powder may cause craving in a cocaine addict; a blue pill may do it to a Valium® addict and a barbecue can cause a recovering alcoholic to crave a beer.

"I had just got a disability check and that check was like a trigger for me. It just sent me into a state of nervousness or anxiety and I didn't know what to do. Today I may not even walk on the same block that I used to walk on because I know if I'm feeling shaky, there could be a possibility that I'll run

into somebody I want to use with, so I have to stay away from those areas."
Recovering 32-year-old crack cocaine abuser

Protracted withdrawal often causes recovering addicts to slip or renew their drug use, generally leading to a full relapse (O'Malley & Volpicelli, 1995). Unfortunately these slips are associated with a greater chance of drug overdose since users are prone to use the same dose they were injecting, smoking, or snorting when they quit. They often forget that their last dose was probably a very high one that they could handle because tolerance had developed. They don't remember that abstinence allowed their bodies to return to a less-tolerant state.

"We cleaned up because we didn't have any connections when we moved. We had about 15 clonidine pills to help us through and I was drinking. Then we shared one bag, one $20 bag of 'cut,' and both of us were on the floor."
33-year-old husband and wife heroin users

Research with animals and interviews with addicts demonstrate that once abstinence is interrupted, both tolerance and tissue dependence develop at a much faster rate than before.

BASIC PHARMACOLOGY

METABOLISM & EXCRETION

"If you want to explain any poison properly, then remember, all things are poison. Nothing is without poison; the dose alone causes a thing to be a poison."
Theophrastus von Hohenhein, aka Paracelsus, 1535

◇ **Metabolism is the body's mechanism for processing, using, and inactivating a foreign substance**, such as a drug or food in the body.

◇ **Excretion is the process of eliminating those foreign substances** and their metabolites from the body.

As a drug exerts its influence upon the body, it is gradually broken down and inactivated, primarily by the liver. It can also be metabolized in the blood, in the lymph fluid, by brain enzymes and chemicals, or by most any body tissue that recognizes the drug as a foreign substance. Drugs can also be inactivated by diverting them to storage in body fat or proteins that absorb and hold the substances to prevent them from acting on body organs.

The **liver is the key metabolic organ** because it has the ability to break down or alter the chemical struc-

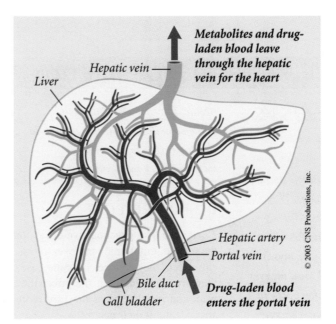

Liver
Hepatic vein
Metabolites and drug-laden blood leave through the hepatic vein for the heart
Hepatic artery
Portal vein
Bile duct
Gall bladder
Drug-laden blood enters the portal vein

© 2003 CNS Productions, Inc.

Figure 2-17•
The liver deactivates a portion of the drug with each recirculation through the circulatory system.

ture of drugs, making them less active or inert. The **kidneys are the key excretory organs** because they filter the metabolites, water, and other waste from the blood and send the resulting urine through the ureter, bladder, and urethra. Drugs can also be excreted out of the body in exhaled breath, in sweat, or in feces.

Metabolic processes generally decrease (but occasionally increase) the effects of psychoactive drugs. For instance, the liver's enzymes help convert alcohol to water and carbon dioxide that are then excreted from the body through the kidneys and urethra, the sweat glands, and the lungs. Some drugs, such as Valium®, are **known as "prodrugs" because they are transformed by the liver's enzymes into three or four other drugs that are also active**.

If a drug is eliminated slowly, as with Valium®, it can affect the body for hours, even days. If it is eliminated quickly, as with smokable cocaine or nitrous oxide, the major actions might last just a few minutes, though other subtle side effects last for days, weeks, or even longer. The following are some other factors that affect the metabolism of drugs.

◇ **Age:** After the age of 30 and with each subsequent year, the liver produces fewer and fewer enzymes capable of metabolizing certain drugs; thus the older the person, the greater the effect. This is especially true with drugs like alcohol and sedative-hypnotics.

◇ **Race:** Different ethnic groups have different levels of enzymes. Over 50% of Asians break down alcohol more slowly than do Caucasians. They suffer more side effects, such as redness of the face, than many other ethnic groups.

◇ **Heredity:** Individuals pass certain traits to their offspring that affect the metabolism of drugs. They can have a low level of enzymes that metabolize the drug; they can have more body fat that will store certain drugs like Valium® or marijuana; or they can have a high metabolic rate that will eliminate drugs more quickly from the body.

◇ **Gender:** Males and females have different body chemistry and different body water volumes. Drugs such as alcohol and barbiturates generally have greater effects in women than in men.

◇ **Health:** Certain medical conditions affect metabolism. Alcohol in a drinker with severe liver damage (hepatitis, cirrhosis) causes more problems than in a drinker with a healthy liver.

◇ **Emotional State:** Anxiety, anger, and other **emotions can exaggerate the effects** of a drug. For example, methamphetamine in an angry person can lead to lashing out and violence.

◇ **Other Drugs: The presence of two or more drugs can exaggerate the effects** by keeping the body so busy metabolizing one that metabolism of the second drug is delayed. For example, the presence of alcohol keeps the liver so busy that Xanax® will remain in the body two or three times longer than normal.

◇ **Exaggerated Reaction:** In some cases the reaction to a drug will be out of proportion to the amount taken. Perhaps the user has an **allergy to the drug** in much the same way a person can go into shock from a single bee sting. For example, a person who lacks the enzyme that metabolizes cocaine can die from exposure to just a tiny amount.

◇ **Other Factors:** In addition factors such as the weight of the user, the level of tolerance, the monthly hormonal cycle for women, and even the weather can affect metabolism of a psychoactive drug.

FROM EXPERIMENTATION TO ADDICTION

DESIRED EFFECTS VS. SIDE EFFECTS

"Let's not kid ourselves. People initially do get something from drugs. They don't say, 'Well, I want to feel miserable so I think I'll swallow this.' They don't think, 'I'm gonna make myself cough by smoking a joint until my eyes become bloodshot.' They don't plan to get hepatitis or AIDS from a shared needle. They get something out of the drug, something desirable enough to throw caution to the wind."
Ian Sholes, Duck's Breath Mystery Theater

DESIRED EFFECTS

People take psychoactive drugs for the mental, emotional, and even physical effects they induce. In some cases they are specific about the effect they want and in other cases they are more abstract about their desires.

Curiosity & Availability

"My first time was when I was in the eighth grade, you know. I got it for free cause, you know, my family, my uncle, and my cousins were like smoking weed and they gave me my first joint and I tried to smoke it but at the time they told me to swallow it and I did, and I got really high, and I couldn't stop laughing."
16-year-old marijuana smoker

To Get High

"It's kind of like life without a coherent thought. It's kind of like an escape. It's like when you go to sleep, you kind of forget about things in your sleep. It's like everything's dreamlike and there's no restraints on anything."
17-year-old heroin user

Self-Medication

"I was very hyperactive, you know. Just always getting into trouble doing things, getting hurt, falling off of things, getting in fights, getting in arguments. And the more I smoked as the years went on, the mellower I got. I stopped getting into trouble."
23-year-old marijuana user

Confidence

"I felt like I was on top of the world and I could accomplish anything. I was self-confident. Just the physical part of staying up so long and being able to feel the freedom of staying up so long was great."
22-year-old recovering meth addict

Energy

"I felt really tingly, excited, sexy. I felt that I had all this energy. I felt like I could do anything. I felt really powerful and I enjoyed that feeling. It made me feel good."
19-year-old recovering male meth addict

Psychological Pain Relief

"Give strong drink to him who is perishing, and wine to those in bitter distress; let them drink and forget their poverty, and remember their misery no more."
The Bible, Proverbs, 31:6-7

Anxiety Control

"It relieved certain anxieties. It alleviated depression, which I had. Lots of depression. You tell the doctor, 'I'm depressed.' 'Okay, take some Valium®.' Now they try to give you antidepressant medications prescribed by the doctor. I'll take the Valium®."
44-year-old Valium® user

To Oblige Friends (internal & external peer pressure)

"If your friends are all getting stoned, then you don't want to just sit there, you know, they're all going to be like having supposedly even more fun because they're stoned, you know. And then they make you look stupid because you feel stupid if you're not."
15-year-old marijuana smoker

Social Confidence

"If you are doing like ecstasy or something, you can just spill your guts to anyone you are with and if you are with a friend or somebody you're dating you can just say whatever you want. It changes everything because you just wake up the next morning and be like, 'Oh God, what did I say last night?' but you remember it."
17-year-old MDMA (ecstasy) user

Boredom Relief

"They tell you you're going to school to get an education so you can get a good job, okay? They told me how to get a job, so that's 8 hours a day. I knew how to sleep, that's 8 hours a day. I had another 8 hours a day that I didn't know how to fill and I used marijuana to fill those 8 hours. Period."
35-year-old recovering marijuana user

Altered Consciousness

"Acid put me in a whole other world, like I don't know, it's hard to explain what it was like. Of course there was the visuals where like everything seemed to either be dripping or like everything would turn into patterns and like I could look at the carpet and just like see like spirals everywhere in it but more so, I used it for kind of a mental and a body high."
18-year-old LSD user

To Deal with Isolation or Life Problems

"When I got addicted to the cocaine, it was because I was being battered and I used that to hide. When I left the cocaine, I used the drinking to hide. When I left the drinking, the cigarettes kicked in. When I left the cigarettes, I began to overeat. It was like I had to fill up that hole with something."
28-year-old recovering compulsive overeater

Oblivion

"On one occasion I was with my friend; we were just sitting in my house just hitting End Dust®, like three cans we killed and then I couldn't, I didn't know what I was doing. I was just sitting there drooling on myself and I passed out. When I woke up I saw him, and then he was talking to himself, and then he spit at me, and then he's like, 'Oh, I thought you were somebody else.'"
Recovering 17-year-old inhalant abuser

Competitive Edge

"I was 125 pounds, not big enough for the team. I started taking steroids, injecting them, that I got from a weightlifter friend down at the gym so I could bulk up. I also started eating like a hungry hog."
19-year-old steroid user

SIDE EFFECTS

"I don't think that a drug is evil in and of itself but just as drugs can be used

to help heal a person, they can result in destroying a life as they did to me. So it really depends on the individual—what and how he chooses and how wisely he uses or chooses not to use medications and drugs."

28-year-old recovering sedative-hypnotic abuser

If drugs did only what people wanted them to and they weren't used to excess, they wouldn't be much of a problem. But drugs not only generate desired emotional and physical effects they also **trigger mild, moderate, dangerous, and sometimes fatal side effects**. This conflict between the emotional/physical effects that users want and those they don't want is one of the main problems with using psychoactive drugs.

A psychoactive drug such as codeine (an opioid-downer) can be prescribed by a physician to relieve pain, to suppress a cough, or to treat severe diarrhea. It also acts as a sedative, gives a feeling of well-being, and induces an emotional numbness. People that self-prescribe codeine just for the feeling of well-being or numbness will have slower reaction time and often become constipated. With moderate use they can also be subject to nausea, pinpoint pupils, dry skin, and slowed respiration. And if users keep using in order to recapture that feeling of well-being over a long period of time, they can become lethargic, lose sexual desire, and even become compulsive users of the drug.

Social side effects of drug use include legal, relationship, financial, and work problems. The more compulsively a person uses, the more severe the various complications.

POLYDRUG ABUSE

Virtually every client who comes in for treatment to a clinic has not confined drug use to just one substance or behavior. For this reason treatment is more complex than just getting a person off one drug. There are a number of reasons a person will resort to polydrug use.

◇ **Replacement:** using another drug when the desired drug is not available, e.g., drinking alcohol when heroin is not available.

◇ **Multiple drug use:** the use of several drugs for different feelings, e.g., taking methamphetamine for stimulation and being bored with it; then using ketamine for a different effect as long as it changes one's mood.

◇ **Cycling:** using drugs intensely for a period of time, abstaining or using another drug to rest the body or lower tolerance and then using again, e.g., taking an anabolic steroid for 2 weeks, then a different steroid for 2 weeks, then nothing for 2 weeks, then back to the original steroid.

◇ **Stacking:** using two or more similar drugs at one time to enhance a specific desired effect, e.g., using alcohol and a benzodiazepine to get to sleep; using MDMA (ecstasy) with methamphetamine to enhance the ecstasy high.

◇ **Mixing:** somewhat similar to stacking, mixing uses drug combinations to induce different effects, e.g., speedballs (cocaine with heroin); lacing a marijuana joint with cocaine; X and L (ecstasy and LSD) to prolong the effects of each; methadone with Klonopin® to mimic the effect of heroin; an antihistamine and a sedative to intensify the downer effects. Some of these combinations are taken intentionally and some unintentionally as when a dealer spikes his drug with a cheaper drug, e.g., PCP is used to spike a marijuana cigarette to mimic a high THC content.

◇ **Sequentialing:** using one drug in an abusive or addictive manner then later on switching to another drug addiction, e.g., a recovering heroin addict who starts using alcohol compulsively; a cocaine addict who switches to methamphetamines. The sequence can also include behavioral addictions, e.g., a recovering alcoholic who becomes a com-

pulsive gambler or a compulsive marijuana smoker who switches to compulsive eating.

◇ **Morphing:** the use of one drug to counteract the unwanted effects of another drug, e.g., a cocaine user so wired he/she has to drink alcohol to come down; the drunk who drinks coffee in an effort to wake up; the heroin addict who uses methamphetamine to function.

LEVELS OF USE

It is important to judge the level at which a person uses drugs and thereby have a benchmark by which to judge whether drug use is accelerating or becoming problematic. To judge a person's level of use it is **necessary to know the amount, frequency, and duration of psychoactive drug use**. These three factors by themselves are not enough to judge the level of use. The second key element is to **know the impact the drug use has on an individual's life**. For example, a man might drink a six-pack of lager beer (amount) twice a week (frequency) and keep it up for 12 years (duration) without developing any problems. Another man might only drink on Fridays but doesn't stop until he passes out. The second man might have more problems regarding relationships, health, the law, or money than the first man who drinks every evening but functions well on the job and works at his relationships.

The following categories can help people judge their level of use.

1. **Abstinence**
2. **Experimentation**
3. **Social/recreational use**
4. **Habituation**
5. **Drug abuse**
6. **Addiction**

The levels of use are presented as distinct categories although the transition from experimentation to habituation or habituation to addiction does not happen so distinctly. Rather it is a continuous process that can ebb and flow. Unfortunately, with most psychoactive drugs **a point is passed where it becomes harder and harder for the person to choose the level at which they want to continue to use**. That point can vary radically from person to person.

ABSTINENCE

Abstinence means people do not use a psychoactive substance except accidentally, e.g., when they drink some alcohol-laced punch, take prescribed medication that has a psychoactive component they don't know about, or are in an unventilated room with smokers. The important fact to remember about abstinence is that even if people have a very strong hereditary and environmental susceptibility to use drugs compulsively, they will never have a problem if they never begin to use. If they never use, there is no possibility of developing drug craving. They might however have a problem with compulsive behaviors, such as gambling, overeating, excessive TV watching, or compulsive sexual behavior.

Recent archival research by the Office of National Drug Control Policy (ONDCP) has shown that those who experiment with alcohol, nicotine, and marijuana between the ages of 10–12 are much more likely to become a heroin or cocaine abuser than those who don't. Further, their research demonstrates that those individuals who never try nicotine before the age of 21 are almost never addicted to tobacco later in life. The same goes for people who don't try any drug until their mid-20s; significantly fewer of them get addicted (Office of National Drug Control Policy [ONDCP], 2001).

"My brother died of alcoholism, so I have never had a drink of alcohol or, for that matter, a puff on a cigarette."
Financier Donald Trump, 1999

EXPERIMENTATION

With experimentation, **people become curious about the effects of a drug** or are influenced by relatives, friends, advertising, or other media and take some when it becomes available to satisfy that curiosity. The feature that distinguishes experimentation from abstinence is the curiosity about drug use and the willingness to act on that curiosity. With experimentation, drug use is limited to only a few exposures. **No pattern of use develops and there are only limited negative consequences in the person's life except if:**

◇ large amounts are used at one time leading to accident, injury, or illness;

◇ the person has an exaggerated reaction to a small amount (e.g., cocaine allergy);

◇ a preexisting physical or mental condition is aggravated (e.g., schizophrenia);

◇ the user is pregnant (e.g., fetal damage);

◇ legal troubles arise (e.g., drug test, possession arrest);

◇ there is a high genetic and/or environmental susceptibility that can lead to compulsive use and addiction;

◇ there is a prior history of addictive behavior with other psychoactive drugs that can lead to a relapse.

Then experimentation can rapidly become a more serious level of drug use.

"A lot of my friends did heroin. I just wanted to try it. It was an experiment. I just wanted to see what it was like. It felt good for a little while; you nod off and you are half-dreaming."
22-year-old polydrug user

SOCIAL/RECREATIONAL

Whether it's a legal six-pack at a party, an illegal joint with a friend, or a couple of lines of cocaine at home, with social/recreational use, the person **seeks out a known drug and wants to experience a known effect but there is no established pattern**. Drug use is irregular, infrequent, and has a relatively small impact on the person's life except if it triggers exaggerated reactions, preexisting mental and physical conditions, an existing addiction, genetic/environmental susceptibility, or legal troubles. Social/recreational use is therefore distinguished from experimental use by the **establishment of drug-seeking behavior**.

"The friends I started hanging out with in school were pretty much the ones that were really rebelling and already knew about cigarettes and pot and so we just started sneaking off and someone would have a joint or something that their dad left around."
24-year-old marijuana smoker

HABITUATION

With habituation **there is a definite pattern of use**, e.g., the TGIF high, the five cups of coffee every day, or the half gram of cocaine most weekends. No matter what happens that day or that week, the person will use that drug. As long as it doesn't affect that person's life in a negative way, it could be called "habituation." Regardless of how frequently or infrequently a drug is used, a definite pattern of use indicates that there is a stronger craving for the drug.

"You would say that I was a habitual user but I don't really think that's the case. So it is a habit. I like a drink. And the question, you know, the question is could I go a day without having a drink? I think so but I've never had a reason to try."
42-year-old habitual drinker

DRUG ABUSE

The definition of drug abuse is **"the continued use of a drug despite negative consequences."** It's the use of cocaine in spite of high blood pressure; the use of LSD though there's a history of mental instability; the alcoholic with diabetes; the two-pack-a-day smoker with emphysema; or the user with a series of arrests for possession. No matter how often a person uses a drug, if negative consequences develop in relationships, social life, finances, legal status, health, work, school, or emotional well-being and drug use continues on a regular basis, then that behavior could be classified as drug abuse.

"I had an EEG and a CAT scan and I was told that I had lowered my seizure threshold by doing so many stimulants but that's not the reason I stopped using them. The reason I actually stopped was because I discovered heroin and I liked it better. I would probably have continued using speed even with the seizures."

36-year-old speed user

ADDICTION

The step between abuse and addiction has to do with compulsion. If users

◇ often use the drug in larger amounts or for longer periods of time than was intended;

◇ unsuccessfully try to cut down or control the drug use;

◇ spend a great deal of time in activities to obtain the substance or recover from its use;

◇ give up or reduce important social, occupational, or recreational activities because of the drug use;

◇ continue use despite knowledge that the drug use is causing physical or psychological problems

then they would be classified as addicted. **These users have lost control of their use of drugs** and those substances have become the most important things in their lives (American Psychiatric Association [APA], 2000).

"The craving was just continuous. It was just like if I was coming off speed, I wanted heroin. If I was coming off heroin, I wanted to snort cocaine. And if I was coming off that, I wanted to stay numb. I wanted to go from one drug to another. If I wanted to stay up all night, I would do speed."

38-year-old recovering polydrug addict

TABLE 2–3   SUMMARY OF THE LEVELS OF DRUG USE

Level of Use	No Risk	Curiosity, Limited Use	Drug-Seeking Behavior	Pattern of Use	Continued Use Despite Negative Consequences	Obsession, Loss of Control
Abstinence	X					
Experimentation		X				
Social/Recreational			X			
Habituation			X	X		
Abuse				X	X	
Addiction				X	X	X

(Courtesy of Tom TenEyck, 2002)

THEORIES OF ADDICTION

For many years there has been an attempt to classify mental and emotional disorders and illnesses. In 1952 the first edition of the American Psychiatric Association's (APA's) *Diagnostic and Statistical Manual of Mental Disorders (DSM)* was published. Besides the standard mental illnesses, such as schizophrenia, depression, and manic-depression (bipolar illness), the manual included classifications of substance-related disorders. These classifications have changed over the years to reflect new research and ideas. In the latest edition *DSM-IV-TR,* **substance-related disorders** are divided into two general categories: substance use disorders and substance-induced disorders.

◇ **Substance use disorders** involve patterns of drug use and are divided into substance dependence and substance abuse. Note that the word "dependence" not "addiction" is used.

● **Substance dependence** is defined in the *DSM-IV-TR* as "a cluster of cognitive, behavioral, and physiological symptoms indicating that the individual continues use of the substance despite significant substance-related problems. There is a pattern of repeated self-administration that can result in tolerance, withdrawal, and compulsive drug-taking behavior."

● **Substance abuse** is defined as "a maladaptive pattern of substance use leading to clinically significant impairment or distress" that results in disruption of work, school, or home obligations, recurrent use in physically hazardous situations, recurrent legal problems, and continued use despite adverse consequences.

◇ **Substance-induced disorders** include conditions that are caused by use of specific substances. Most of these conditions usually disappear after a period of abstinence; however, some of the damage can last weeks, months, years, and even a lifetime. Substance-induced disorders include **intoxication, withdrawal, and certain mental disorders**, e.g., delirium, dementia, anxiety disorder, sexual dysfunction, and sleep disorder. The substances specifically defined in the *DSM-IV-TR* include alcohol, amphetamines, *Cannabis*, cocaine, hallucinogens, inhalants, opioids, PCP, sedative-hypnotics, and even caffeine and nicotine. Polysubstance-related disorders are also included

and probably constitute the majority of substance abusers.

(APA, 2000)

For thousands of years before the classification of mental illnesses and substance-related disorders by the APA's *DSM* in the United States and the World Health Organization's (WHO) International Classification of Diseases (ICD), addiction was most often looked at as a moral failure. However, in the past 5 decades, biological research aided by new imaging techniques, sophisticated epidemiological studies, and careful examination of users' genetic, environmental, and drug use histories has enabled society to understand addiction in a continuously changing light.

"It's just not a physical addiction, it's a spiritual and emotional problem too. It just doesn't encompass your body, your mind is totally off-key. You're just so involved in whatever the addiction is you're not living your life, you're living for the addiction."

43-year-old recovering addict

In addition to a number of psychodynamic concepts of compulsive behaviors, including "regressive behavior caused by unconscious conflicts" and "ego conflicts regarding the environment and inner drives" (Brehm & Khantzian, 1997), there have been three major schools of thought about addiction; some influencing the *DSM* and ICD categories and some influenced by those categories. One school emphasizes the influence of heredity (**addictive disease model**), another the influence of environment and behavior (**behavioral/environmental model**), and the third the influence of the physiological effects of psychoactive drugs (**academic model**).

ADDICTIVE DISEASE MODEL

"Drug addiction is a brain disease— a disease that disrupts the mechanisms responsible for generating,

modulating, and controlling our cognitive, emotional, and social behavior."

Alan Leshner, Ph.D. (Leshner, 1998b)

The addictive disease model, sometimes called the **"medical model," maintains that the disease of addiction is a chronic, progressive, relapsing, incurable, and potentially fatal condition that is mostly a consequence of genetic irregularities in brain chemistry and anatomy that may be activated by the particular drugs** that are abused. It also maintains that addiction is set into motion by experimentation with the **agent** (drug) by a susceptible **host** in an **environment** that is conducive to drug misuse. The susceptible user quickly experiences a compulsion to use, a loss of control, and a determination to continue the use despite negative physical, emotional, or life consequences (Smith & Seymour, 2001).

"The first time I tried it and I got high I said, 'I think I want to use some of this for the rest of my life if I could afford it.' If I could afford this, I would do this everyday for the rest of my life."

43-year-old recovering heroin addict.

Several studies of twins, along with other human and animal studies, strongly support the view that heredity is a powerful influence on uncontrolled compulsive drug use and behavioral addictions (Noble, Blum, Ritchie, Montgomery, & Sheridan, 1991; Blum, Cull, Braverman, & Comings, 1996; Clark et al., 1997; Schuckit, 1986, 2000a; Eisen et al., 1998; Bierut et al., 1998; Raimo, Smith, Danko, Bucholz, & Schuckit, 2000).

Under the addictive disease model, addiction (dependence) is characterized by

◇ compulsive drug abuse marked by use or intoxication throughout the day and an overwhelming need to continue use;

◇ loss of control over the use of a drug with an inability to reduce intake or stop use;

◇ continuation of abuse despite the progressive development of serious

physical, mental, or social disorders aggravated by the use of the substance;

◇ repeated attempts to control use with periods of temporary abstinence interrupted by relapse into compulsive continual drug use;

◇ a progressive escalation of intake and problems. Even in remission, the disease becomes more severe and can be fatal due to overdose, physical deterioration, infected drugs or needles, and a high-risk lifestyle;

◇ being incurable once the user has crossed the line into addictive use. Remission is the object of treatment not cure;

◇ pathological reaction to initial drug use such as increased tolerance, black- or brownouts, dramatic personality and lifestyle changes.

(APA, 2000; Smith & Seymour, 2001)

BEHAVIORAL/ ENVIRONMENTAL MODEL

This theory emphasizes the overriding importance of environmental and developmental influences in leading a user to progress into addictive behavior. As seen in animal and human studies, **environmental factors can change brain chemistry** as surely as drug use or heredity (LeDoux, 1996). Many studies, supported by scans that show brain function, suggest that physical/emotional stress resulting from abuse, anger, peer pressure, and other environmental factors causes people to seek, use, and sustain their continued dependence on drugs (Schroeder, Holahan, Landry, & Kelley, 2000; Griffiths, Bigelow, & Liebson, 1978). For example, chronic stress can decrease brain levels of met-enkephalin (a neurotransmitter) in mice, making normal alcohol-avoiding mice more susceptible to alcohol use (Miczek, Hubbard, & Cantuti-Castelvetri, 1995). Other studies also cite environment as a critical influence (Ciccocioppo, Sanna, & Weiss, 2001; Peele & Brodsky, 1991; Swain, Oetting, Edwards, & Beauvais, 1989; Zinberg, 1984).

The behavioral/environmental model delineates the six levels of drug use:

abstinence, experimentation, social/recreational use, habituation, abuse, and addiction.

ACADEMIC MODEL

In this model, addiction occurs when the **body adapts to the toxic effects of drugs at the biochemical and cellular level** (Spragg, 1940; Tsai, Gastfriend, & Coyle, 1995; Wickelgren, 1998). The principle is that, given sufficient quantities of drugs for an appropriate duration of time, changes in body/brain cells will occur that will lead to addiction. Four physiological changes characterize this process:

◇ **tolerance**—resistance to the drug's effects increase, necessitating larger and larger doses;

◇ **tissue dependence**—actual changes in body cells occur because of excessive use, so the body needs the drug to stay in balance;

◇ **withdrawal syndrome**—physical signs and symptoms appear when drug use is stopped as the body tries to return to normal;

◇ **psychological dependence**—the effects of the drug are desired by the user and these reinforce the desire to keep using.

(Also see Physiological Responses to Drugs in this chapter.)

DIATHESIS-STRESS THEORY OF ADDICTION

All of the existing theories of addiction are true in their own right. It is beneficial however to **integrate these theories and look at addiction as a process that often encompasses a user's life from birth to death**. We have used as a model the diathesis-stress theory of psychological disorders (not addictions).

◇ A diathesis is a constitutional predisposition or vulnerability to develop a given disorder under certain conditions. The genotype may provide a diathesis within the person that leads to the development of the disorder if the person encounters a level of stress that exceeds his or her stress threshold or coping abilities. The diathesis (the biological predisposition or vulnerability) may be so potent that the person will develop the disorder even in the most benign of environments (Nevid, Rathus, & Greene, 1997).

The above theory was originally developed to help explain the causes of schizophrenia (Meehl, 1962; Gottesman, McGuffin, & Farmer, 1987). Our diathesis-stress theory of addiction is similar to the addictive disease model but gives somewhat more flexibility in determining the influence of each of the factors: heredity, environment, and psychoactive drugs.

◇ **A diathesis or predisposition to addiction is the result of genetic and environmental influences, such as stress. When a person is further stressed or challenged by the use of psychoactive drugs or the practice of certain behaviors, then neurochemistry and brain function are further changed to the point that a return to normal use or normal behavior is extremely difficult.** The stronger the diathesis (predisposition), the fewer drugs or less acting out is needed to push the person into addiction; conversely, the weaker the diathesis, the more drugs or behaviors are needed to force a person into addiction.

HEREDITY, ENVIRONMENT, PSYCHOACTIVE DRUGS, & COMPULSIVE BEHAVIORS

Currently it is the belief of more and more researchers in the field of addictionology that **the reasons for drug addiction are indeed a combination of the three factors of heredity, environment, and the use of psychoactive drugs** (DuPont, 1997; Koob, 1998; Leshner, 1998a). Because individual personalities, physiology, and lifestyles vary, each person's resistance or susceptibility to excessive drug use also varies. It is necessary therefore to study the determining factors more closely in order to understand why one person might remain abstinent, another might use drugs sparingly, a third will use for a lifetime and never have problems, and someone else will use and accelerate to addiction within a few months.

HEREDITY

For years scientists have known that **many traits are passed on through generations by genes**, features such as eye and hair color, nose shape, bone structure, and most important, the initial structure and chemistry of the nervous system. In recent years scientists have expanded that list of genetically influenced traits to include more complex physical reactions and diseases such as juvenile diabetes, some forms of Alzheimer's disease, schizophrenia, some forms of depression, and even a tendency to certain cancers. Most surprisingly **many behaviors seem to have an inheritable component** as well, whether it's simply a brain chemistry that results in an exaggerated reaction to alcohol and other psychoactive drugs or a personality that gets a charge from gambling (Noble et al., 1991; Shaffer, 1998).

What is important to remember is that **there isn't just one gene that affects addiction. There are more than 100 that have been associated with drug abuse**, though some are more important than others. These genes can affect receptors, gene transcription factors, enzymes, neuropeptides, G proteins, and transporters, among others (Ikemoto, Glazier, Murphy, & McBride, 1997; Kuhar, Joyce, & Dominguez, 2000). If a person has one or two of these genes, they might have a low propensity to drug dependence whereas if they have a dozen of these genes, they may have a high propensity to addiction. Marc Schuckit, a major researcher in this field, suggests that up to 60% of dependence and addiction to alcohol are due to genetics.

Twin & Retrospective Studies

One set of indicators that a tendency to addiction has an inheritable component is twin studies that have been done in several countries over several decades. Dr. Donald Goodwin of Washington University School of Medicine in St. Louis **looked at identical twins that were adopted into separate foster families** shortly after birth. These studies strongly support genetics and heredity as determining factors in alcohol use. Regardless of the foster parent family environment, adopted children developed alcohol abuse or abstinence patterns similar to their biologic parent's use of alcohol (Goodwin, 1976; Nurnberger et al., 2001).

Other studies have **compared genetic twins (nearly identical genes) and fraternal twins (similar genes)** who are raised in identical environments. In one survey genetics contributed 61% to nicotine dependence and 55% to alcohol dependence (True et al., 1999).

Other evidence of genetic predisposition to alcoholism comes from a **review of the biologic family records of alcoholics** in various treatment programs across the United States (Cloninger, 1987). The data showed that if one biological parent was alcoholic, a male child was about 34% more likely to be an alcoholic than the male child of nonalcoholics. If both biological parents were alcoholic, the child was about 400% more likely to be alcoholic. If both parents and a grandfather were alcoholic, that child was about 900% more likely to develop alcoholism. About 28 million Americans have at least one alcoholic parent (Schuckit, 1986).

"I didn't like the way my father fought with my mother when he drank, so I never drank a drop, not a drop, until I was 27. Then it was like a light got turned on and I tried to make up for lost time."

37-year-old drinker

Alcoholism-Associated Genes

Another breakthrough in this line of inquiry came in 1990 when **a specific gene associated with alcoholism was identified** by Ernest Nobel and Ken Blum, researchers at UCLA and the University of Texas at San Antonio respectively (Noble et al., 1991). Many researchers believe this gene helps indicate a person's susceptibility to compulsive drinking. In some studies this **DRD2 A1 Allele gene was found in more than 70% of severe alcoholics** in treatment but in less than 30% of people who were assessed to be social drinkers or abstainers (Feingold, Ball, Kranzler, & Rounsaville, 1996). What the presence of this gene and other yet-to-be discovered ones means is that when people with these hereditary markers do use alcohol, they are at a much higher risk of becoming alcoholics than drinkers in the general population (Anthenelli & Schuckit, 1998). However if they never drink, problems with alcohol will never occur. Research seems to confirm the role this gene also plays in cocaine addiction (Zhang, Walsh, & Xu, 2000).

Kenneth Blum and fellow researchers believe **this gene indicates a tendency to a number of problematic behaviors**, including gambling, psychoactive drug use, attention-deficit disorder, aberrant sexual behavior, overeating, antisocial personality, and even Tourette's syndrome, not just drinking. **They refer to it as a "compulsivity gene" and call the process "the reward deficiency syndrome"** (Blum et al., 1996; Blum et al., 2000).

In practical terms what genetic markers mean is that these people with one or more marker genes are more susceptible to developing alcoholism (or other compulsive drug use) and that when they begin drinking or using other drugs, they are more likely to do it at a more rapid rate than people without that susceptibility. Though many susceptible people receive an intense reaction from alcohol with their first drinking experience, they also seem to need larger amounts of alcohol than others do to get drunk. So when they reach that intoxicated state it is much more intense than most anything they've felt before and causes greater dysfunction (Cloninger, Bohman, & Sigvardsson, 1986; Cloninger, 1987). Many have

blackouts starting with the first few times they use where they don't remember what happened to them while drunk, or brownouts where they can remember only parts of their drunken experience.

Genes can also help prevent dependence from developing. The DRD4 gene, which signifies an excess of dopamine, has been shown to play a role in the personality trait of spiritual acceptance, a temperament that helps a person develop a lifestyle that doesn't include addiction (Comings, Gonzales, Saucier, Johnson, & MacMurray, 2000).

Another marker for a propensity to alcohol addiction is the P300 ERP (event-related potential) wave that relates to a person's cognition, decision making, and processing of short-term memory. In alcoholics the amplitude of this wave is reduced as it is in their sons, suggesting yet another genetic connection (Begleiter, 1980; Blum et al., 2000; Enoch, White, Harris, Rohrbaugh, & Goldman, 2001).

ENVIRONMENT

The environmental influences that help determine the level at which a person uses drugs can be positive or negative and as varied as **sexual/physical/emotional abuse, stress, love, nutrition, living conditions, family relationships, nutritional balance, health care, neighborhood safety, school quality, peer pressure, and television.** Interactions with the environment, particularly home environment, actually **make new nerve cell connections and alter the neurochemistry a person is born with**, thereby helping to determine how that person will use psychoactive drugs.

Environment & Brain Development

Environmental influences have the greatest impact on the development of the brain. Though we are born with most of the nerve cells we will ever have, about 100 billion neurons in the brain alone, **environment influences the 100 trillion connections that develop between nerve cells.** In this way environment helps mold the brain's architecture and neurochemistry, thus altering the way the brain reacts to outside influences. The growth and alteration are especially influential in the first 10 years of life.

"My mother was addicted to speed and heroin and I grew up with it. Then I was taken away from her. I'd go and visit her, seeing her high, seeing her not high, seeing her high again, coming down the next time, back and forth. And then when I was 11 years old she was shot and killed on Valentine's Day. After that I didn't have anything to look forward to and so I didn't care anymore."
24-year-old heroin addict

The process of making new connections and altering brain chemistry continues after the first 10 years but at an increasingly slower rate. Current evidence indicates that it may take at least 20 years for the brain to get "hard wired" or form all its major and vital connections although recent research shows that the frontal lobe volume increases until age 44 and the temporal lobe until age 47 (Bartzokis et al., 2001). On the other hand we keep making and losing connections until the day we die but the older we are, the more difficult the process.

"Every experience you have matters to your brain. And if you are being bathed with repetitive stress hormones and stress chemicals in your brain, it changes your brain in a negative way and can actually cause your brain to become more at risk for these disorders."
Daniel Amen, M.D., 1998

A common saying is "**Psychology is biology**," meaning that every thought and memory has a physical component. Through subtle chemical, structural, and biological changes, **the brain keeps track of all that happens to a person in his or her lifetime**. The

stronger the environmental influences and the more often thoughts or actions are repeated, the more indelible the imprinting on the brain. If a person uses a certain telephone number again and again, the person memorizes it because the area of the brain responsible for numbers has physiologically written that information on the nerve cells. Because a traumatic experience, such as an accident, a war experience, childhood/domestic abuse, or even addiction, is so emotionally intense, it can leave intense and lasting physical and chemical impressions on the brain (LeDoux, 1996).

"I broke down after about 6 months over in Vietnam and I was in charge of a gun crew. I didn't respond to my duty of opening up an M-60 and some people's lives were lost in my outfit and I'm responsible. They flew me out to the States and I immediately jumped into alcohol and heroin."
Vietnam veteran

Children who are subject to **excessive emotional pain** while growing up in a chaotic household remember that pain and may try different ways to deal with it. They can try to understand why it happened, learn how to face it, find people to help them, and accept what happened or they can run away, become hyperactive, make jokes, **use drugs, gamble, or overeat, anything to temper the pain or discomfort**. If stress continues long enough, the counter-behavior that the child learned also becomes ingrained in the brain (Nestler, 1995). **The brain remembers the counter-behavior just as it remembers the stress and pain.** That addiction memory becomes part of the personality of the user (Boening, 2001). Once connections are made and chemistry altered in response to environmental challenges, they are very difficult to change though not impossible (Bierman, 1995).

"My grandfather was a drunk, and my father was a drunk. That is who

basically beat me up. I figured the more pain he caused me, the more pot I could smoke. Being abused as a kid really scars you for life. So the more pot I could smoke, the more relief I got from the pressure of being abused."
35-year-old male in recovery

Environment can make a person more liable to use and abuse psychoactive substances

◇ if stress is common in the home;
◇ if drinking or other drug use is common in the home;
◇ if healthy ways of reacting to stress or anger aren't learned and self-medication becomes the only solution;
◇ if there are mental health problems triggered by the home environment;
◇ or if one's diet lacks sufficient vitamins and proteins needed to synthesize neurotransmitters and maintain a healthy brain chemistry (e.g., being underweight reduces dopamine levels, possibly leading to amphetamine use to rebalance brain chemistry) (Pothos, 2001).

People can also become more susceptible to use if society tells them in word and deed that drinking, smoking, and using drugs to solve all problems are a normal part of life. Massive advertising campaigns for tobacco or alcohol make people more likely to use. Belonging to a social, business, or peer group where excessive drinking or drug use is considered normal increases use. Living in a community where access to legal and illegal drugs is easy increases use.

"My parents have a glass of wine after they come home from work to relax and unwind. I'm the same way, just with marijuana. It's just kind of a regular thing that I do instead of alcohol or anything else."
23-year-old marijuana smoker

And if, in addition to these environmental stressors and influences, people have a hereditary susceptibility to use,

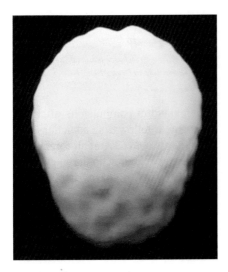

Figure 2-18 •

When the brain is functioning normally, there is an even distribution of function throughout the brain. When drugs are used, many parts of the brain become inactive or occasionally overactive.

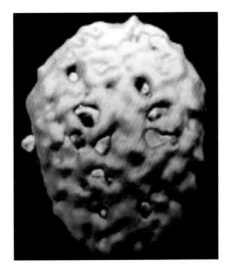

Figure 2-19 •

This is a SPECT scan of a person who has abused methamphetamine for about 8 years. What we see are multiple areas of decreased activity (less than 50% of normal) across the cortical surface of the brain (not real holes in the brain tissue).

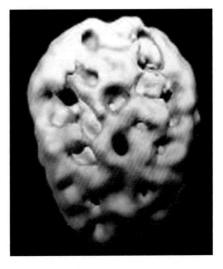

Figure 2-20 •

This SPECT scan shows someone who had been abusing alcohol for about 20 years and what is seen is a dramatic overall shutdown or decreased areas of activity across the brain.

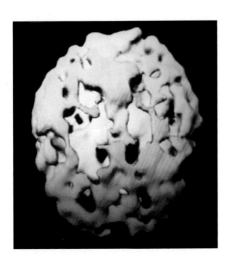

Figure 2-21 •

Heroin gives the classic brain-melt picture—dramatic suppression of overall cerebral activity. In the Amen Clinic for Behavioral Medicine's experience, people treated with methadone show the same brain dysfunction.

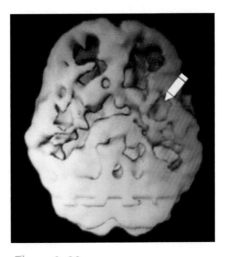

Figure 2-22 •

This SPECT scan shows the brain of a man who had been abusing marijuana heavily for about 12 years. There is a strong suppression of temporal lobe activity on both sides that affects his memory and motivation. Given that he's used for such a long period of time, when he stops using he'll begin to get increased function in his temporal lobes but his brain will never return to normal.

All scans are courtesy of the Amen Clinic for Behavioral Medicine

the chances that they will slide into compulsive use (if they start drinking or taking drugs) greatly increases (DuPont, 1997).

PSYCHOACTIVE DRUGS

The hereditary and environmental influences mean nothing in terms of drug addiction unless the person actually uses psychoactive substances, so the final factor that determines the level at which a person might use drugs is the drugs themselves. Drugs can affect not only susceptible individuals but also those with no predisposing factors. This occurs because, by definition, psychoactive drugs are substances that affect the functioning of the central nervous system. **Excessive, frequent, or prolonged use of alcohol or other drugs inevitably modifies many of the same nerve cells and neurochemistry that are affected by heredity and environment.** This influences not only the person's reaction to those substances when they are used but also the level at which they are used (Hyman, 1998). **Behavioral addictions also alter brain chemistry.**

The development of tolerance, tissue dependence, withdrawal, and psychological dependence are signs that the drugs themselves are causing physical and chemical changes in the body that tend to increase use. For example, in animal experiments the chronic use of THC, the active ingredient in marijuana, increased their vulnerability to amphetamine and heroin (Lamarque, Taghzouti, & Simon, 2001). Several drugs, particularly methamphetamine, kill brain cells through a process called "apoptosis" where damaged cells are programmed to kill themselves (Cadet, Ordonez, & Ordonez, 1997). Nicotine produces immediate and long-term changes in neurotransmitter levels, particularly dopamine and norepinephrine, leading to a faster development of tolerance and dependence (Trauth, Seidler, Ali, & Slotkin, 2001).

Psychoactive drugs and addictive behaviors cause temporary and permanent changes in various parts of the brain that can be imaged. For many years Dr. Daniel Amen has studied these changes in brain function at his behavioral medicine clinics in Fairfield and Newport Beach, California, using **SPECT scans** (single photon emission computerized tomography) of the brain (Amen, 2001). A SPECT scan is a very sophisticated nuclear medicine imaging technique that looks at blood flow and metabolic activity in the brain to show how the brain functions during a given activity, such as taking a psychoactive drug. **PET scans** (photon emission computerized tomography) also show brain function. **CAT scans** (computerized axial tomography-x-ray) or an **MRI** (magnetic resonance imaging), on the other hand, produce anatomical studies of the brain but don't show brain functioning. There is also an **fMRI** (functional magnetic resonance imaging) that traces blood flow to different regions of the brain that give information of motor, sensory, visual, and auditory functions.

Finally, animal studies confirm that **some drugs have greater power to compel continued use than other drugs** (positive reinforcement). For example, cocaine and heroin have a more hypnotizing effect to continue their use than Thorazine® or Tofranil®.

COMPULSIVE BEHAVIORS

There is a growing belief among many researchers that certain behaviors can become compulsive, such as **gambling, sexual activity, and eating, in a way that is extremely similar to compulsive drug use**. Dr. Howard Shaffer, Director of Harvard Medical School's Division on Addictions, told a group of Las Vegas casino executives that the excitement from gambling causes the brain to be rewired, particularly the reward/reinforcement center. He stated that some people can limit their betting while others experience a loss of control, along with increased craving, and they continue to gamble despite adverse consequences (Shaffer, 1998).

"I had given most of the money away and the only money I really did have at that point was our daughter's money and I remember one night—9 months to the night that my husband died—saying screw it, I'm outa here and I sat down in front of a $25 video poker machine and I imagine in 24 hours I went through $10 grand. It just happened to be her college money but, uh, I was always going to get it back."
43-year-old compulsive gambler

PET scans of the brains of compulsive overeaters have shown a lack of dopamine (D_2) receptor sites in the nucleus accumbens, part of the reward/reinforcement center. This is the same area activated by psychoactive drugs (Wang, Volkow, et al., 2001).

"If you have a decrease in dopamine receptors that transmit pleasurable feelings, you become less responsive to the stimuli, such as food or sex, that normally activate them. When you don't reward yourself enough, your brain signals you to do something that will stimulate the circuits sufficiently to create a sense of well-being. Thus an individual who has low sensitivity to normal stimuli learns behaviors,

such as abusing drugs or overeating, that will activate them."
Dr. Nora Volkow, Brookhaven National Laboratories (National Institute on Drug Abuse [NIDA] Notes, 2001)

Behavioral compulsions often accompany or follow drug addictions. For example, 25% to 63% of all compulsive gamblers (depending on the study) have been alcohol or drug dependent (National Research Council [NRC], 1999). Many recovering addicts switched to gambling to pass the time because they thought it was harmless. It is now recognized that **gambling and other compulsive behaviors are actual dysfunctions of brain chemistry in the same way that drugs disrupt brain chemistry** (Potenza, 2001). Psychological and social treatment for these compulsive behaviors are evolving along the same lines and using the same interventions utilized in the treatment of drug addiction.

These compulsive behaviors are different from **obsessive-compulsive disorder** (OCD), e.g., repetitive hand washing, repeated and excessive checking to insure that the door is locked or that the stove is turned off, and compulsive ordering like arranging magazines, books, or objects into a certain order and being upset if they are not in the expected place. OCD has been shown to occur along a different brain and neurotransmitter pathway than that associated with compulsive behaviors. With compulsive behaviors there is an experience of pleasure associated with the action whereas OCD actions are not associated with a pleasurable experience. (OCD is also different than **obsessive-compulsive personality disorder** where a person is preoccupied with details, rules, lists, order, organization, control, and doing things just right to the point that less gets done.)

ALCOHOLIC MICE & SOBER MICE

To better understand the close connection of heredity, environment, psychoactive drugs, and compulsive behaviors and to further visualize the diathesis-stress theory of addiction, it might be helpful to examine a series of classical animal studies done over the past 40 years by Gerald McLaren, T.K. Li, Horace Lo, D. S. Cannon, and other researchers (Li, Lumeng, McBride, Waller, & Murphy, 1986). Animal experiments are often used to help us understand what the effects of a drug would be on human beings. They were first used scientifically by Johann Jakob Wepfer, a seventeenth-century scientist.

The basic experiments are as follows: years ago researchers developed **two genetic strains of mice** (Fig. 2-23a) to help researchers understand alcoholism. **One of the strains of mice loved alcohol.** When given the choice between water and even 70% concentrations of alcohol, these mice went for the alcohol every time. If all they had was water, then they would grudgingly drink water. **The other strain of mice hated alcohol.** Given the same choice, even with concentrations as low as 2% alcohol, the mice always chose the pure water (Cannon & Carrell, 1987).

In one experiment researchers first took a group of the alcohol-hating mice and injected them with high levels of alcohol, the equivalent of what adult human beings would drink if they were heavy drinkers. Within a few weeks **these once-sober mice came to prefer alcohol through overexposure to the drug.** In fact if not stopped, they would drink themselves to death (Fig. 2-23b).

Researchers then took another group of the alcohol-hating mice and subjected them to stress by putting them in very small constrictive tubes for intermittent periods. Within a few weeks this group of sober mice also came to prefer higher and higher concentrations of alcohol to pure water. In essence sober mice had been turned into alcoholic mice, first through applying stress (environment) and then allowing them access to alcohol (exposure to psychoactive drugs) (Fig. 2-23c).

Furthermore researcher Dr. Jorge Madrones, a nutritionist, took another group of alcohol-hating mice and restricted their diet of vitamin B and some essential proteins. This **limited nutrition also resulted in increased alcohol use** after several months (Madrones, 1951) (Fig. 2-23d).

Finally **once the mice whose genetics made them prefer alcohol were given access to alcohol, they drank themselves to death.** Even when they were subjected to electrical shocks aimed at preventing them from drinking the alcohol (aversive therapy), they continued to drink even when the shocks came close to being fatal (Fig. 2-23e). It is important to remember that none of the mice would become alcoholic if they were never given alcohol, even those mice with the highest susceptibility to compulsive drinking.

What was most interesting was that **when the forced drinking, stress induction, and nutritional restrictions were stopped, the genetically sober alcohol-hating mice did not return to their normal nondrinking habits.** They had been transformed into alcohol-loving mice and if given the chance to drink, they would be alcoholic mice.

When the brains of the four groups of mice were examined (the hereditary alcoholic mice, the stress-induced alcoholic mice, the alcohol-induced alcoholic mice, and the nutritionally restricted alcoholic mice), **all had similar brain cell changes and neurotransmitter imbalances that made them prefer alcohol** even though they started with different neurochemical balances. This research suggests that whether the neurochemical disruption can be caused by heredity, environment, psychoactive drugs, nutritional deficiency, or a combination of several of the factors, they can all lead to serious addiction (Li & Lumeng, 1984; Li et al., 1986).

COMPULSION CURVES

Human beings, of course, are different from mice. We are more complex, our brains are more intricate, and our social patterns are much more diverse. We have the power of reason, we have more control of our environment, and we have self-awareness. Yet research, especially over the last 10 years, shows that the **basic drug-craving mechanisms, which reside mostly in**

© 2003 CNS Productions, Inc.

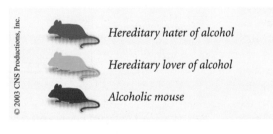

Hereditary hater of alcohol

Hereditary lover of alcohol

Alcoholic mouse

Figure 2-23a • Two strains of mice have been bred to help test theories of addiction, an alcohol-hating mouse and an alcohol-loving mouse.

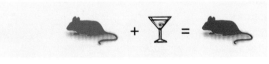

Figure 2-23b • Alcohol-hating mouse is force-fed large quantities of alcohol.

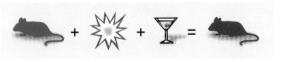

Figure 2-23c • Alcohol-hating mouse is subjected to stress and alcohol is made available.

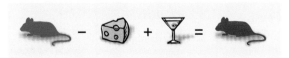

Figure 2-23d • Alcohol-hating mouse is nutritionally deprived and alcohol is made available.

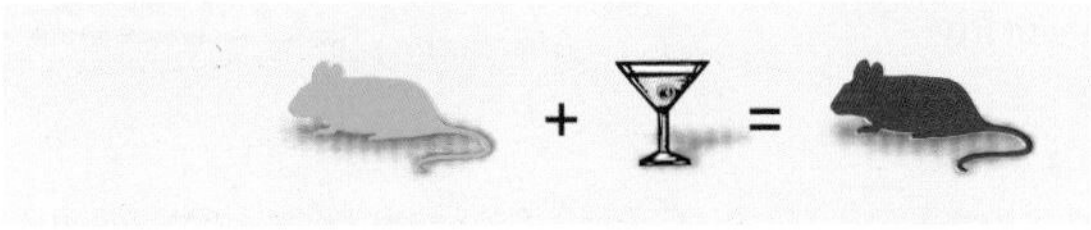

Figure 2-23e • Alcohol is made available to alcohol-loving mouse.

the old brain, are similar to those of most other mammals. The difference is that in humans it usually takes a combination of heredity, environment, and psychoactive drug use to increase compulsive use.

To help understand the interrelationship of heredity, environment, and the use of psychoactive drugs in human beings, we have developed a graphic representation of the ways that a user might advance from experimentation to addiction.

Since every person is unique, **every person starts with a different genetic susceptibility**. Those with low genetic susceptibility or predisposition have more room for drug experimentation or environmental stressors than those with high genetic predisposition. The susceptibility is most often reflected by the brain's structure and neurochemical composition. The important point is that more and more studies confirm that there is at least some heredity influence to any addiction, even compulsive overeating, smoking, and gambling (Brownell & Wadden, 1992; Carmelli, Swan, Robinette, & Fabstiz, 1992; Eisen et al., 1998). The contribution of heredity to drug addiction in our society is only an educated guess but researchers have estimated figures of anywhere from 10% to 60% (Fig. 2-24).

Once a person is born with their genetic makeup, environmental influences, particularly stressors, have the greatest effect on susceptibility. These influences include lack of bonding with a caregiver, physical/emotional/sexual abuse (especially during adolescence), poor nutrition, or societal attitudes that permit drug use (Peele & Brodsky, 1991; Zinberg, 1984). Again, **a person may have experienced low, medium, or high environmental contributions towards drug addiction** (Fig. 2-25).

The **final factor that will push a person to addiction is the use of psychoactive drugs**. The practice of compulsive behaviors, such as gambling, can also push one along the curve (Fig. 2-26). Therefore a person who starts with a low inherited susceptibility and low environmental stress might need

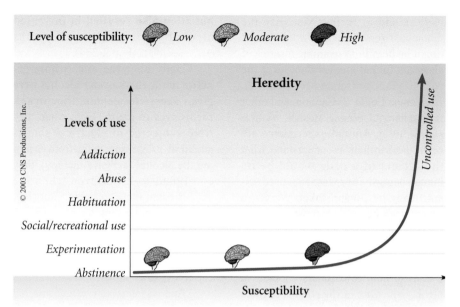

Figure 2-24 • *Initial susceptibility is inherited.*

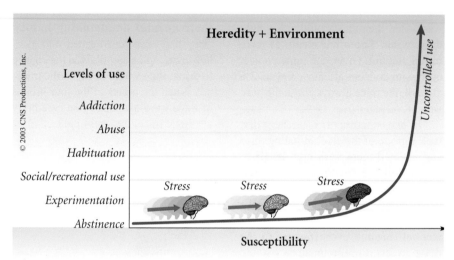

Figure 2-25 • *Susceptibility increases due to environmental stressors.*

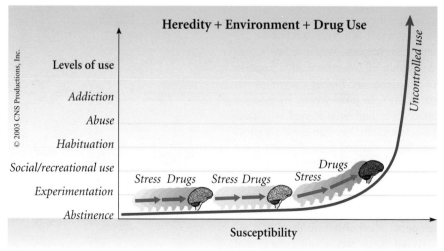

Figure 2-26 • *Susceptibility increases due to drug use. It can progress to abuse and addiction.*

intense use of drugs or behaviors to push him/her into addiction. The greater the environmental stress, the fewer drugs or behaviors needed. Drug use is not just measured by frequency or amount of drug used; drugs have different potencies (heroin vs. alcohol) and different routes of administration (smoking cocaine vs. snorting cocaine).

The drugs that push the hardest and the quickest towards addiction are, in order from fastest to slowest:

> smoking tobacco,
> smoking crack cocaine,
> smoking or injecting heroin,
> injecting methamphetamines,
> snorting cocaine,
> ingesting opioid painkillers,
> ingesting amphetamines,
> ingesting sedative-hypnotics,
> drinking alcohol,
> smoking marijuana,
> ingesting PCP,
> ingesting caffeine,
> ingesting MDMA (ecstasy),
> ingesting LSD,
> ingesting peyote.

If a person starts with a low or even moderate level of inherited susceptibility, it takes a larger amount of environmental influences to push him/her close to the level of critical susceptibility and addiction than someone with a high inherited susceptibility (Fig. 2-27). Depending on the environmental contribution, it then takes a lot more drug use or acting out to push them into uncontrolled use of drugs (or acting out of compulsive behaviors) than someone with high inherited susceptibility.

It might take those with low susceptibility 10 years of drinking to become alcoholics or it might never occur. It might take them 2 years of occasional injection to become a heroin addict or 6 months of smoking to get to a pack of cigarettes a day. People in the middle of the scale, with moderate inherited susceptibility, might need just 2 or 3 years of use to slip into alcohol addiction or 6 months of heroin use to graduate to a $200-a-day habit. People with a high susceptibility might slip into compulsive heavy drinking after

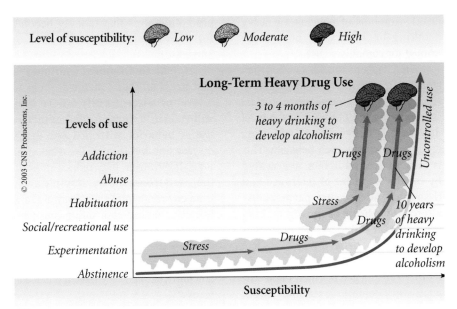

Figure 2-27 • *Addiction develops at different rates.*

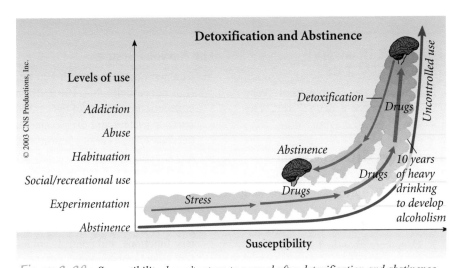

Figure 2-28 • *Susceptibility doesn't return to normal after detoxification and abstinence.*

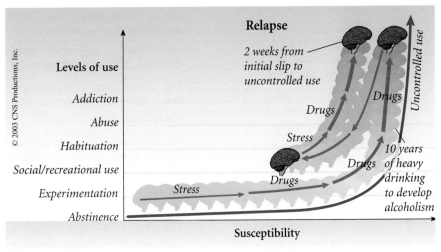

Figure 2-29 • *Users return to addictive use more quickly after relapse.*

just 3–4 months of bingeing or heavy drinking because their bodies are primed for compulsive use.

What happens to addicts when they stop using cocaine or stop gambling (Fig. 2-28)? They drop below critical susceptibility but not back to the level they were at before they started using drugs or practicing their behavior. This is because their **addiction, aggravated by the development of tolerance and tissue dependence, has permanently altered their brain chemistry making them forever liable to trigger uncontrolled use or behavior** quicker than before. Note that their level of use may return to abstinence but their brain susceptibility remains extremely high,

prompting slips that quickly become full-blown relapses (continuous or binge use).

If their environment continues to pile stress on them, they will move to a level of susceptibility where they will return to uncontrolled addictive use or behavior with just one drink or just one bet (Fig. 2-29) (Clark et al., 1997). If, however, they reduce stress in their environment by staying away from environmental cues, learning how to relax, having counseling and support, attending self-help groups, continuing to learn, and overcoming stressful thoughts, memories, and mental conflicts, then they have a chance at recovery.

CONCLUSIONS

The interrelations of heredity, environment, psychoactive drugs, and compulsive behaviors requires that **any study of addiction should focus on the totality of people's lives**: their personality, thinking patterns, relationships, how they live, what they eat, and their family history. In subsequent chapters this book will not only study stimulants, depressants, psychedelics, inhalants, and other drugs but will also look at compulsive behaviors, including compulsive overeating and gambling, whose causes are similar to those that lead to drug use, abuse, or addiction.

CHAPTER SUMMARY

HOW PSYCHOACTIVE DRUGS AFFECT US

1. Research has shifted from "Why do we crave a drug?" to "Why can't we stop craving a drug?"

How Drugs Get to the Brain

2. Method of intake, speed of transit, and affinity for nerve cells and neurotransmitters determine drug effects.

3. Drugs are absorbed into the body in five ways: inhaling (including smoking), injecting (intravenous, intramuscular, subcutaneous), mucous membrane absorption (snorting, under the tongue, next to the cheek, rectally, vaginally), eating or drinking, and contact absorption (e.g., transdermal skin patches).

4. Drugs enter the body and are distributed through the bloodstream where they cause a direct effect, are ignored, are stored, or biotransformed. Eventually they reach the central nervous system (CNS = brain and spinal cord) where they will have the greatest effect.

5. Psychoactive drugs must cross the blood-brain barrier to reach the fatty nerve cells of the brain.

The Nervous System

6. The nervous system, with 100 billion nerve cells and 100 trillion connections, consists of the central nervous system and the peripheral nervous system (PNS = autonomic and somatic systems).

7. The peripheral nervous system connects the senses and organs to the outside world and to the central nervous system, regulates involuntary functions, and controls voluntary muscle movements.

8. The central nervous system receives, analyzes, and responds to messages from the peripheral nervous system. Psychoactive drugs can alter incoming information, disrupt messages, and disrupt thinking.

9. The evolutionary perspective divides the brain into the old brain and the new brain.

10. The old brain controls physiological functions, emotions/feelings, and survival memories. Drug craving and addiction memories reside here.

11. The new brain (neocortex) controls speech, reasoning, creativity, and other memories. Old-brain

craving usually overrides new-brain rational thoughts.

12. A survival mechanism called the "reward/reinforcement center" (mesolimbic dopaminergic reward pathway) gives a surge of pleasure and a drive to repeat an action that is favorable to the organism.

13. The reward/reinforcement center is also activated by psychoactive drugs. This reward system says, "Do it again, do it again" when activated by drugs. It also imprints the memory of euphoria or pain relief. The key part of the system is called the "nucleus accumbens."

14. Satiation switches normally turn off the "do it again" message and stop the craving. Psychoactive drugs and compulsive behaviors are so strong they disrupt the reward/satiation mechanism and sometimes lead to craving, abuse, and addiction.

15. There are a number of theories as to why the on/off switches (of the reward/reinforcement center and satiation network) are disrupted and disabled.

16. Psychoactive drugs affect physiological functions as well as emotions and feelings.

17. The conflict between doing what our old brain tells us and the common sense and morality of our new brain is found in the writings and beliefs of religions and social systems throughout history.

18. Messages are transmitted by nerve cells. A nerve cell (neuron) consists of dendrites, cell body, axon, and terminals. Junctions between nerve cell junctions are called "synapses."

19. Messages travel within a nerve cell as electrical signals. However, at the synapse between most nerve cells there is a synaptic gap or cleft. Messages cross this gap as neurochemicals called "neurotransmitters," which slot into specific receptor sites where the messages are then converted back to electrical signals.

20. Neurotransmitters intensify signals (excitatory), inhibit signals (inhibitory), or a combination of the two.

21. Because neurotransmitters (e.g., dopamine, GABA, serotonin, norepinephrine, endorphins, enkephalins) transmit messages between nerve cells, psychoactive drugs that affect specific neurotransmitters exert an effect on the central and peripheral nervous systems.

22. Psychoactive drugs affect natural functions by increasing (agonist), mimicking, blocking (antagonist), or otherwise disrupting the release of these neurotransmitters, thereby affecting their normal functions.

Physiological Responses to Drugs

23. When a person takes certain drugs over a long period of time, the body becomes used to their effects, so more is needed to achieve the same high. Tolerance develops with all psychoactive drugs. They alter the hedonic set point.

24. There are different kinds of tolerance, e.g., dispositional tolerance and pharmacodynamic tolerance.

25. The tolerance to physical effects can develop at a different rate than the tolerance to psychological effects.

26. The brain and body try to biologically adapt to the increased quantities of drugs by changing their chemical balance and the cellular composition of organs, such as the liver. This results in physical or tissue dependence. The person can come to depend on the drug just to maintain balance.

27. The pleasurable effects of drugs cause an altered state of consciousness and virtually hypnotize the user into continued use (psychological dependence).

28. When a user stops taking a drug after tissue dependence has developed (mostly with opiates, alcohol, and sedative-hypnotics), the body experiences many of the unpleasant sensations and physical changes it was kept from feeling while taking the drug. This backlash and subsequent attempt to try to rebalance itself is known as "withdrawal."

29. There are three types of withdrawal: nonpurposive withdrawal (objective signs of withdrawal), purposive withdrawal (addict manipulation and faked symptoms to get drugs), or protracted withdrawal (remembrance or recurrence of past drug experiences that can cause a person to keep using). Protracted withdrawal is one of the main reasons for relapse.

Basic Pharmacology

30. Metabolism, the body's mechanism for processing, using, and inactivating foreign substances, primarily involves the liver. Excretion, the body's processes to eliminate waste, involves the kidneys, which filter drugs from the blood and excrete them in the urine. The lungs and skin are also involved in excretion.

31. A variety of factors, such as age, race, health, and gender, help determine how fast a drug is metabolized.

FROM EXPERIMENTATION TO ADDICTION

Desired Effects vs. Side Effects

32. People take drugs for many reasons including getting high, self-medicating, building confidence, increasing energy, satisfying curiosity, obliging friends (peer pressure), and avoiding problems.

33. Side effects can be mild, moderate, dangerous, or even fatal and can involve legal, relationship, financial, and work problems.

34. Polydrug abuse is very common. Drug abusers take other drugs to enhance the effect of their primary drug, to counteract unwanted side effects, to act as a substitute for an unavailable drug, and for other reasons.

Levels of Use

35. The level of use is judged first by the amount, frequency, and duration of use then by the effect use has on the individual's life.

36. The six levels of use are abstinence, experimentation, social/recreational use, habituation, abuse, and addiction.

37. The hallmark of drug abuse is continued use despite adverse consequences.

38. The hallmarks of addiction are a loss of control over use and a compulsion to use.

Theories of Addiction

39. The addictive disease model (medical model) says addiction is a chronic, progressive, relapsing, incurable, and potentially fatal condition that is mostly a consequence of genetic irregularities.

40. The behavioral/environmental model says that certain environmental factors can change brain chemistry, e.g., stress, nutrition, abuse, anger, and peer pressure.

41. The academic model says that it's the adaptation to toxic effects of psychoactive drugs that causes the development of tolerance, tissue

dependence, withdrawal, psychological dependence, and ultimately addiction.

42. The diathesis-stress theory states that the combination of heredity and environment creates a predisposition or susceptibility to addiction that can be triggered and aggravated by using psychoactive drugs and/or by acting out certain behaviors.

Heredity, Environment, Psychoactive Drugs, & Compulsive Behaviors

43. Heredity gives people their starting point in life. They begin with a certain inherited susceptibility to use or not use drugs. This susceptibility is reflected in certain neurochemical or neurostructural imbalances. Twin studies, biological family studies, and the discovery of alcoholism-associated genes reinforce these theories.

44. Environment, especially sexual/ physical/emotional abuse, then molds that basic architecture of the nervous system further increasing or decreasing susceptibility to compulsive drug use ("Psychology is biology"). Dietary imbalances also affect the chemistry of the brain.

45. Excessive, frequent, or prolonged use of psychoactive drugs modifies brain chemistry and triggers preexisting hereditary/ environmental susceptibility to abuse and addiction through tolerance and other physiological mechanisms.

46. Compulsive behaviors, such as compulsive gambling, overeating, compulsive sexual activity, and Internet obsession, are similar to drug addictions in that they disrupt brain chemistry and can become addictive.

Alcoholic Mice & Sober Mice

47. Animal experiments with alcohol-loving/alcohol-hating mice demonstrate that compulsive use can be reached through heredity, stress, nutritional restriction, or ingestion of large amounts of alcohol or other drugs that cause similar brain cell changes.

Compulsion Curves

48. In humans it is the combination of heredity, environment, and drug use that can push a person out of experimentation and social/recreational use towards habituation, abuse, and addiction.

Conclusions

49. To understand addiction one has to look at the totality of people's lives not just their drug-seeking behavior.

REFERENCES

Ahmed, S. H., & Koob, G. F. (1998). Transition from moderate to excessive drug intake: Change in hedonic set point. *Science, 282,* 5387.

Amen, D. G. (2001). *Healing ADD.* New York: G. P. Putnam & Sons.

American Psychiatric Association. (2000). *Diagnostic and Statistical Manual of Mental Disorders* (4th ed., text revision [DSM-IV-TR]). Washington, DC: Author

Anthenelli, R. M., & Schuckit, M. A. (1998). Genetic influences in addiction. In A. W. Graham & T. K. Schultz (Eds.), *Principles of Addiction Medicine* (2nd ed., pp. 17–36). Chevy Chase, MD: American Society of Addiction Medicine, Inc.

Bartzokis, G., Beckson, M., Lu, P. H., Nuechterlein, K. H., Edwards, N., & Mintz, J. (2001). Age-related changes in frontal and temporal lobe volumes in men. *Archives of General Psychiatry, 58*(5), 461–465.

Bassareo, V., & Di Chiara, G. (1999). Differential responsiveness of dopamine transmission to food-stimuli in nucleus accumbens shell/core components. *Neuroscience, 89*(3), 637–641.

Begleiter, H. (1980). *Biological Effects of Alcohol.* New York: Plenum Press.

Bierman, K. (1995, October 3). Early violence leaves its mark on the brain. *The New York Times.*

Bierut, L. J., Dinwiddie, S. H., Begleiter, H., Crowe, R. R., Hesselbrock, V., Nurnberger, J. I. Jr., Porjesz, B., Schuckit, M. A., & Reich, T. (1998). Familial transmission of substance dependence: Alcohol, marijuana, cocaine, and habitual smoking: A report from the Collaborative Study on the Genetics of Alcoholism. *Archives of General Psychiatry, 55*(11).

Blum, K., Braverman, E. R., Cull, J. G., Holder, J. M., Luck, R., Lubar, J., Miller, D., & Comings, D. E. (2000). Reward deficiency syndrome (RDS): A biogenetic model for the diagnosis and treatment of impulsive, addictive, and compulsive behaviors. *Journal of Psychoactive Drugs, 32*(1).

Blum, K., Cull, J. G., Braverman, E. R., & Comings, D. E. (1996). Reward deficiency syndrome. *American Scientist, 84,* 132–145.

Boening, J. A. (2001). Neurobiology of an addiction memory. *Journal of Neural Transmission, 108*(6), 755–765.

Brehm, N. M., & Khantzian, E. J. (1997). Psychodynamics. In J. H. Lowinson, P. Ruiz, R. B. Millman, & J. G. Langrod (Eds.), *Substance Abuse: A Comprehensive Textbook* (3rd ed., pp. 91–100). Baltimore: Williams & Wilkins.

Brownell, K. D., & Wadden, T. A. (1992). Etiology and treatment of obesity: Understanding a serious, prevalent, and refractory disorder. *Journal of Consulting and Clinical Psychology, 60,* 505–517.

Cadet, J. L., Ordonez, S. V., & Ordonez, J. V. (1997). Methamphetamine induces apoptosis in immortalized neural cells. Protection by the proto-oncogene, bel-2. *Synapse, 25,* 176–184.

Cannon, D. S., & Carrell, L. E. (1987). Rat strain differences in ethanol self-administration. *Pharmacology of Biochemical Behavior, 28,* 57–63.

Carmelli, D., Swan, G. E., Robinette, D., & Fabstiz, R. (1992). Genetic influences on smoking: A study of male twins. *The New England Journal of Medicine, 327,* 899–933.

Childress, A. R. (1999). Limbic activation during cue-induced cocaine craving.

American Journal of Psychiatry, 156(1), 11–18.

Childress, A. R., McElgin, W., Mozley, D., Reivich, M., & O'Brien, G. (1996). Brain correlates of cue-induced cocaine and opiate craving. *Society for Neuroscience Abstracts, 22,* 365–369.

Ciccocioppo, R., Sanna, P. P., & Weiss, F. (2001). Cocaine-predictive stimulus induces drug-seeking behavior and neural activation in limbic brain regions after multiple months of abstinence: Reversal by D(1) antagonists. *Proceedings of the National Academy of Science, 98*(4).

Clark, D. B., Moss, H. B., Kirisci, L, Mezzich, A. C., Miles, R., & Ott, P. (1997). Psychopathology in preadolescent sons of fathers with substance use disorders. *Journal of the American Academy of Child and Adolescent Psychiatry, 36*(4), 495–502.

Cloninger, C. R. (1987). Neurogenetic adaptive mechanisms in alcoholism. *Science, 236,* 410–416.

Cloninger, C. R., Bohman, M., & Sigvardson, S. (1986). Inheritance of risk to develop alcoholism. In M. C. Braude, & H. M. Chao (Eds.), *Genetic and Biological Markers in Drug Abuse and Alcoholism.* NIDA Research Monograph 66. Rockville, MD: Department of Health and Human Services.

Comings, D. E., Gonzales, N., Saucier, G., Johnson, J. P., & MacMurray, J. P. (2000). The DRD4 gene and the spiritual transcendence scale of the character temperament index. *Psychiatric Genetics, 10*(4).

Denton, D., Shade, R., Zamarippa, F., Egan, G., Blair-West, J., McKinley, M., Lancaster, J., & Fox, P. (1999). Neuroimaging of genesis and satiation of thirst and an interceptor-driven theory of origins of primary consciousness. *Proceedings of the National Academy of Sciences, 96*(9), 5304–5309.

Diagram Group. (1991). *The Brain: A User's Manual.* Rockville Centre, NY: Berkley Press.

DuPont, R. L. (1997). *The Selfish Brain: Learning From Addiction.* Washington, DC: American Psychiatric Press, Inc.

Eisen, S. A., Lin, N., Lyons, M. J., Scherrer, J. F., Kristin, G., True, W. R., Goldberg, J., & Tsuang, M. T. (1998). Familial influences on gambling behavior. *Addiction Magazine, 93,* 1375–1384.

Enoch, M., White, K. V., Harris, D. R., Rohrbaugh, J. W., & Goldman, D. (2001). Alcohol use disorders and anxiety disorders: Relation to the P300 event-related potential. *Alcoholism:*

Clinical and Experimental Research, 25(9), 1293–1301.

Feingold, A., Ball, S. A., Kranzler, H. R., & Rounsaville, B. J. (1996). Generalizability of the type A/type B distinction across different psychoactive substances. *American Journal of Drug and Alcohol Abuse, 22*(n3), 449–463.

Freud, S. (1884/1995). *The Complete Letters of Sigmund Freud to Wilhelm Fleiss.* Cambridge, MA: Harvard University Press.

Goldstein, A. (2001). *Addiction: From Biology to Drug Policy.* New York: Oxford University Press.

Goodwin, D. W. (1976). *Is Alcoholism Hereditary?* New York: Oxford University Press.

Gottesman, I. I., McGuffin, P., & Farmer, A. E. (1987). Clinical clues to the "real" genetics of schizophrenia. *Schizophrenia Bulletin, 13,* 23–47.

Griffiths, R. R., Bigelow, C. E., & Liebson, I. (1978). Experimental drug self-administration: Generality across species and type of drug. *National Institute on Drug Abuse Research. Monograph Series, 20,* 24–43.

Hoffman, B. B., & Taylor, P. (2001). Neurotransmission. In J. G. Hardman, L. E. Limbird, & A. G. Gilman (Eds.), *Goodman & Gilman's: The Pharmacological Basis of Therapeutics* (10th ed., pp. 115–153). New York: McGraw-Hill.

Hyman, S. E. (1996). Shaking out the cause of addiction. *Science, 273*(5275), 611.

Hyman, S. E. (1998, March 30). An interview with Steven Hyman, M.D. [Online]. Available: *http://www.pbs.org/wnet/closetohome/science/html/hyman.html*

Ikemoto, S., Glazier, B. S., Murphy, J. M., & McBride, W. J. (1997). Role of dopamine D_1 and D_2 receptors in the nucleus accumbens in mediating reward. *The Journal of Neuroscience, 17*(21), 8580–8587.

Institute of Medicine. (1999). *Marijuana and Medicine: Assessing the Science Base.* Washington, DC: National Academy Press.

Jaffe, J. H., Knapp, C. M., & Ciraulo, D. A. (1997). Opiates: Clinical aspects. In J. H. Lowinson, P. Ruiz, R. B. Millman, & J. G. Langrod (Eds.), *Substance Abuse: A Comprehensive Textbook* (3rd. ed., pp. 51–84). Baltimore: Williams & Wilkins.

Kandel, E. R., Schwartz, J. H., & Jessell, T. M. (Eds.). (1991). *Principles of Neural Science* (3rd ed.). New York: Elsevier.

Koob, G. F. (1998, March 30). An interview with George Koob, M.D. [Online].

Available: *http://www.pbs.org/wnet/closetohome/science/htm/koob.html*

Koob, G. F., & Le Moal, M. (1997). Drug abuse: Hedonic homeostatic disregulation. *Science, 278,* 52–63.

Koob, G. F., & Le Moal, M. (2001). Drug addiction, disregulation of reward, and allostasis. *Neuropsychopharmacology, 24*(2), 97–129.

Kuhar, M. J., Joyce, A., & Dominguez, G. (2000). Genes in drug abuse. *Drug and Alcohol Dependence, 62,* 157–162.

Lamarque, S., Taghzouti, K., & Simon, H. (2001). Chronic treatment with Delta(9)-tetrahydrocannabinol enhances the locomotor response to amphetamine and heroin. Implications for vulnerability to drug addiction. *Neuropharmacology, 41*(1).

LeDoux, J. E. (1996). *The Emotional Brain.* New York: Simon and Schuster.

Leshner, A. I. (1998a, March 30). An interview with Alan Leshner, Ph.D. [Online]. Available: *http://www.pbs.org/wnet/closetohome/science/html/leshner.html*

Leshner, A. I. (1998b). What we know: Drug addiction is a brain disease. In A. W. Graham & T. K. Schultz (Eds.), *Principles of Addiction Medicine* (2nd ed.) Chevy Chase, MD: American Society of Addiction Medicine, Inc.

Li, T. K., & Lumeng, L. (1984). Alcohol preference and voluntary alcohol intakes of inbred rat strains and the National Institutes of Health heterogeneous stock of rats. *Alcoholism, 8,* 485–486.

Li, T. K., Lumeng, L., McBride, W. J., Waller, M. B., & Murphy, J. M. (1986). Studies on an animal model of alcoholism. In M. C. Braude & H. M. Chao (Eds.), *Genetic and Biological Markers in Drug Abuse and Alcoholism.* NIDA Research Monograph 66. Rockville, MD: Department of Health and Human Services.

Ljungman, G., et al. (2000). Nasal spray using midazolam to calm children undergoing chemotherapy. *Pediatrics,* January, 2000.

Madrones, R. J. (1951). On the relationship between deficiency of B vitamins and alcohol intake in rats. *Quarterly Journal of Studies on Alcoholism, 12,* 563–575.

Meehl, P. E. (1962). Schizotoma, schizolyphy, schizophrenia. *American Psychologist, 17,* 827–838.

Merton, T. (1955). *No Man Is an Island.* New York: Harcourt, Brace & Company.

Miczek, K. A., Hubbard, N., & Cantuti-Castelvetri, I. (1995). Increased cocaine self-administration after social stress. *Neuroscience Abstracts, 21.*

National Institute on Drug Abuse. (2001). Pathological obesity and drug addiction share common brain characteristics. *NIDA Notes*, 16(4).

National Research Council. (1999). *Pathological Gambling: A Critical Review.* Washington, DC: National Research Council.

Nesse, R. M. (1994). An evolutionary perspective on substance abuse. *Etiology and Sociobiology, 15,* (339–348). New York: Elsevier Science, Inc.

Nesse, R. M., & Berridge, K. C. (1997). Psychoactive drug use in evolutionary perspective. *Science, 278,* 63–65.

Nestler, E. J. (1995). Molecular basis of addictive states. *Neuroscientist, 1,* 212–220.

Nestler, E. J. (2001). Total recall—the memory of addiction. *Science Magazine, 292*(5525).

Nestler, E. J., Barrot, M., & Self, D. W. (2001). Delta FosB: A sustained molecular switch for addiction. *Proceedings of the National Academy of Science,* 25:98(20), 11042–6.

Nevid, J. S., Rathus, S. A., & Greene, B. (1997). *Abnormal Psychology in a Changing World.* Upper Saddle River, NJ: Prentice Hall.

Noble, E. P., Blum, K., Ritchie, T., Montgomery, A., & Sheridan, P. J. (1991). Allelic association of the D2 dopamine receptor gene with receptor-binding characteristics in alcoholism. *Archives of General Psychiatry, 48*(7), 648–654.

Numberger, J. I. Jr., Foroud, T., Flury, L., Su, J., Meyer, E. T., Hu, K., Crowe, R., Edenberg, H., Goate, A., Bierut, L., Reich, T., Schuckit, M., & Reich, W. (2001). Evidence for a locus on chromosome 1 that influences vulnerability to alcoholism and affective disorder. *American Journal of Psychiatry, 158*(5).

O'Brien, C. P. (2001). Drug addiction and drug abuse. In J. G. Hardman, L. E. Limbird, & A. G. Gilman (Eds.), *Goodman & Gilman's: The Pharmacological Basis of Therapeutics* (10th ed., pp. 621–641). New York: McGraw-Hill.

Office of National Drug Control Policy. (2001). *National Drug Control Strategy: 2000 Annual Report.* Bethesda, MD: National Drug Clearinghouse.

Olds, J. (1956). Pleasure centers in the brain. *Scientific American, 195*(4), 105–116.

Olds, J., & Milner, P. (1954). Positive reinforcement produced by electrical stimulation of septal area and other regions of rat brain. *Journal of Comprehensive Physiology and Psychology, 47,* 419–427.

O'Malley, S., & Volpicelli, J. (1995). Slip vs. relapse (in-house study). *Haight Ashbury Files.*

Peele, S., & Brodsky, A. (1991). *The Truth About Addiction and Recovery.* New York: Simon & Schuster.

Potenza, M. N. (2001). The neurobiology of pathological gambling. *Seminar in Clinical Neuropsychiatry, 6*(3), 217–226.

Pothos, E. N. (2001). The effects of extreme nutritional conditions on the neurochemistry of reward and addiction. *Acta Astronaut,* 49.

Purves, D., Augustine, G. J., Fitzpatrick, D., Katz, L. C., LaMantia, A., & McNamara, J. O. (1997). *Neuroscience.* Sunderland, MA: Sinauer Associates, Inc.

Raimo, E. B., Smith, T. L., Danko, G. P., Bucholz, K. K., & Schuckit, M. A. (2000). Clinical characteristics and family histories of alcoholics with stimulant dependence. *Journal of Studies of Alcoholism, 61*(5).

Ross, E. M., & Kenakin, T. P. (2001). Pharmacodynamics. In J. G. Hardman, L. E. Limbird, & A. G. Gilman (Eds.), *Goodman & Gilman's: The Pharmacological Basis of Therapeutics* (10th ed., pp.31–43). New York: McGraw-Hill.

Schroeder, B. E., Holahan, M. R., Landry, C. F., & Kelley, A. E. (2000). Morphine-associated environmental cues elicit conditioned gene expression. *Synapse, 37.*

Schuckit, M. A. (1986). Alcoholism and affective disorders: Genetic and clinical implications. *American Journal of Psychiatry, 143,* 140–147.

Schuckit, M. A. (2000a). Genetics of the risk for alcoholism. *American Journal of Addiction, 9*(2).

Schuckit, M. A. (2000b). *Drug and Alcohol Abuse.* New York: Kluwer Academic/Plenum Publishers.

Schuckit, M. A., & Smith, T. L. (2001). The clinical course of alcohol dependence associated with a low level of response to alcohol. *Addiction, 96,* 903–910.

Shaffer, H. (1998, February 28). Lecture to casino executives, Las Vegas gaming convention. *Medford Mail Tribune.* Medford, OR.

Smith, D. E., & Seymour, R.B. (2001). *Clinician's Guide to Substance Abuse.* New York: McGraw-Hill.

Snyder, S. H. (1996). *Drugs and the Brain.* New York: Scientific American Library.

Spragg, S. D. S. (1940). Morphine addiction in chimpanzees. *Comparative Psychology Monograph, 15* (7), 1–132.

Stahl, S. M. (2000). *Essential Psychopharmacology.* Cambridge, England: Cambridge University Press.

Suzuki, D. (Producer). (1994). *The Brain: Our Universe Within.* Maryland: Discovery Channel.

Swain, R. C., Oetting, E. R., Edwards, R. W., & Beauvais, F. (1989). Links from emotional distress to adolescent drug use: A pathological model. *Journal of Consulting and Clinical Psychology, 57,* 227–231.

Trauth, J. A. Seidler, F. J., Ali, S. F., & Slotkin, T. A. (2001). Adolescent nicotine exposure produces immediate and long-term changes in CNS noradrenergic and dopaminergic function. *Brain Research, 892*(2), 269–280.

True, W. R., Xian, H., Scherrer, J. F., Madden, P. A. F., Bucholz, K. K., Heath, A. C., Eisen, S. A., Lyons, M. J., Goldberg, J., & Tsuang, M. (1999). Common genetic vulnerability for nicotine and alcohol dependence in men. *Archives of General Psychiatry, 56*(7).

Tsai, G., Gastfriend, D. R., & Coyle, J. T. (1995). The glutamatergic basis of human alcoholism. *American Journal of Psychiatry, 152,* 332–340.

Volkow, N. D. (2001) Disregulation of orbitofrontal cortex linked with methamphetamine abuse. *American Journal of Psychiatry, 158,* 2015–2021.

Wang, G. J., Volkow, N. D., et al. (2001). Brain dopamine and obesity. *Lancet, 357*(9253), 354–357.

Wickelgren, I. (1998). Teaching the brain to take drugs. *Science, 280,* 2045.

Wilkinson, G. R. (2001). Pharmacokinetics. In J. G. Hardman, L. E. Limbird, & A. G. Gilman (Eds.), *Goodman & Gilman's: The Pharmacological Basis of Therapeutics* (10th ed., pp. 3–29). New York: McGraw-Hill.

Zhang, J., Walsh, R. R., & Xu, M. (2000). Probing the role of the dopamine D1 receptor in psychostimulant addiction. *Annals of the New York Academy of Science, 914,* 13–21.

Zinberg, N. (1984). *Drugs, Set and Setting.* New Haven: Yale University Press.

Uppers

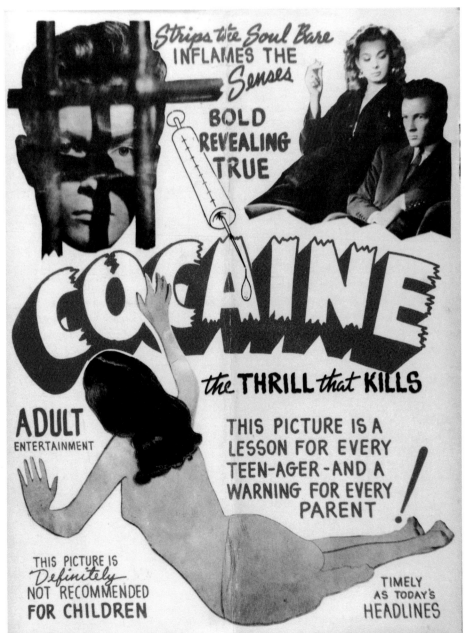

*D*rug exploitation films date back to the beginning of cinema with films such as Dentist Scene about laughing gas (1894), Hasher's Delirium (1906), The Mystery of the Leaping Fish (1916), Reefer Madness (1936), and Cocaine Fiends (1939).

- **General Classification:** Uppers include very strong stimulants (e.g., cocaine, amphetamines), moderate stimulants (e.g., diet pills, Ritalin®), milder plant stimulants (e.g., khat, betel nut, ephedra), and legal mild stimulants (e.g., caffeine, nicotine).

- **General Effects:** Stimulants force the release of the body's own energy chemicals and stimulate the brain's reward/reinforcement center. They also constrict blood vessels, increase heart rate, and raise blood pressure. Prolonged use of the stronger stimulants depletes energy resources, induces paranoia, and triggers intense craving.

- **Cocaine:** Usually injected, snorted, or smoked, cocaine, an extract of the coca leaf, causes the most rapid stimulation and subsequent severe comedown of all the stimulants.

- **Smokable Cocaine (crack, freebase):** The basic effects of smoking cocaine are almost the same as snorting or injecting cocaine. Smoking crack is the most rapid-acting method of use and creates the greatest compulsion.

- **Amphetamines:** Longer lasting and usually cheaper than cocaine, these synthetic stimulants, including methamphetamine (meth, "crank," and "ice"), saw an increase of use in the 1990s. Amphetamine analogues, (especially ecstasy, a psycho-stimulant) witnessed explosive increased use and abuse by the 2000s.

- **Amphetamine Congeners:** Methylphenidate (Ritalin®) is used to treat attention-deficit/hyperactivity disorder (ADHD) in children and adults. Diet pills are used to control weight gain. A popular combination, "fen-phen," was banned because of dangerous cardiovascular effects.

- **Lookalike & Over-the-Counter (OTC) Stimulants:** Counterfeit stimulants, often containing caffeine or other mild stimulants, are falsely advertised as amphetamines, cocaine, or even MDMA (ecstasy). Legal mild over-the-counter stimulants when used to excess can have toxic cardiovascular effects to the system.

- **Miscellaneous Plant Stimulants:** Extracts of plants, like khat, yohimbe, betel nuts, and ephedra, are used worldwide in addition to coffee, tea, or colas. Synthetic versions of plant extracts, e.g., methcathinone, pseudoephedrine, and Pervitine®, have many of the effects of methamphetamine.

- **Caffeine:** Coffee, tea, chocolate, and most soft drinks contain the alkaloid caffeine and can be mildly addicting. Many over-the-counter medications also contain caffeine.

- **Nicotine:** Nicotine is a toxic alkaloid found in tobacco. When tobacco is smoked or chewed, it first stimulates, then relaxes, then, at large doses, it depresses. Hundreds of other by-products and additives in tobacco, like tar and nitrosamines, can cause cancer and respiratory or cardiovascular problems.

- **Conclusions:** Though stimulants initially boost energy and drive, they have a number of side effects, toxic consequences, and addiction problems when they are overused.

GENERAL CLASSIFICATION

"I took it for weight loss 'cause I have a weight problem but I also liked the high. I liked how it made me feel. I liked the rush, the way that you could get everything done, boom, boom, boom. Just like that."

20-year-old female recovering from methamphetamine addiction

In the restless world of the twenty-first century dominated by intense business activity, workers holding two or three jobs, super moms, high stress levels, and millions of dreamers dashing after the brass ring, it seems appropriate that stimulants are so widely used. From powerful illegal stimulants, including cocaine and methamphetamine, to prescription diet aids and drugs to control hyperactivity, down to plant stimulants like ephedra, and finally to the most popular mild legal substances, particularly coffee, caffeinated soft drinks, and cigarettes, uppers are a regular part of life for most human beings. During the past year just in the United States, approximately

◇ 4.2 million Americans used cocaine, including crack;

◇ 2.5 million shot, snorted, ate, or smoked amphetamines (speed, meth, "ice") for nonmedical reasons;

◇ 76.6 million smoked cigarettes;

◇ 200 million drank coffee and tea, along with 100 billion caffeinated soft drinks.

Worldwide the use of stimulants is even more prevalent.

◇ Japan has had a methamphetamine problem since World War II.

◇ Colombia produces much of the world's cocaine but also has a large local addict population.

◇ Two hundred million people use betel nut and its extracts the way others use coffee.

◇ The average daily caffeine consumption worldwide is 70 milligrams (mg) (about 1 cup of coffee) though in some countries it's as high as 400–500 mg a day.

Some stimulants are found in plants: the coca shrub (cocaine), the tobacco plant (nicotine), the khat bush (cathinone), the ephedra bush (ephedrine), the betel nut (arecoline), and the coffee plant (caffeine). **Other stimulants are synthesized** in legal or "street" laboratories. Methamphetamines, diet pills, methylphenidate (Ritalin®), methcathinone, and looka-like stimulants are the most common.

There is also a whole class of designer drugs that are variations of the amphetamine molecule (amphetamine analogues). **Drugs such as MDMA (ecstasy), MDA, MMDA, and MDE are classified as "psycho-stimulants"** and will be covered extensively in Chapter 6. However, it is important to remember that in addition to their psychedelic effects, the drugs are still causing methamphetamine-like physical and mental effects.

GENERAL EFFECTS

Though there is a great difference in strength, **all stimulants increase the chemical and electrical activity in the central nervous system.** In low doses all stimulants boost energy, raise the heart rate and blood pressure, increase respiration, and reduce appetite and thirst. They also make the user more alert, active, confident, anxious, restless, and aggressive. Those effects allow some stimulants to be

◇ **used clinically to treat narcolepsy, obesity, and attention-deficit/ hyperactivity disorder (ADHD);**

◇ **used illegally to keep the user awake and energized, increase confidence, and induce euphoria.**

The major effects of stimulants occur because of the way they manipu-

TABLE 3–1   UPPERS (STIMULANTS)

Drug Name	Some Trade Names	Street or Slang Names
COCAINE (from coca leaf)		
Cocaine HCL (hydrochloride) (Schedule II)	None but it is manufactured and sold legally for medical purposes (topical anesthetic)	Coke, blow, toot, snow, flake, girl, lady, nose candy, big C, la dama blanca
Cocaine freebase (Schedule II but extra legal penalties)	None	Crack, base, rock, basay, boulya, pasta, paste, hubba, basuco, pestillos, primo
AMPHETAMINES (synthetic)		
d,l amphetamine (Schedule II)	Adderall®, Biphetamine®	Crosstops, whites, speed, black beauties, bennies, cartwheels, pep pills
Benzphetamine (Schedule III)	Didrex®	
Dextroamphetamine sulfate (Schedule II)	Dexedrine®	Dexies, Christmas trees, beans
Dextromethamphetamine HCL (Schedule II)	None	Ice, ya ba, yaa baa, yaa maa, glass, batu, shabu, yellow rock
Freebase methamphetamine (Schedule II)	None	Snot
Levo amphetamine (no schedule)	Vick's Inhaler®	
Methamphetamine HCL (Schedule II)	Desoxyn®	Crank, meth, crystal, peanut butter speed, pervitin (overseas)
Methyldioxymethamphetamine (MDMA) & other amphetamine analogues (MDA, MDE, etc.)		*see Chapter 6*
AMPHETAMINE CONGENERS		
Dexfenfluramine (Schedule IV)	Redux® (no longer sold in the United States)	The combination of dexfenfluramine and fenfluramine with phentermine HCL or phentermine resin was called "fen-phen"
Diethylpropion (Schedule IV)	Tenuate®	
Fenfluramine (Schedule IV)	Pondimin®	Fen-phen (in combination)
Methylphenidate (Schedule II)	Ritalin®, Concerta®, Metadate CD®, Methylin®	Pellets
Phendimetrazine (Schedule III)	Bontril®, Prelu-2®	Pink hearts
Pemoline (Schedule II)	Cylert®	Popcorn coke
Phentermine HCL (Schedule IV)	Adipex-P®, Banobese®, Obenix®, Zantryl®	Robin's eggs, black and whites, fen-phen (in combination)
Phentermine resin complex (Schedule IV)	Ionamin®	Part of fen-phen
OTHER DIET PILLS & ATYPICAL STIMULANTS		
Modafinil	Provigil®	
Sibutramine (Schedule IV)	Meridia®	
LOOKALIKE & OVER-THE-COUNTER STIMULANTS		
Can contain caffeine, ephedrine, phenylephrine, phenylpropanolamine (taken off the market), and/or pseudoephedrine	Lookalikes: Super Toot® OTCs: Dexatrim®, Acutrim®, Sudafed®	Legal speed, robin's eggs, black beauties
Herbal caffeine, herbal ephedra	Herbal Ecstasy®, Herbal Nexus®, Cloud Nine®, Nirvana®	Herbal X

continued

TABLE 3–1   (continued)

Drug Name	Some Trade Names	Street or Slang Names
MISCELLANEOUS PLANT STIMULANTS		
Arecoline (betel nut)	None	Areca, supai, pan parag, marg, maag, pinang
Cathinone, cathine (khat bush) (*Catha edulus*) (methcathinone is the synthetic version)	None	Cat, qat, chat, miraa, Arabian tea, catha, goob, ikwa, ischott, khat kaad, kafta, la salade, liss, bathtub speed, wild cat, mulka,
Ephedrine (ephedra bush)	Many commercial products	Ma huang, marwath
Yohimbine (yohimbe tree)	Yohimbi 8®, Manpower®	
CAFFEINE (xanthines)		
Chocolate (cocoa beans)	Hershey®, Nestles®	
Coffee	Colombian, French, espresso	Java, Joe, mud, roast, latte
Colas (from cola nut)	Coca Cola®, Pepsi®	Coke
Over-the-counter stimulants	No Doz®, Alert®, Vivarin®	
Tea	Lipton®, Stash®	Cha, chai
Guarana, maté, yoco	Various	
NICOTINE		
Chewing tobacco	Day's Work®, Beechnut®, Levi-Garrett®, Redman®	Chew, chaw
Cigarettes, cigars	Marlboro®, Kents®, Pall Mall®, American Spirit®	Cancer stick, smoke, butts, toke, coffin nails
Pipe tobacco	Sir Walter Raleigh®	
Snuff	Copenhagen®, Skoal®	Dip

late energy chemicals and trigger the reward/reinforcement center of the brain.

BORROWED ENERGY

The biochemical process that increases energy involves at least two adrenaline-like neurotransmitters:

◇ **epinephrine, which has greater effects on physical energy**;

◇ **norepinephrine, which has greater effects on confidence, motivation, and feelings of well-being.**

Serotonin and dopamine, which also affect energy, are released but to a lesser extent.

Most norepinephrine and epinephrine neurons arise in a small area in the brainstem called the "locus coeruleus." The 3,000 neurons that release these neurotransmitters extend to almost every part of the brain, transmitting

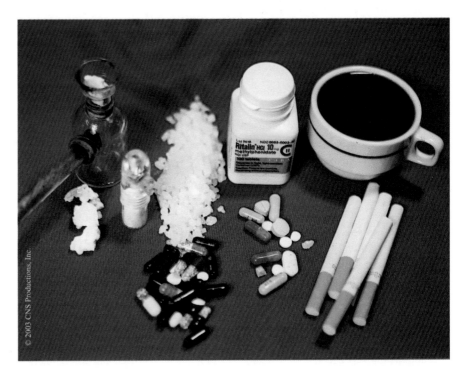

Examples of stimulants are crack cocaine and powdered cocaine, amphetamine pills and methamphetamine powder, amphetamine congeners (e.g., Ritalin®), caffeine, and nicotine.

messages across synaptic gaps reading one-third to one-half of all the cells in the brain (Snyder, 1996; King & Ellinwood, 1997). Remember that a single neuron can have thousands of dendrites and terminals. As expected more of these chemicals are released while we are awake than when we are asleep but the average 24-hour output is fairly constant. In time they are reabsorbed and rereleased when needed or they are metabolized and depleted, signaling the nerve cells to synthesize fresh neurotransmitters.

Sometimes, though, the body needs extra energy or a shot of confidence, e.g., when the person exercises, is scared and needs to flee, is making love, has to give a speech, or is in a fight. At these moments **the nervous system automatically and naturally releases extra amounts of epinephrine, norepinephrine, and other chemicals**. Remember the initial burst of energy the body experiences when you start to exercise? Eventually the extra energy chemicals are reabsorbed or metabolized, allowing the body to return to normal, to calm down.

"The closest thing I've had to a natural high was the rock climb and I was terrified. The adrenaline is just pumping through your system and you're just so high off of that, your heart is pumping and you sit down. We sat up there about 5 minutes after the climb and I never felt so good and alone with myself other than when I was using drugs."
18-year-old recovering cocaine abuser

Stimulants force the release of the energy chemicals and infuse the body with large amounts of extra energy before the body needs it. The user tries to use up the extra energy through activity, movement, talking, and hyperalertness. The effect is multiplied with strong stimulants (cocaine and amphetamines) because they keep the neurotransmitters circulating either by blocking their reabsorption and/or by blocking their metabolism.

"I did it for the adrenaline. I did it to stay awake. I did it 'cause I enjoy life a lot and wanted to get the most out of life. I stayed awake and did it, and did it, and did it."
19-year-old recovering stimulant addict

In summary the **normal progression of events** in regards to energy release is as follows:

◊ the body demands extra energy;

◊ nerve cells and glands release energy chemicals;

◊ the body transforms these chemicals to extra energy;

◊ the person finishes his/her tasks;

◊ most of the extra energy chemicals are reabsorbed.

When a person uses strong stimulants, the process is reversed.

◊ Stimulants are ingested, smoked, injected, or snorted.

◊ The drugs release extra energy chemicals and the user becomes overly active to use up the surplus.

◊ With continued use of stimulants, nerve cells become depleted of their energy chemicals.

◊ The body becomes exhausted and demands extra energy.

◊ The person takes more and more stimulants.

The Crash & Withdrawal

If strong stimulants are only taken occasionally, the body has time to recover. But if they are taken continuously over a long period of time or in large quantities, the **energy supplies become depleted** and the body is left without reserves. It is squeezed dry— exhausted. With stronger stimulants, this crash and its subsequent withdrawal symptoms and **severe depression can last for days or weeks or occasionally months**. Even a mild stimulant like coffee can lower energy supplies as the user builds a tolerance. Six or 8 cups a day will not keep the user awake and alert.

"There is only so much you can do and after a while you don't get high anymore, no matter how much more you do. You just need to crash and the depression is terrible: the fatigue, not even being able to walk, not being able to get out of bed, and just being desperate to sleep. The depression lasts up to 8 days but it is intensely acute for 3 or 4 days in my case."
Recovering 36-year-old female meth addict

It is important to remember that the energy and confidence received from stimulants are not a free gift; they are a loan from the rest of the body and must be repaid by giving the body time to recover.

REWARD/REINFORCEMENT CENTER

Besides the physical stimulation, cocaine, amphetamines, and other strong stimulants disrupt the reward/reinforcement center as explained in Chapter 2. Even the milder stimulants have some effect on this system. Normally **this center that exists in all mammals is a survival mechanism that gives a surge of pleasure when a physiological or psychological need is being satisfied**, e.g., hunger, thirst, sexual desire (Goldstein, 2001). The **stronger stimulants artificially overstimulate this center** and signal the brain that hunger is being satisfied although no food is being eaten; that thirst is being satisfied although no liquid is being drunk; and that sexual desire is being satisfied although there has been no sexual activity. This stimulation is perceived as an overall rush (feelings of well-being and pleasure). As the drug is used more and more, the intensity of this rush diminishes but the emotional memories linger on. **Dopamine is the neurotransmitter most often involved in triggering these feelings.**

National Institute on Drug Abuse (NIDA) researchers have imaged the limbic system of the brain during cocaine craving using a positron emission tomography (PET) scan. They found that cocaine craving activates this circuitry to an exceptionally high level (Childress, McElgin, Mozley, Reivich, & O'Brien, 1996; Childress et al., 1999; Garavan et al., 2000).

WEIGHT LOSS

Since the body is fooled into thinking its basic needs have been satisfied, the user can become dehydrated and malnourished. In fact many long-term users of stimulants develop vitamin and mineral deficiencies that can damage teeth and cause other health problems.

The fact that **stimulants fool the body into thinking it has satisfied hunger without eating and thereby cause weight loss** is one of the main reasons they are used. Even tobacco can decrease appetite because of this effect. The fear of gaining weight causes many cocaine, amphetamine, nicotine, and even caffeine users to maintain their habit.

"I was fat from about the age of 8. My doctor put me on amphetamines when I was 16. Unfortunately they made my heart race, so I gave them up. In my senior year I took up smoking and that kept the weight off 'cause when I gave them up 10 years later, I gained about 30 pounds. In college I started drinking coffee to study for exams. Unfortunately I figure all these stimulants have screwed up my appestat [appetite regulator] or whatever controls appetite 'cause I've kept gaining weight over the years."
57-year-old male recovering compulsive overeater

CARDIOVASCULAR SIDE EFFECTS

Many stimulants, including nicotine and caffeine, **constrict blood vessels** thus decreasing blood flow to tissues and organs including the skin. (Notice the pale pasty complexion of heavy smokers.) Since blood flow is decreased, tissue repair and healing are slowed. In addition **heart rate is in-**creased and, with the stronger stimulants, various heart arrhythmias, including tachycardia, can occur. At the same time **blood pressure increases**, so a ruptured vessel (a stroke if it's in the brain) is possible though unusual during early use. However, the chronic use of these drugs **weakens blood vessels**, also increasing the risk of stroke.

Polydrug use of a stimulant with a depressant can cause additional, unexpected, and possibly fatal cardiovascular effects. Alcohol and cocaine metabolize to cocaethylene, a potent metabolite that can have more serious effects.

EMOTIONAL/MENTAL SIDE EFFECTS

Initial release of extra neurotransmitters by the stronger stimulants tends to **increase confidence** and **induce euphoria**. But as use continues, the imbalance of dopamine, serotonin, epinephrine, norepinephrine, and other neurotransmitters often transforms those feelings into **talkativeness, restlessness, irritability, insomnia**, and eventually, **paranoia, aggressiveness,** and **violence**. Excess use of even milder stimulants, including caffeine, khat, and ephedra, can cause restlessness, talkativeness, insomnia, and irritability.

"It's almost like there's a veneer over the nerves and it takes off that veneer, that coating, and you are just like a live wire. You'll be on a crowded bus and you might go into a rage very spontaneously, without any real cause."
25-year-old meth abuser

High-dose or prolonged methamphetamine/cocaine use can cause **paranoia** and **psychosis** by increasing the level of dopamine in the central nervous system. Even high-dose methylphenidate use can induce paranoia and psychosis. The drug-induced psychosis is hard to distinguish from a real psychosis, such as schizophrenia. Unprovoked violence is also common with excess methamphetamine or cocaine use. During a 2-month period in Japan, 30 of the 60 murder cases that occurred were related to amphetamine/methamphetamine abuse (Schuckit, 2000)

"I used to drive around and hear my motorcycle talking to me and I would see faces come out of the trees and I'd see all kinds of crazy stuff. After 10 days of no sleep it's like living in a dream 'cause I couldn't distinguish reality from what the drug was doing to me. I was that far gone."
22-year-old meth addict living in a therapeutic community

TOLERANCE & ADDICTION LIABILITY

As stimulants force the release of extra neurotransmitters, the central nervous system loses some of its ability to synthesize these chemicals thus contributing to the **rapid development of tolerance**. This causes other physiological changes in the user's neurochemistry that promote the rapid development of physical and psychological dependence. While the physical dependence of extended cocaine and methamphetamine use isn't quite as severe as with heroin, the psychological dependence is just as powerful and causes severe craving during the crash and subsequent withdrawal.

Tolerance and dependence can also develop with amphetamine congeners, caffeine, nicotine, and other milder stimulants. In fact the strongest dependence develops with tobacco.

COCAINE

Cocaine epidemics seem to occur every few generations. The first was at the end of the nineteenth century, the next in the 1920s and 1930s, and then it wasn't until the '70s and '80s that use exploded with the popularization of smokable cocaine. Since then experimentation and casual use have declined somewhat but **hardcore use of cocaine has remained strong into the 2000s.** The average age of those coming into treatment has gone up while the younger generation has turned to MDMA (ecstasy) for their recreational use of a psychoactive stimulant drug. As with any newly discovered drug, cocaine spawned many myths and advocates when it first became popular.

"I have more than once observed that in my second character, my faculties seemed sharpened to a point and my spirits more tensely elastic; thus it came about that, where Jekyll perhaps might have succumbed, Hyde rose to the importance of the moment. My drugs were in one of the presses of my cabinet; how was I to reach them?"

Robert Louis Stevenson, 1886, <u>Dr. Jekyll and Mr. Hyde</u>

There is speculation that Robert Louis Stevenson wrote *Dr. Jekyll and Mr. Hyde* **under the influence of cocaine,** which had recently gained public attention through the works of a number of scientists including Sigmund Freud in 1884 (*Über Coca*). The theme of the novel is about the dramatic transformation of Dr. Jekyll

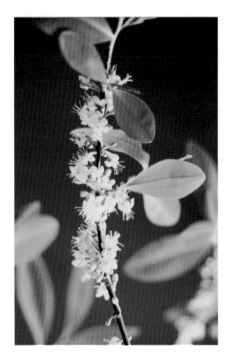

The Erythroxylum *coca plant.*
Courtesy of the Fitz Hugh Ludlow Memorial Library

when he takes an experimental medication and the consequences of this experimentation. The mania of his alter ego, Mr. Hyde, can be likened to some of the effects of intense use of cocaine, particularly if drug-induced psychosis, paranoia, and anger are manifest. This idea of opposites, of ups and downs, of dramatic personality transformations is always present when the effects of cocaine are examined.

"The powers of Hyde seemed to have grown with the sickliness of Jekyll. And certainly the hate that now divided them was equal on each side. . . . He thought of Hyde, for all his energy of life, as of something not only hellish but inorganic."

Robert Louis Stevenson, 1886, <u>Dr. Jekyll and Mr. Hyde</u>

BOTANY, CROP YIELDS, & REFINEMENT

The coca shrub dates back millions of years. One writer half-jokingly speculated that eating the plant caused the extinction of the dinosaurs because of its toxicity. The coca bush, which contains the alkaloid cocaine, grows mainly on the **slopes of the Andes Mountains in South America** (Peru, Bolivia, Ecuador, and Colombia). Lesser amounts are grown in certain parts of the Amazon Jungle and on the island of Java in Indonesia. The South American cultivation of the *Erythroxylum coca* and *Erythroxylum novogranatense* plants accounts for 97% of the world's crop. The green-yellow shrubs, which grow best at altitudes between 1,500 ft. and 5,000 ft., are 6–8 ft. tall. **The leaves of the coca bush contain 0.5% to 1.5% by weight of the alkaloid cocaine.** One acre of coca bushes will yield 1.5–2 kilograms (kg) of cocaine (Grinspoon & Bakalar, 1985).

The **cocaine refinement technique is a 4- or 5-step process** depending on the chemicals used (Karch, 1996).

◇ Soak the leaves in lime (or other alkali) and water for 3 or 4 days.

◇ Add gasoline, kerosene, or acetone to extract nitrogenous alkaloids.

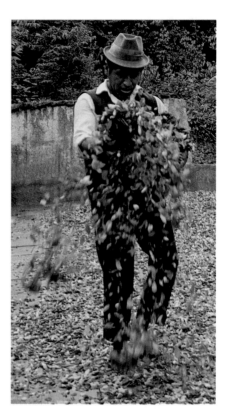

This Bolivian farm worker is sorting coca leaves. It takes 250 kilograms (kg) of leaves to make 1 kg of cocaine.
© Alain Labrousse, 1994

◇ Discard the waste leaves and add sulfuric or hydrochloric acid.

◇ Mix in lime and ammonia to precipitate the basic alkaloids.

◇ Use a number of chemicals to separate the cocaine hydrochloride from the paste.

SMUGGLING & THE STREET TRADE

Since coca leaves are difficult to grow outside of South America and because the extraction process is fairly complex, a highly organized crime cartel developed in Colombia in order to operate the cocaine trade. **These Colombian cartels control cultivation and production in the growing countries and much of the street trade in the United States.** However about two-thirds of the actual smuggling into the United States in recent years has been handled by drug gangs and cartels centered in Mexico. These groups prefer sea routes due to increased surveillance of air space and greater scrutiny of the southern U.S. border due to the September 11, 2001 terrorist attacks on the United States. The Colombian trafficking groups in the United States are based on close-knit criminal cells operating within a given geographic area and since there is minimal contact between cells, the organization is hard to break up (Drug Enforcement Administration [DEA], 2002a).

The United States consumes 70% of the world's cocaine. Although in 2000 the federal government seized more than 103 tons of the refined product (cocaine), an estimated 200–300 metric tons still get through to U.S. markets. The figures for the amount of cocaine produced in Colombia came under question in 1999 because larger acreage of the higher-yielding *Erythroxylum coca* rather than *Erythroxylum novogranatense* had been planted. It was estimated that about 500 metric tons were produced in Colombia instead of the previous estimate of 100 tons (Lichtblau & Schrader, 1999; Office of National Drug Control Policy [ONDCP], 2000). In May of 2001 a single drug bust by the U.S. Coast Guard found 13 tons of cocaine in one Belize-flagged vessel run by a crew of Ukranians and Russians.

The amount of money in the cocaine trade is staggering.

◇ Americans spent an estimated $36.1 billion on cocaine in 2000.

◇ At the wholesale level, cocaine prices varied from $17,000 to $26,000 per kg of refined cocaine with an average purity of 81%.

◇ At the street level, prices varied from $20 to $200 per gram with an average purity of 57%.

◇ "Rocks" of crack cocaine, varying in size from one-tenth to one-half of a gram, sell for $10 to $20 each.

◇ The average hardcore cocaine user spends about $186 a week, about half what was spent by users 10 years ago.

(DEA, 2001)

"I can remember having someone hold a gun to my head and take my money instead of giving me cocaine. At that point I had to go back to the bank, withdraw money, and go right back to the same location hoping that the same person with the gun would not be there."

38-year-old recovering cocaine abuser

Estimates of the number of casual cocaine users and hardcore users vary widely depending on the survey and the definition of hardcore users. Is someone who binges once a month a hardcore user? Once every 2 months? For example, the National Household Survey on Drug Abuse (NHSDA) estimated 445,000 hardcore cocaine users and 2,155,000 occasional users in the United States in 2000. However, the **Drug Use Forecasting (DUF) program**, which questions arrestees in city jails about their drug use and backs up the questions with urinalysis, **estimates 3,103,000 hardcore users**. The DUF data seems closer to the truth since they interview the very population most likely to be involved in hardcore use. What both methods have in common is a consistency of survey methods from year to year, so many surveys are more valuable to judge trends in use rather than absolute numbers (ONDCP, 2000).

HISTORY OF USE (*also see Chapter 1*)

Many landmarks in the history of coca and cocaine use have to do with the changing methods of use and the purity of the substance. The methods include chewing the leaf or chopping it with ash and placing it on the gums; drinking the refined cocaine alkaloid in wine; injecting a solution of the drug in a vein; snorting cocaine hydrochloride; and smoking freebase or crack crystals.

The effects of cocaine are directly related to the blood levels of the drug. The more cocaine that reaches the brain, the more intense the high, the greater the craving, and the more quickly tolerance, craving, abuse, and addiction occur.

Chewing the Leaf

Native cultures in South America have chewed coca leaves for thousands of years for social and religious occasions and to fight off fatigue, lessen hunger, and increase endurance. **The Incas usually chewed the leaf for the juice, adding some lime or ash (from ground shells) to increase absorption by the mucosal tissue in the cheeks and gums, which takes 3–5 minutes.** If the chewer swallows the coca juice, not only does the digestive system break down the drug but it takes longer (about 20–30 minutes) to reach the brain. A habitual user might chew 12–15 grams of leaves 3 or 4 times a day but even so, the maximum amount of cocaine available for absorption would be just 75 mg. The chopped leaves mixed with ash can also be spooned under the tongue for absorption.

The Incas in Peru integrated the use of the coca leaf in every part of their lives much as coffee or tea are part of an American's everyday life. Originally use was generally confined to nobility, priests, and the elite but when the Conquistadors conquered the Inca Empire in the sixteenth century, they greatly increased the cultivation and availability of the leaf. **They grew it for personal profit, to generate government taxes, and to enable the Incas to work more efficiently at high altitudes** digging in the silver mines (Monardes, 1577; Karch, 1997).

Even to this day up to 90% of the Indians living in coca-growing regions chew the leaf. In many native homes in Bolivia visitors are ceremoniously offered pieces of leaves to chew even before refreshments are served. The cocaine blood levels for a coca leaf chewer are about one-fourth of those of smokers and one-seventh of those of IV users (Karch, 1996). A recent political candidate in Bolivia made it to the runoffs in the presidential race on a platform condemning free trade and coca eradication. Evo Morales, an Aymara Indian who leads the farmers and is in favor of agrarian reform, defends coca growing saying it's for traditional purposes, to numb the sensations

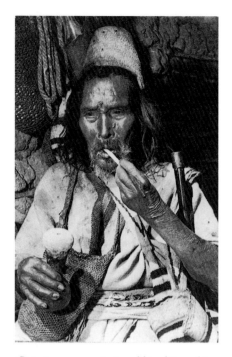

Carrying on a centuries-old tradition, this Colombian coca chewer carries his leaves in a pouch hung on his shoulder. The pop’oro (gourd) in his right hand contains powdered lime (llipta) that he mixes in his mouth with the coca to increase absorption of the coca juice.

Courtesy of the Fitz Hugh Ludlow Memorial Library

● ●

of cold and hunger, and for use in religious ceremonies (Coca Growers, 2002).

In 1861 Albert Nieman, a graduate student in Gottingen, Germany, isolated cocaine from the other chemicals in the coca leaf. This powerful alkaloid, **cocaine hydrochloride, was 200 times more powerful by weight than the coca leaf** thus setting the stage for the widespread use and abuse of the drug. However, it took 20 years before this happened, due in part to the physician Karl Koller who discovered the anesthetic properties of the drug and **Sigmund Freud** who promoted the use of the refined cocaine hydrochloride in his book *Über Coca.* The drug was recommended for a variety of ailments including depression, gastric disorders, asthma, and morphine or alcohol addiction. Its use as a local anesthetic or even as an aphrodisiac was also suggested (Guttmacher, 1885). It was the stimulating and mood-enhancing qualities

that most interested Freud. However, since cocaine was a new drug that hadn't been studied over time, he made a number of errors of judgment.

"Coca is a far more potent and far less harmful stimulant than alcohol and its widespread utilization is hindered at present only by its high cost. . . . I have already stressed the fact that there is no state of depression when the effects of coca have worn off."
Sigmund Freud, 1884

The overly optimistic judgments of Freud and others were made early in the experimental process before dependence and addiction had a chance to develop. When the drug was made more widely available and some people became chronic users, then the true nature and liabilities of refined cocaine became obvious even to Freud and his colleagues.

Drinking Cocaine

The fact that the newly refined cocaine could be dissolved in water or alcohol made other routes of use possible, namely drinking, injecting, and contact absorption. **Beginning in the late 1860s cocaine wines became popular** in France and Italy. However it wasn't until a clever manufacturer and salesman, Angelo Mariani, developed Vin Mariani and promoted its use through the first celebrity endorsements (e.g., Thomas Edison, Robert Louis Stevenson, and Pope Leo XIII) that the first cocaine epidemic began. Although the wine contained only a modest amount of cocaine (2 glasses of wine contained the equivalent of 1 line of cocaine), its effect was more than modest because it was used with alcohol (Karch, 1997). It has been found in recent years that alcohol and cocaine form cocaethylene, a metabolite that has stronger and longer-lasting effects than other cocaine metabolites and causes more intense effects than cocaine hydrochloride by itself. **It takes 15–30 minutes for the metabolites of cocaine to reach the brain after oral ingestion.**

Suddenly in the 1880s and 1890s, patent medicines laced with cocaine, opium, morphine, heroin, *Cannabis*, and alcohol became the rage. They were touted as a cure for any ailment including asthma, hay fever, fatigue, and a dozen other illnesses.

Since these patent medications controlled pain and induced a high, the perception was that they cured illness rather than just controlled the symptoms. **In the late 1800s the prolonged use of cocaine and other prescription medications created a large group of dependent users and addicts, the majority being women.** This was similar to the patent medicine era of addiction 30 years earlier (Aldrich, 1994).

Injecting Cocaine

The **invention of the hypodermic needle in 1857** had a more immediate effect on the use of morphine than on cocaine for two reasons. First, the refinement of morphine from opium occurred 50 years earlier than the refinement of cocaine and second, the use of an opiate painkiller such as morphine had a natural outlet in the Crimean and U.S. Civil Wars and at home as a remedy for dozens of painful illnesses.

Medically the subcutaneous injection or external application of cocaine caused topical anesthesia (useful for minor surgery) and deadened the pain of skin ulcerations. Unfortunately when physicians first began using cocaine medicinally, many were unaware of the drug overdose potential, even from topical use, and a number of deaths occurred. **Injecting cocaine intravenously results in an intense rush within 15–30 seconds and gives the highest blood cocaine level.** The rush is more intense than chewing the leaf, drinking cocaine wine, or snorting cocaine hydrochloride. Since cocaine is rapidly metabolized by the body, IV use means that the rush and subsequent crash will be equally intense. If cocaine is injected **subcutaneously or intramuscularly, the high is delayed 3–5 minutes** and is not quite as intense.

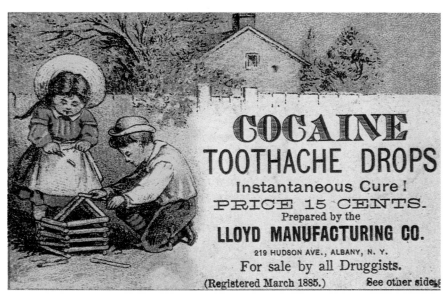

Snorting Cocaine

The early 1900s gave rise to a popular new form of cocaine use, snorting the powder into the nostrils. Called "tooting," "blowing," or "horning," **this method gets the drug to the nasal mucosa and into the brain within 3–5 minutes**. Peak effects take a few more minutes to occur.

"What snorting I have done burns the nose terribly and is very uncomfortable. It's much delayed where shooting is quicker. In fact after 20 minutes I was still getting higher to the point where I did not want to be."
26-year-old recovering cocaine addict

Snorting cocaine is a self-limiting method of using cocaine. This occurs because cocaine constricts the capillaries that absorb the drug, so the more that is snorted, the slower the absorption. The blood level of cocaine is much less than when used intravenously. As the constricting effect of cocaine wears off, **the nasal tissues swell, causing a runny sniffling nose** characteristic of cocaine snorters. In addition chronic use can kill nasal tissues and in a few cases perforate the nasal septum that divides the nostrils (Smith & Seymour, 2001).

Mucosal & Contact Absorption

Besides absorption through mucosa in the nose, gums, and cheeks, cocaine can be **absorbed through mucosal tissue in the rectum and the vagina and act as a topical anesthetic**. Rectal application is used in parts of the gay male community (Karch, 1996). Cocaine can also be absorbed through the outer skin (epidermis) but not at levels high enough to cause effects, merely to be detectable in the bloodstream (and cause problems in drug testing).

Smoking

In 1914 Parke-Davis Pharmaceuticals introduced cigarettes that contained refined cocaine but the high temperature (195°C or 383°F) needed to convert cocaine hydrochloride to smoke resulted in the destruction of many of the psychoactive properties of the drug. Thus chewing, drinking, injecting, and snorting cocaine remained the principal routes of administration until the mid-1970s when street chemists **converted cocaine hy-**drochloride to freebase cocaine. This process lowered the vaporization point to 98°C and made the drug smokable.** Unlike the cocaine hydrochloride cigarettes introduced in 1914, freebase cocaine could be smoked without destroying most of its psychoactive properties. In the early and mid-1980s an easier method of making freebase cocaine (called "dirty basing") was developed setting the stage for another cocaine epidemic. This new form of smokable cocaine was called "crack."

When absorbed through the lungs, cocaine reaches the brain within only 5–8 seconds compared to the 15–30 seconds it takes when injected through the veins. The smokable cocaine reaches the brain so quickly it causes more dramatic effects before it is swiftly metabolized. This up and down rapid roller coaster effect results in intense craving.

"I prefer snorting because it would never get me that far out there. Freebase would get me out there more quickly and I didn't really like that."
17-year-old male recovering crack smoker

PHYSICAL & MENTAL EFFECTS

Metabolism

Because **cocaine is metabolized very quickly by the body, effects disappear faster than with amphetamines** and amphetamine congeners. Cocaine is metabolized to ecgonine methyl ester, benzoylecgonine, and if alcohol is present, cocaethylene. The half-life of cocaine is about 40–60 minutes. This means that half the drug is metabolized to pharmacologically inactive metabolites in that period of time. However, even after the drug has almost disappeared from the blood, effects continue to occur. Cocaine use is detectable in the urine for up to 36 hours.

Medical Use

As the **only naturally occurring topical anesthetic with powerful vasoconstriction effects**, cocaine is

The anesthetic effects of cocaine made the drug a favorite of dentists long before Novocaine® was synthesized.
Courtesy of the National Library of Medicine, Bethesda, MD

used in aerosol form to numb the nasal passages when inserting breathing tubes in a patient, to numb the eye or throat during surgery, and to deaden the pain of chronic sores. (This topical anesthetic effect also numbs the nasal passages when the drug is snorted.) Cocaine receptors are also found on the bronchi and smooth muscles of the lungs, so stimulation causes dilation of bronchi. Because of this effect cocaine was once used to treat asthma. Synthetic topical anesthetics, particularly procaine and lidocaine that mimic the effects of cocaine, are used nowadays for eye surgery, dental procedures, and other minor surgeries because they are much less stimulating to the brain. None of the synthetic anesthetics constrict blood vessels and are therefore combined with epinephrine, a vasoconstrictor, to prevent excess bleeding.

Neurochemistry & the Central Nervous System

Most of cocaine's effects are the result of its influence on catecholamine neurotransmitters. **Cocaine forces the release of these neurotransmitters (norepinephrine, epinephrine, and dopamine) and then blocks their reabsorption**, so more are available for intense stimulation. In an experiment with cocaine users, Dr. Nora Volkow at NIDA's Regional Neuroimaging Center used PET scans to show that **cocaine blocked 60% to 77% of the dopamine reuptake sites**. At least 47% of the sites had to be blocked for users to feel a drug-induced high (Volkow, Fowler, Wang, et al., 1997).

"I felt like I was invincible and I could do whatever I wanted to do. I felt like no one could stop me. That's what it made me feel like. I felt like I could clean the whole house three times in a row, you know, within an hour, and I wouldn't be tired when I was finished."
28-year-old female recovering cocaine addict

The Crash. By blocking the reuptake ports, cocaine leaves those neu-

rotransmitters vulnerable to metabolism by enzymes that live between the brain cells, resulting in their depletion (Smith & Seymour, 2001). Since cocaine is also metabolized so quickly by the body, the initial euphoria, the feeling of confidence, the sense of omnipotence, the surge of energy, and the satisfied feeling disappear as suddenly as they appeared, so **the crash after using cocaine can be particularly depressing**. With cocaine this depression can last a few hours, several days, or even weeks.

"Initially I remember the mood swings but then the swings became further and further apart and the depression got deeper and deeper and deeper and of course eventually it led me to my attempt at suicide, which was my extreme. I really did want to die and that I remember as being way out of proportion to the actual events of my life."
44-year-old recovering cocaine addict

The biological mechanisms of cocaine are quite complex. For example, in an experiment at Massachusetts General Hospital, **brain scans of 10 cocaine addicts just after injection of the drug showed 90 distinct areas of brain activation**, especially the amygdala and nucleus accumbens (Breiter et al., 1997). Recent studies at Yale, Harvard Medical School, and Northwestern University discovered that a protein called "delta-FosB" sensitized mice to the pleasurable and rewarding effects of cocaine, implying that this heightened sensitivity contributes to the intense craving caused by cocaine use (Kelz, Chen, Carlezon, et al., 1999).

Unfortunately the intense stimulation has a price, especially when done frequently. It's like putting 200 volts into a 115-volt light bulb. The bulb burns more brightly but the strain on the filament can eventually burn it out. For example,

◇ **dopamine** coordinates fine motor skills, signals the reward/reinforcement center, and regulates thoughts

but it can also **overstimulate the brain's fright center causing the paranoia** experienced by many stimulant abusers. The fright center is a survival mechanism to warn us of danger but overstimulation causes overreaction or paranoia. A shadow, sudden movement, or loud voice may seem unbearably threatening;

"There was these little nail holes in the door and he swore up and down that someone was looking at us through them. I put my feet down on the bed and just doing something like this and he would slap the shit out of me, 'Bitch who you signaling?' He would get on his knees and look under the bed."
34-year-old recovering crack abuser

◇ **catecholamines** increase confidence and energy and cause a euphoric rush that seems extremely pleasurable. Eventual depletion of the catecholamines causes exhaustion, lethargy, anhedonia (the inability to feel pleasure), and low blood pressure;

◇ **acetylcholine** increases reflexes, alertness, memory, learning, and aggression but that can turn into muscle tremors, memory lapses, mental confusion, and even hallucinations;

◇ **serotonin** initially causes elation, facilitates sleep, raises self-esteem, and increases sexual activity but with excessive use it becomes insomnia, agitation, and severe emotional depression (Uhl et al., 2001).

Sexual Effects

"It makes you feel like, you know, you're really sexy, and you know, makes you feel like you're the best man in the whole world."
36-year-old recovering cocaine addict

Cocaine and amphetamines have similar sexual effects. Cocaine at **low doses enhances sexual desire, delays ejaculation**, and is considered an aphrodisiac by many users. Unfortunately with higher doses and chronic use, **sexual dysfunction becomes more common**, e.g., the inability to achieve an erection.

"After a while when you keep doing it, it's just like you're impotent and you can't . . . it doesn't have no effect. The opposite sex can do anything they want to you and you won't react. Your body doesn't react to it, to any kind of touch or emotion, you know."
36-year-old recovering cocaine addict

In addition the need to raise money plus the disinhibiting effects of cocaine lead to **high-risk sexual behavior** and unusual sexual behavior (Smith & Wesson, 1985).

Aggression, Violence, & Cocaethylene

Disruption of neurotransmitter levels are heavily implicated in the aggression and violence associated with stronger stimulants. When

◇ **inhibitory functions are suppressed** in the anterior cingulate gyrus and temporal lobes,

◇ **emotional triggers are overstimulated** in our amygdala,

◇ **the fright center is hyperactivated** in our limbic system,

◇ **the normal function of our temporal lobes are disrupted,**

then aggression and occasionally violence are often a glance away (Amen, Yantis, Trudeau, Stubblefield, & Halverstadt, 1997).

"I found that using cocaine, mainlining it straight to the nervous system, it's like I want to kill people. It is a very unhealthy state of mind. . . . It is like spinning out of control and all the thoughts are centered around, 'Where should I hit them first?' Damn, I want to hurt people, you know. It is just psychotic thinking."
32-year-old recovering cocaine abuser

In a small study of domestic violence, researchers found that 67% of the perpetrators had used cocaine the day of the incident and virtually all of those had also used alcohol. Interviews and research seem to indicate that **cocaethylene (an active metabolite when cocaine and alcohol are taken together) induces greater agitation, euphoria, and violence** than just cocaine alone (Brookhoff, O'Brien, Cook, Thompson, & Williams, 1997; Landry, 1992).

"When my mate hallucinated from smoking too much, thinking I was trying to do his brothers, and I got my face damaged badly because of the hallucinations. He slammed my face into concrete."
28-year-old female recovering crack abuser

The cocaethylene reaches the brain as easily as the cocaine and has almost identical effects but is somewhat more toxic. **Cocaethylene also seems more likely to induce cardiac conduction abnormalities** compared to cocaine and therefore is more likely to induce a heart attack. Since the half-life of cocaethylene is more than three times that of cocaine by itself (2 hours vs. 38 minutes), its effects, including high blood pressure, last longer (Karch, 1996; Gold & Miller, 1997). Many cocaine abusers are aware of this extended half-life effect and so they "front load" with alcohol to prolong the effects of the more expensive cocaine. However, it is theorized that the extended anxiety and panic attacks that are common with cocaine abusers even after they quit could be attributed to the slow elimination of cocaethylene (Randall, 1992).

"I popped a guy on New Year's Eve. He left me there in the pouring rain on New Year's Eve, so I just turned around and popped him and broke his nose. I popped a lot of guys. I can break doors down with my foot. It is not just a guy thing."
26-year-old female recovering cocaine abuser

The paranoia and dysfunctional lifestyle involved with cocaine use engenders excess violence. Autopsies showed that 31% of all homicide victims in New York in the early 1990s had cocaine in their bodies (1,332 out of 4,298 victims). Two-thirds of those who tested positive were 15–34 years of age, 86% were male and 87% were African American or Latino (Tardiff et al., 1994).

Cardiovascular Effects

"Well there was a heavy beating, tachycardia, a sense of not being able to get my breath, the sensation of everything moving very quickly and very intensely."
34-year-old female recovering cocaine abuser

Physiologically it is the cardiovascular system that is most affected by long-term cocaine use. Cocaine affects the circulatory system by direct contact (due to receptors right on the heart and blood vessels) and by its effect on the autonomic nervous system in the brain. When injected, **cocaine raises the heart rate and constricts blood vessels causing a 20–30 unit rise in blood pressure**, sometimes more. This means that while more blood is available for central blood vessels to energize muscles and increase blood flow to the heart, less is available for the smaller vessels to heal damaged tissues, aid digestion, and infuse other peripheral systems with sufficient oxygen. This leads to cellular changes including **damage to heart muscles, coronary arteries, and other blood vessels**. Recent research showed that when snorted, the mechanism for hypertension (high blood pressure) is different than when injected. The major effect of snorting is on cardiac output rather than blood vessel constriction but the end results are the same (Tuncel et al., 2002).

The raised blood pressure can also **weaken the walls of the blood vessels and cause a stroke**, usually within 3 hours of use. Chronic cocaine use is similar to chronic stress. The hearts of chronic abusers are often slightly enlarged and coronary arterial blood flow

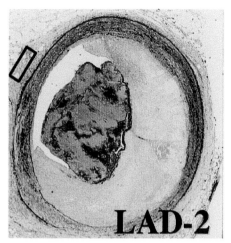
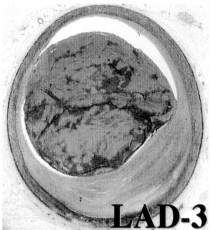

These cross sections of the left anterior descending (LAD) coronary artery are of a 36-year-old long-term IV cocaine user who died from acute myocardial infarction. The thrombus (clot) that caused the heart attack can be seen in both cross sections of the lumen (interior) of the LAD. It overlays the fatty plaque that has built up over the years on the walls of the coronary artery, probably due to the cocaine use.

Courtesy of Dr. Rene Virmani, Chairman, Department of Cardiovascular Pathology, Armed Forces Institute of Pathology

• •

is sluggish. Chronic cocaine use also causes a disorganization in the usual formation of heart muscles and scarring of these muscles known as "constriction bands." This makes chronic users more likely to suffer a cocaine-induced heart attack (Karch, 1996).

Neonatal Effects

"Three of my children have been taken directly from me in the hospital, like directly out of my arms to the nursery, found out they were positive for cocaine and, you know, back to the nursery and I wasn't allowed to like see them without going to the nursery."
30-year-old recovering crack user

Smoked, snorted, or injected, cocaine and amphetamines are of particular danger to the fetus of a pregnant woman. When a pregnant woman uses cocaine, within seconds her **baby will also be exposed to the drug.** Because of the stimulatory effects on the cardiovascular system in particular, the chances of **miscarriage, stroke, and sudden infant death syndrome** (SIDS) due to raised blood pressure and blood vessel malformations are increased (Gold & Miller, 1997).

In a Toronto inner-city hospital 12% to 20% of all newborns had been exposed to cocaine (Foreman, Klein, Barks, et al., 1994). Respiratory ailments were more common in those infants. Infants born cocaine-affected have been called **"jittery babies"** because they are agitated, have higher blood pressure, are more irritable, and are sometimes smaller.

"The first 2 or 3 weeks out of the hospital, the babies are pretty normal and then all of a sudden the chemical that they were born with is out of the system. They go through a couple of weeks of severe withdrawal where they have seizures, tremors, vomiting, diarrhea, screaming, 16 to 20 hours a day. After about 2 weeks of that the brain releases some of that cocaine [actually a metabolite of cocaine] back into that system, then we have a couple of weeks of reprieve, and then that whole process starts over again."
Foster mother who cares for drug-affected babies

Many of the abnormalities in the newborns of drug users have more to do with the mother's lifestyle than the drug itself. For example, amphetamine and cocaine abusers are generally malnourished, so the fetus suffers from malnutrition. The mothers are more likely to smoke tobacco and to have a venereal or IV drug-induced disease, such as hepatitis or AIDS, so the fetus is infected too. A drug-dependent mother is more likely to be indifferent to the daily demands of an infant than a nonuser, so bonding problems, neglect, and emotional deprivation are more likely. For example, in a study of 218 cocaine-exposed babies from high-risk, low-socioeconomic status, the mental retardation rate was five times the rate of the general population but only twice the rate for noncocaine-exposed children of the same socioeconomic group. **The rate of mild or greater mental delays was also double the rate of the nonexposed children** (Singer et al., 2002). However another analysis of 36 studies of physical growth, cognition, language skills, motor skills, and behavior in cocaine-exposed children up to the age of 6 showed minimal effects, suggesting that many children can outgrow some of the effects or develop alternate methods of learning (Frank, 2001).

The public attitude towards drug abuse by pregnant women led to a murder conviction of a mother for killing her unborn child by using crack during pregnancy. The jury in South Carolina found the woman guilty after only 15 minutes of deliberation and the 24-year-old mother was sentenced to 12 years in prison.

Despite the severe problems of cocaine toxicity and withdrawal noted in cocaine-exposed fetuses and babies, there is hope. Demonstration projects like those of the Haight Ashbury Free Clinics' Moving Addicted Mothers Ahead (MAMA) and Ujima House Centers have shown that **good prenatal and postnatal care of these infants,** along with continued excellent pediatric and parenting resources, **results in toddlers who catch up in their emotional and physical development** to noncocaine-exposed children by their 8th to 10th birthdays.

Tolerance

Tolerance to the euphoric effects can begin to develop after the first injection or smoking session. Binge or chronic users have escalated their doses from one-eighth of a gram to 3 grams per day within only a few days while chasing the initial high or the euphoria. Most cocaine users remember their early experiences with cocaine as the most satisfying. The more they use, the less satisfying it becomes.

Withdrawal, Craving, & Relapse

Contrary to notions held by many researchers until the 1980s, **there are true withdrawal symptoms** when cocaine use ceases. Although similar to the crash, withdrawal effects can last months, even years, depending on dosage, frequency, length of use, and any pre-existing mental problems. The major symptoms are

◇ **anhedonia** (the lack of ability to feel pleasure),

◇ **anergia** (a total lack of energy),

◇ **loss of motivation** or initiative,

◇ **emotional depression,**

◇ **vivid and unpleasant dreams,**

◇ **insomnia,**

◇ **increased appetite,**

◇ **psychomotor agitation,**

◇ and an **intense craving** for the drug.

(American Psychiatric Association [APA], 2000; Gold & Herkov, 1998)

"I got shot in the leg. I have a bullet in my leg now. I was bleeding to death and the only thing I wanted to do was smoke. I told my buddy, 'Come on give me a hit, give me a hit.' I am smoking the pipe, the pipe is full of blood, it is full of blood. I am smoking, trying to get high, and here I am about to bleed to death."

65-year-old recovering crack addict

These symptoms are also common in amphetamine withdrawal. It is these symptoms, particularly craving, that generally cause the recovering compul-

sive user to relapse again and again. The time frame for a **typical cycle of compulsive cocaine (or amphetamine) use is** as follows:

◇ immediately after a binge, usually lasting several days, **the user crashes,** sleeps all day long trying to regain energy, and then swears off the drug forever;

◇ a few days later **the user usually feels much better** and may leave or drop out of treatment at this time. This temporary return to normal feelings is called "euthymia";

◇ however about 1 week to 10 days after quitting, the **craving starts to build,** the energy level drops, and the user feels very little pleasure from any surroundings, activities, or friends. Emotional depression begins to increase;

◇ so 2–4 weeks after vowing to abstain, users feel the **craving and depression build to a fever pitch** and unless they are in intensive treatment they will usually relapse.

Overdose

Most drug-related visits to emergency rooms are due to cocaine. About 175,000 visits in major cities involved cocaine with one-fourth of those attributable to crack (Drug Abuse Warning Network [DAWN], 2002). An overdose of cocaine can be caused by as little as $1/50$ of a gram or as much as 1.2 grams. The "caine reaction" is very intense and generally short in duration. **Most often an overdose is not fatal. It only feels like impending death.**

"I almost did too much and I felt after I did it, I felt my knees buckle and I fell on the toilet stool, you know. And I was just shaking, like in a convulsion, you know. And if my buddy wasn't there to grab me and put me in the shower, I don't know what would've happened."

36-year-old cocaine addict

However **in 2,000–3,000 U.S. cases every year, death occurs within 40 minutes to 5 hours after exposure**

(occasionally the next morning). Death usually results from either the initial stimulatory phase of toxicity (seizures, hypertension, stroke, and tachycardia) or the later depression phase terminating in extreme respiratory depression and coma. Heart seizures and death will occasionally occur the morning after heavy use due to cocaethylene that lasts in the blood and brain after the cocaine and alcohol have been metabolized (Landry, 1992; Karch, 1997).

"I have seen a friend go through overdose. His skin was gray-green. His eyes rolled back, his heart stopped, and there was a gurgling sound that is right at death; and I had to bring him back and that's enough to put the fear of God in anybody."

Intravenous cocaine user

First-time users and even those who have used cocaine before can get an exaggerated reaction far beyond what might normally occur or beyond what they have experienced in the past. This is partially due to the phenomenon known as "**inverse tolerance**" or "kindling." As people use cocaine they get more sensitive to its toxic effects rather than less sensitive as one would expect.

Miscellaneous Effects

Formication. A side effect of long-term or high-dose cocaine and amphetamine use is an imbalance in sensory neurons that causes **sensations in the skin that feel like hundreds of tiny bugs** ("coke bugs," "meth bugs," "snow bugs") are crawling under one's skin. Users on coke or "speed runs" have been known to scratch themselves bloody trying to get at the imaginary bugs.

Dental erosions. These frequently occur as a result of either **poor dental hygiene, malnutrition, the erosive effects of acidic cocaine** that has trickled down from the sinuses to the upper front teeth, from repetitive and compulsive overbrushing of the teeth while intoxicated, or from a combination of these effects.

Seizure. This effect is caused by overdose, stroke, or hemorrhage and **occurs in 2% to 10% of regular cocaine users** (Karch, 1996). Three times as many women as men have seizures from cocaine overdoses.

Gastrointestinal complications. Though more unusual than cardiovascular effects, problems such as gastric ulcerations, retroperitoneal fibrosis, visceral infarction, intestinal ischemia, gastrointestinal tract perforation, and colonic ischemia have been observed in heavy cocaine users (Lindner et al., 2000).

Cocaine Psychosis

Schizophrenia is usually caused by hereditary imbalances of brain dopamine in the mesolimbic dopamine pathway. It can also be caused by dis-

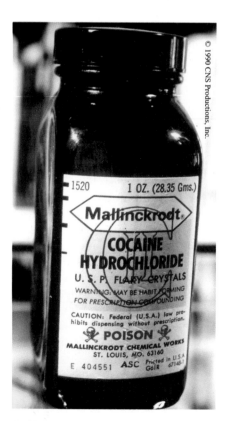

In 2002, 1 ounce (oz.) of cocaine when sold legally in the United States for medicinal purposes cost about $100. When sold illegally, 1 oz. of cocaine cost up to $2,000.

••••••••••••••••••••••••••

eases or drugs that increase dopamine. **Because cocaine increases dopamine, repeated use can trigger stimulant-induced paranoid psychosis/schizophrenia** (Stahl, 2000). This cocaine psychosis was first documented in the late 1880s when intensive cocaine experimentation and abuse began. In the 1970s the progression from euphoria to dysphoria and ultimately to psychosis was observed to be mostly dose related but the setting in which the drug is taken can also affect the quality of the symptoms (Post & Kopanda, 1976). Excessive methamphetamine use is more likely to cause a stimulant psychosis because the drug lasts much longer in the system than cocaine, which is rapidly metabolized and therefore becomes quite expensive to keep using.

Symptoms of cocaine psychosis include prominent auditory, visual, or tactile hallucinations and paranoid delusions (APA, 2000). **It is difficult for clinicians to tell the difference between a preexisting psychosis and cocaine/methamphetamine-induced psychosis.** A thorough psychological and drug history, along with a drug test, are necessary to determine the cause. One of the sure signs is the **symptoms disappear after a period of abstinence from the stimulant**, which may range from a few hours to a few days or occasionally even months (Ziedonis &Wyatt, 1998). Repeated use of cocaine can sensitize the user so that smaller and smaller doses will induce the psychotic symptoms. Milder symptoms of transient paranoia appear in 33% to 50% of chronic cocaine users (Satel & Lieberman, 1991).

OTHER PROBLEMS WITH COCAINE USE

Polydrug Use

Cocaine's stimulating effects can be so intense that the user needs a downer to take the edge off or to get to sleep. The most common drugs used for this purpose are alcohol, heroin, or a sedative-hypnotic such as clonazepam, though any downer will do in a pinch. The combination of cocaine or methamphetamine with heroin or an-

other downer is known as a "speedball." Sometimes the second drug can be more of a problem than the cocaine itself.

"I cured my alcoholism with crack cocaine. I no longer had a desire to drink until I ran out of crack cocaine and was all buzzy and jittery and then I wanted to drink."
38-year-old recovering polydrug abuser

Adulteration & Contamination

Even with the increased supplies coming into the country, the increased purity, and the lower prices, **cocaine at the street level is almost always adulterated**. The street dealer will add an adulterant to lower the purity from 80–90% down to approximately 60% often to pay for his or her own habit or just to make a few extra dollars. Adulteration of cocaine involves dilution with such diverse products as baby laxatives, lactose, vitamin B, aspirin, Mannitol®, sugar, Tetracaine® or Procaine® (topical anesthetics), and even flour or talcum powder (Marnell, 1997).

"I have had lots of problems like veins I've missed and gotten it underneath the skin causing abscesses, hematoma. My veins in certain spots have turned rock hard . . . my arm apparently has some level of vein infection, which I am now on antibiotics for."
27-year-old recovering cocaine abuser

When the drug is used intravenously, not only are **diluents put into the bloodstream but so are bacteria and viruses** from contaminated drugs or needles that can transmit diseases, including blood and heart infections, AIDS, hepatitis B, and especially hepatitis C. The use of other contaminated paraphernalia, such as snorting straws, can also transmit infection.

"There were people like me that would snort coke and would share a straw and those straws cut. You wind up having those straws cut into your

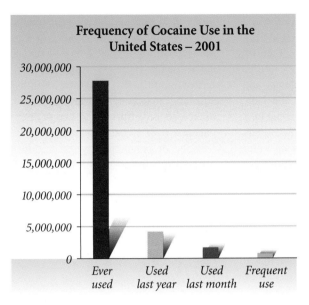

Frequency of Cocaine Use in the United States – 2001

Figure 3-1 •

Of the 28 million Americans who have experimented with cocaine, 4.2 million used it in the past year, 1.7 million used it in the last month, and about 1 million reported cocaine dependence or abuse. Of these figures about one-fourth smoke the drug (crack).

National Household Survey, 2001 (Substance Abuse and Mental Health Services Administration [SAMHSA], 2002)

nasal passage and there is some blood involved and that is enough for a lot of people to actually pass on infections, nevermind the fact that being high on cocaine loosens you up and leads to possible unsafe behavior."

48-year-old HIV and hepatitis C-positive male recovering cocaine abuser

The hepatitis C infection rate for IV drug users is 50% to 90% in most studies. The use of cocaine also seems to aggravate various conditions, especially AIDS, because it increases viral loads and lowers CD_4 counts (Baldwin et al., 2002).

COMPULSION

Considering all the problems with cocaine—the expense, the adulteration, the illegality, the possibility of overdose, the physical and psychological dangers—two questions come to mind, "Why do people use cocaine?" and "Why do they use it so compulsively?"

"At first it was maybe every hour because the feeling would only last that long and the more I did it, the feeling didn't even last that long, and I would eventually get up to about maybe 10 minutes, and maybe every 5 minutes. I would try to pace myself and make

however much I had last as long as I could but it was usually out of control, you know."

26-year-old recovering crack abuser

Why Do People Start Using Cocaine & Amphetamines?

◊ The drugs **mimic pleasurable natural body functions**: adrenal energy rush, confidence, euphoria, increased sensitivity, and stimulation of the reward/reinforcement center.

◊ It is sometimes **easier to get a chemical high** instantly than a natural high over a period of time.

◊ People also use these drugs to **combat boredom**.

◊ People succumb to internal or external **peer pressure**.

◊ People are curious and the **drugs are readily available**.

◊ People use them as a way to **block out personal worries or other effects caused by their environment**: e.g., poverty, hopelessness, and violence.

"I would have to take at least a gram to get through the day, to deal with other people's problems and I spent more time going into the bathroom and less time doing my work. And as

soon as I'd sit down to do my work, I needed to go to the bathroom again to use more."

26-year-old recovering crack abuser

Why Is Cocaine (& Amphetamines) Used So Compulsively?

◊ Users want to **recapture the initial rush** (the energy surge and the stimulation of the reward/reinforcement center, which is extremely intense. Most find that it's hard to reproduce that initial rush but that doesn't stop them from trying.

◊ They want to **avoid the crash** that is inevitable after the intense high. In many cases a user will shoot up or smoke every 20 minutes or even every 10 minutes in a binge episode.

◊ Users want to continuously **avoid life's problems**, such as difficult relationships, lack of confidence, traumatic events, a hated job, or loneliness.

◊ People use in response to their **hereditary predisposition to use**. That is, certain people's natural neurotransmitter balance makes them react more intensely to a drug. They are, in essence, presensitized to the drug.

◊ Cocaine, in and of itself, **changes the neurochemical balance and creates an intense craving** that will cause someone to keep shooting, snorting, or smoking (bingeing) until every last microgram is gone, until he or she passes out, or until an overdose occurs. Even coca leaf chewing is often done in a binge pattern as noted by Johan von Tschudi, an early explorer of the Amazon Basin, in his book *Travels in Peru*.

"They give themselves up for days together to the passionate enjoyment of the leaves . . . it, however, appears that it is not so much a want of sleep or the absence of food, as the want of coca that puts an end to the lengthened debauch."

Von Tschudi, 1854 (Karch, 1996)

SMOKABLE COCAINE (crack, freebase)

"I couldn't bear to be sober. I needed to smoke crack cocaine because smoking crack cocaine takes away all your thoughts. You don't think about reality. You don't think about your bills, 'Oh, I have to pay this tomorrow.' You don't think about yourself. You don't think about nobody around you but crack cocaine."

43-year-old female recovering crack, heroin, and meth addict

Even though smokable cocaine had been around since the mid-1970s in the form of freebase cocaine, **the smokable cocaine epidemic didn't start until around 1981** when a glut of the powder in the Bahamas, the major transshipment point from Colombia, caused the price to drop by 80%. **Dealers made a shrewd marketing decision to convert the powder to crack.** This way they could sell small chunks or "rocks" of it for prices as low as $2.50 a hit. Immigrants to Florida taught the process to young people in Miami, and southern Florida became the main area for conversion laboratories (DEA, 2002b).

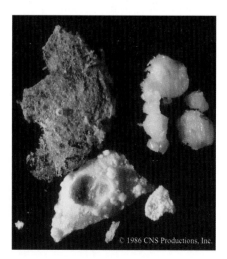

In this collection of crack cocaine samples, each "rock" is made in a slightly different manner. The various colors come from the impurities left after heating the mixture.

The use of crack spread to the rest of the United States supported at first by after-hours cocaine clubs, then by freebase parlors, then by crack houses (1984), and finally by curbside use and distribution (Hamid, 1992). In the New York City area three-fourths of the new users were young white professionals or middle-class youngsters from Long Island, New Jersey, or Westchester County. Because of the low price, it soon spread to less affluent neighborhoods. It was estimated in the late 1980s that 10,000 gang members were dealing cocaine (and other drugs) in some 50 cities across the United States.

Some thought that the spread of crack to the office, factory, schoolyard, ghetto, and barrio was generated by media attention. Others thought that the basic properties of smokable cocaine were the cause of the epidemic. The fact that the use of crack continues to be a severe problem despite vastly curtailed media coverage speaks to the addictive nature of smokable cocaine rather than to the influence of the media.

The words "crack cocaine" didn't appear in the general media until 1985, tentatively at first, as if society was trying out a new nickname. **By 1986 there seemed to be a crack epidemic that crossed all social and economic barriers.** By the '90s the crack epidemic had become ingrained in the American psyche as one of the main causes of society's ills: gang violence, AIDS, crime, and addiction. Then the epidemic began to wane. At the beginning of the twenty-first century, an older smaller core of crack abusers had become entrenched in society, many in lower-income groups. In one study about half of the women seeking treatment in 1999 were 35 or older and 42% had been using for 11 years or more (Substance Abuse and Mental Health Services Administration/Treatment Episode Data Sets [SAMHSA/TEDS], 2000).

PHARMACOLOGY OF SMOKABLE COCAINE

In the early 1970s South American **cocaine refinery workers realized you could smoke cocaine paste**, an in-termediate step in cocaine refinement, and smoking it did not destroy its euphoric and stimulating effects. Chemically, cocaine paste is cocaine freebase. Unfortunately the off-white doughy substance also contains chemicals such as kerosene, sulfuric acid, and sodium carbonate. It is usually smoked with tobacco or marijuana by the middle- and lower-income classes. When smoked in a marijuana joint, it is called "bazooka," "basuco," or "pasta." In a study of 158 "pasta" smokers in Lima, Peru, the effects were reported to be similar to snorted cocaine but more intense and immediate (Jeri, Sanchez, Del Pozo, & Fernandez, 1992).

"After a few minutes of intense enjoyment, they developed anxiety and vehement wishes to continue smoking, leading to repeated or chain smoking. When they run out of 'paste,' they try to obtain or buy more in a state of compulsive anxiety. The user does not sleep, has no appetite, and his/her only wish is to continue smoking. Some patients from the very first puffs experience perceptual disturbances (visual hallucinations)."

(Jeri et al., 1992)

Making cocaine suitable for smoking (freebasing, "basing," "baseballing") involves dissolving cocaine hydrochloride in an alkali solution and heating it to create crystals of freebase cocaine. After the solution is cooled, ether is added to **separate the now fat-soluble freebase from the adulterants in the original cocaine hydrochloride leaving behind pure cocaine freebase crystals.** Unfortunately the flammability of the ether can cause explosions and burns.

"Cheap basing" or "dirty basing" involves dissolving the cocaine in a solution of baking soda and water and heating it until crystals precipitate out. **This method does not remove as many impurities** or residues as the freebasing, so contaminants like talcum powder and especially baking soda remain. The chunks of smokable cocaine made by this method are called "crack" because of the crackling sound that occurs when it is smoked or "rock" because the product looks like little rocks.

"The high almost felt as if I—like I could feel my brain almost frying and when you smoke crack cocaine it's got like a crinkling sound like when you crinkle plastic or something and I felt like I could hear that going on inside my head."
17-year-old recovering cocaine user

The converted freebase cocaine, made by either the "basing" method or the crack method, has four chemical properties sought by users.

◇ **It has a lower melting point than the powdered form** (98°C vs. 195°C), so it can be heated easily in a glass pipe and vaporized to form smoke at a lower temperature. Too high a temperature destroys most of the psychoactive properties of the drug.

◇ Smokable cocaine **reaches the brain faster** than when cocaine hydrochloride is snorted or even when injected since it enters the system directly through the lungs.

◇ Freebase cocaine is **more readily absorbed by fat cells of the brain** since it is more fat-soluble than cocaine hydrochloride thus causing a more intense reaction.

◇ Users are also able to **get a much higher dose of cocaine in their systems over a short period of time** because of the very large surface area in the lungs (about the size of a football field).

Besides the names "crack," "rock," and "freebase," smokable cocaine has also been called "paste," "base," "basay," "hubba," "gravel," "Roxanne," "girl," "fry," and "boulya." There is a frequent misperception that crack and freebase are different drugs than cocaine. They aren't. **Crack and freebase are just a different chemical form of cocaine that make it smokable.** However when talking to users,

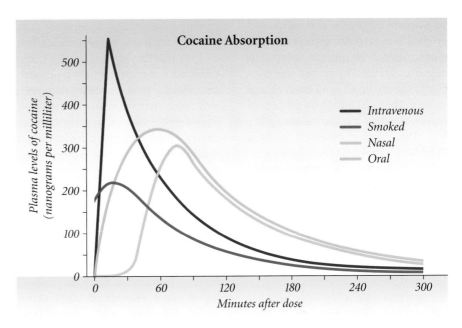

Figure 3-2 •

This graph shows the plasma levels of cocaine after equivalent doses were taken through different methods. While smoking gets cocaine to the brain slightly more rapidly than IV use, injection puts a larger amount into the system at one time. When coca leaves are chewed, peak blood plasma levels are about one-fourth to one-eighth of the levels obtained by smoking.

NIDA Research Monograph 99, Research Findings on Smoking of Abused Substances

crack seems to be the more dangerous drug because the overwhelming craving it produces is much more powerful, blocks out the ability to function normally, and causes a much more rapid downslide. Whether it is the extra additives in "dirty basing," the different social situations in which it is used, the lower price, or other reasons that cause the chaos and disruption of many poorer communities is still not clear.

"It tastes like more because that is all you want, more. Not like if you smoke a joint, you high. You ain't looking for no more but this, this is a trip because this little bitty thing that costs $20 is gone in 3 minutes, maybe 5."
36-year-old recovering female crack user

EFFECTS & SIDE EFFECTS

The effects of smoking crack are almost the same as snorting or injecting cocaine but since smoking cocaine reaches the brain more quickly, the **effects and side effects seem more intense**. Unfortunately for the crack smoker much of the cocaine is lost to the air, about 50% when smoked in a cigarette and about 75% when smoked in a glass pipe (Siegel, 1992). For this reason much **more cocaine has to be smoked than injected to achieve the same effects**. Smoking or using the drug intravenously can produce similar blood levels of cocaine but it is necessary (and easier) to keep smoking the crack again and again to keep the brain reacting.

"The feeling that I had on crack cocaine is entirely different than any other drug I have tried. It was that crack cocaine gives you this high where you just seem like there's no worry in the world whereas with heroin and speed I worried about where my next hit was going to come from."
42-year-old recovering crack smoker

Smoking crack gives a rush that lasts as little as 5–10 seconds and a

subsequent euphoria, excitation, and arousal that lasts for several minutes more. After 5–20 minutes these feelings are replaced by irritability, dysphoria (general feeling of unease), and anxiety. These feelings lead the user to smoke again to try and recapture the high. Thus crack is almost always used in a binge pattern whether smoked, injected, or even snorted. Physical side effects of smokable cocaine include slurred speech, thirst, coughing, dry skin, blurred vision, and tremors. As use becomes chronic, chest pains, sore throat, black or bloody sputum, hypertension, weight loss, insomnia, tremors, and heart damage can occur.

Some of the other more unusual physical side effects include

◊ **crack keratitis** or abrasions of the eye due to the anesthetic effects of cocaine that make the user unaware of damage caused by rubbing the eye too much;

◊ **crack thumb** and **crack hands** that are caused by repetitive use of butane lighters to heat up crack pipes. A callus builds up on the thumb and the hand has multiple burns;

◊ **crack burns** that are superficial burns to the face and hands due to the use of small torches to melt freebase in a short glass pipe. More severe body burns result when the ether explodes during the freebase process.

Unwanted psychological effects of chronic use include paranoia, intense craving, asocial behavior, attention problems, irritability, drug dreams, hyperexcitability, visual and auditory hallucinations, depression, cocaine psychosis, and certain social problems such as high-risk sexual activity (Siegel, 1992; Castilla, Barrio, Belza, & de la Fuente, 1999).

Respiratory Effects

Because a user inhales an extremely harsh substance, smoking cocaine can also cause breathing problems, severe **fever, chest pains, pneumonia, coughs, crack lung, and other respiratory complications**, including hemorrhage, respiratory failure, and death due to the drug's effect on the medullary centers of the brain. Crack lung, a relatively new syndrome, describes the pain, breathing problems, and fever that resemble pneumonia (Gold & Miller, 1997). Crack reduces the ability of the lungs to diffuse carbon dioxide. Many crack smokers smoke the tar-like black residue in crack pipes and overload their lungs with this residue that makes it difficult for the normal clearance mechanisms of the lungs to function, resulting in black or dark brown sputum (Greenbaum, 1993). **All of the respiratory problems are further aggravated since the majority of users also smoke cigarettes.** Irritation, destruction of mucous membranes, and lung cancer can result from the combination.

"I had a lot of coughing after using it and shortness of breath. I didn't really notice it at the time but if I went out to ride my bike or lift weights, I would have a really hard time."
17-year-old male recovering crack smoker

Polydrug Abuse

As with snorted and injected cocaine, the intensive stimulation caused by smokable cocaine increases the potential for the abuse of depressants, especially alcohol, heroin, and sedative-hypnotics.

"Crack was my drug of choice, I would have a drink to mellow myself out. If the drink wouldn't do it I would go get me some hop heroin and snort it. It would make me come down but it would be a whole different high and it would make me sick because I don't do heroin! I am not cool with heroin. I just snort it to come down. That's it, that's all."
36-year-old recovering female crack user

Some smokers combine **freebase and marijuana in a combination called "champagne," "caviar,"** "gremmies," "fry daddies," "cocoa puff,"

"hubba," or "woolies." In addition users are even mixing PCP or ketamine with crack in a nasty mixture called "space basing," "whack," or "tragic magic." Further there is the addition of freebase cocaine to smokable tar heroin to make a **smokable speedball called "hot rocks"** or "Belushi rocks." Finally, crack or cocaine hydrochloride is being used with wine coolers for an oral speedball known as "crack coolers." When crack is not available, users have switched to shooting and even smoking methamphetamine (speed). A mixture of "crank" (methamphetamine sulfate) with crack smoked together is called "super crank."

Overdose

The most frequent symptoms of overdose that people experience when smoking cocaine are on the mild side: **very rapid heartbeat and hyperventilation**. However, these reactions are often accompanied by a feeling of impending death. Although most people survive and only get very sweaty and clammy and feel that they are going to die, several thousand in fact are killed by cocaine overdose every year. There were 4,864 deaths in 2001 due to the direct and indirect effects of cocaine use (DAWN, 2002). The **deaths resulted from cardiac arrest, seizure, stroke, respiratory failure, and even severe hyperthermia** (extra-high body temperature).

"A friend was freebasing heavily and he started going into convulsions and throwing up blood. It was real awful. I was really scared and I thought he was going to die. Me and my other friend, we just kept freebasing . . . and then when he came out of it, he started freebasing again."
Recovering 16-year-old girl

CONSEQUENCES OF CRACK USE

Economic Consequences

The crack trade expanded rapidly in the late 1980s because the dealers used the best sales strategies of a free enterprise system: reduce the price to increase sales; increase the size of the sales force to cover the territory more efficiently; encourage free trade to avoid tariffs and impounding; and **create appealing packaging to make the product attractive to a wider segment of the population** (Wesson, Smith, & Steffens, 1992).

The less expensive sale units of crack cocaine expanded the potential number of users especially among teenagers. **Crack is not cheaper than cocaine hydrochloride; it is just sold in smaller units.** One gram of cocaine hydrochloride is the standard street sale amount going for about $50 to $100. Now one-tenth of a gram that has been converted to crack or "rock" can be bought for $10 to $20, a manageable sum for teenagers and incidentally about twice the price of cocaine hydrochloride when figured on a per-gram basis. The economics of crack cocaine created more dealers and increased the availability of the drug. **There is an addiction to the money and lifestyle that comes from dealing** (Cross, Johnson, Rees Davis, & Liberty, 2001).

"I know it's jive, I know it's negative. I'm trapped in something here. But I'm used to the money. What else can I do? You gonna send me to McDonalds? After I'm generating this kind of money everyday, I can't go back to McDonalds for $6.50—what is it?— $6.75 an hour today, which is still insulting."
16-year-old crack dealer/user

Though a few young dealers buy new cars and show off their wealth, **the majority of the small-time dealers make just enough to support their own habit** or get by. Drug gang homicides are common as local gangs, along with gangs from other countries, vie to control the crack trade (Dunlop & Johnson, 1992). The gangs include the Bloods and the Crips, along with Dominicans, Puerto Ricans, Mexicans, Jamaicans, and especially the Colombians. A number of these gangs have also expanded the trade to smaller cities.

Social Consequences

"It seems like every time I would hit the pipe, my daughter would say, 'Mommy.' And so I would say, 'Why are you bothering me?' It really made me crazy. I mean, my son, he would just pick on things and make noise or something just to bother me because he knew that I was doing this."
Recovering crack user

Because of the compulsive nature of crack, **addictive use of the drug is still having devastating social ramifications** in the United States that include increased rates of abandonment, neglect, and abuse of children by single- or even no-parent families, and the increasing number of burned-out grandmothers caring for their crack-addicted daughter's children. It has also brought about the **formation of an underclass of women who trade sex for crack** at whatever price they can get (Goldstein, Ouellet, & Fendrick, 1992).

"It's two types of women using cocaine. One's a 'tossup' [a woman who trades sex for crack]. They're the ones who are down there. They done lost everything they have. They have no self-respect. Me and my sister, we'd work a brother in a minute to get his dope. Once we got his dope—'Go on, get outta my house.' Me and my sister, we paid our rent, we paid our utilities, we fed our children, we kept clothes on their backs, we kept the house clean. We had not lost our self-esteem. We had not hit rock bottom yet."
24-year-old female recovering crack user

In a study of 283 women who exchanged sex for money or crack, 30% were infected with HIV (Edlin, Irwin, & Faruque, 1994). For many men (particularly in some inner-city African American communities) a major impact on their families and society has occurred because of the **high rate of crime associated with crack use.** There have been high rates of imprisonment, violent deaths, and child abandonment by addicts. In fact about 75% of all inmates in prisons come from single-parent or no-parent homes (Federal Bureau of Prisons, 1997). The disruptive family environment coupled with cocaine use leads to economic and social chaos.

"Well crack is a drug that is so addictive that it takes your money, your furniture, your home, your car, your clothes. . . . And then you have to go to places where they feed the homeless. And it just takes everything. And when I was on heroin and speed, I had money. I kept money. I had an apartment. I paid my rent. But the crack cocaine drug was the most awful, the most terrifying drug that I ever experienced."
42-year-old recovering polydrug abuser

COCAINE VS. AMPHETAMINES

Although all the **physical and mental effects of cocaine and amphetamines are very similar**, there are differences.

The Price. A heavy cocaine user spends $100 to $300 a day whereas a heavy amphetamine user spends about $50 to $100 a day; although if the amphetamine user has developed an intense tolerance, the costs are similar.

Quality of the Rush or the High. When either cocaine or an amphetamine is smoked or injected intravenously, it produces an intense rush followed by a high or euphoria. When either drug is snorted, the intense rush usually doesn't occur, only the euphoria. When an amphetamine or cocaine is drunk, again, there is usually no rush, only the euphoria. Although it is hard to demonstrate experimentally, the majority of users seen at the Haight Ashbury Clinic claim that the rush and high from cocaine is much greater than that from amphetamines but amphetamines release greater amounts of energy.

"Cocaine is more euphoric and not as intense as speed. Speed is very intense and you're going, going, going. The coke is shorter lasting but the cravings are much worse. When I wanted to do speed, it was mainly because I wanted to get things done. I felt speed helped me perform. And the cocaine, I felt like I had absolutely no choice. Cocaine took me down real fast and real hard."
Crack cocaine smoker

Duration of Action. Cocaine's major effects last about 40 minutes; amphetamine's last 4–6 hours.

Manufacture. Cocaine is plant derived; amphetamines are synthetic.

Methods of Use. The most popular ways of using cocaine are snorting, smoking, or shooting. Amphetamines are most often snorted or injected.

Addiction Rate. A survey of clients at one treatment center showed that methamphetamine users fell into addiction more quickly than cocaine users and came into treatment more quickly (Gonzalez Castro, Barrington, Walton, & Rawson, 2000). When crack is involved, the slide to compulsive use is much quicker.

AMPHETAMINES

During 2000, **6,700 illegal methamphetamine laboratories were seized by the DEA and local/state law enforcement agencies** in the United States, a testimony to the growth of this powerful stimulant. In addition new efforts to limit the importation of precursor chemicals has been one of the reasons for the recent decrease in purity from 72% in 1994 to 35% in 2000. The overall supply however remains constant while use continues to spread to other parts of the United States from the West Coast.

CLASSIFICATION

Amphetamines are known as "sympathomimetic agents" because they stimulate the release of neurotransmitters in the brain that activate our sympathetic nervous system, which in turn controls our fight or flight response. They also stimulate the reward/reinforcement center. These amphetamines, known on the street as "uppers," "speed," "meth," "crank," "crystal," "ice," "shabu," and "glass," are a class of **powerful synthetic stimulants with effects very similar to cocaine but much longer lasting and somewhat cheaper to use**. Amphetamines are most often snorted, injected, or taken orally. Recently, smoking methamphetamine has increased in popularity especially with the more readily available methamphetamine called "ice" or "glass."

There are several different types of amphetamines: amphetamine, methamphetamine, dextroamphetamine, and dextro isomer methamphetamine base. The effects of each type are very similar; the major differences being their method of manufacture and their strength. There is also a difference in whether they have stronger psychological or physical effects.

HISTORY OF USE

Discovery

Amphetamine was first synthesized in 1887 in a systematic effort to synthesize ephedrine, a natural extract of the ephedra bush, used to treat asthma. Interestingly the stimulant qualities and medical applications weren't recognized until the 1930s when Methedrine® (methamphetamine) and Benzedrine® (dextroamphetamine) inhalers were marketed as bronchodilators to help asthmatics breathe. Benzedrine® and Methedrine® were also discovered to be stimulants that could **energize the user, counter low blood pressure, reduce the need for sleep,**

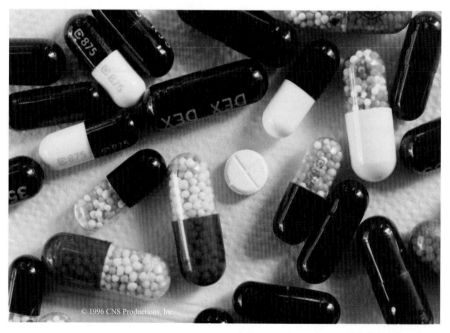

In the past, traditional types of speed diverted to street use or manufactured illegally were small tablets of amphetamine ("crosstops") from Mexico; Biphetamines® ("black beauties"); Dexedrine® ("dexys," "beans"); Benzedrine® ("bennies"), one of the classic "stay awake" amphetamine pills; and Methedrine® (or Ambar®), a methamphetamine. Interestingly the pills and tablets shown here look exactly like the real drugs but are known as "lookalikes" and were falsely sold as the actual drugs.

and suppress appetite. The drugs were also used to treat MBD or minimal brain dysfunction. The inhalers were sold over the counter until 1959 while prescription Methedrine® wasn't taken off the market until 1968.

Amphetamines were also widely used in pill form during World War II by Allied, German, and Japanese forces to keep pilots alert for extended missions and to keep ground troops awake and somewhat more aggressive in battle. An estimated 200 million Benzedrine® tablets were legally dispensed to American GIs during World War II and another 225 million during the Vietnam conflict between 1966 and 1969 (Miller & Kozel, 1995; Grinspoon & Hedblom, 1975).

Amphetamines were also used to **treat narcolepsy (falling asleep sickness), epilepsy (a subtype), and depression**. Concurrently amphetamines came to be abused by students cramming for exams, truckers on long hauls, workers laboring long hours, and soldiers or pilots trying to stay awake for 48 hours straight.

Japanese Epidemic

Abuse of amphetamines in Japan continued after World War II when large stocks of the drug were looted from military supplies and sold on the black market. The enactment of Japan's Stimulant Drug Program in 1951 brought the problem under some control (Fukui, Wada, & Iyo, 1991). However, amphetamine abuse continues and there are still 1–2 million amphetamine users and 15,000–25,000 arrests for dealing and using each year. The Japanese crime syndicates (Yakuza) smuggle the drugs from China or the Philippines and control the sales. One bust alone seized 500 kg of the substance worth over $200 million in retail sales.

Diet Pills

Recognizing the appetite-suppressing properties of amphetamines, pharmaceutical companies in the '50s and '60s promoted their use to a growing segment of society that wanted to lose weight. Their advertising led to huge quantities of amphetamines and methamphetamines, including Dietamine®, Nobese®, Obetrol®, Bar-Dex®, Dexedrine®, and Dexamyl®, flooding the prescription drug market. Worldwide legal production in 1970 was estimated to be 10 billion tablets (Karch, 1996). **In 1970 an estimated 6% to 8% of the American population was using prescription amphetamines mostly for weight loss** (Ellinwood, 1973). The fact that amphetamines also induced euphoria and elation did not hurt the desirability of the stimulants. As early as 1943 over half of Smith, Kline & French Pharmaceuticals® Benzedrine® sales were prescribed for people who wanted to lose weight or counteract depression. It was in fact one of the first antidepressants available to physicians (Grinspoon & Hedblom, 1975).

Street Speed

The 1960s were the peak of the speed craze that was supplied by both diverted and illegally manufactured amphetamines. The power for the "Summer of Love," one of the cornerstones of the hippie movement, was fueled by the energy chemicals released by amphetamines. In a reaction to the speed epidemic, the **Controlled Substance Act of 1970 classified amphetamines as Schedule II drugs** and made it hard to buy them legally in the United States. In addition prescription use of the drugs was more tightly regulated. The street market expanded to fill the need, so instead of buying legally manufactured amphetamines that had been diverted, people bought speed and "crank" that had been manufactured illegally. The purity rose from an average of 30% in the early '70s to 60% by 1983 (King & Ellinwood, 1997).

"I very seldom ran out in the beginning in the '60s and '70s. It was cheap; people gave it away. It wasn't like using dope. You didn't have to get money together every day."
38-year-old female speed user

The most popular form of street speed was the "crosstop." Also called "cartwheels" and "white crosses," these were diverted and smuggled into the United States from Mexico. In the early 1970s they cost $5 to $10 per 100 tablets. In the 1990s the price was $1 to $5 per tablet if they could be found. As of the 2000s what are most often available are bogus (lookalike) "crosstops" that contain either caffeine or ephedrine instead of an amphetamine.

The late '80s and '90s saw a resurgence in the availability and abuse of illicit methamphetamines, particularly **"crank" (methamphetamine sulfate) and "crystal" (methamphetamine hydrochloride)**. Once stymied by the tight control of chemicals needed to produce illegal amphetamines, clever street chemists learned to alter commonly available compounds to produce speed products. However, some of the street meth even in the 1980s was actually lookalike drugs, including phenylpropanolamine (a decongestant), ephedrine, pseudoephedrine, or simply caffeine tablets disguised to look like amphetamine products.

"Ice"

As the 1990s began, a highly potent and **smokable form of methamphetamine**, dextro isomer methamphetamine HCL ("ice," "glass," "batu," or "shabu"), had taken center stage, at least in the press. Besides its smokability, greater strength, and longer duration of effects, "ice" had the appeal of a new fad. As with the spread of smokable crack cocaine, "ice" was initially being marketed as a "newer better amphetamine." It cost 2–3 times as much as methamphetamine, which is surprising because it can be made with a very simple and safe crystallization process.

Surprisingly, perhaps because it is so intense, "ice" did not catch on in the United States as a common drug of abuse except in Hawaii and a few places on the West Coast. However, some Asian countries had a severe "ice" problem. The Philippines was estimated to have 400,000 "shabu" addicts in 1992. The average daily dose was from 1–3 grams at a cost of $10 to $20 per gram (Wesson et al., 1992). Recently though, be-

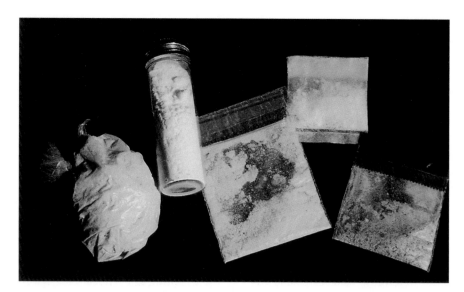

Several street samples of methamphetamines are being manufactured illegally including "crank," "crystal," and a scarce form called "peanut butter meth" on the left. Most methamphetamines on the wholesale level are off-white or yellow. In home labs the methamphetamine can be of almost any color since many small-time street chemists don't really know what they're doing.

Courtesy of Lt. Ed Mayer and JACNET, Jackson County, Oregon

cause of simpler manufacturing techniques, most of the methamphetamine being seized in the United States is, in fact, dextro isomer methamphetamine base ("ice"); although it is not only smoked, it is shot and snorted as well (DEA, 2002a).

Current Use

Licit Use. Amphetamines and methamphetamines are used to **treat attention-deficit/hyperactivity disorder, narcolepsy** (a type of epilepsy), and occasionally **weight control**.

Illicit Use. From 1993 to 2000 the number of people admitted for amphetamine addiction more than doubled, partly due to

◊ the aging of that population,

◊ the extended periods of chronic use,

◊ and the spread of use to other states (DASIS Report, 2001).

The resurgence, particularly in the use of illicit methamphetamines (predominantly "crank" and "crystal meth"), has been signaled by the dramatic increase in the number of methamphetamine labs raided by the authorities, particularly in California, Oregon, Texas, and more recently in the Midwest. While methamphetamine use in 2001 was less than half the peak level of the early 1980s, the current growth is troublesome (SAMHSA, 2002). An additional worry is that the age of first use has dropped. Some 10–13 year-olds are smoking, eating, and snorting "crank." **Some of the reasons for this upsurge are lower prices and increased availability.**

While the use of methamphetamine has dropped, the use of MDMA (ecstasy), a psycho-stimulant, has increased dramatically, fulfilling the stimulant cravings of large numbers of young people although it is often also used to boost the effects of ecstasy (*see Chapter 6*).

"I started shooting speed and I couldn't keep getting $20 bucks from my mom, you know. I had to either start selling it or start stealing stuff 'cause I had a big habit. So I was stealing cars and I was jacking stereos and I would rip

anybody off who gave me money just to get myself high. Incidentally, stealing the car was also a high."
17-year-old recovering IV meth user

The profile of the typical user is a white male between the ages of 19 and 40. Recently there has been increased use among women. Historically, **stimulant epidemics last about 10–15 years** and go in waves from one coast of the United States to the other. Methamphetamine use swept towards the eastern and southern United States in the 1990s and to everywhere else in the 2000s although the heaviest use is still out West. Eventually, **due to the intensity of the high and the severity of the side effects, amphetamine abuse becomes self-limiting** and the rapid growth of use levels out.

Methamphetamine Manufacturing

Over the years **much of the street manufacturing and dealing of methamphetamines was by biker gangs** (Hell's Angels and Gypsy Jokers) because of the money involved and the partiality of bikers to the drug. But there has been an **ever-increasing involvement of Mexican gangs and drug cartels** in the manufacturing and distribution of the drug.

Historically labs made methamphetamines with the P$_2$P method (total synthesis) or by reduction of ephedrine or pseudoephedrine. In raided laboratories, only 3% still used the P$_2$P method. One of the reasons for the resurgence in the use of methamphetamine is new, somewhat safer, cheaper, and almost odor-free manufacturing techniques (Marnell, 1997). **Illicit methamphetamine manufacturing used to be an extremely risky business.** The fumes were toxic and explosions could and did occur if the chemicals were handled improperly. Foul odors that emanated from the "cookers" were of great help to law enforcement agencies in locating methamphetamine labs. Now methamphetamine can even be manufactured on a stove top. The DEA estimates that there are over 300 ways to manufacture methamphetamine (DEA, 1998). A user can go to the hardware store and get items such as rock salt, battery acid, red phosphorous road flares, pool acid, mason jars, coffee filters, and plastic tubing to help in the manufacturing (Keefe, 2001). In 1998 the Methamphetamine Trafficking Penalty Enhancement Act equalized the penalties for methamphetamine with those for crack cocaine while the Methamphetamine Anti-Proliferation Act of 1999 gave increased assistance to the DEA and local officials to fight the spread of methamphetamine.

One of the changes in methamphetamine manufacturing has been due to the restriction in selling certain precursor chemicals. The main precursor, **ephedrine, is mostly smuggled from China to the United States through Mexico or Canada. In China the drug is extracted from the ephedra bush.** Some of the ephedrine comes from Germany where it is synthesized. A small portion is converted to methamphetamine in Mexico but the majority is smuggled into the United States (mainly central and Southern California) and then converted. When ephedrine is not available, pseudoephedrine (found in many OTC cold tablets and medicines) can be used.

The growth of methamphetamine use and manufacturing in the Midwest was emphasized by the 235 labs that were raided just in Missouri. Methamphetamine cases in that state account for 80% of domestic violence cases and police department drug investigations (DEA, 2002c). In the past most of the laboratories were small enterprises capable of producing only a pound or so of methamphetamine a day but those run by Mexican gangs (26% of the total and mostly in the West) can cook 10–150 pounds in just 2 days. The DEA estimates that the Mexican-run labs manufacture three-fourths of the methamphetamine consumed in the United States. One pound of methamphetamine wholesales for $4,000 to $30,000, 1 ounce for $500 to $2,500, and 1 gram for $25 to $150 (DEA, 2002a).

One other problem with the illegal synthesis of methamphetamine is the **environmental danger of the chemicals used in the manufacturing process** even with the newer manufacturing methods. Labs have been found in rented hotel rooms, backyard trailers, apartments, and rented houses. When done making the methamphetamine or when the law is too close, the makers of the drug simply abandon the room or property. Toxins and cancer-causing agents, such as acetone, red phosphorus, hydrochloric acid, benzene, and lead acetate, are left behind or secretly dumped into streams and landfills. It costs thousands of dollars to clean up each raided laboratory.

One of the **recent developments internationally is the use of ya ba**, also called "yaa maa," "yaa baa," and "Nazi speed." Manufactured in Thailand, Laos, and particularly Myanmar (Burma), the little brightly colored pills are being smuggled into the United States in ever-increasing amounts. Ya ba is taken orally or crushed and smoked on a piece of foil. Mostly though, this methamphetamine is abused in Thailand and other Asian countries where it sells for about $2–$3 a pill (Leinwand, 2002a). It is estimated that 1 billion pills were made last year in dozens of secret laboratories on the Myanmar border. It used to be the drug of poor men—taxi drivers and long-distance drivers—to stay awake and keep working but recently, as with other countries, use spread to discotheques and schools. About 700 patients are being treated at the main drug detoxification hospital in Bangkok. Younger and younger people are using the drug as the mid-level dealers enlist poor students to handle low-level distribution (Calvani, 2002). An interesting side note reported in the *Bangkok Post* on July 19, 1996, was that the pills used to be called "yaa maa," which in the Thai language means "horse drug." The government renamed them "yaa baa" or "ya ba" meaning "madness drug" in order to discourage its rural citizens from using the drug because "yaa maa" gave them the impression that it would enable them to work like a horse.

EFFECTS

Routes of Administration

Snorting methamphetamine causes irritation and pain to the nasal mucosa especially when used to excess.

Intravenous use puts large quantities of the drug directly into the bloodstream and causes a more intense high than snorting or swallowing; however it often causes pain in the blood vessels. Also, with injecting, there is the attendant risk of contaminated needles.

Oral ingestion used to be more popular but takes longer to reach the brain. Because of the extremely bitter taste of methamphetamines, they are often put into a gelatin capsule or in a piece of paper when taken orally.

"Smoking methamphetamine gives you a good rush. I mean, it's a lot better than snorting it as far as the rush goes. You breathe out and you feel that feeling. It's kind of like shooting but it's different. It's more mellow and it's a shorter high."

Intravenous methamphetamine user

Because of the dangers in shooting methamphetamine, some users have taken to smoking "crank," "crystal," or "ice." The technique of **smoking "crank" or "ice" is similar to smoking freebase cocaine** (in a pipe). Smoking gets the drug to the brain faster. No matter how the drug is taken, amphetamines last 4–6 hours compared to only 10 minutes to $1\frac{1}{2}$ hours for cocaine. "Ice," the smokable form of methamphetamine, is alleged to last at least 8 hours, some say up to 24 hours, after it is smoked.

Neurochemistry

Use of amphetamines increases the levels of catecholamine neurotransmitters (**epinephrine, norepinephrine, and dopamine**) in three ways as opposed to cocaine, which increases the levels in two ways. Amphetamines and cocaine

◇ **stimulate the release of catecholamines,**

◇ **block their reuptake** in the sending neuron,

◇ but only **amphetamines block their metabolism**.

This means that the excess catecholamines exist in the synapse for a much longer time than cocaine thereby prolonging the effects.

Long-term use of amphetamines causes long-term and even permanent alterations in the ability of the body to produce these vital neurotransmitters. In animal studies norepinephrine levels were depressed 3–6 months after cessation of heavy use (King & Ellinwood, 1997). Dopamine levels also remained depressed after cessation of use. Another study of former methamphetamine abusers compared to a nonusing control group showed a 24% decrease in dopamine transporters thus causing a disruption in movement control and feelings of pleasure (Volkow et al., 2001). This means that the user comes to rely on artificial stimulants to keep their dopamine and norepinephrine activity feeling like normal, let alone raised.

In other words **prolonged amphetamine use, in and of itself, alters brain chemistry in a way that increases craving (endogenous craving)**. This process also occurs with cocaine.

In addition to depleting neurotransmitters, researchers in 1996 demonstrated that high-dose methamphetamine use causes definitive degeneration of serotonin fibers in the brain within hours after use (Zhou & Bledsoe, 1996).

Physical Effects

As with cocaine the initial physiological effects of small-to-moderate doses of amphetamines include **increased heart rate, raised body temperature, rapid respiration, higher blood pressure, extra energy, dilation of bronchial vessels, and appetite suppression**.

"I would inject some speed and right after doing it you get an incredible rush, which some people compare with sexual feelings. And your heart pounds and I've seen people actually pass out from having too much speed. My heart would pound, and I would sweat, and the rush would pass, and then I would just be very high energy."
19-year-old recovering meth user

As with cocaine users **methamphetamine abusers go on binges or "runs," staying up for 3, 4, or even up to 10 days at a time**, putting a severe strain on their bodies, particularly the cardiovascular and nervous systems. During these runs people will try to use their excess energy any way they can—dancing, exercising, cleaning the kitchen at midnight, taking apart a car, or painting the whole house.

"I liked to do little intricate drawings. I would draw for hours, anything small with a lot of detail. I would clean my apartment from top to bottom, even doing my floor with Brillo® pads— my wooden floor—vacuuming my ceiling. If I ran out of stuff to do I would dump out everything in the vacuum cleaner and vacuum it back up. I didn't like to be outside because I would get paranoid."
38-year-old recovering amphetamine user

Tolerance to amphetamines is pronounced. Whereas 15–30 mg per day is the usual prescribed dose, a long-term user might use 5,000 mg or 5 grams over a 24-hour period during a "speed run." This means that extended use (or the use of large quantities) will lead to extreme depression and lethargy.

"If I didn't have speed, if I ran out, I would become depressed, very anxiety-ridden. I had suicidal thoughts and I would sleep for long stretches of time 'till I had more speed. And then I would start the whole process over again."
33-year-old recovering speed user

Long-term use can cause sleep deprivation, heart and blood vessel toxicity, and **severe malnutrition**. The blood vessel toxicity can cause extensive damage to cerebral vasculature resulting in multiple aneurysms (the ballooning out of capillary weak spots). With long-term use and hypertensive episodes, the user can experience a cerebral hemorrhage (stroke) and ar-

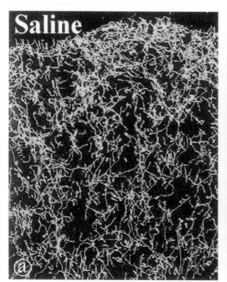
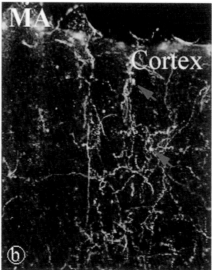

Injection of methamphetamine into normal rat brain tissue (a) causes degeneration of serotonin nerve fibers 5-HTT (b). Fibers were reduced in a number of regions in the brain, including the frontal and parietal cortices (a and b), hippocampus, striatum, and thalamus (Zhou & Bledsoe, 1996). Reprinted by permission, Neuroscience.

rhythmias, possibly caused by myocardial (heart muscle) lesions (King & Ellinwood, 1997). Research also suggests that methamphetamine use after a stroke will increase the amount of damage (Wang, 2001). The malnutrition plus the calcium-leaching effects of **amphetamine overuse often results in bad or rotted teeth**. One of the confirming signs of amphetamine abuse is poor dental health.

Finally, if the user has not built up a tolerance, is unusually sensitive, or takes a very large amount, an **overdose** can occur (convulsions, hyperthermia, stroke, cardiovascular overexcitation, and collapse).

"I shot some speed once and immediately had a seizure. Apparently my heart stopped beating and the person I was with was pounding on my chest. I was real sore and black and blue the next day."
38-year-old meth user

Mental & Emotional Effects

Amphetamines initially **produce a mild-to-intense euphoria and a feeling of well-being. But with prolonged use irritability, paranoia, anxiety, mental confusion, poor judgment, and even hallucinations** can be induced by the unbalanced neurotransmitters.

Amphetamines release neurotransmitters that mimic sexual gratification. Thus they are sometimes used to augment sexual activity and by those prone toward multiple partners and/or prolonged sexual interactions. The drug has also been heavily used in gay populations for sexual endurance. But again, because of the rapid development of tolerance, there is an eventual decrease of sex drive and performance. For many users the rush from shooting or smoking **methamphetamine becomes a substitute for sexual activity**.

"I didn't really go out with anybody when I was using. I chose the drugs over any girl, any time. If I asked a girl out and she told me to meet her somewhere and my dealer told me to meet
him at the same time, I'd go with my dealer and try to score more drugs than go with her. The girls were always last on my list."
Recovering 19-year-old meth abuser

Aggression caused by excessive amphetamine use depends on the dose, the setting, and the preexisting susceptibility to violence in the user. **The increased suspiciousness, paranoia, and overconfidence lead to misinterpretations of others' actions and hence to violent reactions.** Taken to extremes prolonged use can result in violent, suicidal, and even homicidal thoughts. Strangely, in those with hyperactivity disorder, amphetamines can help to control their aggression (King & Ellinwood, 1997).

Amphetamine psychosis can be caused by excessive amphetamine use just as excessive cocaine use can cause cocaine psychosis. And just as with cocaine, **symptoms include hallucinations, loss of contact with reality, and pressed speech that is almost indistinguishable from true schizophrenia or paranoid psychosis**. It is the ability of methamphetamines to release excess dopamine that accounts for most of the symptoms. Conversely drugs that control the symptoms are those that limit or block dopamine release. The amount of amphetamines necessary to precipitate a psychosis has been the subject of several investigations. Early studies reported cases where a mere 55 mg precipitated a psychosis and others where it took 2,000 mg to 5,000 mg. Half the users in one study experienced psychotic episodes within 2 years of beginning use and others took 10 years to react so severely (Grinspoon & Hedblom, 1975).

The first amphetamine psychoses were noted in the late 1930s shortly after the drug came into common usage. Many more cases were noted during World War II and in the '50s and '60s when amphetamines became the drug of choice.

Amphetamine psychosis from excessive use and the listless depression that often comes from withdrawal of high-dose intravenous use or heavy

smoking of "ice" are usually not permanent although recent research may indicate that the depression may indeed be permanent in some users (Zhou & Bledsoe, 1996).

"I just got so sick of it, you know, just being high for so long. It just messes up your mind. I once stayed up for 23 days with no sleep—not 1 hour of sleep, not one wink of sleep. When you stay up for that long, you're just like a pile of mush. Your brain's just nothing, you know. You can't even talk. And it just doesn't even feel good. I don't want that feeling anymore."
17-year-old recovering meth abuser

Upon cessation of use, the disturbed user will usually return to some semblance of normalcy after the brain chemistry has been rebalanced, usually within a week. If there was a pre-existing mental condition, recovery can take a lot longer. Since extended use can also damage nerve cells, a number of the changes in long-term users, even without pre-existing mental problems, can last a lifetime (Richards, Baggot, Sabol, & Seiden, 1999).

Much of the current interest in "crank," "crystal," and "ice" abuse is concentrated among adolescents and older teenagers, particularly among Asian American and Caucasian American youth. There is also a significant abuse of amphetamines by biker gangs and by gay and lesbian subcultures. Recently there has been an increasing abuse of these drugs in the Hispanic community. In addition **the ability of amphetamines to suppress appetite is still one of the main reasons for their current popularity**. The projection of an ideal thin body in advertisements helps promote current abuse, much as it did in the '50s, '60s, and '70s before government regulations limited the legal supply of the drug.

Effects of "Ice"

"Ice" stimulates the brain to a greater degree than the regular methamphetamine but stimulates the heart, blood vessels, and lungs to a lesser degree. The decrease in cardiovascular effects (up to 25% less than that of regular "crank") encourages users to smoke more, resulting in more overdoses and a quicker disruption of neurotransmitters. This disruption means **more "tweaking" or severe paranoid, hallucinatory, and hypervigilant thinking, along with greater suicidal depression and addictive use.** Detoxification from mental and psychotic symptoms of excessive "ice" use usually takes several days longer than detoxifying from regular methamphetamine abuse.

Right-Handed & Left-Handed Molecules

The increasing sophistication of street chemists can be seen in current methamphetamine manufacturing techniques. "Ice" is a specific and subtle form of the methamphetamine molecule known to scientists as an **"optical isomer."** When such a molecule is being formed, nature creates mirror images of atomic bonds such that half of the molecules formed are right-handed isomers and the other half are left-handed isomers (Fig. 3-3).

The amazing feature of this situation is that the two individual isomers often have very different effects on the body. **A dextro (right-handed) isomer methamphetamine base molecule is 2–4 times stronger in stimulating the brain than the levo (left-handed) isomer methamphetamine base.** However, the levo isomer is 2–4 times stronger in stimulating the heart, blood vessels, and nasal sinuses than the dextro isomer. By the late 1980s street chemists learned that if they used pure left-handed pseudoephedrine to make methamphetamine, it would be transformed to pure right-handed or dextro isomer methamphetamine base, which is stronger, lasts longer, and is more smokable than regular "crank" or "crystal meth." It is also less toxic to the cardiovascular system. **In the 2000s much of the methamphetamine sold as meth is actually "ice."** This means that the methamphetamine on the streets has increased in strength over the last 10 years even though the street purity might have remained the same.

AMPHETAMINE CONGENERS

When the prescription use of amphetamines was severely limited because of federal legislation, physicians turned to amphetamine congeners to help treat certain problems that had previously been treated with the stronger stimulants. Amphetamine congeners are stimulant drugs that are chemically dissimilar but pharmacologically related to amphetamines and produce many of the same effects as amphetamines and methamphetamines but are not as strong.

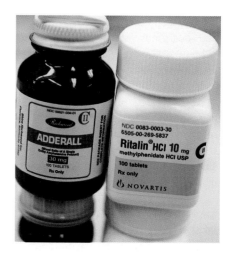

The two most common medications for ADHD are methylphenidate (e.g., Ritalin®, Concerta®) and amphetamine (e.g., Adderall®).

METHYLPHENIDATE (Ritalin®) & ATTENTION-DEFICIT/HYPERACTIVITY DISORDER (ADHD)

Methylphenidate (Ritalin®) is one of the most widely used amphetamine congeners. It is prescribed as a mood elevator or as a treatment for narcolepsy, a sleep disorder. However, it is most often prescribed to deal with attention-deficit/hyperactivity disorder (ADHD) (APA, 2000). Amphetamines are also widely prescribed for ADHD.

Diagnosis of ADHD

Tests for ADHD often rely on diagnostic interview methods but since **there is still no explicit diagnostic test, controversy continues about the extent and the severity of this disorder** (National Institutes of Health [NIH], 1998). Diagnosis is particularly difficult in early childhood because other conditions can cause many of the same symptoms. For example, inattention often occurs among children with a low IQ or those with high intelligence who are placed in understimulating environments. In order to attain more precise diagnoses, Dr. Daniel Amen, an ADHD specialist, and others have used single photon emission computerized tomography (SPECT) scans to pinpoint brain activity that signifies attention-

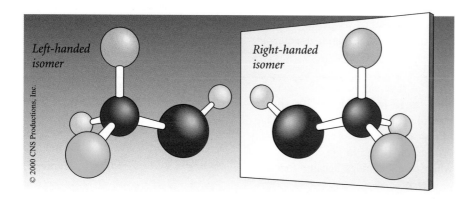

Figure 3-3 •

In this example of right- and left-handed molecules, notice that you need four nonidentical bonds.

© 2000 CNS Productions, Inc.

Left-handed isomer

Right-handed isomer

deficit disorder. In one imaging study part of the corpus callosum in children with ADHD was smaller than in a control group, suggesting dysfunction in self-regulation and attention (Semrud-Clikeman et al., 1994). Recent magnetic resonance imaging (MRI) studies of 152 children with ADHD found that their cerebrums were 3.2% smaller compared to a control group while the underlying white matter was 6% smaller. The smaller brain did not signify lower intelligence (Castellanos et al., 2002). It will still take many years of additional research to be able to diagnose ADHD accurately and then the questions of treatment come to the fore. For this reason the use of medications to treat ADHD remains controversial.

This disease is classified under the *International Classification of Diseases (ICD-10)* of the World Health Organization (WHO) into 3 subtypes: (1) hyperkinetic disorder, (2) disturbance of activity and attention, and (3) hyperkinetic conduct disorder (World Health Organization [WHO], 1998).

In the United States the 3 subtypes of ADHD according to the *DSM-IV-TR Diagnostic Manual of the American Psychiatric Association* are:

1. ADHD, Combined Type
2. ADHD, Predominantly Inattentive Type
3. ADHD, Predominantly Hyperactive-Impulsive Type

The person with **ADHD, Predominantly Inattentive Type** (attention-deficit disorder or ADD) or the **Combined Type** has 6 or more of the following symptoms.

Inattention

a) Displays **inattention to details** that causes careless mistakes in school or at work.
b) Has **difficulty sustaining attention** at work or play.
c) **Doesn't seem to listen** when spoken to directly.
d) **Doesn't follow through** on schoolwork, chores, or duties.
e) Has **difficulty organizing** tasks or activities.

f) **Avoids tasks that require sustained mental effort**.
g) Often **loses things** necessary for tasks or activities.
h) Is often **easily distracted** by extraneous stimuli.
i) Is often **forgetful** in daily activities.

The person with **Predominantly Hyperactive-Impulsive Type** (hyperactivity disorder or HD) or the **Combined Type** has 6 or more of the following symptoms.

Impulsivity

a) Often **fidgets** with hands or feet or squirms in seat.
b) Often **leaves seat**.
c) Often **runs about or climbs excessively** in inappropriate situations.
d) Has **difficulty playing or engaging in leisure activities quietly**.
e) Is often on the go or often **acts as if driven**.
f) Often **talks excessively**.

Hyperactivity

a) Often **blurts out answers** before questions are completed.
b) Often has **difficulty awaiting turn**.
c) **Often interrupts** or intrudes on others.

In diagnosing ADD, HD, or a combination ADHD,

a) some **symptoms must be present before the age of 7**;
b) symptoms should manifest themselves in at least **two different settings**;
c) there must be evidence of **impairment of social functioning**;
d) the symptoms are **not better accounted for by other mental disorders**.

(APA, 2000)

Epidemiology

Since diagnostic judgments are necessarily subjective, estimates of the prevalence of ADHD vary widely.

◇ It is estimated that between **2% and 9.5% of all school-age children worldwide have ADHD**.

◇ Between **3% to 7% of all school-age children in the United States have ADHD** (APA, 2000).

◇ ADHD is at least **three times as prevalent in boys** as in girls (Barkley, 1998). Mood changes, social withdrawal, and fear are more common in girls than the aggressiveness and impulsivity found in boys.

◇ If one examines children receiving psychiatric treatment, about 40% to 70% of inpatients and 30% to 50% of outpatients could be diagnosed with ADHD (Cantwell, 1996; Pliszka, 1998; Biederman, Faraone, et al., 1993).

◇ In addition **10% to 50% of children with ADHD will continue to have symptoms in adulthood** (Weiss, Hechtman, Milroy, & Perlman, 1985; Mannuzza et al., 1991).

Pharmacotherapy for ADHD

It seems a contradiction that many stimulants in small doses have the ability to focus attention and control hyperactivity. It is theorized that **dopamine depletion is one of the main causes for ADHD** and amphetamines or amphetamine congeners force the release of dopamine and prevent its reuptake and metabolism. **Amphetamines are also prescribed for this condition.**

It is estimated that 750,000 to 1 million school children are receiving 20 million prescriptions for stimulants and the figure is growing (IMS Health, 2002). These drugs, such as **methylphenidate (Ritalin®), d-amphetamine (Dexedrine®, Adderall®), or pemoline (Cylert®), seem to work in about 75% of ADHD children**. Pemoline® use is decreasing because of the need to monitor liver function due to a possible complication of toxic hepatitis. Another drug that has been tried is modafinil (Provigil®), a new stimulant that has had some success. Other drugs that that have been tried with varying degrees of success are bupropion (Wellbutrin®) and clonidine (Catapres®). Recently different formulations of methylphenidate have been accepted for the ADHD market including Metadate CD®, Methylin®, and Concerta®, a time-release formulation of the drug. Production of methylphenidate increased more than 10-fold from 1990 to 1998 (DEA, 2002c). However since 1997 the use of stronger stimulants has increased from 15% to 36% for those in treatment. Recently a new drug atomoxetine (Strattea®), a non-stimulant, has been approved for the treatment of ADHD.

In addition to drug therapy other adjunctive or **separate therapies** that are employed **include lifestyle changes, education, behavior modification, psychotherapy, parenting classes, parent support groups, and dietary changes** (Pary, Lewis, Arnp, Matuschka, & Lippman, 2002).

Recent research by the National Institutes of Health studied the effectiveness of methylphenidate by itself, methylphenidate in conjunction with behavior-management therapy, behavior-management therapy alone, and just standard therapy available in the community. The researchers, working at six separate sites, found that **for those with ADHD alone, methylphenidate by itself was as effective as methylphenidate and therapy and more effective than therapy alone**. On the other hand 70% of the children that were studied also had other problems like depression and anxiety. In those cases behavior therapy provided significant benefits especially when used in combination with methylphenidate (Jensen, 1999).

Concerns Regarding ADHD Pharmacotherapy

In November 1999 the Colorado Board of Education **passed a resolution to discourage overprescription of drugs like methylphenidate** (Ritalin®) for ADHD and Luvox® (fluvoxamine maleate), an SSRI antidepressant drug prescribed for obsessive-compulsive disorder. Concerns about methylphenidate include the subjective nature of some ADHD diagnoses and the confusion with symptoms from other disorders or with the natural exuberance of childhood. The concern in some quarters was strong enough for the military to bar anyone who has used methylphenidate in childhood (after the age of 12) from military service. The military services are exempt from the American Disabilities Act, so they can bar potential enlistees because of ADHD. The irony of this stance is the fact that most governments, including the United States, have made amphetamines readily available to soldiers in combat.

Methylphenidate is a Schedule II drug (as are amphetamines), which means it has addiction liability. Users who abuse methylphenidate will develop tolerance quickly and continue to increase dosage. Occasionally they will even switch to snorting or injecting the drug to try to recapture the original effects. Methylphenidate has been **diverted to illegal distribution channels**, sold on the street, and used as a party drug. A few teenagers even appropriate their younger brother's or sister's supply to party with or to sell. When sold on the streets, methylphenidate tablets (called "pellets") sell for $3 to $10 each.

There are also **grave questions about the long-term effects of strong stimulants on children** in general and whether this leads to dependence on these kinds of drugs. Interestingly studies have shown an **increased risk of alcohol and drug abuse among adults with untreated ADHD** but the reasons for this relationship are hard to pinpoint (Biederman, Wilens, Mick, et al., 1997). Finally, in a group of adolescents in treatment for substance abuse disorders, about half also had diagnosable ADHD (Horner & Scheibe, 1997).

The high occurrence of ADHD in drug abusers might have several explanations.

◇ It could be an attempt at **self-medication**.

◇ It could be that **ADHD leads to social alienation and problems with self-esteem**, both of which are predictors of problems with alcohol and other drugs.

◇ It could be that the **pre-existence of a mental condition** makes one more likely to get into compulsive behavior.

◇ It could be that psychoactive stimulants make one more susceptible to drug use because of neurotransmitter disruption or increased **accept-**

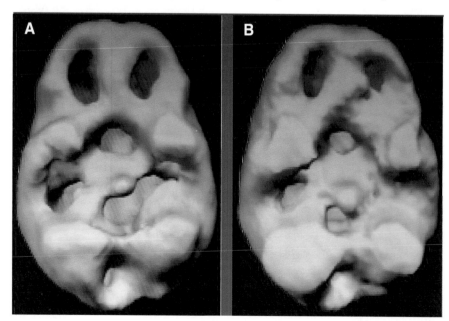

In these SPECT scans of a patient with attention-deficit disorder (A), the holes represent areas of the brain that are underactive (50% of normal or less), especially the area of the prefrontal cortex that controls the executive function (cingulate gyrus). When Ritalin®, is taken (B), it increases dopamine output from the basal ganglia and increases activity in the prefrontal cortex and frontal lobes.

Courtesy of the Amen Clinic for Behavioral Medicine, Fairfield and Newport Beach, CA (Amen, 1999)

ance of the idea of taking drugs to alleviate mental problems.

◇ Finally there could be **genetic factors that are common to both ADHD and substance abuse disorders**. One study found that the chance of an identical twin having the disorder if his brother has the disorder is 11–18 times greater than that of a nontwin sibling (Barkley, 1998). Another study at the University of Oslo found that heritability factors accounted for 80% of the differences between those with the disorder and those without. Other researchers found a strong genetic link between ADHD and other addictions or impulse-control disorders including heavy alcohol and drug use, compulsive overeating, gambling, and even Tourette's syndrome (Miller & Blum, 1996; Comings, Wu, Chiu, et al., 1996; Blum et al., 2000).

Nearly half of these children with ADHD have oppositional defiant disorder, a condition where they overreact to slights, can have outbursts of temper, be stubborn, or act defiant. If left untreated, these can progress to more serious conduct disorders including stealing, vandalism, and arson (National Institute of Mental Health [NIMH], 1999).

On the positive side a study at Harvard Medical School showed that boys (6–17 years old) with ADHD who are treated with stimulants, including Ritalin®, are 84% less likely to abuse drugs and alcohol when they get older compared to those who are not treated (Biederman, Wilens, Mick, Spencer, & Faraone, 1999).

In the last few years attention has focused on the continued presence of ADHD in large numbers of adults. Though earlier research had shown a reduction in the continuation of ADHD symptoms once puberty was reached, the **new research indicates the need to treat some ADHD patients with drugs like methylphenidate throughout their lives**.

DIET PILLS

In 2001 it was estimated that 300 million people worldwide were obese

Diet drug maker settles for $4.8 billion

By Julie Appleby
USA TODAY

American Home Products agreed Thursday to pay up to $4.8 billion over 16 years to settle claims from consumers who took the weight-loss combo known as "fen-phen."

45 days. If not enough people accept the deal, American could walk away from it.
The proposal includes:
▶ A $1 billion fund for medical tests to check for heart damage for anybody who took the drug and to provide treat-

ment if necessary.
▶ $2.3 billion to pay damages to those who now suffer or later develop moderate to severe heart-valve problems. Payment, based on age and severity of condition, ranges from $500 to $1.4 million.

Those with less severe disease could get more money later if their conditions worsen.
▶ Up to $429 million for plaintiffs' lawyers.
A toll-free number for more information and to register for the settlement is 800-386-2070.

and 750 million were overweight; of those about 150 million were in the United States. The market for people who want to lose weight is tremendous and historically there have been pharmaceutical companies selling both prescription and over-the-counter medications to help dieters. Unfortunately **each wave of diet drug use seemed to create problems**. In the '50s, '60s, and '70s, amphetamines and methamphetamines saturated the market but were found to cause heart problems, anorexia, and dependence. Amphetamine congeners were the next wave and those diet pills, with names like Adipex® and Obetrol®, again saturated the market saying they were safer than amphetamines and methamphetamines.

On September 30, 1999, American Home Products, as the defendant in a class-action lawsuit in federal court, agreed to pay $3.75 billion to $4.8 billion to all people who used two amphetamine congener diet pills, fenfluramine (Pondimin®) and dexfenfluramine (Redux®), and suffered or may suffer heart-valve damage. Prescription records show that approximately 5 million Americans have been prescribed Pondimin® or Redux®. Another amphetamine congener implicated in cases of heart-valve damage is phentermine (Ionamin® and Fastin®). The **combination of phentermine and fenfluramine or dexfenfluramine became known as "fen-phen"** and like other diet pill fads a severe price was paid for a pharmacological shortcut to weight loss. In 1997 a report by the Mayo Clinic said that its doctors had found 24 cases of heart-valve damage in "fen-phen" users (all women) (Connolly, Crary, McGoon, et al., 1997; Mayo Clinic, 1999). In September of 1997 the Food and Drug Administration (FDA) announced the withdrawal of fenfluramine and dexfenfluramine from the market in the United States. The law-

suits over this combination of diet pills continue into the 2000s.

Other popular amphetamine congeners used as diet pills include pemoline (Cylert®) and diethylpropion (Tenuate®, Tepanil®). The stimulation, loss of appetite, and mood elevation caused by amphetamine congener diet pills are weaker but similar to the effects of amphetamines with some of the same side effects: excitability, nervousness, and increased blood pressure, heart rate, and respiration. If used to excess, heart irregularities, convulsions, and even stroke, coma, and death can also occur. Despite their widespread use to control appetite and shed weight—there is significant weight loss in the first 4–6 months—users usually regain and even exceed their starting weights.

In general, **diet pills (amphetamines and amphetamine congeners) are only recommended for short-term use**, so careful monitoring by physicians is very important. Long-term and high-dose use of these diet pills has been associated with the development of abuse and addiction.

LOOKALIKE & OVER-THE-COUNTER (OTC) STIMULANTS

LOOKALIKES

The lookalike phenomenon in the 1980s contributed to the abuse of stimulants. By taking advantage of the interest in stimulant drugs, a few legitimate manufacturers began to make legal over-the-counter products that looked identical to prescription stimulants. Their various products **contained ephedrine and occasionally pseudoephedrine (anti-asthmatics),** phenylpropanolamine (PPA, a decongestant and a mild appetite suppressant), and caffeine (a stimulant). These were being combined, packaged, and sold as "legal stimulants" in a deliberate attempt to misrepresent the drugs as controlled drugs (Morgan, Wesson, Puder, & Smith, 1987). The same chemicals were also showing up as illicit amphetamine lookalikes, such as "street speed," "cartwheels," and "crank," and as cocaine lookalikes, such as Supercaine®, Supertoot®, and Snow®. The cocaine lookalikes often added benzocaine or procaine to mimic the numbing effects of the actual drug.

The problem with the lookalike products was their toxicity when overused, particularly when two or more of the drugs were combined. Also an amphetamine-like drug dependence developed in users who chronically abused the drugs (Tinsley & Wadkins, 1998). The physical problems, especially **cardiovascular problems, could be particularly severe since large amounts were required to get a speed- or cocaine-like high**. For these reasons, in the early 1980s the FDA banned the OTC sales of products containing two or more of these ingredients. Since that time the sale of lookalikes persists with individual OTC stimulants being packaged to look like controlled prescription stimulants. Further some manufacturers circumvented the combination ban by combining herbs that contain ephedrine, caffeine, or PPA rather than the drugs themselves. (*See Herbal Ecstasy® and Herbal Nexus® in this chapter.*) In 2000 the FDA put out a warning about using PPA, especially for young women. They recommended using products with pseudoephedrine instead. Many pharmaceutical companies replaced their products that contained PPA with ephedrine and pseudoephedrine. Recently the FDA has issued warnings about ephedra and ephedrine.

OTHER OVER-THE-COUNTER STIMULANTS

Pseudoephedrine and phenylpropanolamine (PPA), which have de-

congestant, mild anorexic, and stimulant effects, also used to be found in hundreds of allergy and cold medications (often in combination with antihistamines, such as Benadryl®) and in over-the-counter diet pills, like Dexadiet® and Dexatrim®. Individuals who ingested these drugs and drank coffee or other caffeinated beverages often experienced anxiety attacks and rapid heartbeats. Caffeine has been sold as an OTC stimulant for years in tablets with trade names such as NoDoz® and Vivarin®. The FDA is continuing to examine all of these products, issuing warnings and sometimes banning them outright. The debate continues.

MISCELLANEOUS PLANT STIMULANTS

Caffeine from the coffee bush and cocaine from the coca bush are often thought of as the principal plant stimulants by Americans, but worldwide dozens of plants or their extracts with stimulant properties have been used for centuries by hundreds of millions of people, often in the Middle East, Far East, and Africa. These plants include the **khat bush, betel nuts, the ephedra bush, and the yohimbe tree**.

KHAT & METHCATHINONE
Khat ("qat," "shat," "miraa")

In 2001 U.S. Customs officials seized 82,000 pounds of khat leaves, a plant stimulant. This hardly compares to the 1.5 million pounds of marijuana seized in the same year but it is a growing problem. Most of the leaves were destined for East African and Middle Eastern immigrants who have large enclaves in New York, Washington, DC, Dallas, and Los Angeles. In those cities khat branches with leaves are sold in bundles in some stores and restaurants (Leinwand, 2002b). Several years ago police arrested a Middle Eastern immigrant who was growing 1,000 plants he claimed were used medicinally to treat his diabetes. However, there is a growing group of teens and young adults who use khat, or its stronger synthetic version methcathinone, as a stimulant and exchange relevant information about using the drug via the Internet.

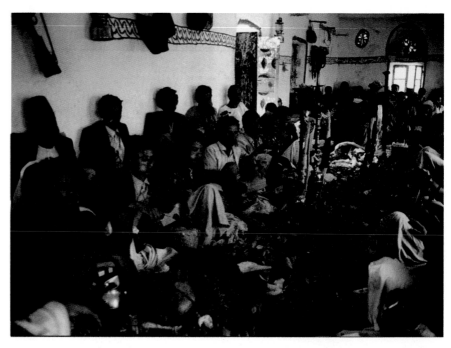

Khat is used socially in many countries in East Africa, southern Arabia, and the Middle East. Notice the piles of khat leaves on the dining table at this wedding in Yemen.
© Alain Labrousse, 1994

Back in 1992 when the United States sent troops to Somalia, the soldiers were surprised to find a large percentage of the population chewing the leaves, twigs, and shoots of the khat shrub (*Catha edulis*) in order to get stimulant sensations somewhere between those of coffee and methamphetamine. In Yemen, another country on the Arabian Peninsula, more than half the population uses khat and it is not unusual for people to spend over one-third of their family income on the drug. **It is the driving economic force in Somalia, Yemen, and a few other countries in East Africa, southern Arabia, and the Middle East.** Such drug usage is not a new development in those countries. References to khat can be found in Arab journals from the thirteenth century. The leaves were used by some physicians as a treatment for depression but **mostly it was and is used in social settings**. Many homes in some Middle Eastern countries actually have a room dedicated to khat chewing, similar to British homes that have a tearoom or parlor. Khat is used mostly by men in the countries where it is cultivated.

The khat shrub is 10–20 ft. tall. Because the main active ingredients can lose potency unless handled quickly, the leaves and sprouts are harvested early in the morning, kept moist, and speedily transported to market where they are sold by noon. **The fresh leaves and tender stems are chewed and the juice swallowed.** Dried leaves and twigs, which are not as potent as the fresh leaves, can be **crushed for tea or made into a chewable paste** (U.S. Department of Justice, 1992).

The **main psychoactive ingredient, cathinone,** only has a half-life of approximately 90 minutes, so the leaf must be chewed continuously to sustain a high. Cathinone is a naturally occurring amphetamine-like substance that produces a similar **mild euphoric effect, along with exhilaration, talkativeness, enhanced self-esteem, hyperactivity, wakefulness, aggressiveness, and loss of appetite.** Unfortunately side effects include anorexia, tachycardia, hypertension, dependence, chronic insomnia, and

gastric disorders (Kalix, 1994). People who use too much khat can become irritable, angry, and often violent.

Chronic khat abuse can result in physical exhaustion and suicidal depression upon withdrawal, symptoms similar to those seen with amphetamine withdrawal. There are also rare reports of paranoid hallucinations and even overdose deaths. In experiments with monkeys where the animals were allowed to self-administer a drug to see if it was addictive, cathinone was shown to have a powerful reinforcing effect. The binge pattern of use found with cocaine and amphetamines was repeated by the monkeys with cathinone use (Goudie & Newton, 1985).

Worldwide **hundreds of millions of dollars are spent on the drug** even in poor countries. The stimulation and subsequent crash caused by khat has had an economic impact on countries, including reduced work hours, decreased production, income loss, and malnutrition (Giannini, Burge, Shaheen, & Price, 1986).

Methcathinone

In the early 1990s in the United States a **synthetic version of cathinone** called "methcathinone" was synthesized in illegal laboratories in the Midwest and sold on the street as a powerful alternative to methamphetamine. It is **usually snorted** but can be taken orally (mixed in a liquid), intravenously, and smoked in a crack pipe, in a cigarette, or in a joint. Since it is cheap to manufacture, a number of labs have sprung up. By the end of 1994, 34 methcathinone laboratories had been raided in Michigan and recently law enforcement officers have found labs in other Midwest states, including 22 in Indiana and 8 in Wisconsin. Like methamphetamine manufacturing, ephedrine is the main raw ingredient for methcathinone synthesis. One gram of the drug sells for $40 to $120 compared to methamphetamine that sells for $40 to $200 (DEA, 2002c).

Methcathinone (also known as "ephedrone") was originally synthesized by Parke-Davis Pharmaceuticals

in 1957 in the United States but rejected for production due to side effects. The formula became widely known in Russia and by the early 1980s methcathinone manufacturing and illicit use was widespread. It has been estimated that 20% of illicit drug abusers in the Russian Republic use methcathinone (Calkins, Alkan, & Hussain, 1995).

Using methcathinone instead of khat is similar to using cocaine instead of the coca leaf. **Methcathinone is much more intense than khat**, so its addictive properties and side effects can be more intense (and quite similar to those of methamphetamines). Side effects include lack of coordination, labored respiration, and nervousness. PET scans of long-term methcathinone users show lasting reductions in dopamine production that can lead to nervous system and muscular problems, such as Parkinsonism (a dopamine deficiency disease) (Ricaurte et al., 1997).

BETEL NUTS

References to the betel nut (**seeds of the betel palm**, *Areca catechu*) date back more than 21 centuries. They have been **widely used in India, Pakistan, the Arab world, Taiwan, Malaysia, the Philippines, New Guinea, Polynesia, southern China, and some countries in Africa**. Marco Polo brought betel nuts back to Europe in 1300. The betel palm is widely cultivated, usually on large plantations, in a number of countries with a tropical climate. Each palm produces about 250 seeds per year.

Today more than **200 million people worldwide use betel nuts** not only as a recreational drug but also as a medication. In Taiwan alone 17% of men and 1% of women, an estimated 2 million people, chew the nut on a regular basis. The main active ingredient, arecoline, increases levels of epinephrine and norepinephrine. The effects of these central nervous system stimulants are similar to those of nicotine or strong coffee and include a **mild euphoria, excitation, and a decrease in fatigue.** Maximum effects occur 6–8 minutes after chewing begins. Some

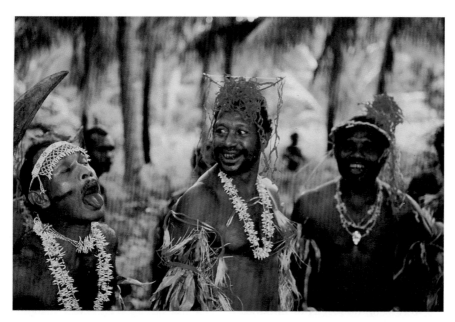

More than 200 million people use the betel nut, often sprinkled with dry coral lime, wrapped in pepper leaves, and then chewed. The betel nut turns the saliva bright red and stains the teeth as it has with these three ceremonial dancers in Port May, Santa Ana, in the Solomon Islands.

Courtesy of Joan Linn Bekins

users claim that betel chewing lowers tension, reduces appetite, and induces a feeling of well-being (Bibra, 1995). Some users chew from morning until night, others use them only in social situations. Some liken the practice to gum chewing or cola drinking in the West. This drug can also produce psychological dependence.

The betel nut (husk and/or meat) is generally chewed in combination with another plant leaf (peppermint, mustard, etc.) and some slaked lime to make it more palatable and increase absorption. The juice of this mixture **stains the teeth and mouth dark red** over time. In high doses arecoline can be toxic. Another substance in betel nuts, muscarine, is epidemiologically linked to esophageal cancer. Up to 7% of regular users have cancer of the mouth and esophagus. **The most common danger has to do with tissue damage to mucosal linings of the mouth and esophagus.** There is even a prominent and identifiable set of withdrawal symptoms similar to those experienced during withdrawal from caffeine.

In the late 1990s a product called "gutkha" was introduced and marketed in India. Gutka is a sweetened mixture of tobacco, betel nut, and betel leaves. It was sold at price even affordable to children (about 40¢ to 50¢) and packaged to attract their attention. The sales of these products have already reached close to $1 billion due to the habituating nature of these substances. Children as young as 12 years old have been diagnosed with precancerous lesions in their mouths due to gutkha use when the product had only been available in India for a few years.

YOHIMBE

Yohimbine, a bitter spicy extract from the African **yohimbe tree** (*Corynanthe yohimbe*), can be brewed into a stimulating tea or used as a medicine. **It is reported to be a mild aphrodisiac.** It seems to increase the activity of the neurotransmitter acetylcholine, which results in more penile blood inflow. It also increases blood pressure and heart rate. Yohimbine has been reported to **produce a mild euphoria and occasional hallucinations but in larger doses it can be toxic** and

even cause death by respiratory paralysis (Marnell, 1997). The bark can be bought at some herbal stores, along with a whole series of medicines for "increasing potency" with names like Male Performance®, Yohimbe Power®, Manpower®, and Aphrodyne® (prescription only).

EPHEDRA (ephedrine)

The **ephedra bush** (*Ephedra equisetina*), found in deserts throughout the world, contains the drug ephedrine. This drug is **a mild-to-moderate stimulant that is used medicinally to treat asthma, narcolepsy, other allergies, and low blood pressure.** Many use it to make tea; the Mormons brewed it as a substitute for coffee that was forbidden by their religion. Ephedrine, also known as "marwath" and "**ma huang**," has been mentioned as a stimulant tonic and medication in China for over 5,000 years and is still sold in herbalists' shops today. Ephedrine was isolated and synthesized in 1885 but then was forgotten for almost 50 years before a scientific paper recommended it for asthma. Its popularity increased dramatically. Up until then epinephrine was the only effective medication used to treat asthma.

Ephedrine has more peripheral effects, such as bronchodilation, and fewer central nervous system effects, like euphoria, than amphetamines but one of the common side effects of excessive ephedrine use is drug-induced psychosis (Karch, 1996). Extract of ephedrine has been **used by athletes for an extra boost but overuse can lead to heart and blood vessel problems.** The cardiovascular dangers moved the National Football League to ban the use of ephedrine by the players. A weightlifter's death in Ohio led to the banning of sales of the extract in that state. Other states have followed suit and banned the sales of all ephedrine-based products. Many lookalike and over-the-counter products that advertise themselves as MDMA, amphetamine substitutes, or other stimulants (e.g., Cloud 9®, Nirvana®) contain ephedrine as the active ingredient.

Natural ephedra, synthetic ephedrine, and pseudoephedrine are also the main ingredients in the synthesis of methamphetamine and methcathinone and because of the demand for them a large illegal trade has sprung up, along with extensive smuggling from China and Germany.

Herbal Ecstasy® & Herbal Nexus®

In an attempt to cater to some people's desire for abusable stimulants and psychedelics, entrepreneurs have introduced stimulant herbal products. These capsules and tablets combine the **herbal form of ephedrine (ephedra), an herbal extract of caffeine (possibly from the kola nut),** with other herbs and vitamins and are advertised as Herbal Ecstasy®, Herbal Nexus®, or other catchy names. The use of herbal substances is an attempt to get around the FDA ban on some combinations of these products and to cash in on the current interest in certain psychoactive drugs including MDMA (ecstasy), nexus (CBR), and other stimulants. Some of these herbal products also contain vitamins and are touted as buffers for the toxic effects of the real ecstasy and nexus. Unfortunately the problems, even with herbal ephedra, have caused several states to go beyond merely limiting the amount that can be bought to placing outright bans on products with any form of ephedra or ephedrine.

CAFFEINE

"Coffee is a great power in my life; I have observed its effects on an epic scale. Many people claim coffee inspires them, but, as everybody knows, coffee only makes boring people more boring."
Honoré De Balzac, 1839, *On Modern Stimulants*

Caffeine is the most popular stimulant in the world. It is found in coffee, tea, chocolate, soft drinks, 60 different plants, and hundreds of over-the-counter or prescription medications. It has be-

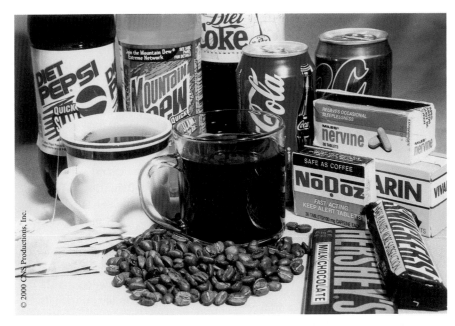

Caffeine concentration in most beverages is only one part in one or two thousand. Pure caffeine extract is a powerful stimulant.

come ingrained in so many cultures that efforts at any kind of prohibition or reduction of use are doomed to failure. **In America 85% of the population consumes substantial amounts of caffeine every day** (Weinberg & Bealer, 2001). There is the morning coffee, the coffee break at work in the morning and afternoon, coffee and colas at meetings and conferences, the tablet of No-Doz® to stay awake on the way home, and even the steaming cup of decaf after dinner to keep the ritual going. As with many psychoactive drugs the ritual surrounding use of coffee or tea is often as important as the stimulation sought. Some of the rituals include selecting the right coffee, grinding the beans, finding a comfortable or "cool" place to drink, collecting dozens of cups, demitasses, or mugs, reading the newspaper, and finding the right pastry or scones to go with the morning brew or the afternoon tea.

HISTORY OF USE

Tea

Tea is the most widely consumed beverage in the world besides water. Tea was thought to have been **present in China as early as 2700 B.C.** but the first written record only dates back to

A.D. 35. It was used in Japan around A.D. 600 but didn't become an important part of the culture until the fifteenth century. **A tea ceremony became an important ritual in Japanese homes and castles.** Tea was introduced into Europe around the end of the sixteenth century and immediately became quite popular, particularly in England and subsequently English colonies like America (Harler, 1984). The Boston Tea Party in 1774, when irate Bostonians threw tea into Boston Harbor to protest a tax on tea, reflected the importance of this psychoactive substance in colonial life. Today the **major exporters of tea are India, China, and Sri Lanka** while the major importers are the United Kingdom, the United States, and Pakistan. About 75% of the world's tea is black tea and 22% is green tea.

Coffee

Coffee was first cultivated in Ethiopia around A.D. 650. Legend says that the stimulant properties of coffee were discovered when Kaldi, an Arab goat herder, noticed the friskiness of his goats when they ate red berries from the coffee bush and tried them himself. Later on, Arabs learned how to prepare a hot drink from the berries rather than just chewing them. Use then spread to Arabia in the thirteenth century and finally to Europe by the fifteenth century. The drink was so stimulating that **many cultures banned it as an intoxicating drug**. In colonial America it was suggested that the use of tea and coffee led to the use of tobacco, alcohol, opium, and other drugs (Greden & Walters, 1997). Fortunately or unfortunately **coffee and tea were also great sources of revenue** and the pressure against prohibition was immense both from governments and the general public.

The use of caffeinated beverages continued to expand until today; in the United States alone each coffee drinker consumes about 20 pounds of coffee per year. There has also been an incredible growth in the number of specialty coffee houses in the United States. Every parking lot and gas station seems to have a coffee kiosk and many discount department stores and grocery chain stores have coffee bars. The number of coffee beverage retailers has grown from 200 in 1989 to more than 20,000 in 2002 and the numbers are accelerating leading to an outcry from neighbors. Starbucks®, the largest of the retailers, had 4,447 stores in 2002 in the United States and 1,242 in other countries with net revenues of approximately $3 billion.

Cocoa

Residue in ancient Mayan pots found in Belize in Central America, dating back to 600 B.C., showed residue of a cocoa beverage (Hurst, Tarka, Powis, Valdez, & Hester, 2002). Cocoa from the roasted and ground beans of the **cacao tree** (*Theobroma cacao*) **was first used in the New World by the Mayan and later Aztec royalty**, mostly as an unsweetened drink or as a spice. It was brought to Europe by Hernando Cortez in 1528. Widespread use didn't occur until the nineteenth century when the first chocolate bars appeared on the market. **There is only a small amount of caffeine in chocolate but the other active ingredient,** theobromine, also has stimulatory effects.

Caffeinated Soft Drinks (colas)

Caffeinated soft drinks (colas) are carbonated beverages that sometimes contain a caffeine extract of the kola nut from the **African kola tree** (*Cola nitida* or *Cola acuminata*) but **mostly they use caffeine extracted from the process of decaffeinating coffee**. The caffeine of the kola nut is released by cracking it into small pieces and then chewing it. The kola nut has been used in some African countries for centuries. The use of the nut for chewing and as a syrup made from powdered kola nut spread to Europe in the mid-1800s. By the late 1800s cola drinks made with carbonated or phosphated liquids, such as Coca Cola®, became popular in the United States (Kuhar, 1995). It is important to note that caffeine is added to other soft drinks and not just colas. Mountain Dew®, orange, and even some lemon-lime sodas now contain this drug.

Other Plants Containing Caffeine

Other plants containing caffeine include guarana, maté (ilex plant), and yoco, found in South America. **Guarana is the national drink of Brazil** made from the guarana shrub. It has more caffeine than coffee and is made into sweet carbonated beverages. **Maté is the most popular caffeine drink in Argentina.** It is a tea-like hot drink made from the leaves of a certain holly plant. Maté leaves can be bought in a number of health food stores (Weil & Rosen, 1993). This is not to be confused with Mate de Coca® that contains coca leaves instead of tea leaves.

PHARMACOLOGY

Caffeine is an alkaloid of the chemical class called "xanthines." It is found in more than 60 plant species such as the *Coffea Arabica* (coffee), *Thea sinensis* (tea), *Theobroma cacao* (chocolate), or *Cola nitida* (cola drinks). The white crystalline bitter-tasting powder ($C_8H_{10}N_4O_2$) was isolated from coffee in 1819 by Friedlieb Ferdinand Runge and from tea 8 years later. Tea leaves contain a higher percentage of caffeine than coffee but less tea is used for the average cup. Caffeine can be used orally, intravenously, intramuscularly, or rectally, though most consumption is by mouth. The half-life of caffeine in the body is 3–7 hours, so **it will take 15–35 hours for 95% of the caffeine to be excreted**. School-age children eliminate caffeine twice as fast as adults (Silverman & Griffiths, 1995a).

In the **United States, per capita consumption of caffeine is 211 mg per day**, about 2 cups of regular coffee plus a cola; in Sweden, 425 mg (85% from coffee); and in the United Kingdom, 445 mg (72% from tea).

◊ About 17% of the per capita daily consumption of caffeine in the United States is from tea, 16% from soft drinks, while 60% is from coffee (National Soft Drink Association, 1999; Silverman & Griffiths, 1995b).

◊ About half of all Americans drink 3.3 cups of coffee on any given day and most of that is regular coffee not the lattes and espressos found in specialty coffees that have exploded in popularity in recent years (Coffee Science Source, 1998).

◊ Twenty percent of adults in the United States consume more than 350 mg of caffeine and 3% consume more than 650 mg per day.

◊ In 2001 **Americans consumed about 540 12-oz. cans of soft drinks per person per year** at a total cost of $54 billion.

◊ There are about 450 different soft drinks available in the United States of which 65% contain caffeine.

"I start in the morning with a double latte. That's 300–400 milligrams of caffeine. I'll have 2 Cokes® for lunch, that's another 100 milligrams. Then a couple of cups of regular coffee in the afternoon—another 200 milligrams. That's 700 milligrams minimum. I

TABLE 3–2   CAFFEINE CONTENT IN VARIOUS SUBSTANCES

Amount of Beverage or Food	Caffeine Content in Milligrams (mg)	
	Average	Range
Coffee (1 cup)		
demitasse espresso (4 oz.)	200 mg	
ercolated coffee (6 oz.)	100 mg	75–150 mg
instant coffee (6 oz.)	75 mg	60–100 mg
decaf coffee (6 oz.)	3 mg	2–4 mg
Tea (6 oz. cup)		
1-minute brew	25 mg	10-40 mg
3-minute brew	40 mg	20-55 mg
5-minute brew	60 mg	25-100 mg
Soft Drinks (1 can)		
Jolt Cola®	70 mg	
Mountain Dew®	54 mg	
Coca-Cola®	46 mg	
Pepsi Cola®	38 mg	
Chocolate		
hot chocolate (6 oz.)	10 mg	
chocolate milk (6 oz.)	4 mg	
milk chocolate (4 oz.)	24 mg	
dark chocolate (4 oz.)	80 mg	
baking chocolate (4 oz.)	140 mg	
M&M's® (1.75 oz.)	15 mg	
Haagen Dazs® coffee ice cream (½ cup)	32 mg	
Medications		
Dexatrim®	200 mg	
No-Doz® (1 tablet)	100 mg	
Vivarin® (1 tablet)	200 mg	
Excedrin® (1 tablet)	65 mg	
Midol® (1 tablet)	32 mg	
Percodan®	32 mg	

know plenty of people at work who will have at least 10 cups of coffee besides the lattes and chocolate bars. They're up to 2,000 milligrams a day. Their tolerance is incredible. They'll drink a cup and fall asleep."

36-year-old caffeinated businessman

PHYSICAL & MENTAL EFFECTS

As with any drug an individual's reaction to caffeine varies widely. They may have an inherited sensitivity due to differences in caffeine metabolism, they may develop a tolerance to the effects, they might have an illness that influences the effects, or they might use other substances, including alcohol, tobacco, or another stimulant, which alters the effects of the caffeine. For these reasons definitive answers about the physical effects of caffeine or any drug can be hard to predict for any given person (Weinberg & Bealer, 2001).

Medically caffeine is used as a bronchodilator in asthma patients. It has been used as an adjunct to pain medication and to counteract a sudden drop in blood pressure. **It is found in a number of over-the-counter prepara-**tions: decongestants, analgesics, alertness aids, appetite suppressants, diuretics, and menstrual pain controllers. Caffeine constricts blood vessels in the brain making it valuable as a **treatment for headaches, especially migraine headaches** (which are caused by dilation of vessels).

Nonmedically caffeine is most widely known and used as a mild stimulant. In low doses (100–200 mg) **caffeine can increase alertness, dissipate drowsiness or fatigue, and help thinking.** Even at doses above 200 mg there can still be increased alertness and performance but, as with any drug, excessive use can cause problems. **The stimulation is caused by caffeine's inhibiting effect on adenosine**, a neuromodulator that normally depresses mood, induces sleep, has anticonvulsant properties, and causes low blood pressure, a slow heart rate, and dilation of blood vessels. When caffeine blocks adenosine, the result is raised mood, wakefulness, high blood pressure, fast heart rate, and vasoconstriction (Weinberg & Bealer, 2001). Since caffeine users' reactions to the drug often depend on heredity, the rise in blood pressure is more pronounced in those prone to high blood pressure (Rachima-Maoz, Peleg, & Rosenthal, 1998).

At doses of more than 350 mg per day (about 3–4 cups of coffee), again depending on the susceptibility and tolerance of the user, **anxiety, insomnia, gastric irritation, high blood pressure, nervousness, and flushed face can occur**. In one study, at doses of 500 mg, stress hormones were elevated about 32% above normal and they persisted hours after use. Coffee drinkers also felt more stressed than on the days they didn't use caffeine (Lane et al., 2002). At doses above 1,000 mg, increased heart rate, palpitations, muscle twitching, rambling thoughts, jumbled speech, sleep difficulties, motor disturbances, ringing in the ears, and even vomiting and convulsions can occur. **Caffeine is lethal at about 10 grams** (100 cups of coffee). Since excessive caffeine use can trigger nervousness, **people who are prone to panic attacks should avoid caffeine** (Greden &

Walters, 1997). A physician or psychiatrist should ask patients who come in with symptoms of anxiety about their caffeine consumption. In fact physicians rarely consider caffeine consumption in their patients with cardiovascular, sleep, gastric, and other problems.

"When I was fourteen, a friend of mine and I got a couple of boxes of NoDoz® and downed the whole 2 boxes of 'em between us. We got way sick, very sick, way more sick than I've ever gotten off of alcohol. The room was spinning, and spinning, and spinning. Caffeine overdose: not fun."
Caffeine abuser

Consuming 350 mg or more of caffeine can lower fertility rates in women and affect fetuses in the womb (e.g., higher blood pressure). A retrospective study at the University of Utah of 2,500 pregnant women found that **6 or more cups of coffee a day almost doubled the risk of miscarriage** compared to women who either didn't drink coffee or only drank 1–2 cups a day (Klebanoff, Levine, DeSimonian, Clemens, & Wilkins, 1999). In addition it is thought by a number of researchers that some susceptible women develop benign lumps in their breasts from drinking too much coffee.

Some researchers also feel that caffeine use makes it harder to lose weight. This difficulty happens because **caffeine stimulates the release of insulin**. Insulin metabolizes sugar thus reducing the level of sugar in the blood and triggering hunger in the user.

Coronary heart disease, ischemic heart disease, heart attacks, intestinal ulcers, diabetes, and some liver problems have been seen in long-term, high-dose caffeine users, more often in countries with very high per capita caffeine consumption.

TOLERANCE, WITHDRAWAL, & ADDICTION

Tolerance to the effects of caffeine does occur although there is a wide variation among the ways differ-

ent people will react to several cups of coffee or tea. Coffee drinkers might eventually need 3 cups to wake up instead of the usual single cup with lots of cream and sugar. For those with a high tolerance, a cup of coffee can even encourage sleep.

"For a week or 2 at most, you can obtain the right amount of stimulation with 1, then 2 cups of coffee brewed from beans that have been crushed with gradually increasing force and infused with hot water. . . . When you have produced the finest grind with the least water possible, you double the dose by drinking 2 cups at a time; particularly vigorous constitutions can tolerate 3 cups. In this manner, one can continue working for several days."
Honoré de Balzac, 1839, On Modern Stimulants

Continuous use of caffeine increases the number of adenosine receptor sites, so it takes more caffeine to block them; this is one of the main mechanisms for the development of tolerance (James, 1991). Withdrawal symptoms do occur after cessation of long-term high-dose use and can occur after levels of use as low as 100 mg per day, which is 1 strong cup of coffee or 2 colas. These symptoms appear within 12–24 hours and peak within 24–48 hours, and last 2 days to a week. **The most prominent withdrawal symptom is a throbbing headache** that is worsened by exercise but of course relieved by having a cup of coffee. **Other symptoms include sleepiness, fatigue, lethargy, depression, decreased alertness, sleep problems, and irritability.** The subjects in one extensive experiment had withdrawal symptoms when ceasing an average intake of 235 mg a day, or 2–3 cups of coffee (Griffiths et al., 1986; Silverman et al., 1992).

"The headache hits me about 5 in the afternoon of the day I quit and stays around through the next day. Then I feel tired and my ass drags for the

next 2 weeks. I'll stay off it for a while and then I'll start with half a cup and pretty soon I got a pot going all the time plus a couple of 6-packs of Diet Coke® in the icebox."
20-year caffeine abuser

Withdrawal symptoms are observed in newborns when their mothers have been drinking 200–1,800 mg a day. Irritability, jitteriness, and vomiting occurred an average of 20 hours after delivery, then disappeared (McGowan et al., 1988).

Dependence can occur with daily intake levels of 500 mg (about 5 cups of coffee, 10 cola drinks, or 8 cups of tea) (Weinberg & Bealer, 2001). Coffee creates a milder dependency than that found with amphetamines and cocaine. It interferes less with daily functioning and is not as expensive as the stronger stimulants. However, two-thirds of those treated for excessive caffeine use (caffeinism) will relapse after treatment.

"I was addicted to caffeine. I don't think I'm addicted any more. When I was in college 18 credits during the summer term, I was taking 8 shots of espresso a day in mochas, double mochas. I couldn't get through the day without it. I really felt like I had to have my coffee or there was no way I'd go to class."
Recovering caffeine addict

Since 70% of the soft drinks sold in the United States contain caffeine, the question comes to mind, why is it put in drinks? It's not for the flavor since one study found that **only 8% of soda drinkers could taste the presence of caffeine**, so it seems that colas, like coca wine, are popular because they stimulate the mind and body (Griffiths & Vernotica, 2000). The concerns about soft drinks loaded not only with caffeine but with large amounts of sugar led a number of school districts, particularly the Los Angeles school district, to restrict soda sales (Severson, 2002). However, earlier in the year the California State

Legislature voted down a statewide measure to restrict soft-drink sales because they felt it would reduce school income by millions of dollars; the San Diego City Unified School District would have lost about $500,000.

NICOTINE

"One of the sounds I remember from growing up in the '40s and '50s was the sound of my dad's cigarette cough. It started deep in the lungs and ended in an explosion of air. I could tell he was approaching from a block away. I just accepted it as a fact of life. He later became Advertising Director for American Tobacco just when the first Surgeon General's Report on Health and Tobacco was released in 1964. He gave up smoking in 1976 after retiring and died of throat cancer 17 years later, caused by his years of smoking (according to his oncologist). Talk about mixed feelings . . . tobacco supported his family then took his life and that of thousands of others."

William Cohen, co-author of Uppers, Downers, All Arounders

Tobacco comes from the leaves and other parts of a plant species belonging to the genus *Nicotiana*, a member of the deadly nightshade family that also includes tomatoes, belladonna, and petunias. There are 64 *Nicotiana* species but **most commercial tobacco comes from the milder broad-leafed *Nicotiana tabacum* plant** and a number of its variants. Though tobacco is available in cigarettes, cigars, pipe tobacco, snuff, and chewing tobacco, **cigarettes account for 90% of all tobacco use in America**. In a country such as India, chewing tobacco (and chewing the betel nut) is more popular (85% of all adult men). Whether it is smoked, chewed, absorbed through the gums, or even used as an enema, this stimulant ultimately affects many of the

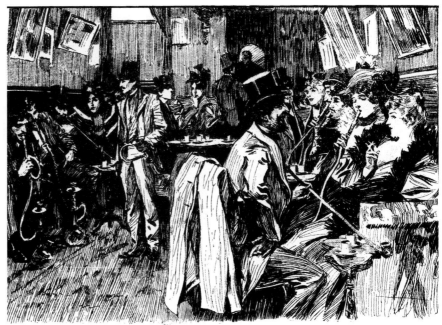

A SCENE IN ONE OF THE RECENTLY OPENED TURKISH SMOKING PARLORS.

At the turn of the twentieth century, tobacco dens were as notorious as the psychedelic clubs of the 1960s and the rave clubs of the 1990s.

same areas of the brain as cocaine and amphetamines though not as intensely.

HISTORY (*also see Chapter 1*)

Native Americans & Tobacco

After several voyages to the New World, Columbus and a number of other French, Portuguese, and Spanish explorers noticed that the Native Americans "drank the smoke" of certain dried leaves and seemed to receive both stimulatory and sedative effects from the process (O'Brien, Cohen, Evans, & Fine, 1992). **Explorers and diplomats introduced tobacco to Europe where it was used for recreation and as a medicine.** It was listed as a cure for almost every known illness including ulcerated abscesses, fistulas, and sores. (In this century it is listed as the cause of just as many diseases.) Use spread to Europe, Russia, Japan, Africa, and China in the 1600s and later on to virtually every country in the world. **Originally smoking tobacco several times a day in a pipe was the most common form of use but in the eighteenth century, chewing tobacco and using snuff became popular** in Europe

and America. This was because a user didn't have to carry or light a pipe, roll a cigarette, or carry the means to light them. Smokeless tobacco remained the preferred method of use until the end of World War I (Benowitz & Fredericks, 1995).

Growth of Cigarette Smoking

As with most other psychoactive drugs, it was technical and social developments that greatly increased the use and ultimately the concentration of the active psychoactive ingredients. These developments were

◊ **improved cigarette-manufacturing technology (cigarette rolling machine),**

◊ **a milder type of tobacco that allowed for deeper inhalation and more continuous use,**

◊ **lower prices due to mass production,**

◊ **increased and more skillful advertising,**

◊ **more aggressive marketing techniques**.

For example, new marketing concepts during World Wars I and II initiated millions of GIs into smoking cigarettes. **Cigarette companies supplied free or cheap cigarettes to the soldiers** in an effort to expand their market. England even stockpiled cigarettes during World War II in case of invasion or an interruption in the supply. Interestingly some of the reasons for the switch to cigarettes were worries about the health risks of smokeless tobacco including the fear that chewing it caused tuberculosis. In the nineteenth and early twentieth centuries, fear of tuberculosis was the equivalent of our present day fear of cancer (O'Brien et al., 1992; Slade, 1992).

If a user smoked 40 cigarettes a year in the late 1800s, it was not nearly the health problem it is today when the **consumption of an average heavy smoker is 30–40 cigarettes a day or more than 10,000 a year**. This new popularity of tobacco not only multiplied the number of smokers, it multiplied the number of dollars made from tobacco. Gross sales of tobacco products in the United States in 2001 were approximately $52 billion (U.S. Surgeon General, 2002). In 2001,

◇ 56.3 million Americans smoked cigarettes in the past month;

◇ 35.4 million smoked cigarettes every day;

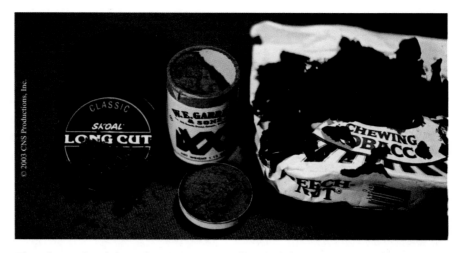

Three forms of smokeless tobacco are moist snuff on the left, white powder snuff in the middle, and loose-leaf on the right. More than 120 million pounds of chewing tobacco and snuff were sold in the United States in 1998—20 pounds per user.

◇ 12.1 million smoked cigars;

◇ 2.3 million smoked tobacco in pipes (SAMHSA, 2002).

Smokeless Tobacco

The **three types of smokeless tobacco, moist snuff, powder snuff, and loose-leaf**, are still popular. A pinch of moist snuff—finely chopped tobacco as found in brands such as Copenhagen® and Skoal®—is stuck in the mouth next to the gums where the nicotine is absorbed into the capillaries. Powder snuff is a fine powder that is most often sniffed into the nose but it is also rubbed on the gums or chewed. Stems and leaves of the tobacco plant are fermented, dried, and then ground into powder. Various scents and flavors are then added to the powder to improve the bitter taste of nicotine. Snuff boxes and this form of tobacco were once considered very chic and fashionable throughout the world. Today sniffing snuff is not nearly as popular as smoking or chewing tobacco. This method of use is irritating to mucosal tissues and deadens the sense of smell.

With loose-leaf chewing tobacco, larger sections of leaf are stuffed into the mouth and chewed to allow the nicotine-laden juice to be absorbed. Brands include Beech Nut® and Red Man®. There were approximately 7.3 million regular smokeless tobacco users in the United States in 2001 with sales over $1 billion (SAMHSA, 2002). The use of chewing tobacco and snuff is prevalent in professional and amateur male athletes in America.

PHARMACOLOGY

Nicotine

Nicotine is the most important ingredient in tobacco in terms of car-

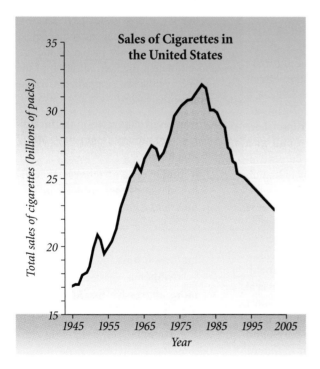

Sales of Cigarettes in the United States

Total sales of cigarettes (billions of packs)

Year

Figure 3-4 •

Sales of cigarettes have climbed from 18 billion packs a year in 1945 to a peak of 32 billion packs a year in 1985. By 2002 U.S. sales had dropped to 22 billion packs.

diovascular and particularly psychoactive effects. The average tobacco leaf (*Nicotiana tabacum*) contains 2% to 5% nicotine. Pure nicotine is colorless, bitter, smelly, and highly poisonous. Mixed in water it is a powerful insecticide. Smoking and inhaling a cigarette delivers nicotine to the brain in 5–8 seconds. Chewing tobacco or placing snuff on the gums delivers the nicotine in 5–8 minutes.

◇ **The average cigarette contains 10 mg of nicotine but only delivers 1–3 mg of that to the lungs** when burned and inhaled. About 70 mg ingested at one time is fatal. Chain smokers might get up to 6 mg in their lungs before rapid distribution and metabolism put a damper on high blood-nicotine levels.

◇ In comparison **one chew of tobacco will deliver approximately 4.5 mg of nicotine and one pinch of snuff about 3.6 mg**.

◇ The actual blood-nicotine level of one cigarette is measured as approximately 25 µg/L or 25 micrograms per liter of blood. The average smoker will maintain a nicotine level of 5–40 µg/L depending on the time of day (Schmitz, Schneider, & Jarvik, 1997).

◇ **The nicotine in the first cigarette of the day raises the heart rate by an average of 10–20 beats per minute and the blood pressure by 5–10 units.**

The effect of nicotine is the main reason for the widespread use of tobacco. **Nicotine, a central nervous system stimulant, disrupts the balance of neurotransmitters (endorphins, epinephrine, dopamine, and particularly acetylcholine).** Acetylcholine affects heart rate, blood pressure, memory, learning, reflexes, aggression, sleep, sexual activity, and mental acuity. What nicotine does is mimic acetylcholine by slotting into nicotinic acetylcholine receptor sites, so those cholinergic effects are exaggerated. The release of dopamine makes a smoker feel satisfied and calm, so **a cigarette both stimulates and calms.**

"When I first started smoking, it was a head rush. It felt really good, I liked it. It made me feel kind of dizzy. Now it makes stress go away, seems to help me concentrate when I'm working, working my computer. Best thing I think I can do if I'm stressed is to smoke a cigarette to calm down."
Two-pack-a-day smoker

Some of the emotional effects are related to the settings where tobacco is used. A person might feel more confident holding a cigarette while starting a conversation or talking on the phone to a client. But after continued use tobacco's effectiveness at calming and relieving anxiety seems more associated with preventing nicotine withdrawal rather than acting as a true sedative. In fact nicotine addicts rarely identify their very first use of tobacco as pleasurable.

Scientists have located one of the key proteins in the nicotine receptor that seems to be responsible for the positive reinforcing properties of nicotine. When the scientists developed a strain of mice without the key protein (1 of the 10 proteins that form the nicotinic receptor), the mice had no desire to self-administer nicotine on a regular basis. Even when injected with nicotine, the level of the calming neurotransmitter dopamine did not increase

(National Institute on Drug Abuse [NIDA], 2000).

In another experiment PET imaging studies found that smokers had lower levels of the enzymes MAO-A and B (monoamine oxidase A and B) that resulted in calming the smoker (Fowler, Volkow, Wang, et al., 1996).

Craving

Besides the mildly pleasurable effects that smokers receive from tobacco, some of the reasons for continuing to smoke include

◇ the **social context**, such as drinking and smoking in bars and at a meal;

◇ the **ritual aspects** of lighting up and smoking;

◇ the perception of smoking as an **adult activity**;

◇ the **desire to manipulate mood**;

◇ the desire to **be rebellious**;

◇ the perception that smoking is **sexually attractive**.

The two most important reasons that people continue to smoke have to do with weight loss and craving. **Nicotine suppresses appetite and increases metabolism.** On average, smokers weigh about 6–9 pounds less than nonsmokers (Klesges, Meyers, Klesges, & LaVasque, 1989; Schmitz et al., 1997). Since withdrawal from smoking is often ac-

TABLE 3–3   SOME INGREDIENTS FOUND IN CIGARETTE SMOKE

Tobacco Smoke	Common Product	Adverse Health Effects
Cadmium	Artists oil paints	Yellow stains on teeth
Hydrogen cyanide	Gas chamber poison	Breathing difficulty
Vinyl chloride	Garbage bags	Whitening of fingers and pain when cold
Toluene	Embalmer's fluid, glue	Inflamed, cracked skin
Benzene	Rubber cement	Drowsiness, dizziness, headaches, nausea
Naphthalene	Paint pigment	Headache, confusion
Arsenic	Rat poison	Pins and needles feeling in hands and feet

(Compiled by the California Department of Health Services)

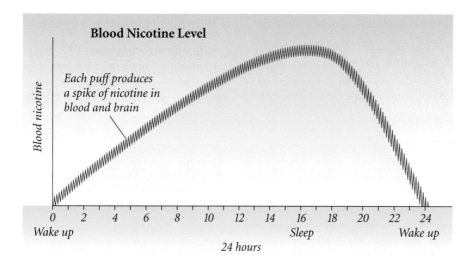

Blood Nicotine Level

*Each puff produces
a spike of nicotine in
blood and brain*

Blood nicotine

0   2   4   6   8   10   12   14   16   18   20   22   24
Wake up   Sleep   Wake up

24 hours

Figure 3-5 •

*This chart shows the change in blood-nicotine levels in a heavy smoker for a 24-hour period.
Notice how the drop in the blood level overnight might lead to that intense craving for a
cigarette and a cup of coffee in the morning.*

companied by weight gain, the **fear of putting on pounds can keep smokers from quitting** or cause relapse when they do quit. A current hypothesis about weight gain is that nicotine raises the metabolic rate to burn more calories and lowers the inherited weight set-point (Perkins, 1993).

Finally the most important reason that people continue to smoke is an intense desire to maintain a certain nicotine level in the blood (and therefore in the brain) in order to avoid withdrawal symptoms. This need to avoid negative effects by continued use is known as "**negative drug reinforcement.**" In addition the authors believe that the very act of relieving withdrawal symptoms can activate the nucleus accumbens inducing a certain sense of pleasure. This same effect has been postulated for heroin or other opioid withdrawal (Goldstein, 2001).

*"It calms me down. Now I think I'm
not sure if it's mostly the calm or just
the fact of getting rid of the stress of
having a nicotine fit . . . keeping the
nicotine levels up to a point where I
don't stress out, or freak out, or bitch
at anybody, or yell, or scratch their
eyes out."*

20-year smoker

TOLERANCE, WITHDRAWAL, & ADDICTION

Tolerance

Physiological adaptation to the initial effects of nicotine develops quite rapidly, some say even faster than with heroin or cocaine. A few hours of smoking are sufficient for the body to begin to learn how to handle these new toxins, probably through neural adaptation. As with users of other drugs, smokers say that the first hit in the morning is the best as they raise their nicotine level back up. Smokers who have quit and then start again feel the dizziness and nausea of a novice user.

*"The first time I smoked it was to im-
press a girl. I got dizzy and high and
had to sit down. A year later my 30th
cigarette of the day only gave me a mild
stimulation, a fit of coughing, and then
a calm. Now all I have left is the cough,
a bunch of smoking rituals, and it
costs about five bucks a pack."*

Two-pack-a-day smoker

Once smokers adapt to the initial effects of tobacco and find a level of smoking that gives them an optimum nicotine level, they can then usually

stick to that level over a long period of time, so the tolerance is not endless as with amphetamines or opioids. One study showed that some regular smokers, if they increased average intake by only 50%, they experienced dizziness, nausea, vomiting, headache, and dysphoria (Collins, 1990).

Withdrawal

Withdrawal from a pack- or two-pack-a-day habit after prolonged use can **cause headaches, nervousness, fatigue, hunger, severe irritability, poor concentration, sleep disturbances, and intense nicotine craving**. It is a true physiological dependence that has been developed through rapid tissue and chemical changes in brain cells. One process that occurs is the creation of more acetylcholine receptors, particularly the nicotinic receptors (Stein, Pankiewicz, Harsch, et al., 1998). When a person tries to stop using tobacco, the activity of acetylcholine is greatly exaggerated by all these extra receptors thus making the user restless, irritable, and discontent. Soon the smoker comes to depend on smoking to stay normal, that is, to avoid these withdrawal effects. Also research has demonstrated that abrupt withdrawal of nicotine resulted in significant decrease of action in the brain's reward function. This effect lasted for days (Epping-Jordan, Watkins, Koob, & Markou, 1998). The resultant lack of a reward function drives a person to crave nicotine when use is discontinued in order to regain the reward function.

The sense of relaxation and well-being that most smokers receive from a cigarette is, in fact, the sensation of the withdrawal symptoms being subdued.

Smokers will try to maintain a constant level of nicotine in the bloodstream and brain. Even when smokers switch to a low tar and nicotine brand, they often increase the number of cigarettes they smoke just to maintain their nicotine target levels. In fact nicotine craving may last a lifetime after withdrawal.

*"I've tried to quit a couple of times. I've
tried the nicotine gum. I've tried quit-*

ting just cold turkey. It doesn't work. There's a lot to be said for living with smokers and trying to quit at the same time. It's almost impossible, just because it permeates the house. It's everywhere whether you want it to be or not."

Two-pack-a-day smoker

Addiction

"I cannot refrain from a few words of protest against the astounding fashion lately introduced from America, a sort of smoke-tippling, which enslaves its victims more completely than any other form of intoxication, old or new. These madmen will swallow and inhale with incredible eagerness, the smoke of a plant they call 'herba Nicotiana', or tobacco."

German Ambassador to The Hague, c. 1627

The use of tobacco is a pure example of the addictive process. The pleasure received from the direct effects of smoking are not as intense as the initial pleasure derived from alcohol, cocaine, or almost any other psychoactive drug. In fact the negative feelings from early tobacco use outweigh any perceived pleasurable ones. Coughing, dizziness, headache, even nausea are experienced by the novice smoker; the cost of a two-pack-a-day habit can run $2,555 a year at $3.50 a pack or in New York City $7.50 a pack or $5,475 a year; the health problems and premature deaths that result from smoking are too numerous to mention and yet people continue to smoke. In fact 80% of smokers believe that cigarette smoking causes cancer, yet they still smoke (Harris Poll, 1999).

One of the strongest indications of the addictive potential of tobacco can be seen when you look at the percentage of casual tobacco users who become compulsive users vs. the percentage of casual users of other psychoactive drugs who become compulsive users of those drugs.

◇ Twenty-three million people have tried cocaine. About 600,000 are weekly users (2.6%) but only a tiny fraction of cocaine users do it on a daily basis.

◇ Seventy-two million people have tried marijuana but only 6.8 million use it weekly (9.4%) and a few percent on a daily basis.

◇ One hundred and seventy-eight million have tried alcohol, yet less than 48 million drink on a weekly basis (27%); 20 million drink on a daily basis (11%).

◇ One hundred and sixty-one million have smoked cigarettes; 66 million of them in the past month (41%); 36 million of them on a daily basis (23%).

(SAMHSA, 2002)

These figures mean that **almost one-third of those who ever tried a cigarette became daily habitual users compared with the 11% of alcohol experimenters who become daily abusers**. And yet people continue to experiment with cigarettes.

Granted you might say that people want to keep using cigarettes because smoking is really pleasurable and that the choice is theirs. According to one survey **80% of smokers interviewed say they want to quit and another 10% say they want to limit the amount they smoke**. That means that 9 out of 10 smokers are unhappy with their smoking and yet they continue to smoke. In the last few years the tobacco companies have started to admit that nicotine is indeed addicting. In a *USA Today* survey 4 out of 5 smokers and nonsmokers alike believed nicotine is an addictive substance.

In many countries the rate of daily use is even higher than in the United States: 50% in China, 40% in England, and 50% in Japan (WHO, 1997). In a British study 90% of teenagers who had smoked just 3–4 cigarettes at the time of the survey were found to be compulsive smokers years later. This statistic means that even the most casual use of tobacco usually leads to compulsive use. And yet people continue to smoke. Globally 12% of women and 47% of men smoke.

It is worth noting here that nicotine craving is much subtler and less noticeable to the user than the other cravings that occur with drugs like cocaine, heroin, or alcohol. However, the craving is nevertheless extremely powerful and may be associated with what is called a "self-determined nicotine state of consciousness" or "state dependence." **State dependence** means that people will try to achieve a certain mental and physical state that may be neither pleasurable nor objectionable

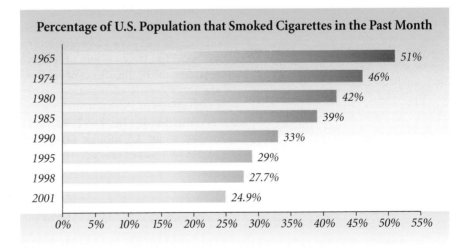

Percentage of U.S. Population that Smoked Cigarettes in the Past Month

Year	Percentage
1965	51%
1974	46%
1980	42%
1985	39%
1990	33%
1995	29%
1998	27.7%
2001	24.9%

Figure 3-6 •

Smoking rates in most other countries are higher than in the United States.

National Household Survey on Drug Abuse, 2001

TABLE 3–4 CIGARETTE USE IN THE UNITED STATES—2001

By Age	Ever Used	Used Past Year	Used Past Month
12-17	7.8 million	4.6 million	3.2 million
18-25	20.3 million	14.3 million	11.4 million
26 & older	123.5 million	46.7 million	41.7 million
Totals	**151.6 million**	**65.6 million**	**56.3 million**

National Household Survey on Drug Abuse, 2001 (SAMHSA, 2002)

TABLE 3–5 SMOKELESS TOBACCO USE IN THE UNITED STATES—2001

By Sex	Ever Used	Used Past Year	Used Past Month
Male	35.1 million	8.9 million	6.7 million
Female	8.0 million	0.9 million	0.6 million
Totals	**43.1 million**	**9.8 million**	**7.3 million**

National Household Survey on Drug Abuse, 2001 (SAMHSA, 2002)

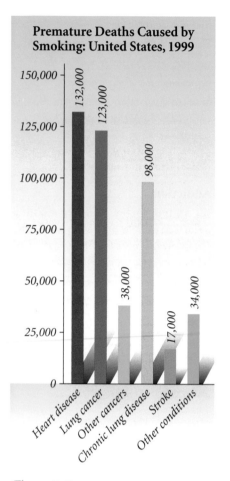

Premature Deaths Caused by Smoking: United States, 1999

Figure 3-7 •

Total estimated premature deaths caused by smoking is 442,000 (CDC, 2002). The average life span of a two-pack-a-day smoker in the United States is 8 years less than a nonsmoker.

but it is a state with which they are familiar and one that they, and not others, have determined.

Recent research indicates that **there may be a genetic predisposition to nicotine addiction that makes tobacco use harder to stop for some than for others.** The suspect gene is the same reward pathway gene, DRD_2 A_1 allele, implicated in predisposition to alcoholism and other drug addictions (Spitz, 1998).

EPIDEMIOLOGY

One interesting note, in 1994 only 5% of Black high school seniors said they smoked on a daily basis compared to 10.6% for Hispanics and 23% for Whites. In focus groups, children said such things as "Smoking hurts stamina for sports," "Boys don't like girls who smoke," and "We believed the media about the dangers of cigarettes." But a 2000 survey found that the rate for Black teenagers had risen to 8.0%, 15.7% for Hispanics, and for Whites, 25.7% (Monitoring the Future, 2002).

SIDE EFFECTS

When tobacco is burned in a cigarette or cigar, the smoke that is created consists of fine particles and droplets of tar. **Tobacco and tobacco smoke contain nicotine and about 4,000 other chemicals**, many created by the burning process. About 400 are classified as toxins and 43 are known carcinogens. For example, some of the major byproducts in a lit cigarette are tobacco tar (a blackish substance that has direct effects on the respiratory system) and nitrosamines (some of which are carcinogenic) (Glantz, 1992).

It is inevitable that some of these ingredients will have adverse effects on the body. The large amount of research regarding the health effects of smoking are second only to research on the health effects of alcohol.

Worldwide **in 1997 tobacco caused about 3.5 million premature deaths or 1 out of every 5.** This figure will increase to 8.4 million annually by 2020. In China alone about 3 million smokers (mostly men) will die prematurely each year by the middle of this century (WHO, 2002).

In the United States it is estimated that 392,000 smokers die prematurely and another 50,000 nonsmokers die from secondhand smoke. That works out to 264,000 deaths in men and more than 178,000 in women. Most of the deaths were from lung cancer, heart disease, and lung disease (Centers for Disease Control [CDC], 2002).

The main reason for the extremely high figures is that often **tobacco takes 20, 30, or even 40 years for its most dangerous effects to become lethal.** Most people who die from smoking have been using for more than 20 years, so the immediate warning signs of overdose—heart palpitations, blackouts, hangovers, rage, paranoia, and nausea—common with other psychoactive drugs are missing. Except for the coughing, dizziness, initial nausea, bad breath, green mucous, lower lung capacity, and lowered energy levels, there are no immediate flashing warning signs. Recognizing the warning signs of cocaine, heroin, or alcohol use is a very visceral very immediate process. Those of tobacco are very subtle and slow. The dangerous side effects weigh directly against the pleasure received. With tobacco that craving can only be countered by an intellectual appreciation of the long-term dangers. In most cases the craving and fear of withdrawal win out over common sense.

According to the Centers for Disease Control (CDC), **smoking costs the United States about $150 billion each year in health costs and lost productivity** or $7.18 for each of the 22 billion packs sold. That works out to about $3,391 per smoker per year.

Longevity

"It might be shortening my life. And I don't breath as well. I love to hike and that's difficult. I get short of breath too easily. Get dizzy. I want to be around when my kids get older, my future grandchild. I'd like to be around and these don't seem to be conducive to that."

20-year smoker

The exceptional 75-year-old smoker who is healthy should not be seen as confirmation that smoking won't shorten life span or impair health. One has to look at the overall statistics. On average, adult male smokers lost 13.2 years of life while adult women smokers lost 14.5 years of life (CDC, 2002). **Internationally and in the United States the average life span loss to those smokers who die in middle age (before the age of 70) will be 22 years** (WHO, 2002).

Almost as important as these premature death statistics is the issue of quality of life. Because of breathing difficulties, poor circulation, and a dozen other imbalances caused by tobacco, a smoker will have more medical complications, be less able to participate in physical activity, and will not be able to live life to the fullest.

Cardiovascular Effects

Smoking accelerates the process of plaque formation and hardening of the arteries (atherosclerosis), the major cause of heart attacks, by increasing low-density fats, increasing blood coagulability, and triggering cardiac arrhythmias (irregular beatings of the heart). The inhaled carbon monoxide created by tobacco combustion also accelerates the process of atherosclerosis. In addition since nicotine constricts blood vessels, it restricts blood flow and raises blood pressure increasing the risk of a stroke (ruptured blood vessel in the brain). The combination of nicotine and carbon monoxide also increases the risk of angina attacks (heart pain).

Respiratory Effects

Cigarette smokers have a much higher rate of bronchopulmonary dis-

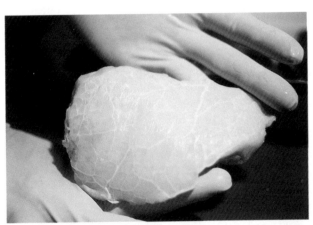

(A)

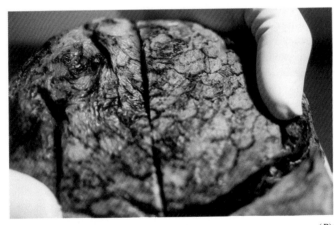

(B)

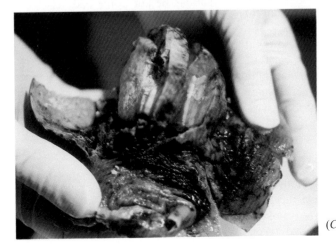

(C)

A normal lung (A) is pink and spongy. It is protected by the rib cage from external damage. Unfortunately smoking deposits tar, other chemicals, and irritants in the alveoli (air sacs) as well as destroying the cilia (fine hairs lining the membranes) that help remove foreign particles. The smoker's lung (B) is blackened by these deposits. Many of the chemicals in tobacco, particularly the tar, cause cancer (C). More than 100,000 people die prematurely from tobacco-induced lung cancer every year.

Courtesy of Leslie Parr, Ph.D.

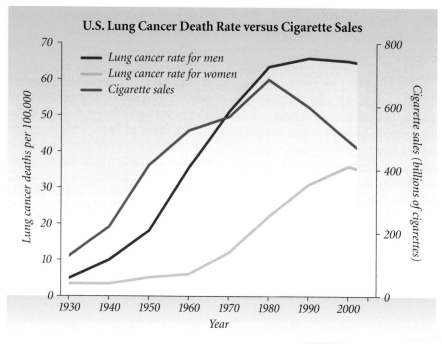

U.S. Lung Cancer Death Rate versus Cigarette Sales

— Lung cancer rate for men
— Lung cancer rate for women
— Cigarette sales

Figure 3-8 •

Since it takes 10–40 years for lung cancer to develop, there is a delay in decreasing rates of lung cancer even though sales among men have been declining for a number of years.

ease, such as **emphysema, chronic bronchitis, and chronic obstructive pulmonary disease**. In addition children who live with smokers have a much higher incidence of asthma, colds, and bronchitis from inhaling secondhand smoke. Finally, environmental pollutants, such as asbestos or volatile chemicals, greatly increase the rates of respiratory illness and cancer in smokers above the levels due to exposure from just smoking alone or just breathing dirty air.

Cancer

The increase in lung cancer since the 1930s when the use of cigarettes started to accelerate is startling. The rate in men has gone up 15-fold and in women 9-fold. In the graph (Fig. 3-8) we have juxtaposed the per capita smoking rate from 1930 to the present next to the per capita death rate from lung cancer. In 1988 lung cancer deaths in women surpassed deaths from breast cancer for the first time in history. According to the American Cancer Society,

◇ **men who smoke are 22 times more likely to develop lung cancer than men who don't;**

◇ **women who smoke are 12 times more likely to develop lung cancer than women who don't;**

◇ **about 85% of men with lung cancer and 75% of women with lung cancer smoke**.

The most likely culprits are the tars and other products of combustion that are inhaled by the smoker.

Studies at the University of California - Los Angeles have shown that precancerous alterations in bronchial epithelium occur not only from habitual cigarette smoking but also from habitual smoking of marijuana and/or crack cocaine (Barsky, Roth, Kleerup, Simmons, & Tashkin, 1998). Pipe and cigar smokers are less likely than cigarette smokers to get lung cancer but more likely than nonsmokers to get not only lung cancer but cancers of the larynx, mouth, and esophagus.

Fetal Effects

When mothers smoke during pregnancy, the newborns have the same nicotine level as grown-up smokers. About 15% of women smoke during

pregnancy, so when they give birth their babies go through withdrawal. The carbon monoxide and nicotine in tobacco smoke reduces the oxygen-carrying capacity of a pregnant mother's blood, so **less oxygen gets to the baby, contributing to a lower birth weight and a higher incidence of crib death** (sudden infant death syndrome - SIDS). Research indicates that women who smoke heavily during pregnancy are **twice as likely to miscarry and have spontaneous abortions as nonsmokers**. In one study the offspring of mothers who smoked during pregnancy were four times more likely to have attention-deficit/hyperactivity disorder (ADHD) (Milberger, Biederman, Faraone, & Jones, 1998). There was also an increased risk of early-onset conduct disorder and even drug dependence (Weissman, Warner, Wickramaratne, & Kandel, 1999).

Smokeless Tobacco Effects

Tobacco is as addicting in its smokeless form as in its smoked form even though the nicotine takes 3–5 minutes to affect the central nervous system when chewed or pouched in the cheek compared to the 7–10 seconds it takes when inhaled from a cigarette. Strangely enough more of the nicotine reaches the bloodstream with smokeless tobacco and the rush is somewhat more intense. The effects of chewing are almost identical to the effects of smoking, including a slight increase in energy, alertness, blood pressure, and heart rate. In the case of tobacco, smoking limits the amount of nicotine that can be put in the body (1–3 mg from a cigarette) as compared to chewing (4 mg or more).

The main advantage of smokeless tobacco over cigarettes is the protection it gives the lungs since no smoke is inhaled. Lung cancer rates and other respiratory problems drop dramatically. Unfortunately there are other problems with smokeless tobacco.

"I can't think of a more disgusting habit than chewing tobacco. I broke up with my boyfriend because he was always dripping tobacco juice, spitting,

and had those awful brown stains on his clothing. Ugh."

17-year-old high school student

Smokeless tobacco is irritating to the tissues of the mouth and the digestive tract. Many users experience leukoplakia, a thickening, whitening, and hardening of tissues in the mouth. **Their gums can become inflamed causing more dental problems** and although the risk of lung cancer is reduced compared to smoking, the risks of oral, pharyngeal, and esophageal cancers are increased. In addition since blood vessels are constricted while either chewing or smoking, circulatory problems, the largest health hazard of smoking, are just as grave with smokeless tobacco. One study found that dry snuff has a higher oral cancer risk than wet snuff and chewing tobacco (Rodu & Cole, 2002).

BENEFITS FROM QUITTING

A number of beneficial physiological changes occur on quitting smoking.

◇ Within 36 hours, blood carbon monoxide levels return to normal.

◇ Within 48 hours, nerve endings adjust to the absence of nicotine and the senses of smell and taste begin to come back.

◇ Within a week, the risk of heart attack drops, breathing improves, and constricted blood vessels begin to relax.

◇ Within 2 weeks to 3 months, **circulation improves, lung function increases up to 30%, and the complexion looks healthy again**.

◇ Within 1–9 months, fatigue, coughing, sinus congestion, and shortness of breath decrease and the lungs increase their ability to handle mucus, thereby helping to clean themselves and reduce infection.

◇ Within 5 years, the heart disease death rate returns to the rate for nonsmokers.

◇ Within 10 years, the lung cancer death rate drops almost to the rate for nonsmokers, precancerous cells

are replaced, and the incidence of other cancers decreases.

◇ **Within 10–15 years, the risk to all major diseases caused by smoking decreases to nearly that of those who have never smoked** (WHO, 1998).

(Adapted from Glantz, 1992)

The potential benefits to the lung by quitting may not be as great for those who started smoking as a teenager. Recent studies by John Wiencke of UC Medical Center in San Francisco showed that smoking in teenagers caused permanent genetic DNA damage to their lung cells leaving them forever at increased risk to lung cancer even if they quit smoking. Such damage was less likely among smokers who started their use in their 20s (Wiencke, Thurston, Kelsey, Varkonyi, & Wain, 1999).

Mentally there are other beneficial changes:

◇ initially there is anxiety, anger, difficulty concentrating, increased ap-

petite, and craving due to withdrawal;

◇ after 2 weeks most of these side effects disappear with the exception of craving and increased appetite.

THE TOBACCO INDUSTRY & TOBACCO ADVERTISING

The Business of Tobacco

Just a handful of companies controls the tobacco market in the United States. Philip Morris (Marlboro®, Virginia Slims®, Basic®), R.J. Reynolds/ Nabisco® (Winston®, Camel®, Salem®), Lorillard (Newport®), American Brands (Carlton®, Lucky Strike®, Pall Mall®), British American Tobacco (Kool®), and U.S. Tobacco (Copenhagen®, Skoal®) account for more than 95% of sales ($46 billion in 1998). **Over the past 25 years there has also been an aggressive expansion into foreign markets** aided by the weakening and dissolution of state-owned and

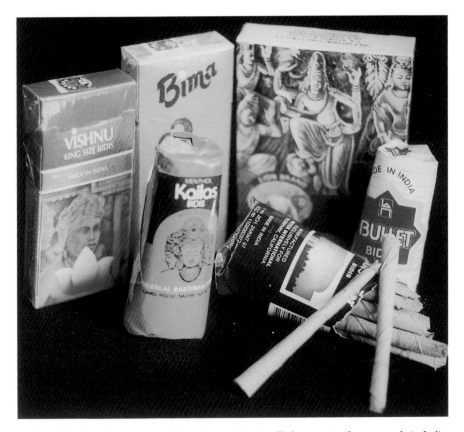

Oddly shaped and brightly colored packages of hand-rolled cigarettes that are made in India are called "bidis."

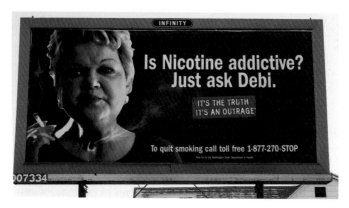
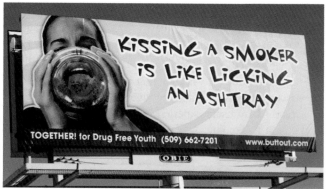

Tobacco advertising can work both ways.

smaller private tobacco companies. Cigarette smoking is growing at a rate of 3% a year in developing countries. **The United States consumes about 440 billion cigarettes annually.** U.S. exports of cigarettes rose to 250 billion by 1996 and have remained over 200 billion since then (U.S. Surgeon General, 2002).

In the 1980s because of the ever-increasing cost of a pack of cigarettes, many manufacturers came out with generic brands that were cheaper, e.g., Basic® by Philip Morris. To win back some of that market, the big manufacturers also lowered the prices on name brands.

Another attempt to expand the market has taken the form of hand-rolled *bidi* cigarettes. These innocuous-looking cigarettes are made in India but are also sold in the United States. The colorful packages seem aimed at children, mainly teenagers, and even come in flavors: grape, chocolate, and root beer to name a few. The dark Indian tobacco contains three times as much nicotine as American-grown tobacco. In one NIDA test *bidi* smokers were found to have a higher blood-nicotine level than conventional smokers. Even carbon monoxide levels were higher in some of the *bidi* smokers. The cigarettes are sold for $1.50 to $3.50 for a pack of 20, often in head shops and health-food stores. In India *bidis* comprise about 70% of the tobacco that is smoked. In the United States the Centers for Disease Control estimate that 2% to 5% of teens have tried *bidis*.

Advertising

Advertising expenditures by the tobacco industry are over $1 billion a year with another $1.5 billion in giveaways, premiums, promotional allowances to retailers, and other items. Advertising works. As a result of the Joe Camel® advertising campaign, sales of Camels® to teenage smokers from the age of 12–18 more than tripled over a 5-year period while the sales to adult Camel® smokers remained the same. The Joe Camel® campaign was finally dropped due to political and social pressure.

However, while the media focused on Joe Camel®, the most popular cigarettes among teenagers have been Marlboro® and Newport®. Among 12–17 year-olds in 1999

◇ 53.5% smoked Marlboro®;
◇ 9.0% smoked Newport®;
◇ 7.8% smoked Camels®.

Ethnically the differences in brand preferences are dramatic among 12–17-year-olds:

◇ **42.2% of Whites preferred Marlboro®** while only 16.5% preferred Newport®;
◇ **59.7% of Hispanics preferred Marlboro®** while only 18.6% preferred Newport®;
◇ **43.9% of Blacks preferred Newport®** while only 8.1% preferred Marlboro®.

(SAMHSA, 2001)

Studies have shown that starting to smoke in the teen years is more addic-

tive to the user than starting to smoke during adulthood. Also smokers who begin young are less likely to break the habit than adult-onset smokers, making the teen market extremely attractive to cigarette manufacturers (Wiencke et al., 1999). **The Centers for Disease Control found that approximately 80% of adult smokers started smoking before the age of 18** (CDC, 2002). The importance of this statistic cannot be overemphasized in terms of prevention and addiction. Proof of this fact can be seen by the tobacco companies' emphasis on appealing to new young smokers. For example, in a confidential memo a number of years ago one tobacco company advised its advertising department as follows:

"Thus, an attempt to reach young smokers, starters, should be based, among others, on the following major parameters:

◇ *Present the cigarette as one of a few initiations into the adult world.*

◇ *Present the cigarette as part of the illicit pleasure category of products and activities.*

◇ *In your ads, create a situation taken from the day-to-day life of the young smoker but in an elegant manner have this situation touch on the basic symbols of the growing-up, maturity process.*

◇ *To the best of your ability (considering some legal constraints), relate the cigarette to 'pot,' wine, beer, sex, etc.*

◇ <u>*Don't [their emphasis]*</u> *communicate health or health-related points."*

Antismoking advertising when done well is extremely effective. In Massachusetts when $70 million was spent in an antitobacco campaign on prime time television, sales of cigarettes dropped 20% compared to a national average drop of 3%. Between 1996 and 1999 current use in grades 7–12 dropped from 30.7% to 23.7% (Soldz, Clark, Stewart, Celebucki, & Klein, 2002).

Lawsuits & Laws

In 2002 a jury in Los Angeles awarded $28 billion to Betty Bullock, a 64-year-old lung cancer sufferer who claimed that Philip Morris, Inc. failed to warn her about the risks of smoking. The jury found the company liable for fraud, negligence, and product liability. The judgment has been appealed and will certainly be reduced. On the same day that Mrs. Bullock won, two more lawsuits were filed against Philip Morris, one for a wrongful death and the other by the smoker herself. **Lawsuits on behalf of dead or living smokers with cancer have been expanding and are being won** (although all judgments are appealed). The newest round of lawsuits are class-action suits against three tobacco giants alleging that cigarette makers used terms such as "light" to mislead smokers into thinking that those brands are safer. As of 2002, suits had been filed in 11 states, including Florida, Illinois, Minnesota, Oregon, and Massachusetts.

Because of the coughing and tearing caused by secondhand smoke, as well as documented actual health problems, numerous laws have been passed at the local, state, and federal levels prohibiting the use of tobacco products in a variety of spaces and buildings (e.g., sections of restaurants, airplanes, some businesses, federal and state buildings).

From indifference to other peoples' habits in the early 1980s, to a powerful crusade in the 1990s, to a growing tide of legislation in the 2000s, public opinion has changed. **Unfortunately tobacco has long been exempt from laws protecting the health of Americans.** The principal law that has been superseded is the one stating that no substance that causes cancer may be sold for human consumption. A special statute was voted by Congress exempting tobacco from this law. In 1997 and 1998 tobacco companies gave $220 million in soft-money political contributions (money given to political parties rather than specific candidates); $138 million to Republicans and $82 million to Democrats (White, 1999). Given the addictive nature of tobacco, some think that such contributions are the equivalent of marijuana or coca growers giving money to politicians to promote drug legalization.

By 1995 the Food and Drug Administration and the Clinton Administration were ready for a full-scale assault on the tobacco industry. The administration said its goal was to cut teenage smoking in half by sharply curtailing "the deadly temptations of tobacco and its skillful marketing" by the industry. **The industry said the real aim of the antismoking forces and the new legislation was to outlaw smoking altogether.** One of the themes of various tobacco industry campaigns was the right to choose. President Bill Clinton gave the FDA authority to regulate cigarettes because of their nicotine content; that is, because nicotine is addictive, it damages people's abilities to choose freely whether they want to smoke or not. The FDA declared cigarettes a drug, releasing material and memos from the tobacco industry itself showing that tobacco companies have long believed cigarettes are addictive, mainly because of nicotine. However, the industry countered FDA control in 1999 by claiming that since tobacco was so dangerous to health [sic], the FDA, which was supposed to regulate drugs beneficial to Americans, had no jurisdiction because, by law, all they could do to such a dangerous substance

would be to outlaw cigarettes. These matters will be in courts for years to come. However, the FDA did succeed in banning the sale of lollipops spiked with nicotine. They were selling for as much as $3 to $4 apiece. They have also banned any lip balm and bottled waters that contain nicotine.

The biggest assault on the tobacco industry has come from a number of state governments that sued or are suing the tobacco companies. Some of the suits are for the extra cost of health care due to smoking. Other suits accuse the tobacco industry of manipulating nicotine levels to keep smokers addicted. Brown and Williamson, the nation's 5th largest manufacturer (Chesterfield®, Eve®), settled a lawsuit in 1996 agreeing to pay 5% of its pretax profits ($50 million a year) toward programs that help people stop smoking.

To resolve two major lawsuits and hopefully forestall further litigation, **the major tobacco companies agreed to $40 billion and $206 billion settlements** to help pay for the medical costs of tobacco-induced illnesses, to finance smoking prevention campaigns (particularly aimed at teenagers), and to support other state programs. The money is to be paid over a period of 25 years. Unfortunately, as a result of reduced state tax income in the early 2000s, **many state governments have redirected the funds away from antismoking campaigns** into general funds. In desperation several states decided to borrow against future moneys thus receiving only a percentage of the settlement. In 2001 each state received an average of $164 million from the settlement but they only distributed 6% to tobacco control programs instead of the 20% to 25% suggested by the Centers for Disease Control. States with the highest smoking rates tended to spend the least on these prevention efforts (Gross, 2002).

Internationally there have been lawsuits for other reasons. The Canadian government tried to sue R.J. Reynolds Tobacco Co. claiming that they avoided taxes by smuggling tobacco into Canada through an Indian reser-

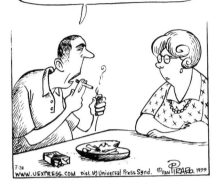

BiZarro   by Dan Piraro

"I'm under too much stress right now. I'll stop smoking after my suit against the tobacco industry is settled."

BIZZARO © 1999 by Dan Piraro. Reprinted by permission of Universal Press Syndicate. All rights reserved.

vation. The suit was thrown out of American courts due to the question of jurisdiction. The Netherlands voted to ban tobacco advertising including nonprint advertising and event sponsorship. Other European nations are battling the tobacco companies in their effort to ban advertising and increase warning labels on tobacco products.

Secondhand Smoke

Besides the issue of the addictive nature of tobacco and nicotine, a main battle over smoking during the 1990s and early 2000s involved the issue of secondhand smoke (the smoke that is inhaled by nonusers in a room with smokers). It is estimated that **one person dies from secondhand smoke (mostly from cardiovascular disease) for every 8 smoker deaths.** When the issue was first raised in the early 1980s, the evidence was scant but since then the U.S. Surgeon General's Office, the National Research Council, the Occupational Safety and Health Administration (OSHA), and the International Agency for Research on Cancer have concluded that secondhand smoke does cause lung cancer and cardiovascular diseases. Other studies have connected

secondhand smoke to other illnesses, including asthma and bronchitis in the children of smokers.

One of the reasons for the danger from secondhand smoke is that the sidestream smoke, mostly from a smoldering cigarette when the user is not inhaling, has higher concentrations of the substances, such as tar, that cause respiratory problems. So while secondhand smoke has small amounts of nicotine, it has 1–40 times the amount of carcinogens found in mainstream (inhaled) smoke.

In 1996 California, Utah, Vermont, Flagstaff, Arizona, New York City, and Boulder, Colorado had banned smoking in all bars and restaurants despite warnings from the owners that business would drop. The results of a study showed that, in fact, revenues increased in four localities, stayed the same in four localities, and in only one did the rate of increase slow down but not decrease (Glantz & Charlesworth, 1999).

THE SURGEON GENERAL'S REPORT ON SMOKING & HEALTH

The Surgeon General's report on smoking and health titled *Reducing*

Tobacco Use and released in 2000, drew a number of conclusions regarding prevention.

1. Efforts to prevent the onset or continuance of tobacco use face the pervasive, countervailing influence of tobacco promotion by the tobacco industry, a promotion that takes place despite overwhelming evidence of adverse health effects from tobacco use.

2. The available approaches to reducing tobacco use—educational, clinical, regulatory, economic, and comprehensive—differ substantially in their techniques and in the metric by which success can be measured. A hierarchy of effectiveness is difficult to construct.

3. Approaches with the largest span of impact (economic, regulatory, and comprehensive) are likely to have the greatest long-term population impact. Those with a smaller span of impact (educational and clinical) are of greater importance in helping persons resist or abandon the use of tobacco.

4. Each of the modalities reviewed provides evidence of effectiveness.

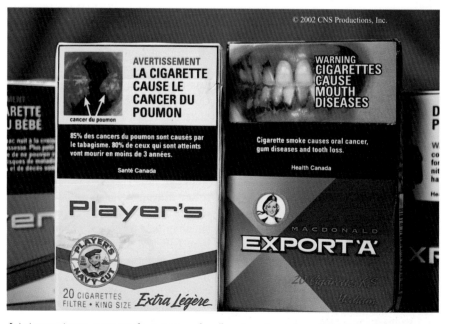

It is interesting to compare the warnings found on American cigarette packages and Canadian cigarette packages. The Canadians are willing to tell the complete truth about tobacco.

◊ Educational strategies, conducted in conjunction with community and media-based activities, can postpone or prevent smoking onset in 20% to 40% of adolescents.

◊ Pharmacological treatment of nicotine addiction, combined with behavioral support will enable 20% to 25% of users to remain abstinent at 1 year post treatment. Even less intense measures, such as physicians advising their patients to quit smoking, can produce cessation proportions of 5% to 10%.

◊ Regulation of advertising and promotion, particularly that directed at young persons, is very likely to reduce both prevalence and uptake of smoking.

◊ Clean air regulations and restriction of minors' access to tobacco products contribute to a changing social norm with regard to smoking and may influence prevalence directly.

(Surgeon General, 2000)

CONCLUSIONS

Stimulants seem like all-American drugs because initially they mimic virtues that are highly prized in our culture: the ability to work hard and stay up late, alertness, confidence, aggression, and mental acuity. Americans want a cup of coffee or a cigarette to wake up; more coffee at work to get going; a cola in the afternoon to carry on; an OTC product or prescription diet pill to hold the appetite down; a snort of methamphetamine to make the work less boring; a daily dose of Ritalin® to hold the kids in line; and a "rock" of crack to bring out the party animal. Instant energy, confidence, and gratification are sought.

Compare the use of stimulants to gain energy and confidence to natural methods where energy supplies are replenished through relaxation, sleep, naps, light morning exercise, meditation, good nutrition, and a healthy lifestyle. The natural methods first create the energy supplies and then let them be spent. The chemical methods drain the body of its energy supplies, so it has to shut down to recover. The natural method works time after time. The chemical method causes tolerance and psychological dependence to develop, so the resulting excess use taxes the body's resources and can damage neurochemistry.

CHAPTER SUMMARY

General Classification

1. Uppers are central nervous system stimulants.

2. The 7 principal stimulants are cocaine (including crack), amphetamines, amphetamine congeners (e.g., Ritalin® and diet pills), look-alike or over-the-counter stimulants, miscellaneous plant stimulants, caffeine, and nicotine.

General Effects

3. By increasing chemical and electrical activity in the central nervous system, stimulants increase energy, raise heart rate, blood pressure, and respiration; they make the user more alert, active, confident, anxious, restless, aggressive, and less hungry.

4. Uppers cause many of their effects by forcing the release of energy chemicals (particularly norepinephrine and epinephrine).

5. Most problems with stimulants occur when the body isn't given time to recover and its energy supply becomes depleted. The user can fall into a severe depression.

6. Cardiovascular side effects can include heart arrhythmias, constricted blood vessels, and heart disease.

7. Another set of problems with the stronger stimulants comes when the stimulated reward/reinforcement center does not signal the need for food, drink, or sexual stimulation, resulting in malnutrition, dehydration, or a reduced sex drive.

8. Since stimulants reduce appetite, almost all of them are used to reduce weight, often causing various health problems.

9. Though stimulants initially increase confidence and induce a certain euphoria, excessive use of the stronger stimulants can cause severe neurotransmitter imbalance. A user can become paranoid, have muscle tremors, become aggressive, and even become psychotic.

10. A major problem with all stimulants is their ability to induce rapid tolerance and ultimately major abuse and addiction problems.

Cocaine

11. Cocaine is noted for the intensity of its stimulation, its high price, and the speed with which it is metabolized in the body. It produces an intense craving and is highly addicting.

12. The coca leaf is chewed and the stimulating juice is absorbed through the buccal mucosa in 3–5 minutes. The refined cocaine hydrochloride can be snorted (2–5 minutes), injected (15–30 seconds), or drunk (15–30 minutes). Cocaine freebase (crack, "rock") is smoked. Smoking is the fastest route to the brain, 7–10 seconds.

13. Cocaine is a topical anesthetic and is used for medical procedures, such as eye surgery, or to desensitize the pain of skin lesions.

14. Cocaine mimics and intensifies natural body functions and highs. The comedown is equally intense,

so the user keeps taking the drug to stay up. The brain becomes sensitized to the memory of the pleasurable effects.

15. Cocaine as well as amphetamines initially delay orgasm and so are taken to try and enhance sexual activity but prolonged use eventually causes sexual dysfunction, including a decrease in orgasm.

16. Cocaine, especially when used in combination with alcohol, can precipitate violence, often domestic violence.

17. Cocaine can also cause heart damage and damage to the fetus of a pregnant user.

18. Tolerance develops rapidly causing severe psychological dependence.

19. An overdose of cocaine can be the result of as little as one-fiftieth of a gram or as much as 1.2 grams or more. Most overdose reactions are not fatal but death can come from cardiac arrest, respiratory depression, and seizures.

20. Cocaine is often used in conjunction with other drugs.

21. The compulsion to use cocaine and methamphetamines is often caused by the desire to experience natural body functions such as extra energy, confidence, alertness, and euphoria artificially. The desire to escape mental pain and overcome a sense of hopelessness also makes a person use. People continue using because body chemistry has been changed by the drug thus creating a compulsion to use.

Smokable Cocaine (crack, freebase)

22. Freebase cocaine and crack are smokable forms of cocaine. Crack has more impurities.

23. Smoking freebase cocaine is more intense than snorting cocaine because when smoked in the freebase form the drug reaches the brain more quickly, can be taken more often, and is more fat-soluble.

24. Crack cocaine causes many problems because of the economics of the drug. It is sold in smaller more affordable units but because of its quick metabolism and rapid addiction, its use quickly accelerates to $100 to $300-a-day amounts.

Amphetamines

25. Amphetamines are very similar to cocaine, the main difference being that they are synthetic, longer acting, and cheaper to buy.

26. Amphetamines were originally prescribed to fight exhaustion, depression, narcolepsy, asthma, some forms of epilepsy, and obesity but were often taken for their mood-elevating and euphoric properties.

27. Prolonged use of amphetamines can induce paranoia, heart and blood vessel problems, twitches, increased body temperature, dehydration, and malnutrition.

28. Tolerance develops rapidly with amphetamines. Amphetamine and cocaine withdrawal causes physical and emotional depression, extreme irritability, nervousness, anergia, anhedonia, and craving.

Amphetamine Congeners

29. Many diet pills and mood elevators mimic the actions of amphetamines but are not quite as strong.

30. Currently congeners like Ritalin® and Cylert® are used in the treatment of attention-deficit/hyperactivity disorders (ADHD). Amphetamines, e.g., Adderall®, are also used.

31. Diet pills can still cause many of the problems found with amphetamines and can be addicting. The diet pill combination of phentermine and fenfluramine or dexfenfluramine, called "fen-phen," was found to cause heart damage and was taken off the market.

Lookalike & Over-The-Counter (OTC) Stimulants

32. Lookalike drugs were popularized to take advantage of the desire for amphetamines and cocaine. They are composed of over-the-counter stimulants. Heavy use can cause heart and blood vessel problems as well as dependence.

Miscellaneous Plant Stimulants

33. Other plant stimulants, such as khat, betel nut, ephedra, and yohimbe, have been used by hundreds of millions of people, particularly in the Middle East and Africa, since ancient times. They are still used today.

34. A synthetic form of khat, methcathinone, is widely used in Russia and is being made in the United States.

Caffeine

35. Caffeine, particularly coffee, is the most popular stimulant in the world. Besides coffee, caffeine is found in tea, chocolate (cocoa), caffeinated soft drinks, and a number of over-the-counter products.

36. Tolerance can develop with caffeine. Withdrawal symptoms such as headaches, depression, sleep problems, and irritability do occur, particularly if consumption is more than 5 cups a day.

Nicotine

37. Nicotine (tobacco) is the most addicting psychoactive drug. In the United States at least 46 million people are addicted to cigarettes compared to the 15 million addicted to alcohol.

38. Nicotine addiction causes more deaths than all the other psychoactive drugs combined.

39. One of the main reasons for tobacco's addictive nature, besides the slight stimulation it gives, is the need for the smoker's body to maintain a certain level of nicotine in the blood to avoid severe withdrawal symptoms.

40. Besides shortening a person's life span, tobacco lowers the quality of life.

41. Smokeless tobacco is as addicting and as damaging as tobacco that is

smoked with the exception of lung damage.

42. Lawsuits brought by local, state, and federal governments in the United States, as well as individual

or class-action suits, are being won against the tobacco companies for increasing the addictive nature of their products and for the health damage caused by smoking.

Conclusions

43. Though stimulants initially boost many of the qualities we admire, they have a full share of side effects that cause damage when the substance is over used.

REFERENCES

Aldrich, M. R. (1994). Historical notes on women addicts. *Journal of Psychoactive Drugs, 26* (1), 61–64.

Amen, D. G. (1999). ADD and the brain. Amen Clinic for Behavioral Medicine [Online]. Available: *http://www.amenclinic.com/ac/amenLA.asp*

Amen, D. G., Yantis, S., Trudeau, J., Stubblefield, M. S., & Halverstadt, J. S. (1997). Visualizing the firestorms in the brain: An inside look at the clinical and physiological connections between drugs and violence using brain SPECT imaging. *Journal of Psychoactive Drugs, 29*(4), 307–320.

American Psychiatric Association. (2000). *Diagnostic and Statistical Manual of Mental Disorders* (4th ed., text revision [DSM-IV-TR]). Washington, DC: Author.

Baldwin, G. C., et al. (2002). Drastic acceleration of HIV progression linked to cocaine use. *Journal of Infectious Diseases, 185,* 701–705.

Barkley, R. A. (1998). Attention-deficit/hyperactivity disorder. *Scientific American,* 1998, September 10.

Barsky, S. H., Roth, M. D., Kleerup, E. C., Simmons, M., & Tashkin, D. P. (1998). Histopathologic and molecular alterations in bronchial epithelium in habitual smokers of marijuana, cocaine, and/or tobacco. *Journal of the National Cancer Institute, 90*(16), 1198–1205.

Benowitz, N. L., & Fredericks, A. (1995). History of tobacco use. *Encyclopedia of Drugs and Alcohol* (Vol. III, pp. 1032–1036). New York: Simon & Shuster MacMillan.

Bibra, E. F. (1995). *Plant Intoxicants: Betel and Related Substances.* Rochester, VT: Healing Arts Press.

Biederman, J., Faraone, S. V., et al. (1993). Patterns of psychiatric co-morbidity, cognition and psychosocial functioning in adults with attention-deficit/hyperactivity disorder. *American Journal of Psychiatry, 150,* 1792–1798.

Biederman, J., Wilens, T., Mick, E., et al. (1997). Is ADHD a risk factor for psychoactive substance use disorders? Findings from a four-year prospective

follow-up study. *Journal of the American Academy of Child and Adolescent Psychiatry, 36*(1), 21–30.

Biederman, J., Wilens, T., Mick, E., Spencer, T., & Faraone, S. V. (1999). Pharmacotherapy of attention-deficit/hyperactivity disorder reduces risk for substance use disorder. *Pediatrics, 104*(2).

Blum, K., Braverman, E. R., Cull, J. G., Holder, J. M., Luck, R., Lubar, J., Miller, D., & Comings, D. E. (2000). "Reward deficiency syndrome" (RDS): A biogenetic model for the diagnosis and treatment of impulsive, addictive, and compulsive behaviors. *Journal of Psychoactive Drugs, 32*(1).

Breiter, H., Gollub, R., Weisskoss, R., Kennedy, D., Makris, N., Berke, J., Goodman, J., Kantor, H., Gastfriend, D., Riorden, J., Mathew, R., Rosen, B., & Hyman, S. (1997). Acute effects of cocaine on human brain activity and emotion. *Neuron, 19,* 591–611.

Brookoff, D., O'Brien, K. K., Cook, C. S., Thompson, T. D., & Williams, C. (1997). Characteristics of participants in domestic violence: Assessment at the scene of domestic assault. *Journal of the American Medical Association (JAMA), 277*(17), 1369–1372.

Calkins, R. F., Aktan, G. B., & Hussain, K. L. (1995). Methcathinone: The next illicit stimulant epidemic? *Journal of Psychoactive Drugs, 27*(3), 277–285.

Calvani, S. (2002). Ya Ba: The medicine which makes you crazy [Online]. Available: *http://www.sandrocalvani.com/interview/yaba.htm*

Cantwell, D. P. (1996). Attention-deficit disorder: A review of the past 10 years. *Journal of the American Academy of Child and Adolescent Psychiatry, 35.*

Castellanos, F. X., Lee, P. L., Sharp, W., Jeffries, N. O., Greenstein, D. K., Clasen, L. A., Blumenthal, J. D., James, R. S., Ebens, C. L., Walter, J. M., Zijdenbox, A. C., Giedd, J. N., & Rapoport, J. L. (2002). Developmental trajectories of brain volume abnormalities in children and adolescents with attention-

deficit/hyperactivity disorder. *Journal of the American Medical Association (JAMA), 288,* 1740–1748.

Castilla, J., Barrio, G., Belza, M., & de la Fuente, L. (1999). Drug and alcohol consumption and sexual risk behavior among young adults: Results from a national survey. *Drug and Alcohol Dependence, 56,* 47–53.

Centers for Disease Control. (2002). Cigarette smoking-related mortality. TIPS, Tobacco Information and Prevention Source [Online]. Available: *http://www.cdc.gov/tobacco.htm*

Childress, A. R., et al. (1999). Limbic activation during cue-induced cocaine craving. *American Journal of Psychiatry, 156*(1), 11–18.

Childress, A. R., McElgin, W., Mozley, D., Reivich, M., & O'Brien, G. (1996). Brain correlates of cue-induced cocaine and opiate craving. *Society for Neuroscience Abstracts, 22:365.5.*

Coca growers' champion wins new era for Indians. (2002, July 16). *San Francisco Chronicle,* p. A6.

Coffee Science Source. (1998). Coffee facts and figures [Online]. Available: *http://www.coffeescience.org/factrend.html*

Collins, A. C. (1990). An analysis of the addiction liability of nicotine. In C. K. Erikson, M. A. Javors, & W. W. Morgan (Eds.), *Addiction Potential of Abused Drugs and Drug Classes.* New York: The Haworth Press.

Comings, D. E., Wu, S., Chiu, C., et al. (1996). Polygenic inheritance of Tourette's syndrome, stuttering, attention-deficit/hyperactivity, conduct, and oppositional defiant disorder: The additive and subtractive effect of the three dopaminergic genes-DRD$_2$, D beta H, and DAT$_1$. *American Journal of Medical Genetics, 6*(3), 264–288.

Connolly, H. M., Crary, J. L., McGoon, M. D., et al. (1997). Valvular heart disease associated with fenfluramine-phentermine. *New England Journal of Medicine, 337*(9).

Cross, J. C., Johnson, B. D., Rees Davis, W., & Liberty, J. J. (2001). Supporting the habit: Income generation activities of frequent crack users compared with frequent users of other hard drugs. *Drug and Alcohol Dependence, 64,* 191–201.

DASIS Report. (2001). Amphetamine treatment admissions increase: 1993–1999 [Online]. Available: *http://www.samhsa.gov/oas/facts/Speed.cfm*

Drug Abuse Warning Network. (2002). Emergency Department trends from DAWN [Online]. Available: *http://www.samhsa.gov*

Drug Enforcement Administration. (2001). Congressional testimony by Errol J. Chavez, Special Agent in Charge, DEA. April 13, 2001 [Online]. Available: *http://www.usdoj.gov/dea/pubs/cngrtest/ct041301.htm*

Drug Enforcement Administration. (2002a). Congressional testimony by Asa Hutchinson, Administrator, DEA. March 13, 2002 [Online]. Available: *http://www.usdoj.gov/dea/pubs/cngrtest/ct031302.html*

Drug Enforcement Administration. (2002b). History of the DEA, 1985–1990 [Online]. Available: *http://www.usdoj.gov/dea/deamuseum/1985_1990.htm*

Drug Enforcement Administration. (2002c). NNICC report on the supply of illicit drugs to the United States [Online]. Available: *http://www.usdoj.gov/dea/concern/drug_trafficking.html*

Dunlop, E., & Johnson, B. D. (1992). The setting for the crack era: Macro forces, micro consequences (1960–1992). *Journal of Psychoactive Drugs, 24*(4), 307–322.

Edlin, B. R., Irwin, K. L., & Faruque, S. (1994). Intersecting epidemics: Crack cocaine use and HIV infection among inner-city young adults. *New England Journal of Medicine, 331,* 1422–1427.

Ellinwood, E. H. (1973). Amphetamine and stimulant drugs. *Drug Use in America: Problem in Perspective. Second report. Marijuana and Drug Abuse Commission,* 140–157.

Epping-Jordan, M. P., Watkins, S. S., Koob, G. F., & Markou, A. (1998). Dramatic decreases in brain reward function during nicotine withdrawal. *Nature, 393*(6680), 76–79.

Federal Bureau of Prisons. (1997). Available: *http://www.bop.gov*

Foreman, R., Klein, J., Barks, J., et al. (1994). Prevalence of fetal exposure to cocaine in Toronto, 1990–1991. *Clinical Investment Medicine, 17*(3), 206–211.

Fowler, J. S., Volkow, N. D., Wang, G. J., et al. (1996). Brain monoamine oxidase A inhibition in cigarette smokers. *Proceedings of the National Academy of Sciences, 93,* 14065–14069.

Frank, D. A. (2001). Cocaine called no more teratogenic than other drugs. *Journal of the American Medical Association (JAMA), 285,* 1613–1627.

Freud, S. (1884). *Über Coca.* In R. Byck (Ed.) (1974), *The Cocaine Papers of Sigmund Freud.* New York: Stonehill.

Fukui, S., Wada, K., & Iyo, M. (1991). History and current use of methamphetamine in Japan. In S. Fukui et al. (Eds.), *Cocaine and Methamphetamine: Behavioral Toxicology, Clinical Pharmacology and Epidemiology.* Tokyo: Drug Abuse Prevention Center.

Garavan, H., Pankiewicz, J., Bloom, A., Cho, J. K., Sperry, L., Ross, T. J., Salmeron, B. J., Risinger, R., Kelley, D., & Stein, E. A. (2000). Cue-induced cocaine craving: Neuroanatomical specificity for drug users and drug stimuli. *American Journal of Psychiatry, 157*(11), 1789–1798.

Giannini, A. J., Burge, H., Shaheen, J. M., & Price, W. A. (1986). Khat: Another drug of abuse. *Journal of Psychoactive Drugs, 18*(2), 155–158.

Glantz, S. A. (1992). *Tobacco: Biology & Politics.* Waco, TX: Health Edco.

Glantz, S. A., & Charlesworth, A. (1999). Tourism and hotel revenues before and after passage of smoke-free restaurant ordinances. *Journal of the American Medical Association (JAMA), 281,* 1911–1918.

Gold, M. S., & Herkov, M. J. (1998). The pharmacology of cocaine, crack and other stimulants. In A. W. Graham & T. K. Schultz, T. K. (Eds.), *Principles of Addiction Medicine* (2nd ed., pp. 137–145). Chevy Chase, MD: American Society of Addiction Medicine, Inc.

Gold, M. S., & Miller, N. S. (1997). Cocaine (and crack): Neurobiology. In J. H. Lowinson, P. Ruiz, R. B. Millman, & J. G. Langrod (Eds.), *Substance Abuse: A Comprehensive Textbook* (3rd ed., pp. 181–198). Baltimore: Williams & Wilkins.

Goldstein, A. (2001). *Addiction: From Biology to Drug Policy* (2nd ed.). New York: Oxford University Press.

Goldstein, P. J., Ouellet, L. J., & Fendrick, M. (1992). From bag brides to skeezers: A historical perspective on sex-for-drugs behavior. *Journal of Psychoactive Drugs, 24*(2), 349–362.

Gonzalez Castro, F., Barrington, E. H., Walton, M. A., & Rawson, R. A. (2000). Cocaine and methamphetamine: Differential addiction rates. *Psychology of Addiction Behavior, 14*(4), 390–396.

Goudie, A., & Newton, T. (1985). The puzzle of drug-induced taste aversion: Comparative studies with cathinone and amphetamine. *Psychopharmacology, 87,* 328–333.

Greden, J. F., & Walters, A. (1997). Caffeine. In J. H. Lowinson, P. Ruiz, R. B. Millman, & J. G. Langrod (Eds.), *Substance Abuse: A Comprehensive Textbook* (3rd ed.). Baltimore: Williams & Wilkins.

Greenbaum, E. (1993). Blackened bronchoalveolar lavage fluid in crack smokers, a preliminary study. *American Journal of Clinical Pathology, 100,* 481–487.

Griffiths, R. R., & Vernotica, E. M. (2000). Is caffeine a flavoring agent in cola soft drinks? *Archives of Family Medicine, 9*(8).

Griffiths, R. R., et al. (1986). Human coffee drinking: Manipulation of concentration and caffeine dose. *Journal of the Experimental Analysis of Behavior, 45,* 133–148.

Grinspoon, L., & Bakalar, J. B. (1985). *Cocaine: A Drug and Its Social Evolution.* New York: Basic Books, Inc.

Grinspoon, L., & Hedblom, P. (1975). *The Speed Culture: Amphetamine Use and Abuse in America.* Cambridge, MA: Harvard University Press.

Gross, C. P. (2002). U.S. States not using tobacco dollars wisely. *New England Journal of Medicine, 347,* 1080–1088, 1106–1108.

Guttmacher, H. (1885). New medications and therapeutic techniques concerning the different cocaine preparations and their effects. In R. Byck (Ed.) (1974), *The Cocaine Papers of Sigmund Freud.* New York: Stonehill.

Hamid, A. (1992). The developmental cycle of a drug epidemic: The cocaine smoking epidemic of 1981–1991. *Journal of Psychoactive Drugs, 24*(4), 337–348.

Harler, C. R. (1984). Tea production. *Encyclopaedia Britannica* (Vol. 18, pp. 16–19). Chicago: Encyclopaedia Britannica.

Harris Poll. (1999). Relapse of smokers. *USA Today.*

Horner, B. R., & Scheibe, K. E. (1997). Prevalence and implications of attention-deficit/hyperactivity disorder among adolescents in treatment for substance abuse. *Journal of the American Academy of Child and Adolescent Psychiatry. 36*(1), 30–36.

Hurst, W. J., Tarka, S. M., Powis, T. G., Valdez, F., & Hester, T. R. (2002). Cacao usage by the earliest Mayan Civilizations. *Nature, 418,* 289–290.

IMS Health. (2002). IMS Health Reports [Online]. Available: *http://www.imshealth.com*

James, J. E. (1991). *Caffeine and Health.* London: Harcourt Brace Jovanovich.

Jensen, P., et al. (1999). A 14-month randomized clinical trial of treatment strategies for attention-deficit/hyperactivity disorder. *Archives of General Psychiatry, 56*(12), 1073–1086.

Jeri, F. R., Sanchez, C., Del Pozo, T., & Fernandez, M. (1992). The syndrome of coca paste. *Journal of Psychoactive Drugs, 24*(2). 173–182.

Kalix, P. (1994). Khat, an amphetamine-like stimulant. *Journal of Psychoactive Drugs, 26*(1), 69–73.

Karch, S. B. (1996). *The Pathology of Drug Abuse.* Boca Raton, FL: CRC Press.

Karch, S. B. (1997). *A Brief History of Cocaine.* Boca Raton, FL: CRC Press.

Keefe, J. D. (2001). Clandestine methamphetamine laboratories. DEA congressional testimony by Joseph D. Keefe, Chief of Operations, DEA. July 12, 2001 [Online]. Available: *http://www.usdoj.gov/dea/pubs/cngrtest/ct071201.htm*

Kelz, M. B., Chen, J., Carlezon, W. A., et al. (1999). Expression of the transcription factor DFosB in the brain controls sensitivity to cocaine. *Nature, 401,* 272–276.

King, G. R., & Ellinwood, E. H. (1997). Amphetamines and other stimulants. In J. H. Lowinson, P. Ruiz, R. B. Millman, & J. G. Langrod (Eds.), *Substance Abuse: A Comprehensive Textbook* (3rd ed.). Baltimore: Williams & Wilkins.

Klebanoff, M. A., Levine, R. J., DeSimonian, R., Clemens, J. D., & Wilkins, D. G. (1999). Maternal serum paraxanthine, a caffeine metabolite, and the risk of spontaneous abortion. *New England Journal of Medicine, 341*(22), 1639–1644.

Klesges, R. C., Meyers, A. W., Klesges, L. M., & LaVasque, M. E. (1989). Smoking, body weight, and their effects on smoking behavior: A comprehensive review of the literature. *Psychological Bulletin, 106,* 204–230.

Kuhar, M. J. (1995). Cola/Cola Drinks. In J. H. Jaffe (Ed.), *Encyclopedia of Drugs and Alcohol* (Vol. I, pp. 251–252). New York: Simon & Shuster MacMillan.

Landry, M. (1992). An overview of cocaethylene. *Journal of Psychoactive Drugs, 24*(3), 273–276.

Lane, J. D., et al. (2002). Caffeine elevates stress throughout the day. *Psychosomatic Medicine, 64,* 593–603.

Leinwand, D. (2002a, August 21). 10 held in smuggling of "Nazi Speed." *USA Today,* p.1.

Leinwand, D. (2002b, August 23). U.S. seizures of narcotic shrub on the rise. *USA Today,* p.1.

Lichtblau, E., & Schrader, E. (1999, December 1). U.S. fears it badly under-estimated cocaine production in Colombia. *Los Angeles Times.*

Lindner, J. D., Monkemuller, K. E., Raijman, I., Johnson, L., Lazenby, A. J., & Wilcox, M. (2000). Cocaine-associated ischemic colitis. *Southern Medical Journal, 93*(9), 909–913.

Mannuzza, S., et al. (1991). Hyperactive boys almost grown up. *Archives of General Psychiatry, 48,* 565–576.

Marnell, T. (Ed.). (1997). *Drug Identification Bible.* Denver: Drug Identification Bible.

Mayo Clinic. (1999). New fen-phen study finds heart-valve disease may improve after stopping drugs. Mayo Clinic Proceedings [Online]. Available: *http://www.mayo.edu/proceedings/1999/dec1999.htm*

McGowan, J. D., et al. (1988). Neonatal withdrawal symptoms after chronic ingestion of caffeine. *Southern Medical Journal, 81,* 1092–1094.

Milberger, S., Biederman, J., Faraone, S. V., & Jones, J. (1998). Further evidence of an association between maternal smoking during pregnancy and attention-deficit/hyperactivity disorder: Findings from a high-risk sample of siblings. *Journal of Clinical Child Psychology, 27,* 352–358.

Miller, D., & Blum, K. (1996). *Overload: Attention-Deficit Disorder and the Addictive Brain.* Kansas City: Andrews and McMeel.

Miller, M., & Kozel, N. (1995). Amphetamine epidemics. In J. H. Jaffee (Ed.), *Encyclopedia of Drugs and Alcohol* (Vol. I, pp. 110–117). New York: Simon & Shuster MacMillan.

Monardes, N. (1577). *Joyfull Newes Out of the Newe Founde Worlde.* Translated by Frampton, J. Reprinted in 1967. New York: AMS Press, Inc.

Monitoring the Future. (2002). Cigarette brands smoked by American teens [Online]. Available: *http://www.umich.edu/~newsinfor/*

Morgan, J. P., Wesson, D. R., Puder, K. S., & Smith, D. E. (1987). Duplicitous drugs: The history and recent status of lookalike drugs. *Journal of Psychoactive Drugs, 19*(1), 21–31.

National Institute on Drug Abuse. (1998). Current trends in drug use worldwide. *NIDA Notes, 13*(2).

National Institute on Drug Abuse. (2000). Nicotine and dopamine. *NIDA Notes, 15*(2).

National Institutes of Health. (1998). Diagnosis and treatment of attention-deficit/hyperactivity disorder: Consensus development conference statement [Online]. Available: *http://odp.od.nih.gov/consensus/cons/110/110_statement.htm*

National Institute of Mental Health. (1999). Attention-Deficit/Hyperactivity Disorder. *NIH Publication No. 96–357.2.*

National Soft Drink Association. (1999). Soft drink facts [Online]. Available: *http://www.mariec@nsda.com*

O'Brien, R., Cohen, S., Evans, G., & Fine, J. (1992). *The Encyclopedia of Drug Abuse* (2nd ed.). New York: Facts On File.

Office of National Drug Control Policy. (2000). What America's users spend on illegal drugs [Online]. Available: *http://www.whitehousedrugpolicy.gov*

Pary, R., Lewis, S., Arnp, C. S., Matuschka, P. R., & Lippmann, S. (2002). Attention-deficit/hyperactivity disorder: An update. *Southern Medical Journal, 95*(7), 743–749.

Perkins, K. A. (1993). Weight gain following smoking cessation. *Journal of Consulting Clinical Psychology, 61,* 768–777.

Pliszka, S. R. (1998). Comorbidity of attention-deficit/hyperactivity disorder in children. *Journal of Clinical Psychiatry, 59* (Suppl. 7), 50–58.

Post, R. M., & Kopanda, R. T. (1976). Cocaine, kindling, and psychosis. *American Journal of Psychiatry, 133,* 627–634.

Rachima-Maoz, C., Peleg, E., & Rosenthal, T. (1998). The effect of caffeine on ambulatory blood pressure in hypertensive patients. *American Journal of Hypertension, 11,* 1426–1432.

Randall, T. (1992). Cocaine, alcohol mix in body to form even longer lasting, more lethal drugs. *Journal of the American Medical Association (JAMA), 267,* 1043–1044.

Ricaurte, B., et al. (1997). Reductions in brain dopamine and serotonin transporters detected in humans previously exposed to repeated high doses of methcathinone using PET. *Society for Neuroscience Abstracts, 22,* 1915. Also in *NIDA Notes, 11*(5).

Richards, J. B., Baggot, M. J., Sabol, K. E., & Seiden, L. S. (1999). A high-dose methamphetamine regimen results in long-lasting deficits on performance. *Journal of Psychoactive Drugs, 31*(4).

Rodu, B., & Cole, P. (2002). Smokeless tobacco use and cancer of the upper respiratory tract. Dry snuff has a higher cancer risk. *Journal of Oral Surgery, Oral Medicine, Oral Pathology, Oral Radiology, and Endodontics, 93*(5), 511-515.

Satel, J. A., & Lieberman, J. A. (1991). Schizophrenia and substance abuse. *Psychiatric Clinics of North America, 16*(2), 401–412.

Schmitz, J. M., Schneider, N. G., & Jarvik, M. E. (1997). Nicotine. In J. H. Lowinson, P. Ruiz, R. B. Millman, & J. G. Langrod (Eds.), *Substance Abuse: A Comprehensive Textbook* (3rd ed., pp. 276–290). Baltimore, MD: Williams & Wilkins.

Schuckit, M. (2000). *Drug and Alcohol Abuse* (5th ed.). New York: Kluwer Academic/Plenum Publishers.

Semrud-Clikeman, M., Filipek, P. A., Biederman, J., Steingard, R., Kennedy, D., Renshaw, P., & Bekken, K. (1994). Attention-deficit/hyperactivity disorder: Magnet resonance imaging morphometric analysis of the corpus callosum. *Journal of the American Academy of Child Adolescent Psychiatry, 33*(6), 875–881.

Severson, K. (2002, September 29). L.A. school district officials vote to restrict soda sales. *San Francisco Chronicle.*

Siegel, R. K. (1992). Cocaine freebase use: A new smoking disorder. *Journal of Psychoactive Drugs, 24*(2), 183–209.

Silverman, K., et al. (1992). Withdrawal syndrome after the double-blind cessation of caffeine consumption. *New England Journal of Medicine, 327,* 1109–1114.

Silverman, K., & Griffiths, R. R. (1995a). Coffee. In J. H. Jaffee (Ed.), *Encyclopedia of Drugs and Alcohol* (Vol. I, pp. 250–251). New York: Simon & Shuster MacMillan.

Silverman, K., & Griffiths, R. R. (1995b). Tea. In J. H. Jaffee (Ed.), *Encyclopedia of Drugs and Alcohol* (Vol. III, pp. 1018–1019). New York: Simon & Shuster MacMillan.

Singer, K, T., Arendt, R., Minnes, S., Farkas, K., Salvator, A., Kirchner, H. L., & Kliegman, R. (2002). Cognitive and motor outcomes of cocaine-exposed infants. *Journal of the American Medical Association (JAMA), 287,* 1952-1960.

Slade, J. (1992). The tobacco epidemic: Lessons from history. *Journal of Psychoactive Drugs, 24*(2), 99–110.

Smith, D. E., & Seymour, R. B. (2001). *Clinician's Guide to Substance Abuse.* New York: McGraw-Hill.

Smith, D. E., & Wesson, D. R. (1985). *Treating the Cocaine Abuser.* Center City, MN: Hazelden.

Snyder, S. H. (1996). *Drugs and the Brain.* New York: W. H. Freeman and Sons.

Soldz, S., Clark, T. W., Stewart, E., Celebucki, C., & Klein, W. D. (2002). Decreased youth tobacco use in Massachusetts 1996 to 1999: Evidence of tobacco control effectiveness. *Tobacco Control* (Suppl. 2), II14 –II19.

Spitz, M. (1998, March 5). Gene can help smokers kick the habit. *San Francisco Chronicle,* p. A4.

Stahl, S. M. (2000). *Essential Psychopharmacology.* Cambridge, England: Cambridge University Press.

Stein, E. A., Pankiewicz, J., Harsch, H. H., et al. (1998). Nicotine-induced limbic cortical activation in the human brain: A functional MRI study. *American Journal of Psychiatry, 155*(8), 1009–1015.

Substance Abuse and Mental Health Services Administration. (2001). *Tobacco Use in America: Findings from the 1999 National Household Survey on Drug Abuse.* Rockville, MD: SAMHSA, Office of Applied Studies.

Substance Abuse and Mental Health Services Administration. (2002). *National Household Survey on Drug Abuse, 2001.* Rockville, MD: SAMHSA, Office of Applied Studies.

Substance Abuse and Mental Health Services Administration/Treatment Episode Data Sets. (2000). *SAMHSA/TEDS, 1999.* Rockville, MD: SAMHSA, Office of Applied Studies.

Surgeon General. (2000). Reducing tobacco use: A report to the Surgeon General [Online]. Available: *http://www.cdc.gov/tobacco/sgr_tobacco_use.htm*

Tardiff, K., Marzuk, P. M., Leon, A. C., Hirsch, C. S., Stajic, M., Portera, L., & Hartwell, N. (1994). Homicide in New York City: Cocaine use and firearms. *Journal of the American Medical Association (JAMA), 272,* 43–46.

Tinsley, J. A., & Wadkins, D. D. (1998). Over-the-counter stimulants: Abuse and addiction. *Mayo Clinic Proceedings, 73*(10), 977–982.

Tuncel, M., Zhongyun, W., Arbiquew, D., Fadel, P. J., Victor, R. G., & Vongpatanasin, W. (2002). Mechanism of the blood pressure-raising effect of cocaine in humans. *Circulation, 105,* 1054–1059.

U.S. Department of Justice. (1992). Khat factsheet. Drug Enforcement Administration, Intelligence Division [Online]. Available: *http://usdoj.gov/dea/concern/khat.html*

U.S. Surgeon General. (2002). U.S. tobacco fact sheets [Online]. Available: *http://www.cdc.gov/tobacco/sgr/sgr_2000/USTobaccoExports.pdf*

Uhl, G., et al. (2001, April 23). Study clarifies brain mechanisms of cocaine's high. *NIDA News Release.*

Volkow, N. D., et al. (2001). Methamphetamine abuse leads to long-lasting changes in the human brain that are linked to impaired coordination and memory. *American Journal of Psychiatry, 158*(3), 377–382, 383–389.

Volkow, N. D., Fowler, J. S., Wang, G. J., et al. (1997). Relationship between subjective effects of cocaine and dopamine transporter occupancy. *Nature, 386,* 827–830.

Wang, Y. (2001). Study finds that methamphetamine use can increase stroke-related brain damage. *Stroke, 23*(3).

Weil, A., & Rosen, W. (1993). *From Chocolate to Morphine.* Boston: Houghton Mifflin Company.

Weinberg, B. A., & Bealer, B. K. (2001). *The World of Caffeine.* New York: Rutledge.

Weiss, R. D., Hechtman, L., Milroy, T., & Perlman, T. (1985). Psychiatric status of hyperactives as adults: A controlled prospective 15-year follow-up of 63 hyperactive children. *Journal of the American Academy of Child Psychiatry, 24,* 211–220.

Weissman, M. M., Warner, V., Wickramaratne, P. J., & Kandel, D. B. (1999). Maternal smoking during pregnancy and psychopathology in offspring followed to adulthood. *Journal of the American Academy of Child and Adolescent Psychiatry, 38,* 892–899.

Wesson, D. R., Smith, D. E., & Steffens, S. C. (1992). *Crack and Ice: Treating Smokable Stimulant Abuse.* Center City, MN: Hazelden.

White, B. (1999, January 11). Soft money donations soared despite ongoing investigations. *Washington Post,* p. A17.

Wiencke, J. K., Thurston, S. W., Kelsey, K. T., Varkonyi, A., & Wain, J. C. (1999). Early age at smoking initiation and tobacco carcinogen DNA damage in the lung. *Journal of the National Cancer Institute, 91*(7), 614–619.

World Health Organization. (1997). The smoking epidemic: A fire in the global village. WHO Press Release [Online]. Available: *http://www.who.int/archives/inf-pr-1997/en/pr97-61.html*

World Health Organization. (1998). International Classification of Diseases (ICD-10). Author.

World Health Organization. (2002). Tobacco epidemic: Health dimensions. WHO Fact Sheet [Online]. Available: *http://www5.who.int/tobacco/page.cfm?sid=47*

Zhou, F. C., & Bledsoe, S. (1996). Methamphetamine causes rapid varicosis, perforation and definitive degeneration of serotonin fibers: An immunocytochemical study of serotonin transporter. *Neuroscience Net, Vol. 1,* Article #00009.

Ziedonis, D., & Wyatt, S. (1998). Psychotic disorders. In A. W. Graham & T. K. Schultz (Eds.), *Principles of Addiction Medicine* (2nd ed., pp. 1007–1027). Chevy Chase, MD: American Society of Addiction Medicine, Inc.

Downers:
Opiates/Opioids &
Sedative-Hypnotics

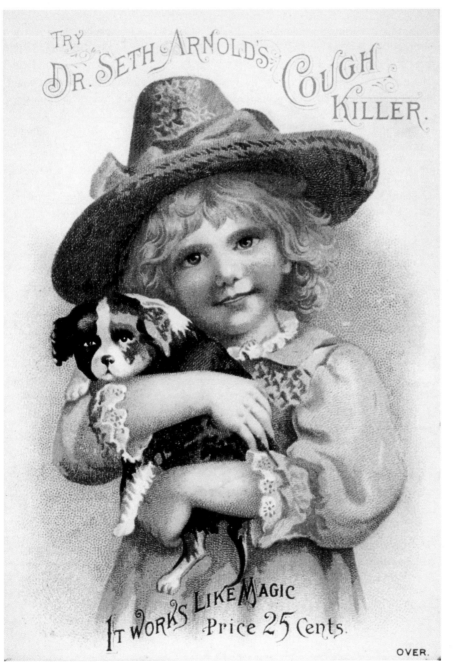

*M*any patent medicines and cure-alls contained opium as the main active ingredient. Although the ingredients were not disclosed, opium, codeine, and morphine were used in many cough syrups, such as Dr. Seth Arnold's Cough Killer and Mrs. Winslow's Soothing Syrup.
Courtesy of the National Library of Medicine, Bethesda, MD

GENERAL CLASSIFICATION

- **Major Depressants:** The three major downers (depressants) are opiates/opioids, sedative-hypnotics, and alcohol (*see Chapter 5*).
- **Minor Depressants:** The four minor downers are skeletal muscle relaxants, antihistamines, over-the-counter depressants, and lookalike depressants.

OPIATES/OPIOIDS

- **Classification:** Opiates are natural or semisynthetic derivatives of the opium poppy. Opioids are synthetic versions of opiates.
- **History of Use (*see Chapter 1*):** The efficiency of different routes of administration helps determine the intensity of effects and abuse potential.
- **Effects of Opioids:** Most opiates and opioids, such as opium, morphine, heroin, and hydrocodone, control pain and possibly induce pleasure. The drugs also suppress coughs and control diarrhea. Opioids' manipulation of naturally occurring neurotransmitters causes most of these effects.
- **Side Effects of Opioids:** These drugs create problems, e.g., depressed respiration and heart rate, constipation, and slurred speech, often due to increasing side effects, increasing tolerance, tissue dependence, and development of withdrawal symptoms.
- **Additional Problems with Heroin & Other Opioids:** Dangerous fetal effects, overdose, drug contamination, dirty needles, high cost, sexually transmitted diseases, abscesses, polydrug use problems, and especially addiction often occur with these drugs.
- **Morphine & Other Opioids:** Morphine is the standard drug used for pain relief; heroin causes the most social and health problems. Codeine, hydrocodone (Vicodin®), oxycodone (OxyContin®), methadone, meperidine (Demerol®), and other opioid analgesics (painkillers) are widely used.

SEDATIVE-HYPNOTICS

- **Classification:** Benzodiazepines, e.g., alprazolam (Xanax®) and clonazepam (Klonopin®), are the most frequently prescribed sedative-hypnotics. Sedatives are calming drugs whereas hypnotics are sleep-inducing drugs.
- **History:** Calming and sleep-inducing drugs have always been desired. Sedative-hypnotics have ranged from bromides and chloral hydrate to barbiturates and benzodiazepines.
- **Use, Misuse, Abuse, & Addiction:** Society's attitudes towards sedative-hypnotics swing between avid acceptance and wariness of addictive potential. Misuse and abuse of sedative-hypnotics occur due to a variety of reasons.
- **Benzodiazepines:** These sedative-hypnotics were developed as safe alternatives to barbiturates but tolerance, addiction, withdrawal, and overdose still occur. These drugs can impair memory.
- **Barbiturates:** Since 1900 more than 2,500 barbiturate compounds were developed (e.g., Seconal®, phenobarbital); they were widely used and abused until the introduction of benzodiazepines.
- **Other Sedative-Hypnotics:** These drugs, prescribed for anxiety and other problems, were also abused for their psychic effects. GHB has been abused at rave and dance parties.

OTHER PROBLEMS WITH DEPRESSANTS

- **Drug Interactions:** Using two or more downers at one time can lead to overdose, especially respiratory depression. Cross-tolerance and cross-dependence also develop.
- **Misuse & Diversion:** Two hundred million doses of prescription drugs are diverted to illicit channels each year in the United States. Besides diversion there are problems such as polydrug use and synergism.
- **Prescription Drugs & the Pharmaceutical Industry:** Americans spent $154.5 billion on prescription drugs in 2002. Of the 3.1 billion prescriptions written, approximately 250 million were for psychoactive drugs, mostly downers. In addition Americans spent $15–$20 billion each year on over-the-counter medications. Some of the most common are antihistamines, sleep aids, nondepressant analgesics, and anti-inflammatories (IMS Health, 2002).

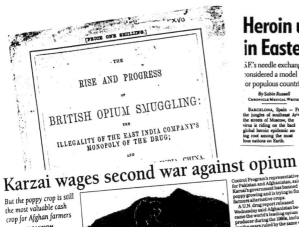

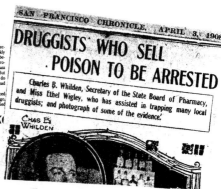

Heroin users spread HIV in Eastern Europe, Asia

Karzai wages second war against opium

But the poppy crop is still the most valuable cash crop for Afghan farmers

Drugstore robbers take painkiller OxyContin

BOSTON — Armed robbers looking for the powerful painkiller OxyContin have hit dozen drug stores around

Doctor charged with writing prescriptions to drug ring

BY BARRY MEIER
The New York Times

An Indiana doctor described as a paid speaker for the manufacturer of the painkiller OxyContin was under arrest yesterday on federal

in federal court for the southern district of Indiana.

This year, Lievertz wrote Oxy-Contin prescriptions worth $130,000 to a patient who was part of a ring that sold the narcotic on

OxyContin, made by Purdue Pharma of Stamford, Conn., was thought to be a narcotic painkiller less prone to abuse because its active ingredient was in a time-release mechanism.

GENERAL CLASSIFICATION

"Not only did nothing feel bad, everything felt good; I mean no physical pain; nothing on my mind weighing me down. Everything was just light, fluffy, and warm."
20-year-old male heroin addict

In the 2000s

◇ a synthetic opiate painkiller (depressant) called **"OxyContin®"** was declared the cause of a new drug epidemic when in fact it was an old problem, such as when Egyptian and other ancient cultures used opium as a medicine and euphoriant;

◇ the National Institute on Drug Abuse (NIDA) issued a number of warnings and papers about the **increase in prescription drug abuse**, particularly sedative-hypnotics and opioids, reminiscent of the overprescription and overuse of opiates and stimulants at the end of the nineteenth century (NIDA, 2001);

◇ and finally continuing research regarding factors such as **alcohol's**

cardiovascular benefits vs. long-term health consequences of binge drinking highlighted the ancient debate of alcohol's role in society.

In general, **downers, which are central nervous system depressants, depress the overall functioning of the central nervous system** to induce sedation, muscle relaxation, drowsiness, and even coma (if used to excess). They also often cause disinhibition of impulses and emotions. Unlike uppers that release and enhance the body's natural stimulatory neurochemicals, depressants produce their effects through a wide range of biochemical processes at different sites in the brain and spinal cord and other organs or systems (e.g., cardiovascular, respiratory).

Some depressants mimic the body's natural sedating or inhibiting neurotransmitters (e.g., endorphins, enkephalins, GABA) whereas others directly suppress the stimulation centers of the brain. Still others work in ways scientists haven't yet fully un-

derstood. Because of these variations, the depressants are grouped into a number of sub-classes based on their chemistry, medical use, and legal classification.

◇ **The three major classes of depressants are opiates/opioids, sedative-hypnotics, and alcohol.**

◇ **The four minor classes of depressants are skeletal muscle relaxants, antihistamines, over-the-counter downers, and lookalike downers.**

MAJOR DEPRESSANTS

OPIATES/OPIOIDS

Refinements and synthetic versions of the opium poppy, such as morphine, codeine, hydrocodone (Vicodin®), oxycodone (OxyContin®), methadone, and even heroin, were developed for the treatment of acute pain, diarrhea, coughs, and a number of other illnesses. Most illicit users take these opiate/opioid drugs to experience euphoric effects, to avoid emotional and physical pain, and to suppress withdrawal symptoms.

SEDATIVE-HYPNOTICS

Sedative-hypnotics represent **a wide range of synthetic chemical substances developed to treat anxiety and insomnia**. The first, barbituric acid, was created in 1864 by Dr. Adolph Von Bayer. Other barbiturates followed (phenobarbital, Seconal®) until more than 2,500 had been created. Bromides, paraldehyde, and chloral hydrate were also widely used until the late 1940s. Since 1950 dozens of different sedative-hypnotics, such as Miltown® (meprobamate), Doriden®, methaqualone (Quaalude® - only available overseas), flunitrazepam (Rohypnol® - only available overseas), GHB, and especially benzodiazepines, e.g., Valium® and Xanax®, have been created. All have toxic side effects when misused and can cause tissue dependence. Benzodiazepines are the most widely used prescription drugs although antidepressants, such as Prozac®, have taken over a substantial share of the market.

ALCOHOL (*see Chapter 5*)

Alcohol, the natural by-product of fermented plant sugars or starches, is the oldest psychoactive drug in the world. It has been widely used over the centuries for social, cultural, spiritual, and religious occasions. It is used for a number of medical remedies from sterilizing wounds to lessening the risk of heart attacks. Abuse also makes alcohol the world's second most destructive drug in terms of health consequences (after tobacco) and social consequences.

MINOR DEPRESSANTS

SKELETAL MUSCLE RELAXANTS

Centrally acting skeletal muscle relaxants include carisoprodol (Soma®), chlorzoxazone (Parafon Forte®), cyclobenzaprine (Flexeril®), and methocarbamol (Robaxin®). **They are synthetically developed central nervous system depressants aimed at areas of the brain responsible for muscle coordination and activity.** They are used to treat muscle spasms and pain. Whereas abuse of these products has been rare, their overall depressant effects on all parts of the central nervous system produce reactions similar to those caused by other abused depressants.

Recently **carisoprodol (Soma®)** has shown up in drug-screening urine tests of a small number of addicts, often in combination with other drugs, particularly benzodiazepines. In San Francisco it is used as a recreational drug of abuse among young Asians. It seems that carisoprodol (an unscheduled drug) is metabolized to meprobamate (a Schedule IV sedative-hypnotic drug) that has anxiolytic, anticonvulsant, and muscle-relaxing properties. Because of the drug's abuse potential, some states have rescheduled carisoprodol to Schedule IV. Besides the young Asians, users are typically White men or women (in equal numbers) in their early 40s (Bailey & Briggs, 2002).

ANTIHISTAMINES

Antihistamines, **found in hundreds of prescription and over-the-counter cold and allergy medicines** (including Benadryl®, Actifed®, and Tylenol P.M. Extra®), are synthetic drugs that were developed during the 1930s and 1940s for treatment of allergic reactions, prevention of ulcers, shock, rashes, motion sickness, and even symptoms of Parkinson's disease (Physicians' Desk Reference [PDR], 2002). In addition to blocking the release of histamine, these drugs cross the blood-brain barrier to induce the common and oftentimes potent side effect of depression of the central nervous system resulting in drowsiness. Even antihistamines are occasionally abused for their depressant effects.

OVER-THE-COUNTER DOWNERS

Depressants, such as Nytol®, Sleep-Eze®, and Sominex®, are sold legally in stores without the need for a prescription. Depressants that were used in the 1880s became marketed as **sleep aids or sedatives** in the twentieth century. Scopolamine in low doses, antihistamines, bromide derivatives, and even alcohol constitute the active sedating components in many of these products. As with other depressant drugs, these products are occasionally abused for their sedating effects.

LOOKALIKE DOWNERS

Lookalike depressants were advertised along with lookalike stimulants in the early 1980s. The great commercial success of the lookalike stimulants encouraged exploitative drug manufacturers to sell **products that looked like prescription downers**. These companies took legally available antihistamines and packaged them in tablets that resembled restricted depressants, such as Quaalude®, Valium®, and Seconal®. As with the other antihistamines, lookalike downers cause drowsiness as a side effect thereby mimicking some of the effects of more potent downers. They are rarely found nowadays except in a few magazine ads for legal downers.

OPIATES/OPIOIDS

In the 2000s most of the headlines concerning opiates/opioids have involved either the use of OxyContin®, the use of a powerful opioid-based gas (fentanyl) to disable terrorists in Russia, or the growing or eradication of opium poppy fields in Afghanistan. To a lesser extent media attention has focused on the treatment of pain in a clinical setting and the need to use sufficient opiates/opioids to block pain without fear of addicting the patient. In terms of treatment for opioid dependence, attention has focused on making therapeutic drugs such **as buprenorphine available through physicians' offices** not just in drug treatment clinics.

Opiates/opioids, some of the **oldest and best-documented groups of drugs,** have not only been the principal drugs used to treat pain (analgesic), diarrhea, and coughs but have also been the source of continual and occasionally explosive worldwide problems, e.g., nineteenth-century Opium Wars, the rise of drug crime cartels, and the spread of AIDS and hepatitis C from shared infected needles. Heroin receives the most publicity but other opiates/opioids also create problems and can be used compulsively.

Since the 1970s **the discovery of the body's own natural painkillers, endorphins and enkephalins, significantly changed our understanding of opiates/opioids** as well as the whole field of addictionology, biochemical research, and pain management (Goldstein, 2001).

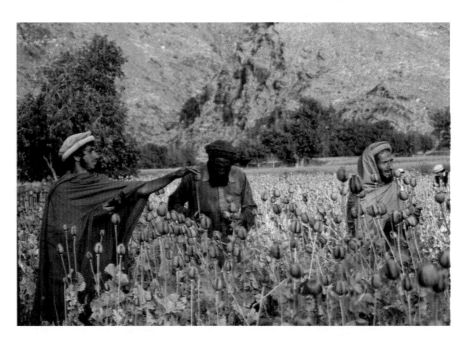

Afghan militia men tend their field of opium poppies. Many militias around the world fund their military operations with money from growing and trafficking drugs.
© 1990 Alain Labrousse

CLASSIFICATION

OPIUM, OPIATES, & OPIOIDS

Opium is processed from the milky fluid of the unripe seed pod of the opium poppy plant (*Papaver somniferum*). The white fluid coagulates and turns brown or black when exposed to air. Opium can also be extracted from the rest of the plant (called "poppy straw"). There are other poppy plants but only the *Papaver somniferum*, which is 1–5 ft. tall, produces opium. There are over 25 known alkaloids in opium but the 2 most prevalent, called "opiates," are **morphine (10–20% of the milky fluid) and codeine (0.7–2.5%)** (Karch, 1996; Marnell, 1997). Although a small amount of opium is used to make antidiarrheal preparations, e.g., tincture of opium and paregoric, virtually all the opium coming into this country is refined into

morphine, codeine, and thebaine. The main reason for the decline in the popularity of opium is the availability of semisynthetic and synthetic prescription opioids.

◇ **Opium poppy extracts** include morphine, codeine, and thebaine.

◇ **Semisynthetic opiates,** e.g., heroin, hydrocodone (Vicodin®), oxycodone (OxyContin®, Percodan®), and hydromorphone (Dilaudid®), are made from the three opium poppy extracts (alkaloids).

◇ **Fully synthetic opiate-like drugs** include meperidine (Demerol®), methadone, and propoxyphene (Darvon®).

◇ **Synthetic opioid antagonists** (naloxone and naltrexone) block the effects of opiates and opioids.

HISTORY OF USE
(see Chapter 1)

The regular use of opium poppies began in ancient Mesopotamia, Egypt,

and Greece and spread eastward to Asia. The ancient Sumerians and Egyptians recorded the paradoxical nature of opium in their medical texts listing it as a **cure for all illnesses, a pleasure-inducing substance, and a poison.** When Socrates was ordered to commit suicide, he drank from a cup that contained not only poisonous hemlock but also opium to dull the pain of dying. Ironically, modern day euthanasia or assisted-suicide formulas often include morphine or other opioids. Greek writings told of the gods' use of opium for mystical or mythical purposes—Greek heroes, such as Jason, used opium to sedate monsters. Hippocrates, the Father of Medicine, prescribed it for sleep, internal ills, and epidemics (Hoffman, 1990; Latimer & Goldberg, 1981).

Over the centuries

◇ experimentation with **different methods of use,**

◇ development of **new refinements of the drug,**

◇ **synthesis of molecules** that act like the natural opiates,

TABLE 4–1   OPIATES/OPIOIDS

Generic Drug Name	Trade Names	Street Names
OPIATES (opium poppy extracts)		
Opium (Schedule II)	Pantopon®, Laudanum®	"O," op, poppy
Diluted opium, (Schedule III)	Paregoric®	
Morphine (Schedule II)	Infumorph®, Kadian®, Roxanol®, MS Contin®	Murphy, morph, "M," Miss Emma
Codeine (Schedule III) (also called "methylmorphine") (usually w/aspirin or Tylenol®)	Empirin® w/codeine, Tylenol® w/codeine Doriden® w/codeine	Number 4s (1 grain), Number 3s ($\frac{1}{2}$ grain) Loads, sets, 4s & doors
Thebaine (Schedule II)	None	None
SEMISYNTHETIC OPIATES		
Diacetylmorphine (Schedule I)	Heroin	Smack, junk, tar (chiva, puro, goma, puta, chapapote), Mexican brown, China white, Harry, skag, shit, Rufus, Perze, "H," horse, dava, boy
Hydrocodone (Schedule III)	Vicodin®, Hycodan®, Lortab®, Lorcet®, Zydone®, Norco®, Tussend®	
Hydromorphone (Schedule II)	Dilaudid®	Dillies, drugstore heroin
Oxycodone (Schedule II)	OxyContin®, Percodan®, Tylox®	Percs, hillbilly heroin, ocs, oxy, o'coffin
SYNTHETIC OPIATES (opioids)		
Buprenorphine (Schedule V)	Buprenex®, Subotex®, Suboxone® (w/naloxone)	
Butorphanol (Schedule IV)	Stadol®	
Fentanyl (Schedule II)	Sublimaze®, Duragesic®, Actiq®	Street derivatives are misrepresented as China white
Levomethadyl acetate (Schedule II) (long-acting methadone)	LAAM®	Lam
Levorphanol (Schedule II)	Levo-Dromoran®	
Meperidine (Schedule II)	Demerol®, Mepergan®, Pethidine®	
Methadone (Schedule II)	Dolophine®	Juice
Oxymorphone (Schedule II)	Numorphan®	
Pentazocine (Schedule IV)	Talwin®	Part of Ts and blues
Propoxyphene (Schedule IV)	Darvon®, Darvocet-N®, Wygesic®, Propacet®	Pink ladies, pumpkin seeds
Tramadol	Ultram®, Ultracet®	
OPIOID ANTAGONISTS		
Naloxone	Narcan®	
Naltrexone	Revia®	

and **time-release versions** of the drugs have slowly increased not only the benefits of these substances but also their potential for abuse.

ORAL INGESTION

Opium, from the Greek word "*opòs*" meaning "juice" or "sap," was originally **chewed, eaten, or blended in various liquids and drunk**. Though the drug was used extensively, the abuse potential of opium was relatively low because it had a **bitter taste, a low concentration of active ingredients, and the supplies were limited**. When taken orally, the drug must go through the digestive system before it enters the bloodstream and makes its way to the brain 20 or 30 minutes later.

The use of opium in medications and potions continued through the Middle Ages and into the Renaissance (in the early 1500s) when it was repopularized by the **Swiss alchemist**

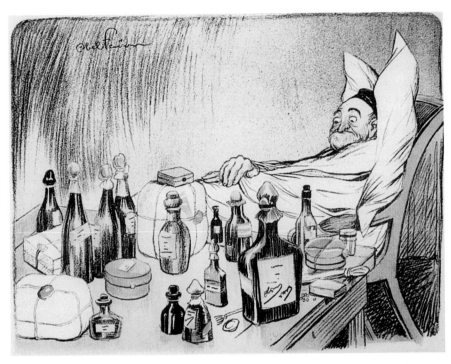

In the nineteenth century, patent medicines laced with morphine, opium, cocaine, and Cannabis *could be bought anywhere. Physicians prescribed opiates as freely as aspirin and as a result physician-induced addiction (iatrogenic addiction) became common, especially among women.*

Courtesy of the National Library of Medicine, Bethesda, MD

Paracelsus who concocted laudanum, a tincture of opium (powdered opium in alcohol), that he prescribed for dysentery, pain, diarrhea, and coughs (O'Brien, Cohen, Evans, & Fine, 1992). Over the next 3 centuries other opium mixtures were developed, especially **paregoric (opium in alcohol plus camphor),** for the treatment of diarrhea. Paregoric is still available as a prescription drug.

SMOKING

In the sixteenth century, opium smoking via the **introduction of the pipe from North America to Europe and Asia** by Portuguese traders **set the stage for the widespread nonmedical use of opium.** Smoking puts more of the active ingredients of the drug into the bloodstream by way of the lungs; the vaporized opium reaches the brain in 7–10 seconds. The higher concentration of the opiate produces a stronger sense of euphoria, relaxation, and well-being than when the drug is ingested, thereby encouraging abuse.

Although opium smoking was initially limited to the middle and upper classes in China (because of the high cost of the drug), it became such a large problem that it was banned in 1729. However, the opium trade had become so lucrative that it was impossible to shut it off. In the early 1800s when prohibition was again tried, the powerful trading companies of the West, e.g., the East India Company of England, along with their governments, forced the Chinese government, through the **Opium Wars,** to continue the trade and to cede Hong Kong to the British (Latimer & Goldberg, 1981).

As the supplies became more plentiful, use increased. **Opium smoking was introduced to the United States by some of the 70,000 Chinese workers who were brought over to build the railroads and mine gold, copper, and mercury.** The biased and bigoted reaction to these Asian immigrants produced headlines that screamed "yellow fiends" and "seducers of white women" resulting in a spate of pro-

hibitory laws that often focused on opium smoking.

One of the current methods of smoking heroin is to heat some on tin foil and inhale the fumes through a straw. This method is called "chasing the dragon." The abuse potential is extremely high.

"I had a very close friend who I was associated with who was smoking a pretty vast quantity every day . . . a half a gram to a gram every day and he used to really get on me and tell me that I was a junkie because I was putting a needle in my arm. And I would tell him, 'Hey, okay, my method is different but you're a junkie, too. You have a habit.'"

34-year-old recovering heroin addict

REFINEMENT OF MORPHINE, CODEINE, & HEROIN

In 1805 the German pharmacist **Frederick W. Serturner isolated morphine from opium.** He found it to be **10 times as strong as opium** and therefore a much better pain reliever. Morphine benefited wounded soldiers beginning with the Crimean War and the U.S. Civil War. Unfortunately its greater strength increased the potential for opiate addiction or morphinism.

In 1832 codeine, the other major component of opium, was isolated. It got its name from the Greek word *"kodeia,"* which means "poppyhead." It was only **twice as strong as opium,** so it was often used in cough syrups and patent medicines.

In 1874 the British chemist **C. R. Alder Wright refined heroin (diacetylmorphine) from morphine** in an attempt to find a more effective painkiller that didn't have addictive properties. This powerful opiate stayed on the shelf until 1898 when an employee of Bayer and Company® thought it should be promoted for coughs, chest pain, tuberculosis, and pneumonia (Trebach, 1981). Unfortunately since heroin crossed the blood-brain barrier much more rapidly than morphine, **the rush and subsequent euphoria came on more quickly and was more intense** (Karch, 1996). **The new drug created a subculture of compulsive heroin users** in the twentieth century. It was estimated that there were between 250,000 and 1 million opium, morphine, and heroin abusers in the United States shortly after the turn of the century.

IV USE

Another major development of the nineteenth century regarding opiate use was **the development of the hypodermic needle in 1853**. Initially drugs were only injected subcutaneously but users found that intravenous use could **inject high concentrations of the drug directly into the bloodstream** through the veins. It takes 15–30 seconds for an injected opiate or opioid to affect the central nervous system. If the drug is injected just under the skin or in a muscle ("skin popping" or "muscling"), the effects are delayed by 5–8 minutes. Until the development of the hypodermic needle, oral use of morphine and smoking of opium induced a certain euphoria and relief from physical and emotional pain but with IV use an **intense rush** also occurred. The intensity of the rush made compulsive drug-seeking behavior more likely.

PATENT MEDICINES

During the mid- to late 1800s opiates became so popular that **hundreds of tonics and medications**, such as Mrs. Winslow's Soothing Syrup or McMunn's Elixir of Opium, came on the market to treat everything from tired blood to coughs, diarrhea, and toothaches (Armstrong & Armstrong, 1991). Just before the turn of the century the use of opioids for nervousness and pleasure (recreational use) by the middle and upper classes also came into vogue as the number of opium parlors and the use of opium increased. Physicians were not fully aware of the addictive potential of opiate drugs and so **iatrogenic (physician-induced) addiction** was a common problem. In fact

4–8 times as many opiate prescriptions per capita were written back then compared to the present day. IV morphine was prescribed for anemia, asthma, cholera, nervous dyspepsia, insanity, neuralgia, and vomiting. Surveys in the 1880s showed that **between 56% and 71% of opium addicts were women** (Hoffman, 1990). Some of the more famous female opiate users were the writers Elizabeth Barrett Browning, Charlotte Bronte, and Louisa May Alcott, the pioneering social worker Jane Addams, and the well-known actress Sarah Bernhardt. Male writers and poets were not immune to the drug. Samuel Coleridge, Charles Baudelaire, Lord Byron, John Keats, Edgar Allan Poe, and Algernon Swinburne used laudanum and other opiates (Aldrich, 1994; Zackon, 1992).

"I arrived on the stage in a semiconscious state, yet delighted with the applause I received."
Sara Bernhardt, 1890 (Palmer & Horowitz, 1982)

SNORTING

In addition to drinking, eating, smoking, and injecting opiates, new immigrants from Europe introduced the habit of sniffing or snorting heroin (also called "insufflation" and "intranasal use"). It takes 5–8 minutes for the drug to enter the nasal capillaries and reach the central nervous system. From the turn of the century until the 1920s, heroin addicts were split evenly between "sniffers" and "shooters" (Karch, 1996). Since more of the drug is needed when snorted to get the same high as when injected, low prices of heroin encouraged insufflation especially for those who were afraid of the needle. This route was popular with heroin-using GIs in Vietnam because of the easy availability and high purity of the drug. **More than half of all heroin addicts entering treatment began their heroin use by insufflation** (Casriel, Rockwell, & Stepherson, 1988; Substance Abuse and Mental Health Services Administration/Treatment Episode Data Sets [SAMHSA/TEDS], 2002).

TWENTIETH CENTURY

Rising concern over the problems caused by use and abuse of opium, morphine, and especially heroin spurred various governments to action. Casual nonmedical use of opiates was **declared illegal at the beginning of the twentieth century** by the international community through The Hague Resolutions and by the United States through **The Pure Food and Drug Act in 1906 and the Harrison Narcotics Act in 1914**. In 1924 production of heroin in the United States was prohibited. The gradual proliferation of laws also increased the jail population. Commitments to federal prisons for violations of the narcotics law rose from 63 in 1915 to 2,529 in 1928 (about one-third of all federal prisoners) (Musto, 1973).

In the first two decades of the twentieth century, opioid addiction was considered a medical problem and was treated by physicians. Even though alcoholism was considered more debilitating and certainly more expensive than opioid addiction, a number of heroin treatment centers were opened.

The availability or prohibition of different opiates/opioids shifted methods of use. When the importation of smokable opium was banned in 1909, it produced a shift to heroin (Zule, Vogtsberger, & Desmond, 1997).

Because these restrictions limited supplies and made opium and heroin valuable commodities, **growing, processing, and distributing opiates/opioids, especially heroin, became major sources of revenue for criminal organizations worldwide.** These groups have included the Chinese Triads, the Mafia and the French Connection, Mexican narcoficantes, African traffickers, the Russian Mafia, and most recently the Colombian Cartel.

In addition **diversion of legal prescription opiates/opioids**, such as hydrocodone, cough syrups, and oxycodone (OxyContin®), through theft, bogus purchases, and forged prescriptions created an illegal market of pills and injectables.

"I went to different physicians. I would rip off prescription pads and since I worked in the medical field, writing my own prescriptions was no problem except that I committed a felony every time I did it, which was once a week. I never got caught but I always lived in mortal fear that they would get me."
Recovering Darvon® (propoxyphene) abuser

Currently an estimated **3.5 million Americans use prescription opiates/opioids illicitly every month** compared to 120,000 to 800,000 heroin abusers. (The estimates of heroin users vary radically. For example, New York City alone is estimated to have 200,000 heroin addicts.) Approximately 3.1 million Americans have tried heroin (SAMHSA, 2002). In 2000 there were approximately equal numbers of injectors and snorters with a much smaller percentage of smokers (NIDA, 2000). Recently smoking and snorting heroin have increased in popularity in the United States due to an influx of white and tar heroin from Colombia and tar heroin from Mexico. Larger percentages of sniffers and smokers are more likely to be found in the eastern half of the United States. Some of the snorters mix tar heroin with water and snort it out of a Visine® spray bottle.

HEROIN - A WORLD VIEW

Since 1992 there has been a steady increase in heroin use worldwide due mostly to increased supplies and decreased cost. There are **5–10 million regular heroin users worldwide** while a dozen countries are battling the growth, use, smuggling, and exportation of heroin on their own soil. Since 1986 worldwide production of illicit opium, the raw ingredient to make heroin, has more than doubled. Even with the increase in supplies, **the United States consumes only 3% (10–15 metric tons) of the world's heroin supply**.

The major opium-growing areas are the Golden Crescent (Afghanistan and Pakistan) and the Golden Triangle (Myanmar [Burma], Thai-

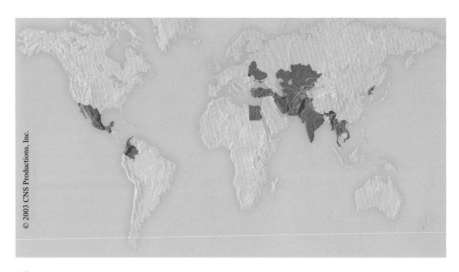

Figure 4-1 •

This map shows the heroin-growing countries in red. About 90% of the world's illegal opium is grown in Myanmar (Burma) and Afghanistan. Though Mexico, Central America, and Colombia grow less than 7% of the world's opium, they supply the majority of heroin to the United States.

land, and Laos). Other countries grow heroin but their markets are more regional. For example, other Southeast Asian types of heroin include Cambodian and Malaysian or Sri Lankan pink heroin. Several ex-Soviet republics, especially Tajikstan and Turkmenistan, also qualify as "narco-states." India is the largest legal grower of opium but the trade is highly regulated and the vast majority of the crop is used for medical purposes. **In the United States most heroin comes from Mexico and Colombia** (DEA, 2002a).

In the 1990s Afghanistan grew more than 70% of the world's supply of illicit opium. The events of September 11, 2001, and the subsequent overthrow of the Taliban government has confused the picture of how much is grown and who is growing it. While Afghan opium produced only 10% of all heroin consumed in the United States, it was **80% of Europe's supply**. Before September 11, 2001, Afghan opium/heroin was not seen as a direct threat to the United States but since then there is the recognition that drug money is used to help finance terrorist activities. Unfortunately one problem is that the Northern Alliance of leaders that helped the United States overthrow the Taliban have often relied on opium growing to finance their regimes. It is

likely that opium will continue to come out of Afghanistan for many years to come.

Southwest Asian heroin from Iran, Turkey, and Lebanon as well as Afghanistan and Pakistan is often known as smokable "Persian brown" or "Perze," which can be more than 90% pure. Several of these countries that grow opium now also have exploding addict populations. There are an estimated 1.9 million opioid users in Pakistan alone.

The Golden Triangle, the second largest producer and exporter of illegal opium and heroin, is also one of the largest-using areas, about 25% of its own crop. Thailand and Burma have $^{1}/_{2}$ million addicts each. The raw opium sells for $150 to $350 per kilogram (kg). In 2000 a $1^{1}/_{2}$ lb. unit of Asian heroin on the East Coast of the United States cost $60,000 to $70,000 and resold in 50-milligram (mg) dime bags for $10. Golden Triangle heroin, known on the street as **"China white"** in its exportable form, can be up to 99% pure (DEA, 2001b).

Attempts to control or limit the growing and refining operations in the Golden Triangle are difficult and dangerous. The following is a description of some of the jungle refining operations.

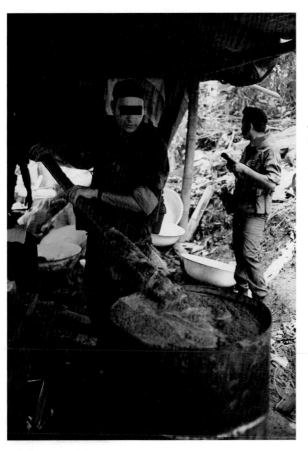

A DEA agent and Thai soldier stand at an illegal opium jungle laboratory in Thailand that has just been raided. The 55-gallon barrel is filled with cooked opium ready to be transformed into 20 kg of morphine and then into an equal weight of heroin. A small jungle laboratory such as this can process 60 kg of heroin every 4 days.
Courtesy of George Skaggard
· ·

"The Golden Triangle is an area of constant motion as far as the narcotics trade is concerned. From year to year, the different insurgent groups are continually forming new alliances and dissolving old ones based on the economics of the narcotic trade rather than the ideologies of the different groups. The groups have their own armies, often containing 3,000 to 7,000 men. Golden Triangle opium is grown by ethnic hill tribes. Ethnic Chinese in the area contract the opium growing by providing the tribes with seeds and cash. The Chinese middlemen collect the opium on a cash basis from the growers and refine it into the world's purest heroin in nearby jungle refineries. The refineries are of two types: those run by large organized insurgent groups or small independently syndicated groups. Large laboratories, usually found on the Burmese

side of the border, make 200 kilograms of heroin at a time. Extraction of morphine from opium takes from 1–2 days and heroin synthesis requires an additional 12–14 hours. There are about 200 of these large laboratories. The smaller laboratories on the Thai side of the border refine about 60 kilograms at a time. Those were the only ones we could raid because of political considerations. The work force of the larger labs includes 10 guards and 20 lab technicians. Security is usually provided by ex-military insurgents armed with M-16 rifles, machine guns, and grenade launchers.

After processing, the heroin is stored in the jungle until it is marketed in nearby Thai border towns to buyers from various countries. Initially the drugs are hauled by pack-mule or horse caravans carrying up to 3,000 kilograms at a time. The heroin finally

arrives in Malaysia, Singapore, or Hong Kong where it is smuggled to the rest of the world's markets, including the United States."
International narcotics agent working in the Golden Triangle

Since the 1940s Mexico has been a major supplier of heroin to the United States. Perhaps the 2,000-mile long U.S./Mexican border is more porous than other routes. Mexico became the number one supplier when the Turkish opium fields dried up in the early 1970s. Most of the heroin was light or dark brown and not as pure as Golden Triangle white heroin. Many of the present day gangs, based mostly in the Mexican States of Durango, Michoacan, Nuevo Leon, and Sinoloa, have been in operation for more than 20 years.

In the 1980s a relatively new form of **Mexican heroin, known as "tar" or "black tar,"** took over a large part of the market in the western United States although it is still only 5% of U.S. heroin seizures. Tar heroin is potent, 40% to 80% pure, but it also has more plant impurities than the Asian refinement of the drug. A small chunk (black or brown) the size of a match head, which is enough for 2–5 doses, costs about $20 to $25. Tar heroin, also called "chapapote," "puta," "goma," "chiva," and "puro," is unique in that it's sold as a gummy pasty substance rather than in the usual powder form. Tar heroin dissolves easily in water and is also more likely to be smoked than other types of heroin.

"I came from the Midwest where we mostly get China white and that to me is a whole lot cleaner than tar. I'd never seen an abscess or anything like that. People on the West Coast have abscesses all the time because here it is black tar. The stuff I see when I break it down, there's so much crap in it. It's like, yuck, I can't believe I put that 'shit' in my veins but I do it anyway."
27-year-old female heroin addict

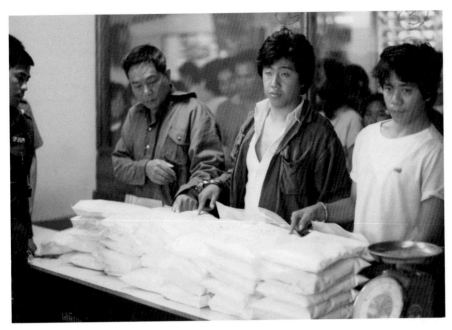

Three heroin drug smugglers in Thailand are posed with their dope. Under Thai law the jail sentence is tied to the number of grams found on them. For over 400 grams, the sentence is 66 years. If they plead guilty, their sentence is cut in half. Unfortunately the severity of the sentences leads to bribery and corruption.

Courtesy of George Skaggard

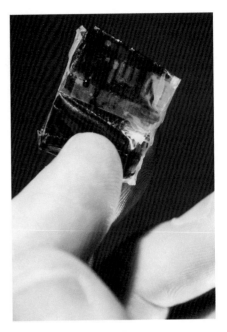

A small sample of Mexican tar heroin, the most common type of heroin sold in the United States, is packed in a little plastic bag.

Courtesy of JACNET, Jackson County, Oregon

In addition to countries that grow, refine, and sell the drug, several countries **have major refining facilities or act as transshipment points** for heroin. These transshipment countries include the Netherlands, Canada, Italy (especially Sicily), France, and Nigeria (the latter also produces its own heroin). Also many ex-Soviet republics and satellites (e.g., Armenia, Uzbekistan, Kazakhstan, Turkmenistan) are involved in transshipment as well as production of heroin (DEA, 2002b).

Alarmingly in the early 1990s a number of **Colombian cocaine cartels diversified and started to grow and distribute opium/heroin** (in addition to their fields of coca shrubs) in an effort to cash in on the growing heroin market. Their existing cocaine distribution channels enabled them to expand rapidly. They also sold purer and cheaper heroin to compete with the China white imported by the Mafia and Asian gangs. The Colombian cartels manufacture large amounts and smuggle it in small units (¹/₂–1 kg) mostly on the east coast in New York, Newark, Boston, and Philadelphia (DEA, 2001a).

(NOTE: For the rest of this chapter, we will use the generic term OPIOIDS to denote both natural and semisynthetic OPIATES and synthetic OPIOIDS.)

EFFECTS OF OPIOIDS

Medically physicians most often prescribe opioids to

◇ **deaden pain,**

◇ **control coughing,**

◇ **stop diarrhea.**

Nonmedically users self-prescribe opioids to

◇ **drown out emotional pain,**

◇ **get a rush,**

◇ **induce euphoria,**

◇ **prevent withdrawal symptoms.**

But to truly comprehend opioids, it is important to understand how pain and pleasure are connected to the nervous system.

PAIN

Whether caused by a wound, a disease, or a nerve problem, **pain is a warning signal that tells us whether we are being damaged physically**. Injury sends a message to the spinal cord and on to the brainstem and medial portion of the thalamus in our brain that in turn tells the body to protect itself from further damage (Jaffe, Knapp, & Ciraulo, 1997). The pain message is transmitted from nerve cell to nerve cell by a neurotransmitter called "substance P." This neuropeptide, first discovered in 1931, signals the intensity of painful stimuli.

If the pain is too intense, the body tries to protect itself by softening the pain signals. It does this by flooding the brain and spinal cord with endorphins and enkephalins. These neurotransmitters attach themselves to opioid mu and kappa receptor sites on the membranes of sending nerve cells telling them not to send substance "P" (Fig. 4-2) (DeVane, 2001). However, many signals still get through.

If the pain remains unbearable, opioid medications can be used to relieve

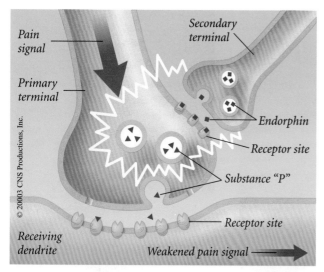

Figure 4-2 •

This diagram of a synapse shows that when pain signals are being transmitted through the nervous system, a secondary terminal releases endorphins that then slot into receptor sites on the primary terminal and limit the release of the pain neurotransmitter substance "P."

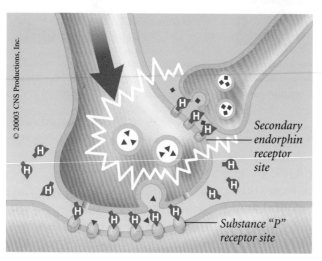

Figure 4-3 •

Heroin (or any opioid) slots into the secondary endorphin receptor sites limiting the release of substance "P." It also blocks most of the substance "P" that gets through by slotting into the primary substance "P" receptor sites on the receiving dendrite of the next neuron.

the agony. **These drugs are effective because they act like the body's endogenous (naturally occurring) painkillers (endorphins and enkephalins).** Opioid medications (exogenous or external opioids) not only limit the release of substance "P," they also help block what little does get through to the receiving neurons (Fig. 4-3).

Pain control is not only limited to physical pain. Decreased anxiety, a sense of detachment, drowsiness, and a deadening of unwanted emotions are often experienced by opioid users. This is due to the drug's inhibiting effect on the locus coeruleus on top of the brainstem and its influence on the dopaminergic reward pathway. Experiments have shown that **severe stress alone can activate natural endorphins to mitigate emotional pain** (Goldstein, 2001). In one animal experiment the greater the stress

relief, the more the use of morphine was remembered, thus imprinting and reinforcing the concept that emotional agitation can be relieved by drugs (Will, Watkins, & Maier, 1998). This negative reinforcement uses many of the same brain mechanisms that cause positive reinforcement of drug-seeking behavior.

"When you are loaded on heroin, you can watch your best friend get hit by a car, all your friends could be dying, your dog could come down with rabies, and you could get AIDS, herpes, and cancer all at once and you don't care. You're separated from it and blocked off from your emotions."
18-year-old female heroin addict

The pain-relieving effects of the various opioids are similar to each

other. The differences have to do with how long the drug lasts, how strong it is per gram, and how toxic it is to the body. For example, heroin, codeine, and Darvon® will relieve pain from 4–6 hours while fentanyl will barely last 1 hour but it is strong enough to be used as an anesthetic during surgery.

PLEASURE

The other major effect of opioids involves endorphins, dopamine, and the mesolimbic dopaminergic reward pathway or the reward/reinforcement center, which includes the nucleus accumbens. As described in Chapter 2 this system, through a variety of mechanisms, **positively reinforces actions that are good for the body's survival.** The normal activation of this system **gives a surge of pleasure that encourages repetition of an action,** such as eating or having sex. Animal research suggests that, in addition to giving a surge of positive reinforcement, **dopamine release in this pathway helps the brain remember (unconsciously) what was done,** so it can be done again in the future (Wickelgren, 1998).

"The last shot is never good enough. You're always looking for a certain shot. You're looking for the same shot you had when you first did the drug, which you'll never get again."
22-year-old recovering heroin addict

Searching for a high (or relief from pain, which can both feel the same), some people try opioids because these drugs also activate this reward pathway. Opioids affect this pathway by

◇ **slotting into the receptor sites meant for endorphins/enkephalins;**

◇ **inhibiting the action of GABA** resulting in increased activation of the reward pathway (Nutt, 1998);

◇ **triggering glutamate receptors** that enhance responsiveness of dopamine neurons resulting in activation of the reward pathway (Carlezon et al., 1997);

◇ **reducing the number of dopamine receptors** (down regulation)

thereby releasing more dopamine to try to overactivate the pathway.

Of the various opioids, **heroin has the strongest effect on the reward pathway**.

"It's like putting all your troubles in one bag and you have a solution for it and that's heroin. Your one problem is to worry about getting your heroin every day."
72-year-old recovering heroin addict

When the natural (endogenous) endorphins and enkephalins give a surge of pleasure (positive reinforcement), various cells in the brain monitor the action and **when the need is filled, the cutoff signal goes out, "you can stop now,"** "mission accomplished," "that's enough." Powerful psychoactive drugs, including **heroin, can disrupt this cutoff switch** in a variety of ways and reinforce the desire to continue the behavior. Genetically some people are more susceptible to disruption of the switch. In others, excessive drug use is the more powerful factor. The more frequently this circuit is overloaded by heroin or other powerful opioids, the greater the malfunction of the satiation switch (Hyman, 1998).

FROM PLEASURE TO PAIN

As we've seen, people use an opioid to either

◇ alleviate emotional/mental/physical pain or

◇ induce a good feeling/rush/high.

What is interesting is that **the area of the brain that signals pleasure/reward is the same area that signals alleviation of pain** (Goldstein, 2001). And since one of the functions of the reward pathway is to encourage us to repeat whatever action activated it, the nucleus accumbens interprets the opioid that caused the rush or the pain alleviation as something that is good for the body. **Drug abusers will keep using past the point of pain relief while nonabusers stop at pain relief.** For example, nonusers and some users will

perceive that chronic heroin users don't get a rush or high after chronic use and their body merely returns to a nonwithdrawal or almost normal state when they shoot up or snort. What the nonaddict doesn't know is that in fact the heroin is now working on a subconscious level in their more primitive survival brain. **The user is activating the nucleus accumbens that then says to do more heroin.**

Another cause of continued use in addicts is the relief from the pain of withdrawal symptoms. In an experiment at the University of Cambridge, England, researchers found in animal experiments that **the relief of withdrawal symptoms functioned as a much more effective incentive for self-administration of the drug** and the longer the heroin was used, the greater the incentive to use during withdrawal (Hutcheson, Everitt, Robbins, & Dickinson, 2001).

"Heroin lasts, like the part where you're getting high, lasts for maybe a couple of months tops and then I don't remember exactly but it seems it was like all of a sudden like a maintenance kind of thing."
26-year-old heroin addict

RECEPTOR SITES

There are actually **multiple natural opioid receptor sites** for the body's own opioids (endorphins, enkephalins, and dynorphins). The main receptors are mu, delta, kappa, and possibly sigma. They are found in the brain, the spinal cord, the digestive track, various organs, and a dozen other sites. **Opioid drugs slot into these same receptor sites** but cause more intense reactions than the body's own (endogenous) opioids. Each opioid drug has a unique affinity for each site. At one synapse the drug might act like an agonist and trigger effects; at another it might act as an antagonist, blocking changes; at a third it might work as a combination agonist and antagonist. For example:

◇ mu receptors trigger the reward/ reinforcement center, block pain

transmission, and depress the autonomic nervous system, including respiration, blood pressure, and pupil contraction;

◇ kappa receptors seem to induce dysphoria rather than euphoria as well as mediate (control) pain at the spinal cord level (Jaffe et al., 1997; Simon, 1997; Gold, 1998).

So one drug, such as fentanyl, will affect pain more than heroin that has a greater influence on the rush and euphoria.

COUGH SUPPRESSION & DIARRHEA CONTROL

Besides pain control and pleasure, opioids are used to suppress coughs and control diarrhea. They suppress coughs by **controlling activation of the cough center in the brainstem** that signals the body to cough when the respiratory tract is irritated. Currently codeine- and hydrocodone-based cough medications are still widely prescribed, e.g., Robitussin A-C® and Hycodan Syrup®.

Diarrhea is also controlled because opioids affect areas in the brainstem that **inhibit gastric secretions and depress activity of intestinal muscles**. Constipation can be a severe problem in surgical patients or in those with intractable pain who use opioids over a long period.

SIDE EFFECTS OF OPIOIDS

PHYSICAL SIDE EFFECTS

Opioids, particularly heroin, **affect almost every part of the body**: heart, lungs, brain, eyes, voice box (larynx), muscles, cough and nausea centers, reproductive system, digestive system, excretory system, and the immune system. Some of the major side effects of heroin are

◇ **insensitivity to warning pain signals**, which is a desired effect but

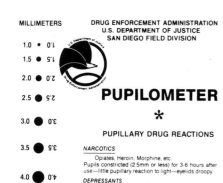

MILLIMETERS

1.0 • 1.0
1.5 • 1.5
2.0 ● 2.0
2.5 ● 2.5
3.0 ● 3.0
3.5 ● 3.5
4.0 ● 4.0
4.5 ● 4.5

DRUG ENFORCEMENT ADMINISTRATION
U.S. DEPARTMENT OF JUSTICE
SAN DIEGO FIELD DIVISION

PUPILOMETER
*

PUPILLARY DRUG REACTIONS

NARCOTICS
Opiates, Heroin, Morphine, etc.
Pupils constricted (2.5mm or less) for 3-6 hours after use—little pupillary reaction to light—eyelids droopy
DEPRESSANTS
Barbiturates etc.
No significant pupillary size change—check for bilateral nystagmus (bouncing of eyes)

A pupilometer is held up to the eyes of a suspected drug user in order to compare the size of pupils against normal standards. Since opioids contract pupils, pupil size is a strong indicator of drug use. (Cocaine and methamphetamines dilate pupils.)

• •

can keep a user from treating a damaging ailment such as abscesses;

◊ **lowered blood pressure;**

◊ **lowered pulse and respiration rate;**

◊ **confusion.**

Some of the **other side effects of the stronger opioids are quite identifiable** in the heavier user, particularly with heroin:

◊ **eyelids droop and the head nods forward;**

◊ **speech becomes slurred, slowed, and raspy or hoarse;**

◊ **the walking gait and coordination are slowed;**

◊ **pupils become pinpoint** and do not react to light;

◊ skin dries out and **itching increases.**

Some of the desired medicinal effects can also become problems:

◊ suppression of the cough center in the brain can **hinder clearance of phlegm** in those users with respiratory ailments such as emphysema and tuberculosis;

◊ opioids can **trigger the nausea center;** some heroin addicts know a batch of heroin is good if it makes them vomit;

"It hit from the feet going up to the head. I was yelling at him to take the needle out and I was on the toilet seat. I mean I hugged that toilet bowl for hours, vomiting."
23-year-old heroin user

◊ opioids are used to stop diarrhea but they **cause severe constipation** with chronic use;

"I'd go to the bathroom maybe about once a week but it didn't bother me because I was on painkillers, so it wasn't really an issue."
28-year-old recovering heroin abuser

◊ and finally opioids affect the hormonal system; a **woman's period is delayed** and a man produces less testosterone while **sexual desire is dulled** often to the point of indifference.

"When I'm on heroin, I can't have an orgasm. It's just one of those things. I can have sex for hours and it starts to get painful. Heroin makes my whole body numb; I don't want to move around and I don't want to have sex when I'm high."
24-year-old dealer/heroin addict

TOLERANCE, TISSUE DEPENDENCE, & WITHDRAWAL

The desire for relief from pain and the experiencing of pleasure combined with **tolerance, tissue dependence, and withdrawal are the main reasons for the addictive nature of opioids.**

"Since the first day I started using heroin, I was using it every day. I thought it was a joke that people wouldn't get addicted the first time but I went ahead and did it anyway. After about 2 weeks of use, I ran out of money and I found out how bad I could get sick. I wish I wasn't sick any of the

time but it's kind of like a requirement. Once you're a junkie, you've got to be sick."
27-year-old female heroin addict

Tolerance

Tolerance **occurs when the body tries to neutralize the heroin** (or any other psychoactive drug) by a variety of methods. It may

◊ **speed up the metabolism,** particularly in the liver;

◊ **desensitize the nerve cells** to the drug's effects;

◊ **excrete the drug more rapidly** out of the body through urine, feces, and sweat;

◊ **alter the brain and body chemistry** to compensate for the effects of the drug.

The body's adjustment requires the user to increase dosage if the same effects are desired. Since tolerance occurs rapidly with opioids, users might need 10 times as much drug (e.g., morphine) in as little as 10 days (O'Brien, 2001). **There is almost no limit to the development of opioid tolerance** (Goldstein, 2001). After a year of opioid use one terminal cancer patient was using 5 fentanyl patches, 20 Demerol® tablets, and continuous morphine suppositories. This limitless tolerance compares to a drug such as nicotine where 3 packs a day are usually the limit.

"After a while they [#4 codeine tablets] didn't really have any effect on me and the pain was taking over with the drug, so I started taking more codeine. And I took more and more and finally I was going through like two bottles of codeine a week."
Recovering codeine abuser

Tolerance develops at different rates for different body systems. High tolerance will develop for the opioid effects on pain relief, respiratory depression, sedation, vomiting, and euphoria. However there's little tolerance for constriction of pupils or for constipation (Jaffe et al., 1997).

Tissue Dependence

The adaptation of the body to the effects of **a strong opioid will temporarily and sometimes permanently alter brain chemistry.** An animal study by Dr. Eric Nestler and colleagues at Yale University showed that chronic administration of morphine to rats actually reduced the size of dopamine-producing cells (in the ventral tegmental area) by one-fourth (Nestler & Agajanian, 1997; Sklair-Tavron et al., 1996). This means that **when chronic morphine (or heroin) use is stopped, the body has less ability to produce its own dopamine and therefore less ability to feel elated or even normal. This depletion intensifies the desire to use the drug again.**

This and many other changes in body chemistry result in tissue or physical dependence since **the body relies on the drug to stay normal.** Researchers also found that animals that became physically dependent, then were withdrawn from the drug, and then readministered the drug would redevelop tissue dependence more rapidly.

Tolerance and physical dependence can extend to other opioids. That is, if users build a tolerance and a physical dependence to heroin, they will also have a tissue dependence and tolerance to morphine, codeine, and other opioids (cross-dependence).

"My tolerance to Demerol®, morphine, and things like that was tremendous. I had to have tons of the stuff. I went to have a local surgery and they were like, 'Okay, how's that?' and I was like, 'Is this just a test or what?'"
35-year-old recovering opioid addict

This **cross-dependence** is the basis for methadone maintenance treatment in which one opioid (heroin) is replaced by another less-damaging one. However, tolerance and physical dependence appear to be receptor specific, so an opioid, such as heroin, that works at the mu receptors will not create as much tolerance as one that works at kappa receptors (Jaffe et al., 1997). This is known as **"select tolerance."**

Withdrawal

For powerful opioids there are two withdrawal phases:

◊ acute withdrawal (detoxification),

◊ protracted withdrawal.

Acute withdrawal occurs when tissue dependence has developed after chronic use and the person suddenly stops using. The physiology has changed enough to trigger this rebounding effect as **the body tries to return to normal too quickly.**

"Your muscles are like wrenching, your entire digestive tract is going crazy. Stomach cramps—but not just stomach cramps, also diarrhea. Everything that can go wrong with your intestinal tract happens. Your legs, you kick constantly; that's why I think they call it 'kicking.' Your legs will jerk and kick uncontrollably. You have insomnia. You vomit, have sweats, and what else, oh yeah, the craziness, delirium."
27-year-old female heroin user

Protracted withdrawal (extended withdrawal symptoms) lasts for months after abstinence has begun. Initially symptoms such as mild increases in blood pressure, body temperature, respiration, and pupil size occur from week 4 up to week 10. A later phase that can last 30 weeks or more also shows a decrease in blood pressure, body temperature, and respiration, along with a general unease. The discomfort and other psychological factors play a significant role in long-term relapse (Schuckit, 2000). Protracted withdrawal is **also the occasional recurrence of withdrawal symptoms brought about by an environmental trigger** (sight, odor, neighborhood, etc.) that stimulates an addict's past memory of using or getting high. Known also as "environmentally cued" or "triggered" craving, this phenomenon can persist for several decades after stopping use.

In general

◊ **short-acting opioids, like heroin, morphine, and Dilaudid®, result in more acute withdrawal symptoms that begin within 8–12 hours** after cessation of chronic use, reach peak intensity within 48 hours, and then subside over a period of 5–7 days;

◊ **long-acting opioids, like methadone, will delay the withdrawal symptoms from 36–72 hours,** reach peak intensity in 4–6 days, and persist for 14 days or more (Jaffe et al., 1997; Schuckit, 2000);

◊ other opioids, such as codeine, Percodan®, and Darvon®, have withdrawal phenomena somewhere between those two extremes.

TABLE 4–2   OPIOID WITHDRAWAL SYMPTIONS

Bone, joint, and muscular pain	Insomnia
Anxiety	Sweating
Runny nose	Diarrhea
Rapid pulseand tachycardia	High blood pressure
Coughing	Dilated pupils
Hyper-reflexes and muscle cramps	Yawning
Anorexia	Chills and goose bumps
Teary eyes	Vomiting
Fever	Stomach cramps

One reason the hyperactivity of withdrawal occurs is the sudden release of excess norepinephrine that has been produced but not released during use of the opioid because the drug inhibits the release of these neurotransmitters in the locus coeruleus (Gold, 1998).

It is important to remember that although acute heroin withdrawal feels like an incredibly bad case of the flu, **it is almost never life threatening** as is acute withdrawal from alcohol or sedative-hypnotics. Unfortunately since acute opioid withdrawal symptoms can be painful and seem so frightening or create so much anxiety, **the fear of withdrawal becomes a greater trigger for continued use** than even the desire to repeat the rush.

"I have at times wished I was dead. That's how severe it would be. I've seen people in jail try to hang themselves. I've seen people in jail shoot their own urine to try and get the heroin out of the urine that's left in there."
72-year-old recovering heroin addict

ADDITIONAL PROBLEMS WITH HEROIN & OTHER OPIOIDS

NEONATAL EFFECTS

Most opioids, especially heroin and morphine, quickly **cross the placental barrier** between the fetus and the mother thereby sending large doses of the drug to the developing infant. Pregnant heroin users have a greater risk of miscarriage, placental separation, premature labor, breech birth, stillbirth, and eclampsia (uterine contractions). **When born to an addicted mother, the baby is also addicted** and since they are much smaller than adults, the tissue dependence and withdrawal symptoms are more severe. These neonatal withdrawal symptoms include low birth weight, a high-pitched cry, irritability, tremors, exag-

gerated reflexes, diarrhea, rapid breathing, sweating, and vomiting, along with sneezing, yawning, and hiccuping (Finnegan & Kandall, 1997). These symptoms can last 5–8 weeks and unlike adults, **babies in withdrawal can die.**

"The two infants that I had that were heroin affected . . . heroin addicted at birth . . . were managed on morphine for 3 months and then continued to do withdrawal for another 3–6 months before the chemicals were out of their bodies. While they're going through withdrawal, they are not developing. They are not rolling over, they are not sitting, they are not playing with toys."
36-year-old foster mother of children born to drug-using mothers

Infants born addicted often have to be medically managed. The opiate paregoric seems to decrease seizure activity, increase sucking coordination, and decrease the incidence of explosive stools. Phenobarbital is also used. In addition to using drugs for detoxification, a restful comforting environment is soothing to the withdrawing infant (Kandall, 1993).

OVERDOSE

About half of all heroin users will experience a clinically significant toxic overdose (McGregor, Darke, Ali, & Christie, 1998). **Most overdoses are accidental** particularly if the user is unsure of the purity of the heroin. Blood pressure drops, the heart beats too weakly to circulate blood, and lungs labor and fill with fluid. The victim often has blue lips and a pale or blue body, pinpoint pupils, fresh needle marks, gasping or rattling respirations, cardiac arrhythmias, and convulsions.

"I've seen her go out like twice and I had to revive her once and that was the most terrifying moment of my entire life, like seeing her on the bed, pretty much dead, and having to shake her, and beat her, and pick her up, and drop her until she like came to 'cause I

didn't know CPR. And she didn't remember anything of it. When she woke up she said, 'Why the hell are you screaming, you're going to freak out our parents.' She had no idea."
26-year-old heroin addict

Severe respiratory depression is the major cause of death with heroin overdose. The person passes out and unless quickly revived will slip into a coma and die. It is estimated that 3,000–4,000 people die from heroin overdoses each year (NIDA, 2000). There were about 97,287 emergency room visits for heroin overdose in 2000 compared to 174,896 for cocaine. These figures for heroin have almost tripled in the past 10 years (Drug Abuse Warning Network [DAWN], 2002b; Cham, Hall, Ernst, & Weiss, 2002).

"You know, people who do heroin aren't worried about dying because like if three people die from a new batch of heroin, everybody wants to know where they are getting that heroin so they can go get some because it's the best and they figure they will just do a little less."
41-year-old recovering heroin addict

After establishing an airway, checking heartbeat, and preventing aspiration, a heroin overdose can be counteracted by a shot of an **opioid antagonist, naloxone (Narcan®), to block and reverse the life-threatening effects** of too much drug (Schuckit, 2000). The Narcan® also obliterates the high and will cause severe withdrawal effects if the overdose victim is an addict.

DIRTY & SHARED NEEDLES

Of the 180,000 treatment admissions for primary injection drug abuse and 34,000 admissions for secondary injection drug abuse, 83% were principally opioid users. The opioid users had been using for an average of 14 years before coming in for treatment (SAMHSA/TEDS, 2002). This excessive use of the injection method for opioids

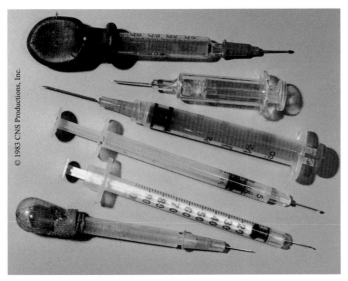

© 1983 CNS Productions, Inc.

Addicts will use diabetics' syringes, eyedroppers, veterinary needles, and anything else that's handy to inject their heroin or other opioids.
••••••••••••••

is important because the most dangerous problem with heroin, the one that causes the most illness and death, is dirty or shared needles. Needles put a large amount of the drug into the bloodstream at one time but unfortunately **users can also unknowingly inject adulterants**. Adulterants range from powdered milk to baby laxatives. **Infectious bacteria and viruses can also be transmitted** including those that cause hepatitis B or C, endocarditis, malaria, syphilis, flesh-eating bacteria, gangrene, and the HIV virus that causes AIDS.

Hepatitis C & HIV

Various studies have shown that **50% to 90% of all needle-using heroin addicts carry hepatitis C.** Even those with less than 1 year of IV drug use had a positive rate of 71.4%. Once infected 20% to 40% will develop liver disease and 4% to 16% will develop liver cancer (Payte & Zweben, 1998). Since the hepatitis C virus (HCV) was identified in 1988 and a test devised for it, the number of cases of HCV caused by transfusion has dropped dramatically but IV drug use transmission remains high. IV users have created a well of infection to be spread to their partners or co-users.

"I watched somebody who refused to wash the syringe out after I had it and I told him I had AIDS, I'm positive, I have the disease. And he said, 'I really don't care.' Didn't wash it out and you could see when he pulled back and the outfit was clear and it had blood in it and he shot it up. I mean I hope the man's alive."
29-year-old recovering heroin addict with AIDS

The transmission of HIV by IV drug use is also substantial. More than half of IV drug users carry the HIV virus although the percentages vary radically from city to city. In San Francisco 4.3% of IV drug users are HIV positive while in New York the figure is as high as 80% because of needle sharing. It is estimated that

◇ 25% of all U.S. AIDS cases (197,091 of 793,026) were transmitted to an IV drug user by a contaminated needle (about three-fourths are male);

◇ 10.5% (69,886) were transmitted to heterosexual or homosexual partners of IV drug users through sexual contact;

◇ 70% of children infected with HIV had mothers who were IV drug users or had sexual contact with IV drug users (Centers for Disease Control, 2002).

Internationally the figures are worse. In Burma the World Health Organization has estimated that between 74% and 91% of the country's IV heroin addicts are HIV positive. It is estimated by the United Nations that **worldwide, 42 million are HIV positive** (from all causes), half of them women. Almost two-thirds of those infected are from Sub-Saharan Africa.

Abscesses & Other Infections

Excess needle use continually traumatizes the blood vessels often causing them to collapse. This is why injection drug users are forced to switch to locations other than the ante cubital fossa opposite the elbow. Injection sites include the wrist, between the toes, in the neck, or even in the dorsal vein of the penis.

Septic abscesses and ulcerations caused by **soft tissue infections are common in IV drug users** since most heroin abusers will shoot up 4–6 times a day often with a contaminated needle. The most common infectious organisms are *staphylococcus aureus* and *beta-hemolytic streptococci* (Orangio, Pitlick, & Latta, 1984). If the infection is too deep or too far along, often part of the flesh has to be cut away. In addition adulterants such as cotton can lodge in or under the skin. **Other signs of IV drug use are lesions or "tracks,"** which are scars on the skin often caused by constant inflammation at the injection site and hyperpigmentation. Sterile abscesses can be caused by irritation not just bacteria. Cellulitis (deep inflammation of soft or connective tissue) can be caused either by bacteria or by irritation from repeated use.

"They can be life threatening if you let them go to a point . . . but I've also lost all my veins. I've hit nerves, I've hit arteries. If you should shoot into an artery, it's extremely painful. Having to wear long-sleeved shirts to work is like an inconvenient thing about shooting up."
40-year-old recovering heroin addict

One of the worst infections is **necrotizing fasciitis, an infection that destroys fascia and subcutaneous tissue** but is not immediately visible on the

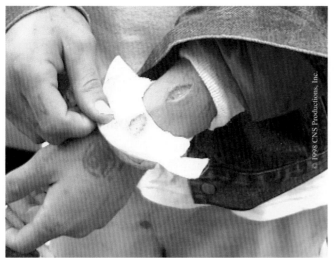

This abscess in the arm of a 25-year-old heroin addict occurred because of infectious organisms that were transmitted by contaminated needles or drugs. Abscesses are more common in opioid abusers than in stimulant abusers even though stimulant abusers shoot up more often.

surface. Bacteria like *clostridium perfinges* and variant strains of *streptococcus* and *staphylococcus* cause this condition known as "flesh-eating disease."

Endocarditis, an infection of heart valves, is found more often in IV drug users. Research points to a variety of organisms (including those involved in abscesses) that are dislodged from the injection site and lodge in heart valves.

Cotton fever, caused by endotoxins (which thrive in cotton), is another illness found more frequently in IV drug users. The term "cotton fever" is also used by addicts to describe any short-term bacterial infection or pyrogen reaction resulting in fever, chills, tremors, aches, and pains.

DILUTION & ADULTERATION

One of the reasons an overdose occurs is that **street drugs can vary radically in purity**. Street heroin varies from 0% to 99% pure, so if a user is expecting 3% heroin and gets 30%, the results could be fatal. Dilution of an expensive item like heroin with a cheap substitute, e.g., starch, sugar (dextrose, lactose), aspirin, Ajax®, quinine, caffeine, or talcum powder, is extremely common. According to the DEA, heroin purity for retail-level sale is 10% to 70% compared to 1% to 10% just 15 years ago. **Part of the reason for the increased purity is the influx of large amounts of unadulterated Southeast Asian and South American**

heroin (DEA, 2002a). Because of increased production and a proliferation of street chemists, it is also much easier to come across synthetic high-potency opioids.

COST

Contrary to popular belief promoted by television and movies that show heroin addicts as derelicts, criminals, and people who have a mental illness, **a majority of heroin users (73%) are gainfully employed** (Office of National Drug Control Policy [ONDCP], 2000a). However because of the buildup of tolerance and the high cost of heroin, a great many users must turn to illegal methods to pay for their habits. **The cost of a heroin habit can range from $20 to $200 a day** depending on the level of use. It is estimated that Americans spend about $12 billion a year on heroin (compared to $42 billion on cocaine).

"When we were really strung out, we were spending $150 to $200 a day to feel normal. It's one thing to spend that kind of money and get loaded but when you're spending that kind of money to just function as a human being, it's irritating."
32-year-old recovering heroin addict

The overwhelming need to support an opioid habit makes antisocial behaviors, such as robbery, and eventual involvement with the legal system almost inevitable. It is estimated that **60% of the cost of supporting a habit is gotten through consensual crime, including prostitution and drug dealing**, and supplemented by welfare payments or occasional work. Most of the remaining 40% comes from shoplifting and burglary.

POLYDRUG USE

Multiple Drug Use: A heroin user might start with heroin in the morning to stop withdrawal symptoms and calm down. Later he might take some speed to get energetic and in the evening use marijuana to relax.

Mixing: A common polydrug combination is cocaine or amphetamine with heroin. This **upper/downer combination, called a "speedball,"** can enhance the euphoric and the painkilling effects of both drugs (Karch, 1996). It can also be dangerous since the user doesn't know which drug will kick in. Many methadone users take clonazepam (Klonopin®) to enhance their methadone because the combination feels somewhat like a heroin high. Some dealers are spiking poor quality marijuana with heroin to give it an extra kick and sell it as high quality pot. Opioids can have additive and synergistic effects when used with most depressant drugs, especially alcohol and benzodiazepines. **These opioid/downer combinations increase the potential for respiratory depression**, lethargy, possible overdose, and even death.

"I'd be waiting and waiting and during the time that I was waiting, I'd be getting drunk. By the time I got around to doing my shot, I was already drunk. I'd hit up and boom, I'd be on the floor."
36-year-old male heroin user in treatment

Morphing: To counter the depressant effects of heroin, addicts might use uppers to change their mood. They then might get so wired from the cocaine or methamphetamine that they will use alcohol or heroin again to come down.

"Before I was using heroin I was a heavy heavy speed user and I started using heroin to come down from speed and then the heroin gradually took over and I stopped using speed entirely and then about 4 months ago I started using crack on top of the heroin. It was a great combination because like crack will take up all of your money real quick and I had to like do a lot more people harm to get my money than I did before."

34-year-old recovering heroin addict

Cycling: A number of heroin addicts will go off their drug for several weeks and switch to a cheaper high to give the body a chance to lower its tolerance and tissue dependence often in an attempt to reduce the cost of their addiction. They might switch to alcohol, benzodiazepines, or marijuana in the interim and then cycle on and off heroin for the next few months.

Sequentialing: This is a long-term consequence of using drugs. Someone might use heroin for several years and then switch to alcohol because they can't stand the IV drug user's lifestyle. After a few years of alcohol and a bloated liver, they might then switch to marijuana only to switch back to heroin once again a few years later.

FROM EXPERIMENTATION TO ADDICTION

The number of people admitted for heroin treatment has gone up in the last 10 years. **The majority (66%) of those entering treatment had been injecting heroin.** However, first time admissions involved more smokers, snorters, and sniffers than injectors (SAMHSA/TEDS, 2002).

Experimentation with alcohol, marijuana, and tobacco begins much earlier than experimentation with heroin. The mean age of first heroin use was about 22.3 years of age in 2000 compared to 17.5 for first marijuana use, 15.9 for tobacco, and 15.8 for alco-

hol (SAMHSA, 2002). **It takes an average of 1 year of sporadic heroin use for someone to develop a daily habit** although some users with a predisposition to opioid addiction might jump to daily use within 15 days.

"I'd wake up in the morning and before I'd go to work (when I was working), I'd have to do a hit of dope just to function. I'd have to do a hit of dope just to get out of bed. I'd have to do a hit of dope to go to the bathroom. It wasn't a matter of getting high anymore, it was a matter of getting functional."

Recovering 38-year-old male heroin abuser

After a while the pain of not using often becomes greater than the pain the user might have been trying to avoid. The pain relief offered by the heroin becomes greater than the pleasure. It's as if the user unconsciously learns that **by creating more pain and then using heroin, the relief and subsequent activation of the reward/reinforcement center is a repeatable way of getting a rush.**

"After a while you're not just killing your pain, you start to kill your feelings, any feelings you might have regardless of whether you're having pain. It's not the pain that you're killing. It's never really the pain."

36-year-old recovering heroin abuser

If an opioid user has passed from experimentation to abuse or addiction, **treatment becomes a physiological as well as a psychological process. Physically the addict has to be detoxified from the heroin** or other opioid, often with the use of medications such as Darvon® (a milder opioid than heroin), methadone (a long-lasting opioid), LAAM® (a very long-lasting opioid), or buprenorphine (a powerful opiate agonist at low doses and an antagonist at high doses). In addition cravings have to be controlled to maintain abstinence. Psychologi-

cally the addict has to learn a new way of living because emotional and environmental cues often lead to relapse (*see Chapter 9*).

A comprehensive long-term study of 582 heroin-addicted criminal offenders over a period of 33 years showed that their lives were characterized by repeated cycles of drug abuse and abstinence interspersed with health and social problems. Over half had died (overdose, accidental poisoning, homicide, suicide, accident, liver disease, etc.) and of the remaining 242 still living, 40% had used heroin in the past year. Their death rate was 50–100 times the rate among the general population of men in the same age range (Hser, Hoffman, Grella, & Anglin, 2001).

The Vietnam Experience

The road from experimentation to addiction can be better understood by looking at the use of heroin in Vietnam by U.S. soldiers from 1967 to the end of the war in 1973. Dr. Lee N. Robins (a psychiatrist at Harvard) and others tested several groups of GIs, first while still stationed in Vietnam and then after they had been returned to the United States. Almost half the GIs had experimented with opium or heroin. Twenty percent had been addicted at one time and reported withdrawal symptoms. Since heroin was so readily available, experimentation was easy even for those who were too young to drink. So the usual progression from alcohol, cigarettes, and marijuana to heroin or cocaine was reversed. According to Robins, the most startling part of the study was that **only 5% of those who had become addicted in Vietnam relapsed within 10 months after they returned to the United States** and only 12% relapsed even briefly within 3 years. Most of the returning GIs didn't even go through treatment (Robins, 1994). This seems to suggest that even though tissue dependence caused by use of drugs can be powerful, other factors, especially preexisting sensitivity determined by heredity and environment, have a greater influence.

DOONESBURY/ by Garry Trudeau

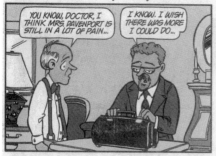
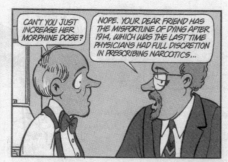
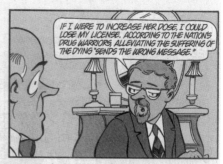
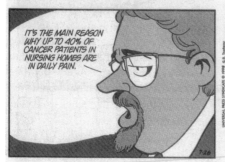
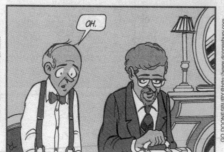
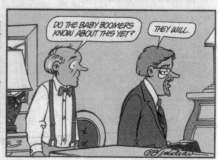

DOONESBURY © 1998, G. B. Trudeau. Reprinted, by permission, Universal Press Syndicate. All rights reserved.

MORPHINE & OTHER OPIOIDS

MORPHINE

When Frederick Serturner isolated morphine in 1805, this truly effective painkiller was embraced by physicians and its sales soared in the mid- to late 1800s. Profits from this revolutionary new medicine established a number of drug companies. It wasn't until 1952 that researchers were able to fully synthesize morphine. It remains **the standard by which effective pain relief is measured**. Morphine is processed from opium into white crystal hypodermic tablets, capsules, suppositories, oral solutions, and injectable solutions. This analgesic may be drunk, eaten, absorbed under the tongue, absorbed rectally by suppository, or injected into a vein, a muscle, or under the skin. Different routes of administration have different effects. For example, 3–6 times more morphine must be taken orally to achieve the same effects as injecting.

The liver is the principal site of metabolism and, along with other tissues, converts the morphine into metabolites that more readily cross the blood-brain barrier and are possibly more potent than the morphine itself (Karch, 1996). Some of the morphine is excreted quickly in the urine while some remains in measurable amounts in the plasma for 4–6 hours and can be detectable in the urine for several days.

Therapeutic Pain Control

"My nurse told me, 'You don't need extra pain medication. I've been through this a hundred times before and I know you're not in pain.'"
Patient in burn treatment unit

Pain is certainly a subjective judgment by the patient and so it can be difficult to know what a patient feels. Physicians and nurses ask patients to self-rate their pain on a 1 to 10 scale with 10 being the worst. The prescribing of morphine, different opioids, or other painkillers is partly based on this rating. In addition several other concerns affect the amount of medication prescribed:

◊ **fear that tissue dependence and addiction might develop**;

◊ concern that the opioid will **mask clues to a serious disease**;

◊ concern that the **patient may be faking symptoms** in order to get drugs to supply a habit (purposive withdrawal).

These three concerns might keep some physicians from prescribing sufficient pain medications even when appropriate. The current problems with OxyContin® and hydrocodone and past problems with drugs such as codeine, Percodan®, and Dilaudid® have made adherence to medically sound prescribing practices difficult. To help establish a better policy to guide the physician, the State Federation of Medical Boards, the American Society of Addiction Medicine (ASAM), and others have adopted model guidelines for the use of controlled substances in treating pain.

For example, a **Pain Patient's Bill of Rights** was enacted into law in California. It states that

◊ inadequate treatment of acute and chronic pain is a significant health problem;

◊ a physician should prescribe in conformance with the provisions of the

California Intractable Pain Treatment Act;

◊ the physician may refuse to prescribe opiate medication for a patient who requests the treatment for severe chronic intractable pain; however that physician shall inform the patient that there are physicians who specialize in treating that kind of pain with methods that include the use of opioids.

ASAM guidelines, issued in 1997, recommended that the physicians use more of their own judgment in prescribing and that they should not be held responsible if the patient cons them into prescribing unneeded opioids. However they also suggest that continuing overprescription practices as well as underprescribing that keeps a legitimate patient in pain should both be remedied by education first rather than sanctions that might interfere with the practice of good medicine (California Society of Addiction Medicine, 1997).

In general, iatrogenic (physician-induced) addiction is unusual nowadays unlike the turn of the twentieth century when physicians were not as knowledgeable about the risks of long-term opioid use. Most of the problems with moderate-strength prescription opioids (e.g. hydrocodone, codeine) come from long-term use. It seems that by relying on the drug to relieve the pain, **the patient becomes more sensitive to pain because the body produces fewer of its own painkillers** and down regulates its own opioid receptors.

"I had been masking the pain for so long that I didn't know how much pain I had or didn't have and when I didn't really have pain, per se, that was pathological. I couldn't deal with the slightest little thing."
37-year-old recovering prescription opioid addict

Since some level of tissue adaptation occurs with even the initial dose of an opioid, some care does need to be taken in prescribing. **The physician needs to learn about risk factors for addiction** such as

◊ physical health, e.g., kidney and liver function;

◊ drug abuse history, medical drug use history, and mental health history;

◊ possible hereditary factors that make the patient more susceptible.

In addition the physician has to

◊ develop a working diagnosis and treatment plan;

◊ discuss risks vs. benefits and compliance with the patient;

◊ keep up-to-date on recent trials of medications or consult with someone familiar with the drugs;

◊ get constant feedback from the patient as to effects, efficacy, and side effects;

◊ be willing to modify the type of medication and dosages;

◊ keep accurate records concerning effects and patient reaction (Verhaag & Ikeda, 1991).

CODEINE

"For me, codeine is just weak heroin. It doesn't do much for me. Codeine just stops the pain and stops your nose from running. It just gets you able to function enough in order to go get you some heroin."
42-year-old male recovering heroin user

Codeine is extracted directly from opium or refined from morphine. Also known as "methylmorphine," it is about one-fifth as strong as morphine and is generally used for the relief of moderate pain. The most common drugs mixed with codeine are aspirin or acetaminophen because of synergistic analgesia (the drugs compliment each other's strength). Codeine is also **commonly used to control severe coughs** (Robitussin A-C®, Cheracol®). It is a Schedule V drug in cough syrups and is even sold over the counter in some states. It is a Schedule II drug by itself or Schedule III when mixed with other drugs and used for analgesia. **Codeine used to be the most widely prescribed and abused prescription**

opioid in the United States and other countries but hydrocodone (Vicodin®) has taken over that dubious honor. Some addicts drink large amounts of codeine-based cough syrup to relieve heroin withdrawal symptoms or just to get slightly loaded. One of the problems with codeine, as with many opioids, is that it triggers nausea. Many physicians switched to hydrocodone for moderate pain relief because it is more effective. The half-life of codeine is about 3 hours and the drug will be detectable in the blood for up to 24 hours and in the urine for up to 2 or 3 days. If physical dependence develops, withdrawal symptoms can begin within a few hours and peak within 36–72 hours.

HYDROCODONE (Vicodin®, Hycodan®, Tussend®, Norco®)

A number of headlines concerning opioids refer to movie, television, or sports stars who developed a dependence on the Schedule II opioid hydrocodone (Vicodin®). It often followed prolonged prescriptive use for chronic pain, especially back pain and pinched nerves. More than 36 million prescriptions were written for hydrocodone in 2001 (IMS Health, 2002). This **most widely prescribed opioid** (semisynthetic) has many of the same actions as codeine but produces less nausea. Four times as many hydrocodone prescriptions for analgesia are written as compared to codeine. It is also used in cough preparations, called "antitussives," e.g., Hycomin Syrup®. As with other opioids, respiratory depression and masking of illness can be dangerous especially when other depressants are used at the same time. There have been reports that abuse of hydrocodone (more than 20 pills a day for at least 2 months) can precipitate a sudden hearing loss. The House Ear Institute in Los Angeles and several other medical centers have identified at least 48 patients with this condition (Marsa, 2001). Further research of this serious side effect is needed.

About 350 deaths are reported each year due to hydrocodone overdose although more occur when used with other depressants (DAWN, 2002a). Seventeen out of 20 DEA field divisions mentioned hydrocodone abuse as a problem (DEA, 1999).

"I injured myself and I was on hydrocodone, you know. I'd take one, next hour and a half I'd be real sleepy and lightheaded... be dizzy. It's like being drunk. I developed a small addiction to it, you know. It was an easy escape; pop a pill, drink some water, drown my fears away, drown the pain away— feel good for a while."

24-year-old weightlifter

METHADONE (Dolophine®)

Methadone was developed during World War II by the Germans to supplement their limited supplies of morphine (O'Brien et al., 1992).

Methadone is a **legally authorized opioid used to treat heroin addiction** through a program known as "methadone maintenance" (*see Chapter 9*). Under this harm reduction program started in New York in 1965, methadone is used as a legally dispensed substitute for heroin (Payte, 1997). The addict comes into the clinic every day to receive a dose (usually mixed with fruit juice). On a few occasions (e.g., when the methadone user has to go out of town) a take-home dose is given in tablet form. There are **approximately 205,000 heroin addicts involved in methadone treatment in more than 950 methadone treatment programs nationwide** (American Association for the Treatment of Opioid Dependence, 2002). Methadone can also be used to detoxify a heroin abuser who has become physically dependent.

Because this long-acting synthetic opioid **reduces drug craving and blocks withdrawal symptoms for 24–72 hours**, it diminishes the craving for heroin, which has a shorter duration of action, causes more intense highs and lows, and is illegal. The disappearance of the intense need to use heroin again and again and come up with increasing amounts of money has led to a

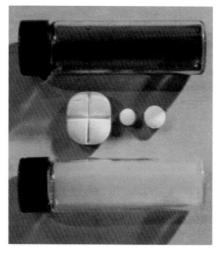

Methadone, a bitter-tasting white powder, can be mixed with orange juice for use at a methadone clinic or it can be dispensed in tablets for take-home doses. It also comes in injectable form for pain management.
Courtesy of the Drug Enforcement Administration

• •

dramatic decrease in crime among those in methadone maintenance (Bell, Mattick, Hay, Chan, & Hall, 1997). Like any opioid, methadone also has painkilling and depressant effects that can be used in clinical situations. The analgesic effects only last 4–6 hours.

Like heroin, **methadone is addicting** and must be monitored closely to prevent diversion into illegal channels. Despite heavy regulation of methadone clinics and tight controls of the supply, methadone is still sold on the street, abused, and responsible for a number of overdoses every year—560 in 2001 (DAWN, 2002a,b). Addicts will combine methadone with other drugs, such as clonazepam (Klonopin®), clonidine (Catapres®), carisoprodol (Soma®), and alprazolam (Xanax®), in order to intensify the high and make it resemble the feeling they get from heroin.

Recently there have been proposals, research, and trials by the U.S. Department of Health and Human Services among others to make methadone treatment more convenient and bring it into the mainstream of health care. Rather than have recovering addicts get their methadone only from methadone clinics, the drug would also be available through certified physi-

cians and nonmethadone drug clinics. There is also a proposal to move methadone treatment out from the scrutiny of the Food and Drug Administration (FDA) to the oversight of the Substance Abuse and Mental Health Services Administration (SAMHSA). This would decrease the amount of regulations that cover its use. There is still much controversy in the treatment community about the overall efficacy of methadone maintenance and other drug replacement therapies.

HYDROMORPHONE (Dilaudid®)

Hydromorphone, a short-acting semisynthetic opioid, can be taken orally or injected. Hydromorphone is refined from morphine through a process that makes it **7–10 times more potent on a gram-for-gram basis than morphine**. Hydromorphone is used as an alternative to morphine for the treatment of moderate-to-severe pain. Since it is more potent, it has a higher abuse potential than morphine. Illegally diverted Dilaudid® is becoming increasingly attractive to cocaine users for the drug combination known as a "speedball" (hydromorphone and cocaine or methamphetamine). A 4 mg tablet of Dilaudid® sold on the street ranges in price from $30 to $70. Though it is quite potent, just a few deaths from overdose are reported each year.

OXYCODONE (OxyContin®, Percodan®)

This semisynthetic derivative of codeine is used for the relief of moderate-to-severe pain. Oxycodone in standard form (Percodan®) is usually taken orally, often in combination with aspirin or acetaminophen. By this route it usually takes about 30 minutes before the effects appear that then last from 4–6 hours. Its pain-relieving effect is **much stronger than codeine but weaker than that of morphine or Dilaudid®**.

Recently the abuse of the time-release version of oxycodone, OxyContin®, has increased—7.2 million prescriptions were written for this analgesic in 2001. Purdue Pharma introduced the long-acting formulation in 1995 for the treatment of severe chronic pain. What some people have been doing **with OxyContin® is chewing, crushing and injecting, or crushing and sniffing the time-release formulation** that holds the oxycodone. **This destroys the time-release effect** so a much larger blood level of oxycodone is achieved. Heroin or other **opioid abusers describe the high as somewhat similar to heroin** and so they try to get the drug prescribed to them or they divert legal supplies. According to the DEA, the abuse of OxyContin® has caused more than 400 deaths although Purdue Pharma called the DEA report flawed (National Council on Alcohol and Drug Dependence, 2002). A number of the deaths involved more than one drug, particularly alcohol.

The introduction of this powerful time-release analgesic occurred at the same time that the medical community was increasing its emphasis on the proper treatment of acute and chronic pain. Because of this new emphasis, long-acting medications gained favor due to better compliance rates, better long-term control of pain, and fewer side effects when compared to short-acting narcotics (when used as directed).

A year after its introduction, reports of increased illicit use started coming in. The drug, which was also called "ocs" "oxy," "o'cotton," and "hillbilly heroin," originally came in 10 mg, 20 mg, 40 mg, 80 mg, and 160 mg tablets. The large tablets were known as "blue bombers" and "o'coffins" due to a high rate of overdose. Shipments of the 160 mg tablets were suspended by the manufacturer. Street prices have averaged about $1 per mg or $10 for the smallest-dose tablets.

As with other desired opioids that were available in pharmacies, drugstore robberies and diversion of legitimate supplies increased.

◇ Some legitimate prescribers wanting to treat pain more humanely were easily duped into writing prescriptions.

◇ Some physicians and pharmacists tried to make money by writing prescriptions for bogus patients (100 of the 40 mg tablets could bring in $4,000).

◇ Legitimate patients sold their supplies to others.

In addition overblown media coverage not only increased general knowledge of the drug but also caused legitimate prescribers to limit treatment of real chronic pain.

MEPERIDINE (Demerol®, Pethidine®, Mepergan®)

A synthetic phenylpiperidine derivative, this short-acting opioid is **one of the most widely used analgesics** for moderate-to-severe pain though it is only one-sixth the strength of morphine. It is most often injected but can also be taken orally. This drug can be neurotoxic in large doses. Demerol® affects the brain in such a way that **it causes as much sedation and euphoria than morphine but less constipation and cough suppression**. Since it is eliminated by the kidneys, patients with impaired kidneys should avoid the drug. Though less potent by weight than morphine, it is often the opioid most often abused by medical professionals.

PENTAZOCINE (Talwin NX®)

Talwin NX®, prescribed for chronic or acute pain, comes in tablets or as an injectable liquid. It has a fraction of the potency of morphine and **acts as a weak opioid antagonist as well as an opioid agonist**. This drug was frequently combined and injected with an antihistamine drug ("Ts and blues") for the heroin-like high. Increased vigilance and reformulation of Talwin® (including the addition of naloxone, a more powerful opioid antagonist) by its manufacturer have almost stopped these problems although some people still abuse Talwin NX® orally by itself. There are no current emergency room reports of pentazocine overdoses perhaps because of its reformulation.

PROPOXYPHENE (Darvon®, Darvocet®, Propacet®, Wygesic®)

Used for the **relief of mild-to-moderate pain**, this odorless white crystalline powder is often prescribed by dentists. More than 20 million prescriptions were written for propoxyphene in 2001 (Scott-Lewin, 2002). It is taken orally for moderate pain with the effects lasting 4–6 hours. Propoxyphene is occasionally used as an alternative to methadone maintenance and **for heroin detoxification**, especially for younger addicts, because it has only one-half to two-thirds the potency of codeine. Although it has abuse potential, Darvon® (and especially Darvon-N®, a napsylate salt) continues to be used successfully in the detoxification of heroin addicts. The older the user, the slower the metabolism, so the drug is more potent in seniors. Misuse of this drug makes someone susceptible to overdose or addiction. Only about 4% of opioid fatalities involve propoxyphene (usually in combination with alcohol).

"After 7 years of doing Darvon®, I started having withdrawals after 3 to 4 hours from the last pill that I had taken, so I was addicted to my watch. Then it got to where it was like 2 hours, so I needed like 14 or 16 Darvons to get through the day."
Recovering 43-year-old female Darvon® abuser

FENTANYL (Sublimaze®)

In September of 2002 Chechen rebels took over a theatre in Russia, holding 500 patrons hostage and threatening to kill them if their demands were not met. Russian troops used a gas to knock out the rebels and unfortunately the hostages. The gas used was based on fentanyl, so those inside the theater essentially were knocked out by the equivalent of an opioid overdose and since no one knew how potent the drug would be, 119 hostages died, along with 50 rebels. Most died of respiratory depression and heart failure. Halothane, a powerful anesthetic used in surgery, was also found in the blood of some victims.

Russians name gas used in raid

German doctor found a second anesthetic

By Craig Nelson
Cox News Service

Moscow — Ending days of intense speculation, Russia's health minister said Wednesday that the gas used in the siege of a Moscow theater was based on fentanyl, a fast-acting, opiate-based narcotic often used as an anesthetic.

United States and Western governments whose citizens were among the hundreds of hostages poisoned.

"To neutralize the terrorists, a substance based on fentanyl derivatives was used," Health Minister Yuri Shevchenko said in comments broadcast on Russian television.

Shevchenko said that the gas itself was not lethal. He admitted, however, that it had proved fatal to those hostages who were in poor health or who had been weakened by the squalid conditions of their captivity. Most died of respiratory and heart failure.

pacitating gas probably contained other substances as well.

Fentanyl belongs to a group of medications called narcotic analgesics, which act on the central nervous system to relief pain. It is often used for general anesthesia and in treatment for cancer. In high enough doses, it can cause dizziness, respiratory difficulties and death.

The health minister's disclosure followed critical remarks Tuesday by the U.S. ambassador to Russia, Alexander Vershbow, who said that with a little more information about the gas, "at least a few more of the hostages

used during the special operation," Shevchenko said.

Moscow health officials said Wednesday that two more former hostages had died, raising the death toll to 119, including one American.

All 50 Chechen separatists were killed in the raid, which climaxed a 58-hour siege.

As of late Wednesday, 152 former hostages remained hospitalized, the Itar-Tass news agency reported.

A day after Russian police detained 30 people suspected of aiding the Chechen rebels, Danish

Even in its milder therapeutic formulation, fentanyl, introduced in 1968, is **the most powerful of the opioids** (50–100 times as strong as morphine on a weight-for-weight basis). It is used intravenously during and after surgery for severe pain. Structurally this synthetic phenylpiperidine derivative is related to meperidine (Demerol®). It is also available in a skin patch to give steady pain relief for patients with intractable pain. A fentanyl lollipop was introduced in 1994 to be used by children for postoperative pain. Recently an oral-transmucosal version (Actiq®) was developed to be dissolved slowly in the mouth. Unfortunately fentanyl is favored as a drug of abuse by some surgical assistants and anesthesiologists due to its availability and strength.

DESIGNER HEROIN

There are street versions of fentanyl (alpha, 3-methyl) and meperidine (MPPP) manufactured in illegal laboratories. They are **extremely potent**, often more than the drugs they are imitating. Sold as "China white," these drugs bear witness to a growing sophistication of street chemists who now can bypass the traditional smuggling and trafficking routes of heroin. Since these designer drugs are made without controls on purity or dosage, they represent a tremendous health threat to the opioid-abusing community. There have been numerous outbreaks of overdose deaths due to ultrapotent fentanyl being sold as normal-potency heroin.

"When I first got out here on the West Coast, I found out that it [China

white] wasn't white dope at all, it was fentanyl. And it wasn't even pharmaceutical fentanyl, it was bathtub fentanyl and people were dying on it."
Dealer/heroin user

If improperly made, street Demerol® (MPPP) can contain the chemical MPTP that destroys dopamine-producing brain cells that control voluntary muscular movement. The subsequent loss of control mimics the degenerative nerve condition known as "Parkinson's disease." This degeneration causes a condition known as the "frozen addict" in which the addict loses the ability to make any physical movements for the rest of his or her life.

LAAM® (levomethadyl acetate)

LAAM® is another **long-acting opioid that is used for heroin replacement therapy** similar to methadone maintenance. It prevents withdrawal symptoms and lasts for about 2–3 days compared to methadone's duration of action of 1–2 days. This reduces visits to the clinic for the drug to every other day or 3 days a week. It also reduces the need for take-home doses thereby reducing the potential of street trade with the drug. The half-life of LAAM® is 48 hours and the half-life of active LAAM® metabolites is 96 hours. Though the drug was developed in the late 1940s as a possible substitute for morphine, the slow onset and long duration of action made it **unsuitable for pain management**. It has been studied since the mid-1960s as a treatment for opioid-

dependent individuals but it wasn't until 1993 that the FDA made LAAM® available for clinical use.

The main detriment to the use of LAAM®, according to a survey of LAAM® clinics, seems to be the complicated paperwork and regulatory hurdles involved with use, along with staff attitude towards the drug (Rawson, Hasson, Huber, McCann, & Ling, 1998). The drug itself seems to work as well as methadone. In 1999 a proposal was made to move the monitoring of LAAM® (as well as methadone) out of the FDA and into SAMHSA in an effort to decrease the bureaucratic paperwork associated with the drugs' use.

NALOXONE (Narcan®) & NALTREXONE (Revia®)

Naloxone and naltrexone are **opioid antagonists**. They block the effects of endogenous as well as exogenous opioids.

Naloxone (Narcan®) is effective in treating heroin or opioid drug overdose. When a heroin overdose victim is injected with the drug, opioid effects (e.g., respiratory depression, low blood pressure, sedation) are immediately halted or reversed and the person snaps back to consciousness in a matter of seconds up to 2 minutes (PDR, 2002). However when the naloxone wears off, the patient can fall back into a coma because the heroin is still in the system and the dangerous effects can return. Often naloxone needs to be injected repeatedly until the heroin is completely metabolized from the body. Naloxone itself will not cause dangerous effects when the heroin has left the body.

"I just remember finding a vein finally and then waking up with a plastic tube in my nose, getting hit in the chest by a paramedic. Then everything went from black to light and they're standing over me and I was really pissed off at them for killing my buzz. And they're like, 'We just saved your life,' and I said, 'Maybe I didn't want you to. You just wasted $20.' But after

a while I thought about it and I know I could have died."

20-year-old male heroin addict in recovery

Naltrexone (Revia®) is used to prevent relapse and help to break the cycle of addiction for opioids. Taking naltrexone daily effectively **blocks the effects of heroin and any other opioid**. Its blocking mechanism will last up to 72 hours. Some clients will take it daily for 3 months or longer while others will only use it when the cravings get strong. Naltrexone is also being used to **reduce cravings for alcohol and cocaine** in support of detoxification and abstinence. A time-release version of naltrexone (Naltrel®) is being developed that would only need to be injected once a month. Naltrexone is not addicting in itself; however if someone is using opioids for pain relief, the naltrexone will make them ineffective. Side effects are usually minimal but can include nausea, irritability, headache, fatigue, and dizziness (Volpicelli, Pettinati, McLellan, & O'Brien, 2001). Naltrexone has also been proven effective in smoking cessation programs particularly among female smokers (Gold et al., 2002).

BUPRENORPHINE (Buprenex®, Subutex®, Suboxone®)

Buprenorphine is **a powerful opioid agonist at low doses and an opiate antagonist at high doses**. In low doses it is used as an analgesic alternative to morphine. It has been approved as **an alternative to methadone for detoxi-**

fication and induction of methadone maintenance because it is more attractive to addicts and limits their supplementary use of heroin or other opioids. Buprenorphine has a high degree of safety, long duration of action, flexible dosing, milder withdrawal effects, and a more acceptable reputation in the treatment community.

The exact dosage used for detoxification varies from patient to patient with the average term of use lasting from 3–21 days. The drug continues to block the effects of morphine and heroin for about 30 hours after use (Strain, Walls, Pristine, Liebson, & Bigelow, 1997). However there is an abuse potential when the drug is used in low doses, so some researchers, treatment physicians, and a pharmaceutical company (Reckitt, Benckiser [a British company]) are combining buprenorphine with naloxone to diminish the opiate agonist effects of the drug (Strain, Stoller, Walsh, et al., 2000). In Europe, Nepal, and India the abuse of buprenorphine is widespread.

Two drugs, Subutex® and Suboxone®, were approved in 2002 for treatment of patients with opioid dependence. Subutex® only contains buprenorphine while Suboxone® combines buprenorphine and naloxone. The important part of the FDA approval is that buprenorphine may now be prescribed by qualified physicians in their offices rather than only at a drug treatment clinic. The theory is that many addicts do not have access to methadone clinics or other treatment facilities, so mak-

ing this milder drug more widely available will increase options for the heroin addict. Unfortunately it also has an abuse potential.

CLONIDINE (Catapres®)

This nonopioid, originally prescribed for the treatment of hypertension, is often **used to diminish opioid withdrawal symptoms** such as nausea, anxiety, and diarrhea. It also seems to alleviate opioid craving. Since it acts on norepinephrine receptors to control their overactivity, one of the main causes of severe withdrawal symptoms, it shortens withdrawal time from almost 1 month down to a couple of weeks in some cases. When used in combination with naltrexone, it shortens severe withdrawal symptoms to about 5 days in a process called "rapid opioid detoxification."

ULTRARAPID OPIOID DETOXIFICATION

In this medically supervised process the patient is given naltrexone orally or naloxone intravenously while heavily sedated or even under general anesthesia to **avoid the pain of acute withdrawal symptoms** precipitated by the opioid antagonist. There is much controversy to this process, along with fatal complications if mistakes are made. Some say that even if the physical withdrawal is treated, the psychological addiction will continue and eventually cause a relapse (Smith & Seymour, 2001) (*see Chapter 9*).

SEDATIVE-HYPNOTICS

CLASSIFICATION

Americans filled more than 3.1 billion prescriptions in 2001 or an average of $49.84 per prescription. More than **60 million of those prescriptions were written for sedative-hypnotics** (mostly benzodiazepines). Their use in other countries is also widespread

(Scott-Lewin, 2002). Many more prescriptions used to be written for sedative-hypnotics in the '60s, '70s, and '80s but the use of **psychiatric medications for depression has taken over a significant part of sedative-hypnotics' share of the market** with tricyclic antidepressants and the newer SSRI antidepressants, e.g., Prozac® (fluoxetine), Paxil® (paroxetine), and Zoloft® (sertra-

line). At least 98 million prescriptions were written in 2001 for psychiatric medications, 45 million for antidepressants alone (Drug Benefit Trends, 2001, 2002).

Almost all sedative-hypnotics are available as pills, capsules, or tablets though some, such as diazepam (Valium®) and lorazepam (Ativan®), are used intravenously for more immediate

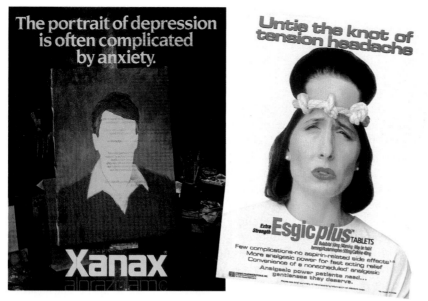

The market for sedative-hypnotics is in the billions of dollars. Advertising used to be directed at those with prescriptive authority but recently prescription drug advertisements in print and on television have directed their message at the consumer so they will "suggest" a certain drug to their doctor.

treatment in seizures and panic attacks. **The two main groups of sedative-hypnotics are benzodiazepines and barbiturates.** There are also a number of nonbenzodiazepine-nonbarbiturate sedative-hypnotics.

The **effects of sedative-hypnotics are generally similar to the effects of alcohol** (e.g., lowered inhibitions, physical depression, sedation, muscular relaxation) and like alcohol, sedative-hypnotic drugs can cause memory loss, tolerance, tissue dependence, withdrawal symptoms, and addiction. The obvious basic difference between the two depressants is their potency. On a gram-by-gram basis, sedative-hypnotics are much more potent than alcohol.

Sedatives are calming drugs, e.g., alprazolam (Xanax®), diazepam (Valium®), and meprobamate (Miltown®). They are also called "minor tranquilizers." A number of benzodiazepines act on the neurotransmitters GABA (gamma amino butyric acid), serotonin, and dopamine to help control anxiety and restlessness. Sedatives are also capable of causing muscular relaxation, body heat loss, lowered inhibitions, reduced intensity of physical sensations,

and reduced muscular coordination in speech, movement, and manual dexterity. They are also used to help with alcohol or heroin detoxification and to control seizures.

Hypnotics are sleep inducers, i.e., short-acting barbiturates and benzodi-

azepines such as Halcion® that work on the brainstem. They also depress most body functions, including breathing and muscular coordination. Some sedatives are used as hypnotics and some hypnotics are used as sedatives, so it is sometimes difficult to separate the two functions.

HISTORY

Calming and sleep-inducing drugs have been around for millennia. The ones used in ancient cultures were natural plant-derived substances (especially opium) that were discovered through self-experimentation. In the last 150 years with the increasing sophistication of chemical processes, virtually all of the sedative-hypnotics have been developed in the laboratory.

At the turn of the century, bromides, paraldehyde, and chloral hydrate were commonly used. Though chemically quite different, they all depressed the central nervous system.

◊ **Bromides**, used as sedatives or anticonvulsants, were first introduced in the 1850s and often sold over the counter but they had a long half-life

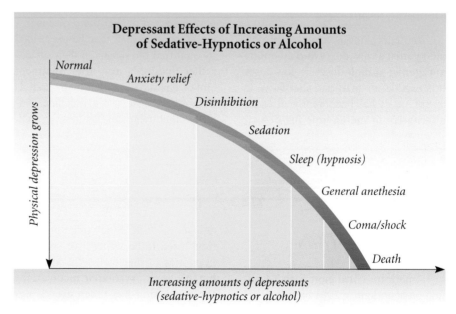

Figure 4-4 •

As this chart shows, the different strengths of sedative-hypnotics can be used simply to calm or to anesthetize for surgery. When users self-medicate with sedative-hypnotics and/or alcohol, they often lose track of where they will end up on the scale.

TABLE 4–3   SEDATIVE-HYPNOTICS

Name	Trade Name	Street Name
BENZODIAZEPINES		
Very Long-Acting		
Flurazepam	Dalmane®	
Halazepam	Paxipam®	
Prazepam	Centrax®	
Quazepam	Doral®	
Intermediate-Acting		
Chlordiazepoxide	Librium® Libritabs®, Limbitrol®	Libs
Clonazepam	Klonopin®	
Clorazepate	Tranxene®	
Diazepam	Valium®	Vals
Short-Acting		
Alprazolam	Xanax®	
Lorazepam	Ativan®	
Midazolam	Versed®	
Oxazepam	Serax®	
Temazepam	Restoril®	
Very Short-Acting		
Estazolam	Pro-Som®	
Triazolam	Halcion®	
Banned in the United States		
Flunitrazepam	Rohypnol®	Ruffies, roofies, roachies
BARBITURATES		
Long-Acting		
Phenobarbital	Luminal®	Phenos
Mephobarbital	Mebaral®	
Intermediate-Acting		
Amobarbital	Amytal®	Blue heaven
Aprobarbital	Alurate®	
Butabarbital	Barbased®, Butisol®	
Talbutal	Lotusate®	
Equal parts secobarbital & amobarbital	Tuinal®	Rainbows, tuies, double trouble
Short-Acting		
Butalbital	Esgic®, Fiorinal®	
Hexobarbital	Sombulex®	
Pentobarbital	Nembutal®	Yellows, yellow
Secobarbital	Seconal®	Reds, red devils, F-40s jackets, nebbies
Very Short-Acting		
Methohexital	Brevital®	
Thiamylal sodium	Surital®	
Thiopental sodium	Pentothal®	
NONBENZODIAZEPINE, NONBARBITURATE SEDATIVE-HYPNOTICS		
Bromides		
Chloral hydrate	Noctec®, Somnos®	Jelly beans, Mickeys, knockout drops
Ethchlorvynol	Placidyl®	Green weenies
GHB (gammahydroxybutyrate)	Xyrem®	Grievous bodily harm, liquid E, fantasy, Georgia home boy
GBL (gamma butyl lactone)	Blue Nitro®, Revivarant®, Insom-X®, Revivarant G®, Gamma G®, GH Revitalizer®, Remforce®	
Glutethimide (obsolete)	Doriden®	Goofballs, goofers
Glutethimide & codeine	Doriden® & codeine	Loads, sets, setups, hits, C&C, fours & doors
Meprobamate	Equinil®, Miltown®, Meprotabs®, Deprol®	Mother's little helper
Methaprylon	Noludar®	Noodlelars
Methaqualone (only illegal forms)	Quaalude® Soper®, Somnafac®, Parest® Optimil®	Ludes, sopes, sopers, Q
Paraldehyde	Paral®	
Zolpidem	Ambien®	

and so prolonged or nonsupervised use could build up toxic doses in the body.

◇ **Chloral hydrate** could be purchased at many drugstores in 1869; it was used both as a sedative and as a hypnotic. It relieved tension and pain and helped treat alcoholics' insomnia. It was often prescribed for women, to treat delirium tremens and to help pregnant women cope (Kandall, 1993). When slipped into a drink, it was the original "Mickey" used to knockout and shanghai sailors. It is still sometimes used because the margin of safety is better for sleep problems than are barbiturates.

◇ **Paraldehyde** (developed in 1882) was used to control the symptoms of alcohol withdrawal. Despite its offensive odor and tendency to become addictive, it is still occasionally used to treat alcohol withdrawal (Hollister, 1983).

◇ **Barbiturates** were first developed at the end of the nineteenth century and slowly grew in popularity; they peaked in the 1930s and 1940s. Phenobarbital, secobarbital, and pentobarbital were among the hundreds of compounds synthesized from barbituric acid. Appreciation of the toxic potential of barbiturates due to a low margin of safety, low degree of selectivity, along with a high dependence and addictive potential, instilled an apprehension of use and encouraged researchers to look for new classes of sedative-hypnotics.

◇ **Meprobamate (Miltown®)** was developed in the late '40s and '50s. Known as "mother's little helper," this long-acting sedative replaced many long-acting barbiturates including phenobarbital. Its popularity peaked from 1955 to 1961 when benzodiazepines took center stage.

◇ **Glutethimide (Doriden®)** was tried as a barbiturate substitute but it seemed to have many of the same disadvantages without enough advantages. It was also weaker than phenobarbital and subject to abuse when it was used in combination with codeine ("loads," "sets," and "setups") in order to potentiate the effects of both drugs. It is no longer manufactured in the United States.

◇ **Benzodiazepines** were discovered in 1957 at Roche Laboratories in a deliberate search for a safer class of sedative-hypnotics. When Librium® (chlordiazepoxide) and Valium® (diazepam) were synthesized and marketed in 1960 and 1963 respectively, they quickly became immensely popular because they were less toxic than barbiturates, meprobamate, and glutethimide although many of the sites of action in the central nervous system were similar to those of barbiturates. Over the years more than 3,000 compounds were developed but only 20 or so were marketed and released (Sternbach, 1983). To this day benzodiazepines dominate the market for sedative-hypnotics. Though they are less toxic than other sedatives, benzodiazepines can be addictive and have dangerous withdrawal symptoms.

USE, MISUSE, ABUSE, & ADDICTION

In the twentieth century, society's attitude towards the use of sedative-hypnotics and psychiatric medications swung like a pendulum. The liberal use of barbiturates in the '30s and '40s, along with the vision of a drug-controlled society as written about in Aldous Huxley's futuristic novel *Brave New World*, led to a search for nonaddictive alternatives. But the widespread use of Miltown® in the '50s, which eventually led to an attitude of "better living through chemistry" in the '60s, seemed to confirm Huxley's fears. Subsequently **benzodiazepines were hailed as miracle drugs and prescribed in huge amounts** (100 million prescriptions per year in the United States by 1975) and again fear of becoming a drug-dependent society came to the fore. As a result a turf war has developed that pits some of those in the medical and treatment communities who want to have the freedom to prescribe benzodiazepines as they see fit against others who feel that overuse of prescription drugs needs to be brought under control. Even within some drug companies, there is a conflict between the research/development departments that want to develop drugs with very targeted effects and the marketing departments that would like to have their drugs approved for as many conditions as possible and used for extended periods of time.

When used properly, sedative-hypnotics can be beneficial therapeutic adjuncts for treatment of a variety of psychological and physical conditions. When misused they can cause undesirable side effects, dependence, abuse, addiction, and even death.

"You don't think that a pill is going to make you go after more and more and more pills like a fix of heroin. And then it becomes a habit. It becomes as hideous as any illicit drug habit. It can become more dangerous actually. I've had a more dangerous time with the taking care of my [pill] habit."
43-year-old recovering benzodiazepine abuser

Sedative-hypnotic (as well as opioid) misuse can occur through several mechanisms:

◇ when **patients overuse the drugs** prescribed by the physician;

◇ when patients **use them in combination with other psychoactive drugs** to potentiate or counteract effects;

◇ when they **borrow the drugs from a friend** to self-medicate;

◇ when they **divert the drugs from legal sources** through forged prescriptions, buying on the black market, or stealing to get high or medicate emotional pain.

Over the years in popular and scientific literature and movies, **sedative-**

TABLE 4–4   MENTIONS OF DRUG PROBLEMS IN U.S. EMERGENCY ROOMS – 2000

(More than one drug is found in many incoming patients.)

Drugs	Number of Drug Mentions
Alcohol in combination with other drugs	204,510
Cocaine	174,881
Heroin	94,804
Marijuana	96,426
Benzodiazepines (Xanax®, Klonopin®, etc.)	91,078
Aspirin, acetaminophen, ibuprofen, NSAIDs, & other OTC pain relievers	83,244
Narcotic analgesics (morphine, (hydrocodone, OxyContin®, etc.)	82,373
Antidepressants (Zoloft®, Trazadone®, etc.)	60,576
Amphetamines & methamphetamines	30,639
Other sedative-hypnotics & anxiolytics	25,675
Antipsychotics	20,097
Barbiturates	7,102
Ketamine & PCP	5,667
GHB	4,969
MDMA	4,511
LSD	4,016
Other hallucinogens	1,849
Inhalants	1,522
All other medications	105,421
Total Drug Abuse Mentions	**1,099,360**

(DAWN, 2002b)

hypnotics have been associated with both accidental and intentional drug overdoses. Many movies use the image of an empty vial of prescription drugs to indicate a suicide attempt or the need for stomach pumps.

In the *Annual Emergency Room Data Survey*, physicians list which drugs cause medical problems severe enough to make people seek medical attention. Table 4-4 shows which drugs are reported most often. Overall there are more than $^3/_4$ million visits to emergency rooms for drug problems such as overdose, dependence, withdrawal syndrome, and drug interactions.

Studies of sedative-hypnotic drug misuse and overdose conducted by the National Institute on Drug Abuse (NIDA) reveal some factors that contribute to abuse or overdose with these drugs.

◇ Since sedatives impair memory, awareness, and judgment, **individuals forget how many sedatives they have ingested** to help them get to sleep or to relieve stress. Rather than waiting long enough for the full dosage of the drug to affect them, they continue to take more of the drug and accidentally reach a toxic state. This effect has been called "drug automatism."

◇ **Ignorance of additive and synergistic effects** resulting from combining these drugs with alcohol or other sedatives is widespread.

◇ **Selective tolerance to some effects of the drug** but not to its toxic effects results in a narrowing window of safety where the amount needed to produce a high comes closer to the lethal dose of the drug.

◇ **Adolescent attitudes of invulnerability** promote risk-taking behavior in respect to the amount of drug ingested when used illicitly.

(NIDA, 2001)

BENZODIAZEPINES

Benzodiazepines are **the most widely used sedative-hypnotics in the United States**. This class of drugs was developed in the 1940s and 1950s as an alternative to barbiturates. Since benzodiazepines have a fairly large margin of safety, many health care professionals initially overlooked their peculiarities, e.g., the length of time they last in body tissues, their ability to induce tissue dependence at low levels of use, and the severity of withdrawal from the drug. For these reasons almost all recommendations for benzodiazepine use today emphasize that **they should be used short term and for specific conditions not as long-term medications**.

MEDICAL USE OF BENZODIAZEPINES

Medically benzodiazepines are used to

◇ provide short-term treatment for the symptoms of **anxiety and panic disorders**;

◇ control anxiety and **apprehension** in surgical patients and diminish traumatic memories of the procedure;

◇ treat **sleep problems**;

◇ control **skeletal muscular spasms**;

◇ elevate the seizure threshold (anticonvulsant) and control **seizures**;

◇ control **acute alcohol withdrawal symptoms**, e.g., severe agitation, tremors, impending acute delirium tremens, and hallucinosis.

"The enclosed space of the MRI machine they were going to slip me into really triggered one of my claustrophobic panic attacks, so we couldn't finish. I was yelling, 'get me outta here,' along

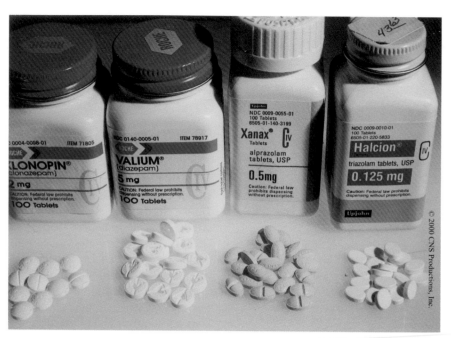

Some of the main benzodiazepines include alprazolam (Xanax®), diazepam (Valium®), clonazepam (Klonopin®), and triazolam (Halcion®).

● ●

with some nasty threats to do them bodily harm. The next time, they gave me some Valium® and though I still felt nervous, it did calm me enough so I could have the scan done. It seemed like a dream."

50-year-old female without any drug problem

NONMEDICAL USE OF BENZODIAZEPINES

Since the desirable **emotional and physical effects of benzodiazepines are very similar to alcohol,** they are sometimes used for the same reasons a person drinks. A double-blind study on nondrug addicts compared the effects of low-dose diazepam injections and alcohol injections. The subjects found the highs from each of the drugs to be extremely similar; however higher-dose diazepam produced more physical impairment (Schuckit, Greenblatt, Gold, & Irwin, 1991).

Benzodiazepines alone can be abused but they are **most often abused in conjunction with other drugs.** Methamphetamine and cocaine abusers often take a benzodiazepine to come down from excess stimulation. Heroin addicts frequently take a benzodi-

azepine when they can't get their drug of choice and alcoholics use them or are given them to prevent convulsions and other life-threatening withdrawal symptoms. For example, depending on the study, 20% to 40% of alcoholics and 25% to 50% of heroin or methadone-maintained addicts abused benzodiazepines (Miller & Gold, 1990). In another study at a treatment center 10% of polydrug clients abused benzodiazepines. In one older study almost 100% of benzodiazepine addicts reported dependence on or addiction to other drugs (Busto, Sellers, Naranjo, et al., 1986). **Benzodiazepine abusers are more likely to be older than 30 years of age, White, well-educated, and female.**

"If I threw down 10 Valium®, I didn't really feel that much. It wasn't like taking Nembutal® or other barbiturates where you get a real rush. I would have to take an awful lot to feel anything. It relieved certain anxieties; it alleviated depression. You tell the doctor, 'I'm depressed.' 'Okay, take some Valium®.'"

48-year-old recovering female benzodiazepine abuser

NEUROCHEMISTRY & GABA

Benzodiazepines have been shown to exert their sedative effects in the brain by potentiating (increasing the effects of) a naturally occurring neurotransmitter, called "GABA" (gamma amino butyric acid), in the cerebellum, cerebral cortex, and limbic system (Potokar & Nutt, 1994). **GABA is recognized as the most important inhibitory neurotransmitter,** so when a drug, like alprazolam (Xanax®), greatly increases the actions of GABA, it subsequently decreases anxiety-producing thoughts and over-stimulating neural messages (Stahl, 2000). Other sedating neurotransmitters, such as serotonin and dopamine, are also increased.

Most benzodiazepines are prodrugs. This means that the liver converts a certain percentage of a drug, like diazepam (Valium®), to a psychoactive metabolite (e.g., nordiazepam). **The metabolites can be as active or even more active than the original drug itself.** Nordiazepam can be further converted to temazepam and oxazepam (Jenkins & Cone, 1998). (These last two active metabolites are also manufactured separately by pharmaceutical companies as Restoril® and Serax®.) The metabolites, along with the original drug, are very fat-soluble (lipophilic) and therefore stay in the body for a long time.

Specific benzodiazepines have been developed to treat specific conditions. For example,

◇ short-term alprazolam (Xanax®) is used for immediate relief of the symptoms of generalized anxiety disorder, panic disorder, and depression resulting from anxiety (many patients are prescribed alprazolam just for depression);

◇ triazolam (Halcion®) is used for short-term (7–10 days) treatment of insomnia;

◇ diazepam (Valium®) is used to gain relief from skeletal muscle spasms caused by inflammation of the muscles and joints or to control seizures such as those that occur during severe alcohol or barbiturate withdrawal;

◇ intravenous Valium® is used as a sedative just before surgery.

TOLERANCE, TISSUE DEPENDENCE, & WITHDRAWAL

Tolerance

Tolerance to benzodiazepines develops as **the liver becomes more efficient in processing the drug.** However, age-dependent reverse tolerance also occurs with these drugs meaning that **a younger person can tolerate higher doses of benzodiazepines than someone older.** The effect of a dose on a 50-year-old first-time user can be 2 or 4 times stronger than the same dose on a 20-year-old.

"I was unhappy and I wanted the easy way out. I'm unhappy. I will go back to the same psychiatrist and get a prescription of Xanax®. It starts out at 25 milligrams and I ended up doing between 800 to 1,000 milligrams a day."
43-year-old recovering benzodiazepine abuser

Tissue Dependence

Physical addiction to a benzodiazepine can develop if the patient takes 10–20 times the normal dose daily for a couple of months or longer or takes a normal dose for a year or more. Since many benzodiazepines are slowly deactivated by the body over a period of several days, **even low-dose use can lead to tissue dependence and addiction** when these drugs are taken daily over a number of years. In addition the pleasant mental effects and hypnotizing aspects of the drugs (reinforcement) can result in a mental or psychological dependence.

Withdrawal

After high-dose continuous use for about 1–3 months or lower-dose use for at least 1–2 years, **withdrawal symptoms can be severe.** It can take a dependent benzodiazepine user **several months to taper from the drug** and allow the body to return to normal. If tapering isn't carefully monitored,

withdrawal seizures can occur, sometimes with fatal outcomes.

"Benzo detox in the morning is very frightening because your mind is just telling your body that 'we are not connected.' It took maybe 10 days before the manic depressive state of the detox finally started to show some light at the end of the tunnel."
34-year-old recovering benzodiazepine abuser

Withdrawal symptoms can include

◇ recurrence of the original symptoms that were being treated with the benzodiazepine;

◇ magnification of the symptoms that were being treated;

◇ pseudowithdrawal in which the user exaggerates the recurrence of symptoms;

◇ true withdrawal in a patient who has become physically dependent, often caused by low GABA and excess epinephrine and norepinephrine.

The drug is long lasting, so with true withdrawal the onset of symptoms is delayed—about 1 day for short-acting and up to 5 days for long-acting benzodiazepines. **The symptoms can last 7–20 days for short-acting and up to 28 days for long-acting benzodiazepines** (Eickelberg & Mayo-Smith, 1998).

Since many of the symptoms of true withdrawal are similar to the symptoms of an anxiety or depressive disorder, it can be **hard to judge the level of dependence.** First a craving for the drug occurs to avoid the withdrawal symptoms, followed by tremors, muscle twitches, nausea and vomiting, anxiety, restlessness, yawning, tachycardia, cramping, hypertension, inability to focus, sleep disturbances, and dizziness. Some people even experience a temporary loss of vision, hearing, or smell and other sensory impairments while in withdrawal; occasionally they have hallucinations (Miller & Gold, 1990; Eickelberg & Mayo-Smith, 1998). The symptoms continue and peak in the first through third weeks. These symptoms occasionally include multiple seizures and convulsions that can be fatal.

"I stopped taking them and on the third day, I remember I was sweating. I changed the sheets on the bed. I took a shower. I was fairly relaxed and I went into a convulsion. I don't remember what happened. All I can remember is waking up and all my front teeth were knocked out. I ended up going through about 80 convulsions."
Recovering Valium® abuser

The persistence of benzodiazepines (Fig. 4-5) in the body from low- or

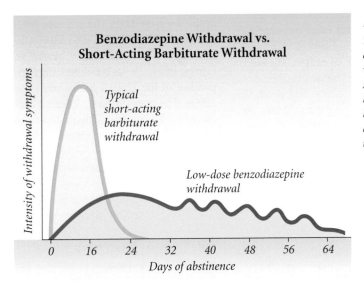

Benzodiazepine Withdrawal vs. Short-Acting Barbiturate Withdrawal

Intensity of withdrawal symptoms

Typical short-acting barbiturate withdrawal

Low-dose benzodiazepine withdrawal

0   16   24   32   40   48   56   64

Days of abstinence

Figure 4-5 •
The delay in the occurrence of withdrawal symptoms can be dangerous to benzodiazepine abusers who stop using abruptly.

regular-dose use taken over a long period of time results not only in prolonged withdrawal symptoms but in **symptoms that erratically come and go in cycles separated by 2–10 days**. These symptoms are sometimes bizarre, sometimes life threatening, and all are complicated by the cyclical nature of benzodiazepine withdrawal. Short-acting barbiturates, on the other hand, follow a fairly predictable course where the symptoms come and then go and do not return. Called "**protracted withdrawal**," the symptoms of benzodiazepine withdrawal may persist for several months after the drug has been terminated.

BENZODIAZEPINE OVERDOSE

The reason actual overdoses and suicides have decreased with the increased use of benzodiazepines and decreased use of barbiturates is that the benzodiazepines have a much greater therapeutic index (the lethal dose of a drug divided by its therapeutic effective dose). The therapeutic index of barbiturates is 10 to 1 while the therapeutic index of benzodiazepines is 700 to 1. With barbiturates it means that 10 times a therapeutic dose in an individual who has not developed tolerance can be fatal. For benzodiazepines 700 times the therapeutic dose can be fatal. **This margin of safety is tremendously diminished when benzodiazepines are taken in combination with alcohol**, other benzodiazepines, phenothiazines, MAO inhibitors, barbiturates, opioids, and other antidepressants (PDR, 2002).

Symptoms of overdose include drowsiness, loss of consciousness, depressed breathing, coma, and death if left untreated; however it might take 50 or 100 pills to cause a serious overdose. Yet street versions of the drug, often misrepresented and sold as Quaaludes®, are so strong that only 5 or 10 pills can cause severe reactions.

MEMORY IMPAIRMENT & ROHYPNOL®

Benzodiazepines impair the ability to learn new information. They disrupt the transfer of information from short- to long-term memory (Juergens & Cowley, 1998; American Psychiatric Association, 1990). The amnestic effect of benzodiazepines (medically known as both **"retrograde" and "anterograde amnesia"**), also commonly called a drug "black out" or "brown out," helps patients forget traumatic surgical and other medical procedures. This effect has unfortunately been **used by a few sexual predators** to cause a victim to forget they were sexually assaulted.

"They took advantage when I passed out at a party and I was sleeping on a couch and I woke up and they were doing stuff to me that they shouldn't have. And I remember running into the bathroom and throwing up and then sleeping on the floor that night. I'm careful now about my surroundings. If it's a safe place where I know I can have a few beers and have fun with my friends, I'll do it but I'm a little bit wary of where I drink or whatever just because of that experience."
20-year-old woman

The drug most associated with date rape is the benzodiazepine Rohypnol® (flunitrazepam). Like other benzodiazepines it also causes relaxation and sedation. Rohypnol® (or another very short-acting benzodiazepine) is slipped into an alcoholic beverage and when drunk **incapacitates the person, lowers inhibitions, and disrupts the memory**. This illicit use began in Europe in the 1970s but didn't start appearing in the United States until the 1990s. The manufacturer, Roche Pharmaceuticals, recently added a blue dye to the tablet to make it more detectable when put into a drink.

Rohypnol® is 10 times more potent by weight than Valium® and is short acting (2–3 hours). It has a long half-life (15–35 hours), so frequent use will cause a build-up of the drug in the body's tissues. When taken with alcohol, the safety margin is greatly reduced. It used to be possible to fill a Rohypnol® prescription in Mexico (25–30¢ per pill) and then bring it into the United States for street sale ($1–5 per pill). **But in 1996 the FDA banned all imports of the drug** even for personal use. Special laws adding 20 more years to the sentence of anyone convicted of using Rohypnol®, GHB, or any drug to sexually assault someone or commit violence were enacted in 1996 (*see GHB in this chapter*).

BARBITURATES

Though barbituric acid was first synthesized in 1863, it remained a medical curiosity until 1903 when it was synthesized to **barbital (Veronal®)**. The chemical modification made it possible for the drug to enter the nervous system and induce sedation. It was originally believed to be free of the addictive propensities of opiates and opioids. Phenobarbital came next in 1913 and since then about 50 of the **2,000 other barbiturates** that have been created have been marketed. By the time there had been extensive clinical experience with these drugs, many dangers such as overdose, severe withdrawal symptoms, dependence, and addiction had become apparent (Lukas, 1995). Since the peak of their use in the '40s and '50s and their abuse in the '50s, '60s, and '70s, their **licit and illicit use has declined dramatically**.

EFFECTS

◊ The **long-acting barbiturates**, such as phenobarbital, last 12–24 hours and are used mostly as daytime sedatives or to control epileptic seizures.

◊ The **intermediate-acting** barbiturates, such as butabarbital, are used as **longer-acting sedatives** and last 6–12 hours.

◊ The **short-acting** compounds, including butalbital and in the past, Seconal® ("reds") and Nembutal® ("yellows"), last 3–6 hours and are used to **induce sleep**. They can cause pleasant feelings along with the sedation (at least initially), so they are more likely to be abused.

◊ The **very short-acting** barbiturates, such as Pentothal®, are used mostly for **anesthesia** and can cause immediate unconsciousness. The high potency of these barbiturates makes them extremely dangerous if abused.

As with benzodiazepines, barbiturates affect GABA, therefore acting as a brake on inhibitions, anxiety, and restlessness. Because they can **induce a feeling of disinhibitory euphoria**, barbiturates seem to have an initial stimulatory effect but the drugs eventually become sedating. To an even greater extent than with benzodiazepines, the effects of barbiturates are very similar to the effects of alcohol. Excessive or long-term use can lead to changes in personality and emotional stability including mood swings, depression, irritability, and boisterous behavior (Lukas, 1995).

The effects of barbiturates often depend on the mood of the user and the setting where taken. An agitated barbiturate user might become combative whereas a tired barbiturate user in a quiet setting might go to sleep.

TOLERANCE, TISSUE DEPENDENCE, & WITHDRAWAL

Tolerance to barbiturates develops in a variety of ways. The most dramatic tolerance, dispositional tolerance (metabolic tolerance), results from the physiologic **conversion of liver cells to more efficient cells that metabolize or destroy barbiturates more quickly.** The other process, pharmacodynamic tolerance, **causes affected nerve cells and tissues to become less sensitive.**

Tissue dependence to barbiturates occurs when 8–10 times the normal dose is taken daily for 30 days or more.

Within 6–8 hours after stopping use of short-acting barbiturates, users will begin to experience **withdrawal symptoms such as anxiety, agitation, loss of appetite, nausea, vomiting, increased heart rate, excessive sweat-** ing, abdominal cramps, and tremulousness. The symptoms tend to peak on the second or third day. The more intense the use, the more severe the symptoms. Withdrawal symptoms resulting from heavy tissue dependence are **very dangerous and can result in convulsions within 12 hours to 1 week from the last dose**.

OTHER SEDATIVE-HYPNOTICS

GHB (gamma hydroxybutyrate)

GHB is a rapidly acting strong central nervous system depressant. The drug was initially available in health food stores or by mail order and described as a nutrient rather than a sedative. It is an amino acid that is naturally occurring in all mammalian brains and is structurally related to GABA and glutamic acid. Its own receptor site is yet to be discovered. GHB was used as a **sleep inducer** in the 1960s and 1970s. By the '90s this slightly salty-tasting white powder, which is taken orally, had also become popular among bodybuilders because it changed the ratio of muscle to fat and was **thought to increase the body's levels of human growth hormone (HGH). It also induces effects similar to alcohol (sedation, disinhibition), ecstasy (empathy, sensory enhancement) or even heroin intoxication (euphoria)**—and so in recent years it became popular, along with other club drugs like LSD, ecstasy, ketamine, and Rohypnol®. Ecstasy and alcohol are the two drugs that are most often taken with GHB. Both enhance the euphoric feelings experienced from GHB while their own effects are enhanced as well.

GHB has been called "liquid ecstasy," "scoop," "Georgia home boy," "easy lay," or "grievous bodily harm" (NIDA, 1999). Because of the wide availability of GHB analogs and precursors, along with the large number of manufacturing kits and recipes available on the Internet, adulteration or misrepre- sentation does not seem to be a problem with knowledgeable buyers. However when bought on the street, dosage and purity are major problems. By the '90s the FDA decided there were enough health risks to take it off the market. Congress added GHB to the Controlled Substances Act in the year 2000. Street chemists have since rushed to fill the void.

"I remember like for the first hour I just felt really woozy and then all of a sudden I like—it started to build and about an hour later like I couldn't move. Like I felt like my head was gonna detach from my body and I just couldn't move my arms and I just stayed that way for about 4 hours I think it was, maybe longer."
19-year-old club drug user

Despite its abuse GHB was researched and found to be safe and effective for the treatment of narcolepsy (involuntary sleep episode) and cataplexy (transient loss of muscle strength) leading to it being approved as the prescription drug Xyrem® in 2002.

GHB is usually dissolved in water or alcohol by the capful or teaspoonful or as a premixed solution. It is most often dissolved into commercial mineral waters so it can be brought into rave events or music festivals without being detected. A dose costs $5 to $10 and **the effects last 3–6 hours**.

◊ With 1 gram there is a feeling of relaxation.

◊ With 2 grams the relaxation increases while heart rate and respiration fall. Balance, coordination, and circulation are disrupted (2.5 grams or a level teaspoon is the preferred amount).

◊ With 2–4 grams coordination and speech become impaired.

◊ Despite a very steep dose-response curve, the rapid development of tolerance has enabled some individuals to take as much as 30 grams in 1 day. High doses result in a longer duration of action.

Depending on the susceptibility of the user, side effects include nausea, vomiting (which are signs of an impending overdose), depression, delusions, hallucinations, seizures, amnesia, respiratory depression, and coma with a greatly reduced heart rate (ONDCP, 2002; Nicholson & Balster, 2001). GHB is thought to lower dopamine levels in the brain by inhibiting its release. This can induce a deep sleep in a GHB user who will then awaken very aroused and active. This may be due to the drug's capacity to cause an accumulation and then a sudden release of the dopamine.

In 2002 as many emergency room visits were due to GHB as to ecstasy, a significant increase since 1994 (DAWN, 2002b). Most of the problems seem to occur with naïve users who become anxious that the first dose isn't working and keep using until they feel something but by then, they've taken too much.

Because GHB causes a mild euphoria and lowers inhibitions, **it has been used by sexual predators to lower the defenses of women.** These effects, along with its ability to induce coma and amnesia, added its name to the list of date-rape drugs (El Sohly & Salamone, 1999). GHB's use spurred the passage of the Drug-Induced Rape Prevention and Punishment Act of 1996 that increased federal penalties for use of any controlled substance to aid in sexual assault or violence.

Case histories of GHB abuse indicate that because of the significant degree of tolerance that occurs with its use, it can be addicting. High daily prolonged use results in severe and difficult to treat sedative-like drug withdrawal symptoms upon cessation that may even result in dangerous withdrawal seizures (Sivilotti et al., 2001).

GBL (gamma butyrolactone or 2[3H]-furanone dihydro) & BD (1,3 butanediol)

Increased legal scrutiny of GHB has resulted in the abuse of GBL and BD. **GBL and BD are prodrugs (they are metabolized to GHB in the body).** They are also ingredients in liquid paint strippers and available through chemical suppliers in the United States and on the Internet. GBL and BD were quickly formulated into mint-flavored elixirs for the rave club scene. These elixirs are sold under the trade names of Blue Nitro®, Revivarant®, Gamma G®, Remforce®, and Insom-X®. Some abusers have even drunk diluted paint stripper or "huffed" the hardware store products containing GBL. Many states are now urging the FDA to take regulatory action against GBL.

METHAQUALONE (Quaalude®, Mandrax®)

Methaqualone was developed in India in 1955 as a safe **barbiturate substitute** and originally marketed in Japan and Europe. In 1965 it was the most commonly prescribed sedative-hypnotic in England. The reasons for the popularity of methaqualone were its overall sedative effect and the prolonged period of mild euphoria caused by suppression of inhibitions. **This disinhibitory effect is similar to that caused by alcohol and can last 60–90 minutes while the sedating effects last 6–10 hours.** Larger doses can bring about depression, irrational behavior, poor reflexes, slurred speech, reduced respiration and heart rate. Tolerance to methaqualone develops quickly.

Although widely used at one time as a sleep aid, the heavy nonmedical abuse of Quaalude® led to the withdrawal of this product from the legitimate U.S. market. **In 1984 it was made a Schedule I drug.** This change led to a tremendous increase in the illicit production of Quaalude® (known as bootleg "ludes" that look identical to the original prescription drug). The active chemical in Quaalude®, methaqualone, is manufactured by street chemists or smuggled in from Europe, South Africa, or Colombia. In Europe and other countries, Mandrax® (methaqualone and an antihistamine) had great popularity in the '70s and '80s. The antihistamine exaggerated the effect of the methaqualone.

Today South Africa still has many Mandrax® abusers. There is no guarantee that the street versions of Quaalude® contain actual methaqualone and even when they do, the dosage may vary dramatically making an overdose more likely.

ZOLPIDEM (Ambien®)

This **short-acting hypnotic** with a 2.5 hour half-life has a lower risk of addiction than most benzodiazepines, so it is prescribed for some sleep disorders. Excess use can cause nausea, diarrhea, headaches, dizziness, and drowsiness the following day. As with benzodiazepines, **zolpidem can cause memory, performance, and learning impairment.** By itself zolpidem rarely causes overdose deaths except in combination with other depressants. Withdrawal effects peak within 24–36 hours and include tremors, cramps, insomnia, anxiety, confusion, rigidity of limbs, and possible hallucinations and seizures.

ETHCHLOVYNOL (Placidyl®)

Called "green weenies" on the street, Placidyl® is **one of the older sedative-hypnotics.** It is still a controlled prescription drug and is subject to limited abuse. Placidyl® is about the equivalent of Doriden® in potency with similar toxic and addictive effects but is shorter acting.

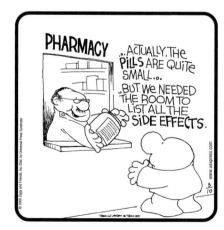

OTHER PROBLEMS WITH DEPRESSANTS

DRUG INTERACTIONS

SYNERGISM

If more than one depressant drug is used, **the polydrug combination can cause a much greater reaction than simply the sum of the effects**. One of the reasons for this synergistic effect lies in the chemistry of the liver.

For example, if alcohol and Valium® (diazepam) are taken together, **the liver becomes busy metabolizing the alcohol**, so the sedative-hypnotic passes through the body at full strength. Alcohol also dissolves the Valium® more readily than stomach fluid, allowing more Valium® to be absorbed rapidly into the body. Valium® exerts its depressant effects on parts of the brain different from those affected by alcohol. Thus when combined, alcohol and Valium® cause more problems than if they were taken at different times. **Exaggerated respiratory depression is the biggest danger** with the use of alcohol and another depressant. This combination also causes more blackouts (a period of amnesia or loss of memory while intoxicated).

"I took my little medication with me one night, drinking in the bar. I played some pool and that's all I remember. This was on a Sunday. When I woke up, it was Wednesday."
Recovering polydrug abuser

Synergistic effects cause **4,000 deaths a year**. In addition almost **50,000 people are treated in emergency rooms** because of adverse reactions to multiple drug use.

CROSS-TOLERANCE & CROSS-DEPENDENCE

Cross-tolerance is the development of tolerance to other drugs by the continued exposure and development of tolerance to the initial drug. For example, a barbiturate addict who develops a tolerance to a high dose of Seconal® is also tolerant to and can withstand high doses of Nembutal®, phenobarbital, anesthetics, opiates, alcohol, Valium®, and even blood-thinning medication. One explanation of cross-tolerance is that many drugs are metabolized or broken down by the same body enzymes. As one continues to take barbiturates, the liver creates more enzymes to rid the body of these toxins. The unusually high levels of these enzymes result in tolerance to all barbiturates as well as to other drugs also metabolized by those same enzymes.

Cross-dependence occurs when an individual becomes addicted or tissue dependent on one drug resulting in biochemical and cellular changes that support an addiction to other drugs. A heroin addict, for example, has altered body chemistry such that he or she is also likely to be addicted to another opiate/opioid, e.g., hydrocodone, oxycodone, meperidine, morphine, codeine, methadone, or propoxyphene (Darvon®). As in this example, cross-dependence most often occurs with different drugs in the same chemical family. A diazepam (Valium®) addict is also tissue dependent on alprazolam, lorazepam, and other benzodiazepines. A heavy butalbital user is also tissue dependent on phenobarbital. Cross-dependence has also been documented to some extent with opiates/opioids and alcohol, cocaine and alcohol, and benzodiazepines and alcohol.

MISUSE & DIVERSION

"I would go over and visit people and the first thing, within 5 minutes, I would go to the bathroom, go over into the medicine cabinet and flush the toilet so no one in the other room would hear me. I'd trash the medicine cabinet and if I didn't find anything there, I'd go through the drawers."
43-year-old recovering prescription drug abuser

As a class, sedative-hypnotic drugs and prescription opioids are frequently misused and **diverted to abuse from legitimate prescribing practices**. Unfortunately, unscrupulous, addicted, or out-of-date medical professionals also participate in unethical, criminal, or inappropriate prescribing practices.

One pattern of illicit use with sedatives and opioids results when a patient is treated for multiple medical complaints by many **different physicians and each prescribes a different sedative or opioid** that is then dispensed by different pharmacies. For example, Dalmane® will be prescribed for sleep, Serax® for anxiety, Xanax® for depression, Valium® for muscle spasms, and Librax® for stomach problems. Each prescription, in and of itself, may be at a nonaddictive level but all these prescriptions together result in a large enough dose of benzodiazepines to create tissue dependence.

"This doctor and I parted paths when I found another doctor who was in the business of prescribing whatever medication you wanted. You know you pay him and he will take care of your pharmaceutical needs, so to speak."
38-year-old recovering sedative-hypnotic abuser

Because of their widespread use for a variety of medical indications, sedative-hypnotics and opioids are also subject to **forged prescriptions or prescription manipulations** (photocopying or changing dosage or number of refills) that provide an abuser with enough drugs for diversion to illicit street sales or to feed an addiction. To combat this problem, many states have mandated triplicate prescriptions for benzodiazepines and added other stringent mechanisms to prevent diversion, much as they have done for opioids. Many physicians and psychiatrists see triplicate prescriptions for benzodiazepines as an intrusion into their practice of medicine.

Another form of diversion is **smuggling drugs and drug precursors that**

are legal outside the United States. Rohypnol®, which is banned in the United States, is smuggled in from Europe or Mexico. Ephedrine is smuggled through Canada or Mexico to make methamphetamine.

Misuse and diversion aren't the only ways that overuse of drugs leading to bad reactions and physical problems can occur. A study led by Dr. Bruce Pomeranz at the University of Toronto estimated that **each year between 76,000 and 137,000 Americans die and an additional 1.6–2.6 million are injured due to bad reactions from legally prescribed drugs and over-the-counter medications**. The figures do not include drug abuse or prescribing errors. While some disagree with the magnitude of the numbers, they do agree that the problem is very real and unfortunately common.

Some of the actions that could help control prescription drug abuse as described by Drs. Peter Lurie and Philip R. Lee at the University of California Medical Center in San Francisco are

◇ better education of physicians regarding pharmacotherapy and the effects of drugs;

◇ better education and research regarding pain control and the use of opioids;

◇ more accurate information regarding drugs rather than just inserts or overdone PDR information;

◇ limited interaction between drug company detailers (salesman) and medical personnel;

◇ increased role for the pharmacist in identifying drug interactions and inappropriate prescribing;

◇ more careful prescribing in hospitals and nursing homes;

◇ greater patient participation in deciding which drug to use;

◇ more attention to patient feedback to judge the effectiveness of drugs;

◇ more testing in geriatric populations to make sure prescribed drugs are not debilitating;

◇ limited prescribing of certain powerful drugs to specialists;

◇ limited prescribing of psychoactive drugs (e.g., duplicate and triplicate prescriptions for scheduled drugs);

◇ less drug advertising in medical journals;

◇ more peer scrutiny of prescribing practices of fellow physicians (Lurie & Lee, 1991).

PRESCRIPTION DRUGS & THE PHARMACEUTICAL INDUSTRY

In 2002 Americans spent about $154.5 billion or 9% of their total medical expenditures of $1.5 trillion on prescription medications. This was almost half of the world's total expenditures for prescription drugs (IMS Health, 2002). It was also twice as much as was spent just 4 years before in the United States. Americans also spent more than $20 billion on over-the-counter drugs such as aspirin, laxatives, and vitamins. At the current rates of growth, both figures will double over the next 10–15 years. Recently there has been a significant increase in the use of prescription medications for children. ADHD drugs and antidepressants, along with more and more therapeutic medications, have caused an increase of 28% in prescriptions issued for those under 19 years old (Agovino, 2002).

In contrast to the $154.5 billion spent on prescription drugs, about

◇ $60–65 billion were spent on illegal drugs,

◇ $70–80 billion on tobacco,

◇ $140–150 billion on alcohol.

(ONDCP, 2000b)

Legal psychoactive drugs, including psychiatric medications, account for approximately 10% to 12% of prescriptions written in the United States. The other prescriptions include cardiovascular medications, antibiotics, menopause medications, hormones, birth-control pills, ulcer medications, diabetes-control medications, antihistamines, thyroid drugs, and bronchodilators.

One of the recent trends has been the **vast increase in television advertisements for prescription drugs**, something that was unheard of just a few years ago. According to the National Institute for Health Care Management (NIHCM) Research and Educational Foundation, sales of the 50 most heavily advertised drugs in 2000 were responsible for almost one-half (47.8%) of the $20.8 billion increase in retail spending on prescription drugs over the past year. The sales increase was due primarily to an increase in the number of prescriptions not to an increase in drug prices. In 2000 overall promotional expenditures rose to $15.7 billion, up from $13.9 billion in 1999 and $9.2 billion in 1996, while spending on direct-to-consumer ads increased to $2.5 billion in 2000, up from $1.85 billion in 1999 (Drug Benefit Trends, 2002).

CHAPTER SUMMARY

GENERAL CLASSIFICATION

1. Downers are central nervous system depressants.

Major Depressants

2. The three major downers are opiates/opioids, sedative-hypnotics, and alcohol.

Minor Depressants

3. The four minor downers are skeletal muscle relaxants, antihistamines, over-the-counter depressants, and lookalike depressants.

OPIATES/OPIOIDS

Classification

4. Opiates (from the opium poppy and semisynthetic versions) and opioids (synthetic versions of opiates) were developed for the treatment of acute pain, to control diarrhea, and to suppress coughs.

5. Opiates include opium, morphine, codeine, heroin, hydrocodone, hydromorphone (Dilaudid®), and oxycodone (OxyContin®). Opioids include methadone, propoxyphene (Darvon®), meperidine (Demerol®), and fentanyl.

History of Use (*see Chapter 1*)

6. The change in routes of administration (from ingesting, to smoking, to injecting, to snorting), along with refinement and synthesis of stronger opioids (from opium, to morphine, to heroin, to fentanyl), has increased the effectiveness as well as the addiction liability of opioids.

7. Opium and morphine were very popular in patent medicines, in prescription medicines, and as recreational drugs. Women addicts outnumbered male addicts in the late 1800s and early 1900s.

8. Drug laws and regulations in the twentieth century limited the supplies but created a criminal subculture that grew, processed, and distributed heroin and other drugs worldwide.

9. The major opium-growing areas are the Golden Crescent (Afghanistan and Pakistan) and the Golden Triangle (Myanmar [Burma], Thailand, and Laos). Most heroin sold in the United States comes from Mexico (black tar heroin and brown heroin) and most recently from Colombia (black tar heroin and white heroin).

Effects of Opioids

10. Pain is normally a warning signal of physical or mental damage. The body's own natural painkillers, endorphins and enkephalins, are mimicked by opioids. These analgesic drugs block the transmission of pain messages to the brain by substance "P."

11. Opioids can also cause pleasure and euphoria by stimulating the dopaminergic reward/reinforcement center.

12. The satiation or on/off switch can be disrupted by opioids.

13. The alleviation of pain activates the same area of the brain that causes euphoria.

14. These drugs also control diarrhea and suppress the cough mechanism.

Side Effects of Opioids

15. Opioids mask pain signals, depress heart rate, slow respiration rate, depress muscular coordination, increase nausea, induce pinpoint pupils, cause itching, delay a woman's period, and create mental confusion.

16. A physical tolerance to opioids develops rapidly, increasing the rate at which the body tissues become physically dependent on the drug.

17. Acute withdrawal from opioids is like an extreme case of the flu, e.g., stomach cramps, diarrhea, and twitching, but is rarely life threatening.

18. Protracted withdrawal can last for months, even years, causing relapses.

Additional Problems with Heroin & Other Opioids

19. Opioids cross the placental barrier and affect fetuses. Babies can be born addicted and can die from opioid withdrawal.

20. Overdose kills 3,000–4,000 heroin users each year mostly through extreme respiratory depression. It can be counteracted by the opioid antagonist, naloxone (Narcan®).

21. Contaminated needles transmit hepatitis C and HIV. Injecting heroin also causes abscesses (skin infections), endocarditis, cotton fever, and flesh-eating disease.

22. Adulteration of drugs, the high cost of an addiction (up to $200 a day), increased crime, and the dangers of polydrug use (e.g., speedballs) add to the complications.

23. The progression from experimentation to physical dependence can occur in a month or in a year or more depending on the user's susceptibility. Pain relief can create the desire to continue use.

24. Addiction depends on factors such as genetics and early environment.

25. Most returning Vietnam veterans who had developed physical dependence on heroin while in Vietnam did not continue use showing that addiction results from many factors.

Morphine & Other Opioids

26. Morphine, the standard drug used for severe pain relief, can be taken by mouth, by injection, or by suppository. The therapeutic use of opioids for pain is subject to much controversy. Some doctors underprescribe due to fear of patient addiction and other reasons.

27. Codeine, which is refined directly from opium, used to be the most widely used and abused prescription opioid for moderate pain and cough control.

28. Hydrocodone (Vicodin®), a synthetic version of codeine, has become the most widely used and abused prescription opioid.

29. Methadone is a long-lasting opioid that heroin addicts use (methadone maintenance) to avoid withdrawal and the addicting highs caused by heroin use.

30. A number of synthetic and semisynthetic opioids, such as hydromorphone (Dilaudid®), oxycodone (Percodan®, OxyContin®), meperidine (Demerol®), propoxyphene (Darvon®), and fentanyl, have made their way to the illicit market. Recently OxyContin®, a time-release version of oxycodone, has been abused by crushing the pills and injecting or snorting the drug.

31. Highly potent synthetic heroin designer drugs (fentanyl and Demerol® derivatives) have appeared on the street, thus increasing the danger of overdose and other toxic problems.

32. Other drugs used to treat opioid addiction are LAAM® (a long-acting opioid), naloxone and naltrexone (opioid antagonists), buprenorphine (Subotex® and Suboxone®), propoxyphene (Darvon®), and clonidine.

SEDATIVE-HYPNOTICS

Classification

33. Sixty million prescriptions were written for sedative-hypnotics although psychiatric medications, e.g., antidepressants, have taken over a large share of this prescription drug market.

34. The effects of sedative-hypnotics are similar to the effects of alcohol.

35. Sedatives (minor tranquilizers) are calming drugs used mostly to treat anxiety. Hypnotics are mainly used to induce sleep.

History

36. Early civilizations used opioids as calming drugs but over the last 150 years sedative-hypnotics have included bromides, chloral hydrate, paraldehyde, barbiturates, Miltown®, and benzodiazepines.

Use, Misuse, Abuse, & Addiction

37. Societal acceptance of sedative-hypnotics has varied from decade to decade from avid acceptance to fear of overuse. They are usually prescribed to control anxiety, induce sleep, relax muscles, and act as mild tranquilizers but many physicians are afraid of physical dependence and addiction.

38. Overdosing and severe withdrawal symptoms have been associated with both barbiturate and benzodiazepine abuse.

39. Overdose is commonly accepted as the main danger of sedative-hypnotics, particularly when used with other depressants such as alcohol.

Benzodiazepines

40. Benzodiazepines, the most widely used sedative-hypnotics, include alprazolam (Xanax®), diazepam (Valium®), clonazepam (Klonopin®), temazepam (Restoril®), and lorazepam (Ativan®).

41. Benzodiazepines are usually used medically to manage anxiety, treat sleep problems, control muscular spasms and seizures, and subdue the symptoms of alcohol withdrawal. They are used nonmedically to relieve agitation, induce a mild euphoria, and lower inhibitions.

42. Benzodiazepines work on the inhibitory transmitter GABA as well as serotonin and dopamine.

43. Benzodiazepines can stay in the body for days, even weeks. When tolerance and tissue dependence have developed, withdrawal symptoms can occur several days after ceasing use.

44. Although it is a most often abused as a recreational drug, Rohypnol® is also used as a date-rape drug.

Barbiturates

45. More than 2,000 barbiturates have been developed over the last 100 years but only 50 or so have been marketed.

46. Barbiturates include butalbital, Nembutal® ("yellows"), Tuinal® ("rainbows"), and phenobarbital.

47. These drugs are mostly used to control seizures, induce sleep, and lessen anxiety but benzodiazepines and other psychiatric drugs have replaced their use over the past 40 years.

Other Sedative-Hypnotics

48. GHB, a strong depressant, has become popular in the party scene.

Effects include sedation and euphoria. GBL is also used in the same way as GHB. These drugs, like Rohypnol®, have been used by sexual predators.

49. Other nonbarbiturate sedative-hypnotics include street methaqualone (Quaalude®), meprobamate (Equanil®), and ethchlorvynol (Placidyl®).

OTHER PROBLEMS WITH DEPRESSANTS

Drug Interactions

50. Alcohol and sedative-hypnotics used together can be especially life threatening. They cause a synergistic (exaggerated) effect that can suppress respiration and heart functions.

51. Cross-tolerance and cross-dependence occur within the sedative-hypnotic class of drugs, within the opioid class of drugs, and to a lesser extent among sedative-hypnotics, opioids, and alcohol.

Misuse & Diversion

52. Hundreds of millions of doses and prescriptions of sedative-hypnotics and prescription opioids are diverted to illicit channels each year through smuggling, conning of physicians, and forgery.

Prescription Drugs & the Pharmaceutical Industry

53. Over $154.5 billion are spent by Americans on prescription drugs. Of the 3.1 billion prescriptions written each year, 250 million were for psychoactive drugs, particularly opioids, sedative-hypnotics, skeletal muscle relaxants, and psychiatric drugs (antidepressants and antipsychotics).

REFERENCES

Agovino, T. (2002, August 11). Kids use more prescription drugs. *The Associated Press.*

Aldrich, M. R. (1994). Historical notes on women addicts. *Journal of Psychoactive Drugs, 26*(1), 61–64.

American Association for the Treatment of Opioid Dependence (2002). AMTA. 217 Broadway, New York, NY, 10007.

American Psychiatric Association. (1990). *Task Force Report on Benzodiazepines.* Washington, DC: American Psychiatric Association Press.

Armstrong, D., & Armstrong, E.M. (1991). *The Great American Medicine Show.* New York: Prentice Hall.

Bailey, D. N., & Briggs, J. R. (2002). Carisoprodol: An unrecognized drug of abuse. *American Journal of Clinical Pathology, 117*(3), 396–400.

Bell, J., Mattick, R., Hay, A., Chan, J., & Hall, W. (1997). Methadone maintenance and drug-related crime. *Journal of Substance Abuse, 9,* 15–25.

Busto, U., Sellers, E. M., Naranjo, C. A., et al. (1986). Withdrawal reaction after long-term therapeutic use of benzodiazepines. *The New England Journal of Medicine, 315,* 854–859.

California Society of Addiction Medicine. (1997). *CSAM Newsletter, 24*(2).

Carlezon, W. A. Jr., Boundy, V. A., Haile, C. N., Lane, S. B., Kalb, R. G., Neve, R. L., & Nestler, E. J. (1997). Sensitization to morphine induced by mediated gene transfer. *Science, 277*(5327), 812–814.

Casriel, C., Rockwell, R., & Stepherson, B. (1988). Heroin sniffers: Between two worlds. *Journal of Psychoactive Drugs, 20*(4).

Centers for Disease Control. (2002). National Center for HIV, STD and TB Prevention [Online]. Available: *http://www.cdc.gov/hiv/stats.htm*

Cham, E., Hall, L., Ernst, A. A., & Weiss, S. J. (2002) Awareness and use of over-the-counter pain medications: A survey of emergency department patients. *Southern Medical Journal, 95*(5), 529–535.

DeVane, C. L. (2001). Substance P: A new era, a new role. *Pharmacotherapy, 21*(9), 1061–1069.

Drug Abuse Warning Network. (2002a). *Drug Abuse Warning Network Annual Medical Examiner Data from DAWN, 2001.* Rockville, MD: Substance Abuse and Mental Health Services Administration (SAMHSA).

Drug Abuse Warning Network. (2002b). *Mid-Year 2002 Preliminary Emergency Department Data from DAWN.* Rockville, MD: Substance Abuse and Mental Health Services Administration (SAMHSA).

Drug Benefit Trends. (2001). Drugs take bigger slice of total health care expenditures. *Drug Benefit Trends, 13*(8).

Drug Benefit Trends. (2002). Advertised prescription drugs are the hot sellers. *Drug Benefit Trends, 14*(4).

Drug Enforcement Administration. (1999). *Heroin Abuse and Addiction.* Bethesda, MD: DEA Publications.

Drug Enforcement Administration. (2000). A pharmacists guide to prescription fraud [Online]. Available: *http://www. deadiversion.usdoj.gov/pubs/brochures/pharmguide.htm*

Drug Enforcement Administration. (2001a). Congressional testimony by Donnie R. Marshall, DEA Administrator [Online]. Available: *http://www.usdoj.gov/dea/pubs/cngrtest/ct050301.htm*

Drug Enforcement Administration. (2001b). The price dynamics of Southeast Asian heroin. Drug Intelligence Brief [Online]. Available: *http://www.usdoj.gov/dea/pubs/intel/01004-intell-brief.pdf*

Drug Enforcement Administration. (2002a). Drug trafficking in the United States [Online]. Available: *http://www.usdoj.gov/dea/concern/drug_trafficking.html*

Drug Enforcement Administration. (2002b). Heroin [Online]. Available: *http://www.dea.gov/concern/heroin.html*

Eickelberg, S. J., & Mayo-Smith, M. F. (1998). Management of sedative-hypnotic intoxication and withdrawal. In A. W. Graham & T. K. Schultz (Eds.), *Principles of Addiction Medicine* (2nd ed., pp. 441–456). Chevy Chase, MD: American Society of Addiction Medicine, Inc.

El Sohly, M. A., & Salamone, S. J. (1999). Prevalence of drugs used in cases of alleged sexual assault. *Journal of Analytical Toxicology, 23,* 141–146.

Finnegan, L. P., & Kandall, S. R. (1997). Maternal and neonatal effects of alcohol and drugs. In J. H. Lowinson, P. Ruiz, R. B. Millman, & J. G. Langrod (Eds.), *Substance Abuse: A Comprehensive Textbook* (2nd ed., pp. 513–534). Baltimore: Williams & Wilkins.

Gold, M. S. (1990). Benzodiazepines: Tolerance, dependence, abuse, and addiction. *Journal of Psychoactive Drugs, 22*(1), 23–34.

Gold, M. S. (1998). The pharmacology of opioids. In A. W. Graham & T. K. Schultz (Eds.), *Principles of Addiction Medicine* (2nd ed.). Chevy Chase, MD: American Society of Addiction Medicine, Inc.

Gold, M. S., Jacobs, W. S., McGhee, D. L., McGraw, D. C., Grost-Pineda, K., & Croop, R. (2002, April 25). *Naltrexone augments the effects of nicotine replacement therapy in female smokers.* Paper presented at the 33rd annual meeting of the American Society of Addiction Medicine, Inc.

Goldstein, A. (2001). *Addiction: From Biology to Drug Policy.* New York: W.H. Freeman and Company.

Hoffman, J. P. (1990). The historical shift in the perception of opiates: From medicine to social medicine. *Journal of Psychoactive Drugs, 22*(1), 53–62.

Hollister, L. E. (1983). The pre-benzodiazepine era. *Journal of Psychoactive Drugs, 15*(1–2), 9–13.

Hser, Y.-I., Hoffman, V., Grella, C. E., & Anglin, M. D. (2001). A 33-year follow-up of narcotics addicts. *Archives of General Psychiatry, 58*(5), 503–508.

Hutcheson, D. M., Everitt, B. J., Robbins, T. W., & Dickinson, A. (2001). The role of withdrawal in heroin addiction: Enhances reward or promotes avoidance. *Nature Neuroscience, 4*(9), 943–947.

Hyman, S. E. (1998, March 30). An interview with Steven Hyman, M.D., Close to Home [Online]. Available: *http://www.pbs.org/wnet/closetohome/science/html/hyman.html*

IMS Health. (2002). IMS Health Reports [Online]. Available: *http://www.imshealth.com*

Jaffe, J. H., Knapp, C. M., & Ciraulo, D. A. (1997). Opiates: Clinical aspects. In J. H. Lowinson, P. Ruiz, R. B. Millman, & J. G. Langrod (Eds.), *Substance Abuse: A Comprehensive Textbook* (2nd ed., pp. 51–84). Baltimore: Williams & Wilkins.

Jenkins, A. J., & Cone, E. J. (1998). Pharmacokinetics: Drug absorption, distribution, and elimination. In S. B. Karch (Ed.), *Drug Abuse Handbook* (pp. 181–184). Boca Raton, FL: CRC Press.

Juergens, S. M., & Cowley, D. R. (1998). The pharmacology of sedative-hypnotics. In A. W. Graham & T. K. Schultz (Eds.), *Principles of Addiction Medicine* (2nd ed., pp. 117–130). Chevy Chase, MD: American Society of Addiction Medicine, Inc.

Kandall, S. R. (1993). *Improving Treatment for Drug Exposed Infants.* U.S. Department of Health and Human Services Administration: DHHS Publication no. (SMA) 93-2011.

Karch, S. B. (1996). *The Pathology of Drug Abuse.* Boca Raton, FL: CRC Press.

Latimer, D., & Goldberg, J. (1981). *Flowers in the Blood: The Story of Opium.* New York: Franklin Watts.

Lukas, S. E. (1995). Barbiturates. In J. H. Jaffe (Ed.), *Encyclopedia of Drugs and Alcohol* (Vol. I, pp. 141–146). New York: Simon & Schuster Macmillan.

Lurie, P., & Lee, P. R. (1991). Fifteen solutions to the problems of prescription drug abuse. *Journal of Psychoactive Drugs, 23*(4), 349–357.

Marnell, T. (Ed.). (1997). *Drug Identification Bible.* Denver, CO: Drug Identification Bible.

Marsa, L. (2001, September 10). Misuse of pain drug linked to hearing loss. *Los Angeles Times.*

McGregor, C., Darke, S., Ali, R., & Christie, P. (1998). Experience of non-fatal overdose among heroin users in Adelaide, Australia: Circumstances and risk perceptions. *Addiction, 93*(5), 701–711.

Miller, N. S., & Gold, M. S. (1990). Benzodiazepines: Tolerance, dependence, abuse, and addiction. *Journal of Psychoactive Drugs, 22*(1).

Musto, D. F. (1973). *The American Disease: Origins of Narcotic Control.* New Haven, CT: Yale University Press.

National Council on Alcohol and Drug Dependence. (2002, April 16). OxyContin deaths higher than expected. *Reuters.*

National Institute on Drug Abuse. (1999). Rohypnol and GHB. NIDA InfoFacts [Online]. Available: *http://www.nida.nih.gov/Infofax/RohypnolGHB.html*

National Institute on Drug Abuse. (2000). Heroin abuse and addiction. Research Report Series [Online]. Available: *http://www.nida.nih.gov/ResearchReports/Heroin/Heroin.html*

National Institute on Drug Abuse. (2001). Prescription drugs abuse and addiction. Research Report Series [Online]. Available: *http://www.nida.nih.gov/ResearchReports/Prescription/Prescription.html*

Nestler, E. J., & Aghajanian, G. K. (1997). Molecular and cellular basis of addiction. *Science, 278,* 58–63.

Nicholson, K. L., & Balster, R. L. (2001). GHB: A new and novel drug of abuse. *Drug and Alcohol Dependence, 63,* 1–22.

Nutt, D. J. (1998). The neurochemistry of addiction. In A. W. Graham & T. K. Schultz (Eds.), *Principles of Addiction Medicine* (2nd ed., pp. 51–56). Chevy Chase, MD: American Society of Addiction Medicine, Inc.

O'Brien, C. P. (2001). Drug addiction and drug abuse. In J. G. Hardman & L. E. Limbird (Eds.), *Goodman & Gilman's The Pharmacological Basis of Therapeutics* (10th ed., pp. 621–641). New York: McGraw Hill.

O'Brien, R., Cohen, S., Evans, G., & Fine, J. (1992). *The Encyclopedia of Drug Abuse.* New York: Facts on File.

Office of National Drug Control Policy. (2000a). *National Drug Control Strategy: 2000 Annual Report.* Bethesda, MD: National Drug Clearinghouse.

Office of National Drug Control Policy. (2000b). *What America's Users Spend on Illegal Drugs, 1988-1998.* Bethesda, MD: ONDCP.

Office of National Drug Control Policy. (2002). Gamma hydroxybutyrate (GHB). ONDCP Drug Policy Information Clearinghouse Fact Sheet [Online]. Available: *http://www.whitehousedrugpolicy.gov/publications/factsht/gamma/index.html*

Orangio, G. L., Pitlick, S., & Latta, P. (1984). Soft tissue infections in par-

enteral drug abusers. *Annals of Surgery, 199,* 97–100.

Palmer, C., & Horowitz, M. (Eds.). (1982). *Shaman Woman, Mainline Lady: Women's Writings on the Drug Experience.* New York: Quill, Inc.

Payte, J. T. (1997). Methadone maintenance treatment: The first thirty years. *Journal of Psychoactive Drugs, 29*(2).

Payte, J. T., & Zweben, J. E. (1998). Opioid maintenance therapies. In A. W. Graham & T. K. Schultz (Eds.), *Principles of Addiction Medicine* (2nd ed., pp. 557–570). Chevy Chase, MD: American Society of Addiction Medicine, Inc.

Physicians' Desk Reference. (2002). *Physicians' Desk Reference* (PDR, 56th ed.). Montvale, NJ: Medical Economics Company.

PhRMA. (2002). Industry Profile, 2002. PhRMA (Pharmaceutical Research and Manufacturers of America Publications) [Online]. Available: *http://www.phrma.org*

Potokar, J., & Nutt, D. J. (1994). Anxiolytic potential of benzodiazepine receptor partial agonists. *CNS Drugs, 1,* 305–315.

Rawson, R. A., Hasson, A. L., Huber, A. M., McCann, M. J., & Ling, W. (1998). A 3-year progress report on the implementation of LAAM in the United States. *Addiction, 93*(4), 533–540.

Robins, L. N. (1994). Lessons from the Vietnam heroin experience. The Harvard Mental Health Letter [Online]. Available: *http://www.mentalhealth.com/mag1/p5h-sb03.htm*

Schuckit, M. A. (2000). *Drug and Alcohol Abuse.* New York: Kluwer Academic/Plenum Publishers.

Schuckit, M. A., Greenblatt, D., Gold, E., & Irwin, M. (1991). Reactions to ethanol and diazepam in healthy young men. *Journal Study of Alcohol, 52*(2), 180–187.

Scott-Lewin, Inc. (2002). Top 200 generic drugs by retail sales in 2001 [Online]. Available: *http://www.drugtopics.com*

Simon, E. J. (1997). Opiates: Neurobiology. In J. H. Lowinson, P. Ruiz, R. B. Millman, & J. G. Langrod (Eds.), *Substance Abuse: A Comprehensive Textbook* (2nd ed., pp. 148–156). Baltimore: Williams & Wilkins.

Sivilotti, M. L., et al. (2001). Discontinuation of GBL can result in severe withdrawal syndrome. *Annals of Emergency Medicine, 38,* 660–665.

Sklair-Tavron, L., Shi, W. X., Lane, S. B., Harris, H. W., Bunny, B. S., & Nestler, E. J. (1996). Chronic morphine induces visible changes in the morphology of

mesolimbic dopamine neurons. *Proceedings of the National Academy of Sciences, 93,* 11202–11207.

Smith, D. E., & Seymour, R. B. (2001). *Clinician's Guide to Substance Abuse.* New York: McGraw-Hill.

Stahl, S. M. (2000). *Essential Psychopharmacology.* Cambridge, England: Cambridge University Press.

Sternbach, L. H. (1983). The benzodiazepine story. *Journal of Psychoactive Drugs, 15*(1–2), 15–17.

Strain, E. C., Stoller, K., Walsh, S. L., et al. (2000). Effects of buprenorphine versus buprenorphine/naloxone tablets in non-dependent opioid abusers. *Psychopharmacology, 148,* 374–383.

Strain, E. C., Walls, S. L., Pristine, K. L., Liebson, I. A., & Bigelow, G. E. (1997). The effects of buprenorphine in buprenorphine-maintained volunteers. *Psychopharmacology, 16,* 59–67.

Substance Abuse and Mental Health Services Administration. (2002). *National Household Survey on Drug Abuse, 2001.* Rockville, MD: SAMHSA, Office of Applied Studies.

Substance Abuse and Mental Health Services Administration/Treatment Episode Data Sets. (2002). Treatment Episode Data Sets (TEDS) for 1999 [Online]. Available: *http://www.samhsa.gov/centers/clearinghouse/clearinghouses.html*

Trebach, A. (1981). *The Heroin Solution.* New Haven, CT: Yale University Press.

Verhaag, D. A., & Ikeda, R. M. (1991). Prescribing for chronic pain. *Journal of Psychoactive Drugs, 23*(4).

Volpicelli, J., Pettinati, H., McLellan, A. T., & O'Brien, C. (2001). *Combining Medication and Psychosocial Treatments for Addictions.* New York: Guilford Publications.

Wickelgren, I. (1998). Teaching the brain to take drugs. *Science, 280,* 2045.

Will, M. J., Watkins, L. R., & Maier, S. F. (1998). Uncontrollable stress potentiates morphine's rewarding properties. *Pharmacology, Biochemistry, and Behavior, 60*(3), 655–664.

Zackon, F. (1992). *The Encyclopedia of Psychoactive Drugs: Heroin, the Street Narcotic.* New York: Chelsea House Publishers.

Zule, W. A., Vogtsberger, K. N., & Desmond, D. P. (1997). The intravenous injection of illicit drugs and needle sharing: An historical perspective. *Journal of Psychoactive Drugs, 29*(2).

Downers:
Alcohol

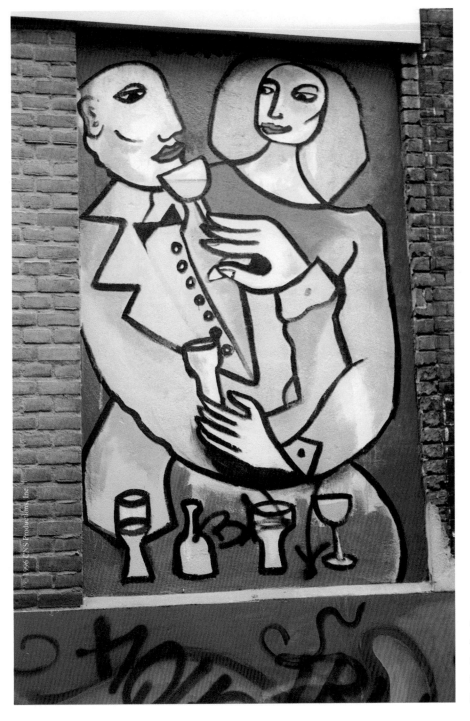

A wall painting in Holland is a reminder that alcohol is part of the great majority of cultures worldwide.

© 1996 CNS Productions, Inc.

- **Overview:** Alcohol is the oldest and most widely used psychoactive drug and is legal in most countries. About 113 million Americans drank alcohol last month and 12–14 million Americans have a drinking problem. About 10,000 years ago, grain was cultivated for bread and alcohol. Mead (fermented honey), beer (fermented barley), wine (fermented grapes and fruit), and finally distilled spirits (usually made from grain) were discovered by succeeding generations. Throughout history societies' laws and morals regarding alcohol have wavered from prohibition and temperance to unrestricted drinking.

- **Alcoholic Beverages:** Alcohol is fermented from the sugar or carbohydrates found in grapes and other fruits, vegetables, or grains. Ethyl alcohol (ethanol) is the main psychoactive component in all alcoholic beverages. Beer is about 5% alcohol, wine is about 12% alcohol, and distilled liquor is about 40% alcohol.

- **Absorption, Distribution, & Metabolism:** Though alcohol is absorbed by the body at different rates depending on weight, gender, age, and a dozen other factors, it is metabolized at a steady rate, mostly by the liver, and subsequently excreted through urine, sweat, and breath. The higher the blood alcohol concentration (BAC), the more severe the effects. A BAC of .08 to .10 signifies legal intoxication or impairment in the United States.

- **Desired Effects, Side Effects, & Health Consequences:**
  ◊ **Levels of Use:** Alcohol use, as with other drugs, ranges from abstinence, experimentation, and social/recreational use to habitual use, abuse, and addiction (alcoholism).
  ◊ **Low-to-Moderate-Dose Episodes:** If a person is not at risk, e.g., genetically susceptible, pregnant, in recovery, etc., there are some documented health benefits from light alcohol use. In general, sedation, muscle relaxation, and lowered inhibitions accompany low-dose use. The disinhibitory neurotransmitter GABA is most affected by alcohol.
  ◊ **High-Dose Episodes:** A range of effects occurs from decreased alertness and exaggerated emotions up to shock, coma, and death. Effects are directly related to the amount, frequency, and duration of use. They also depend on the tolerance to alcohol developed by the user. Blackouts (retrograde amnesia) are common.
  ◊ **Chronic High-Dose Use:** Depending on a drinker's habits and susceptibility, organ damage (particularly liver damage), cardiovascular problems, nervous system damage, gastrointestinal damage, reproductive disruption, cancer, and impairment of mental and emotional processes are common.
  ◊ **Mortality:** Chronic high-dose drinkers are likely to die 15 years earlier than the general population.

- **Addiction (alcohol dependence, alcoholism):** Historically there have been many attempts to classify alcoholism (alcohol dependence) as a disease. Heredity and environment, along with the use of alcohol and other psychoactive drugs, help determine a person's susceptibility to abuse and addiction. The development of tolerance and the presence of withdrawal symptoms advance a user from experimentation to abuse and alcohol dependence (addiction). Much of the current research in the field of alcohol dependence involves identifying the precise biological mechanisms involved in the development of addiction.

- **Other Problems With Alcohol:** Polydrug abuse, mental problems, fetal damage during pregnancy, excess aggression and violence, and driving-related accidents can happen at many levels of alcohol use.

- **Epidemiology:** The culture of the drinker (e.g., wet cultures vs. dry cultures), ethnic background, gender, age, and socioeconomic factors help determine how a person drinks.

- **Conclusions:** Since alcoholism can take anywhere from 3 months to 30 years to develop, it is important for drinkers to assess their susceptibility to compulsive use and their present level of use.

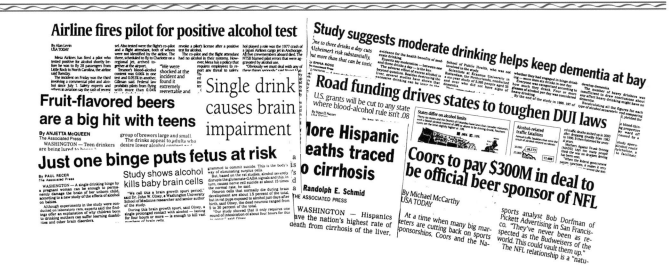

OVERVIEW

INTRODUCTION

"A pragmatic race, the Japanese appear to have decided long ago that the only reason for drinking alcohol is to become intoxicated and therefore drink only when they wish to be drunk."

William Gibson in *Tokyo Pastoral*

"To drink in the French style, moderately and with meals, being afraid for one's health is to limit too much the favors of Bacchus, that god. In any case, getting drunk is almost the only pleasure revealed to us by the passing of the years."

Anonymous

"Everyone thinks that Australians drink just beer and during the day that's pretty much true; when you go out in the afternoon, you have a beer. But at night, like nightclub hours, you drink hard alcohol, that's it."

Australian bartender

Worldwide

◇ **the majority of people in most countries, except mainly Islamic countries, drink alcoholic beverages.**

In the last 15 years in Asia

◇ India's alcohol consumption has almost doubled;

◇ Japan's alcohol consumption has remained the same.

Last month in Europe

◇ 23% of English boys and 27% of English girls 15–16 years old were drunk 3 times or more;

◇ Russian men consumed the equivalent of 6 to 7 bottles of vodka per capita.

Last month in the United States

◇ **about 109 million Americans (48% of the population) had at least 1 beer, 1 glass of wine, or 1 cocktail; 13 million of this group are considered heavy drinkers (5 or more drinks in one sitting at least 5 times in the past month);**

◇ about two-thirds of the 11 million college students (at 4-year colleges) had 1 drink and more than two-thirds of those drinkers were binge drinkers;

◇ about 6.7% of 8th grade students, 18.3% of 10th grade students, and 30.3% of 12th grade students had been drunk.

Yesterday in the United States

◇ about $240 million were spent at bars, restaurants, and liquor stores for alcoholic drinks;

◇ champagne toasts were made to 7,500 brides and grooms.

Also yesterday in the United States, unfortunately

◇ **from 25–30% of hospital admissions were due to direct or indirect medical complications from alcohol;**

◇ about one-half of the murder victims and one-half of the murderers drank alcohol;

◇ more than one-half of the 300 rapes that occurred involved alcohol.

And yesterday in Europe, unfortunately

◇ between 4 and 7 million European children woke up in homes with parents who were problem drinkers;

◇ almost 6 million French men had 4 or more drinks and 2.25 million French women had 2 or more drinks.

And yesterday in Asia, unfortunately

◇ 75,000 alcoholics were homeless in Japan (there are about 100,000 homeless in Japan).

And last year in the United States, unfortunately

◇ more than one-half of American adults had a close family member who has or has had alcoholism;

◇ 2.7 million crime victims reported that the offender had been drinking alcohol prior to committing the crime;

◇ alcohol abuse and addiction cost businesses, the judicial system, medical facilities, and the United States $184 billion or $638 for every man, woman, and child.

And worldwide last year, unfortunately

◇ **over 2 million people died due to alcohol;**

◇ approximately 10% of all diseases and injuries were a direct result of alcohol abuse.

(World Health Organization [WHO], 2003; Bellandi, 2003; Eurocare, 2003; Internal Revenue Service, 2002; Wechsler, Lee, Kuo, Seibring, Nelson, & Lee, 2002; University of Michigan, 2002; Substance Abuse and Mental Health Services Administration [SAMHSA], 2002; Harwood et al., 2000; National Institute on Alcohol Abuse and Alcoholism [NIAAA], 2000; National Clearinghouse on Alcohol and Drug Information [NCADI], 1999; Dawson & Grant, 1998; U.S. Department of Justice, 1998)

HISTORY (*also see Chapter 1*)

Alcohol is the oldest known and most widely used psychoactive drug in the world. It has presumably been present since airborne yeast spores started fermenting plants into alcohol about 1½ billion years ago.

The mists of prehistory cloak our ancient ancestors' discovery of the first psychoactive drug. Perhaps **alcohol was initially found by accident** when a bunch of grapes or a batch of plums was left standing in the sun, allowing the fruit sugar to ferment into alcohol (O'Brien & Chafetz, 1991). Perhaps some wild honey that had fermented was found, diluted with water, and sampled. This drink would later be called "mead" (Waugh, 1968). People enjoyed the taste, the mood-altering effects, or both. Curiosity was followed by experimentation and it was discovered that the starch in potatoes, rice, corn, fruit, and grains could also be fermented into alcohol. Further experimentation found the value of alcohol as a solvent for medicines and as a medicine or tonic in and of itself.

The desire to have ready access to the pleasurable effects as well as the health benefits of beer and wine led humans to search out the raw ingredients with which to manufacture alcoholic beverages and produce them systematically. Some historians believe that **the first civilized settlements were created to ensure a regular supply of grapes for wine, grain for beer and food, and poppies for opium** (Keller, 1984).

We know that ancient societies were using alcohol about the same time that agriculture developed, around 8000 B.C. Archeologists have found a recipe for beer as well as alcohol residues in clay pots in Mesopotamia and Iran dating from 5400–3500 B.C. (Goodwin & Gabrielli, 1997). The use of alcohol is documented in almost all civilized societies throughout history, in myths, religions, rituals, stories, hieroglyphs, sacred writings, songs, or in commercial records written on papyrus scrolls or clay tablets. The Babylonian *Epic of Gilgamesh* says wine grapes were given to the earth as a memorial to fallen gods. The *Bible* contains more than 150 references to wine, some positive, some negative (O'Brien & Chafetz, 1991).

"God give you of the dew of the sky, of the fatness of the earth, and plenty of grain and new wine."
Genesis 27:28, The *Bible*

"And don't get drunk with wine, which leads to reckless actions, but be filled with the Spirit: speaking to one another in psalms, hymns, and spiritual songs, singing and making music to the Lord in your heart."
Ephesians 5:18, 19, The *Bible*

THE LEGAL DRUG

Historically the acceptability of alcohol has been intertwined with cultural, social, and financial imperatives. It has been used as a **reward** for pyramid workers, as a **food** (grain-rich beer) for peasants, as a solvent for opium in the eighteenth-century **cure-all** known as "laudanum," as a **sacrament** for Jewish or Christian religious ceremonies, as a **water substitute** for contaminated wells, as a **social lubricant** for all classes, as a **tranquilizer**, and as a **source of taxes**. Because beer, wine, and liquor are so widely available and legal in most societies (except Muslim-governed countries) and because they are promoted by custom and advertising, many people do not think of alcohol as a drug. Whether it's been used for those desirable reasons or as the focus of prohibition forces, alcohol will continue to be the object of desire or of vilification depending on moral attitude, social acceptability, and the politics of the prevailing government.

Almost every country has had periods in their history where alcohol use was restricted or banned completely. Those prohibitions were usually rescinded (Langton, 1995).

◇ The *Chinese Canon of History,* written about 650 B.C., recognized that complete prohibition was almost impossible because men loved their beer (Keller, 1984).

◇ The Greek writer Anacharsis wrote in 600 B.C. that, "The vine bears three kinds of grapes; the first of pleasure, the next of intoxication, and the third of disgust."

◇ Many Buddhist sects in India prohibited alcohol starting in 500 B.C. and continuing to the present day.

◇ In ancient Persia alcohol was prohibited by the ruling Islamic culture because of widespread health problems such as malnutrition caused by excess consumption; overindulgence was common in the upper classes.

◇ When alcohol began to be distilled around A.D. 800, medicinal uses of the drug were reemphasized; the increased concentration led to more intense physiological and psychological effects.

◇ In Sub-Saharan Africa the idea of banning alcohol was usually avoided because home-brewed beers had great nutritional value.

◊ In the Middle Ages in Europe drinking was tolerated by all classes and drunkenness was often reserved for festive or religious occasions. Pubs and drinking establishments were sometimes thought to be places where sedition or heresy could arise, so the more notorious establishments were closed down (Heath, 1995).

◊ The **Gin Epidemic in England** in the 1700s emphasized that unrestricted use, poverty, and industrial despair coupled with the higher concentration of the alcohol soon led to abuse and addiction. The unrestricted sales of gin (20 million gallons per year in England alone) and the resulting problems of public inebriation, illness, and death subsequently led to increased taxes and severe restrictions on its manufacture just a few decades after its use was promoted by the English government (O'Brien & Chafetz, 1991).

◊ **In Colonial America alcohol was an everyday part of life**: the Pilgrims on the Mayflower regarded it as an "essential victual"; the cultivation, manufacture, sale, and taxation of whiskey and rum helped finance the American Revolution and the slave trade.

◊ Attempts at temperance and treatment were tried by groups such as the Washington Temperance Society in the 1840s, the Oxford Group in the 1920s, and Alcoholics Anonymous in the 1930s, the latter which believed in the **concept of solving alcohol abuse and addiction through personal spiritual change** (Alcoholics Anonymous, 1934, 1976; Nace, 1997; Miller, 1998).

◊ Official prohibition of alcohol by the government of the United States started in 1920 but widespread flouting of the law, criminalization of the manufacturing and distribution system, and **pressure by those who wanted to drink, including the Wet Party, led to the repeal of Prohibition** 13 years later.

◊ The industrial revolution that freed people from the land and expanded leisure time also led to the increased recreational use of alcoholic beverages. Globally alcoholism and problem drinking are always more prevalent in developed countries than in the developing countries (WHO, 1999).

One reason that many restrictions, and even prohibition, have been overturned is alcohol's value as **a major source of revenue for corporations and excise taxes for governments**. Currently the federal government collects $13.50 per proof gallon that's shipped from distilleries while state governments collect up to $6.50 a gallon.

Because alcohol has played a central economic and social role since colonial times in America (and even further back in other countries' cultures) contemporary society's view of the heavy drinker is more forgiving than its view of even an occasional cocaine, heroin, or LSD user. The contradictions surrounding alcohol's accepted place in society and the disfavor in which most other psychoactive drugs are held are not lost on the younger generation.

"Alcohol is heavily social, so one of the problems that I have with prohibition attitudes is that society drinks as much as we do. And because it is legal, I feel I am still part of society even when drunk, whereas with illicit drugs like marijuana, I feel I am stepping outside of what is acceptable."
19-year-old college freshman

ALCOHOLIC BEVERAGES

THE CHEMISTRY OF ALCOHOL

There are **hundreds of different alcohols**. Some are made naturally through fermentation while most that are used industrially are synthesized. Some of the more familiar alcohols include

◊ ethyl alcohol (ethanol, grain alcohol), the main psychoactive component in all alcoholic beverages;

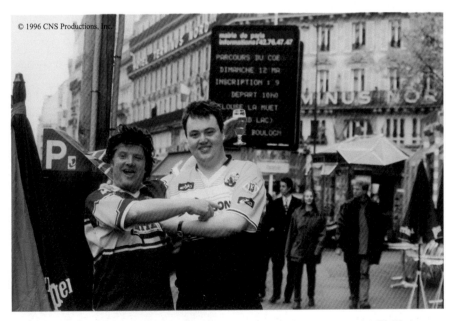

© 1996 CNS Productions, Inc.

Alcohol is a legal drug in most countries. The preference for beer, wine, or distilled liquors depends on the country's culture, on the availability of certain kinds of beverages, and on the specific occasion. These soccer fans are consoling themselves after their team's defeat. It is of interest to note that they would be in the same place, doing the same drinking to celebrate a victory rather than a loss.

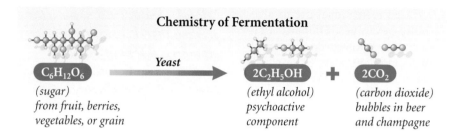

Chemistry of Fermentation

$$C_6H_{12}O_6 \xrightarrow{\text{Yeast}} 2C_2H_5OH + 2CO_2$$

(sugar)
from fruit, berries,
vegetables, or grain

(ethyl alcohol)
psychoactive
component

(carbon dioxide)
bubbles in beer
and champagne

Figure 5-1 •

Yeast feeds on sugar and excretes alcohol and carbon dioxide.

◊ methyl alcohol (methanol or wood alcohol), a toxic industrial solvent;

◊ isopropyl alcohol (propanol or rubbing alcohol), used in shaving lotion, shellac, antifreeze, antiseptics, and lacquer;

◊ butyl alcohol (butanol), used in many industrial processes (O'Brien & Chafetz, 1991).

Ethyl alcohol is the least toxic of the alcohols. Few people drink pure ethyl alcohol because it is too strong and fiery tasting. By convention any beverage with an alcohol content greater than 2% is considered an alcoholic beverage.

Alcoholic beverages also include trace amounts of other alcohols, such as amyl, butyl, and propyl alcohol, that result from the production process and storage (e.g., in wooden barrels). Other components produced during fermentation are called "**congeners.**" Congeners include acids, aldehydes, esters, ketones, phenols, and tannins. They **contribute to the distinctive tastes, aromas, and colors** of the various alcoholic beverages. Beer and vodka have a relatively low concentration of congeners; aged whiskies and brandy have a relatively high concentration (Lichine, 1990). It is thought that congeners may contribute to the severity of hangovers and other toxic problems of drinking, though the main culprit is the ethyl alcohol.

Alcohol occurs in nature when airborne **yeast feeds on the sugars** in honey or any watery mishmash of overripe fruit, berries, vegetables, or grain. **The fermentation process results in ethyl alcohol and carbon dioxide.**

Elephants, bears, and deer as well as birds and insects have been observed in a state of intoxication, exhibiting unsteady and erratic behavior after eating fermented mixtures.

TYPES OF ALCOHOLIC BEVERAGES

The principle categories of alcoholic beverages are beer, wine, and distilled spirits.

◊ **Wine** is produced when **fruits** ferment.

◊ **Beer** is produced when **grains** ferment.

◊ **Distilled spirits** with different concentrations of alcohol can be made

from **fermented grains, roots, vegetables, and other plants**. They can also be **distilled from wine or other fermented beverages**.

Each country seems to have its national or local drinks: Mexican pulque made from cactus, Russian kvass made from cereal or bread, Asian kumiss made from mare's milk, and even California garlic wine. The actual consumption of beer vs. wine vs. distilled alcohol depends very much on the culture of a country. For example, Germans drink 6 times as much beer per capita as they do wine; the French drink 8 times as much wine per capita as Americans (Eurocare, 2003).

Beer

Beer brewing and bread making were probably started about 8000 B.C. in Neolithic times. The raw ingredients (usually grain) were produced in cultivated fields. Some of the first written records concerning beer were found in Mesopotamian ruins dating back to about 5400–3500 B.C. The Mesopotamians taught the Greeks how to brew beer and Europeans in turn learned from the Greeks.

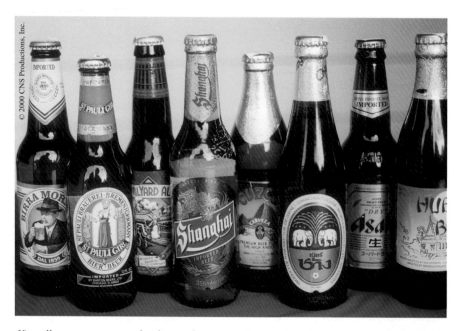

Virtually every country makes beer either as a national enterprise or a local business. These beers and ales come from Italy, Germany, United States, China, Peru, Thailand, Japan, and Vietnam.

TABLE 5–1　PRODUCTION & CONSUMPTION OF BEER & WINE IN EUROPE & THE UNITED STATES

	Beer Production in Hectoliters	Beer Consumption in Liters per Capita	Wine Consumption in Liters per Capita
Germany	114,800	131.7	22
England	59,139	103.6	13
United States	200,000	95.0	20
France	19,493	39.6	60
Italy	11,455	103.6	59

The United States produces the most beer but Germany and England have a higher per capita consumption (Eurocare, 2003).

One hectoliter = 26.4 gallons　　One liter = .2642 gallons

Beer is produced by first allowing cereal grains, usually barley, to sprout in a tub of water where an enzyme called "amylase" is released. After the barley malt is crushed, the amylase helps convert the starches to sugar. This crushed malt is boiled into a liquid mash. It is then filtered, mixed with some hops (an aromatic herb first used around A.D. 1000–1500) and yeast, and allowed to ferment. **Beer includes ale, stout, porter, malt liquor, lager, and bock beer.** The difference among beers has to do mainly with the type of grain used, the fermentation time, and whether they are top-fermenting beers (those that rise in the vat) or bottom-fermenting beers. The top-fermenting beers are more flavorful and include ales, stouts, porters, and wheat beers. The bottom-fermenting beers include the most popular pale lager beers, e.g., Budweiser® and Coors® (Lukas, 1995). Traditional home-brewed beers are dark and full of sediment, minerals, vitamins (especially B vitamins), and amino acids and thus have appreciable food value, unlike modern commercial beers that are highly filtered.

The **alcohol content of most lager beers is 4–5%**; ales, 5–6%; ice beers, 5–7%; malt liquors, 6–9%; while light beers are only 3.4–4.2% alcohol.

Wine

In some early cultures **beer was the alcoholic beverage of the com-mon people and wine was the drink of the priests and nobles** possibly because vineyards were more difficult to establish and cultivate. In Egypt however, pharaohs did have beer entombed with them in their pyramids to sustain them on their afterlife journeys and to offer a gift to the gods. Ancient Greek and Roman cultures seem to have preferred wine; the ruling class kept the best vintages for themselves (Heath, 1995). They also cultivated vineyards in many of their colonies. After the fall of the Roman Empire, many monasteries in Germany, France, Austria, and Italy carried on the cultivation of grapes and even hybridized new species.

Wines are usually made from grapes though some are made from berries, other fruits (e.g., peach wine, plum wine), and even starchy grains (e.g., Japanese saké rice wine). Generally grapes with a high sugar content are preferred. A disease-resistant hybrid of *Vitas vinifera* grafted onto several American species was heavily planted worldwide particularly in temperate climates found in France, Italy, California, New York, Argentina, and Spain. Wine had a short shelf life until the 1860s when Louis Pasteur showed that heating it would halt microbial activity and keep the wine from turning into vinegar (pasteurization).

Grapes are crushed to extract their juices. Either the grapes contain their own yeast or yeast is added and fermentation begins. The kind of wine produced depends on the variety of grape used, the quality of the soil, the ripeness of the grapes, the climate and weather, and the balance between acidity and sugar. White wines typically are aged from 6–12 months and red wines from 2–4 years. Once bottled many wines, particularly some red wines, continue to age and improve in taste although some are drunk "young," such as Beaujolais Nouveau and Chianti.

European wines contain from 8–12% alcohol whereas **U.S. wines have a 12–14% alcohol content.** Wines with higher than 14% alcohol content are called "fortified wines" because they have had pure alcohol or brandy added during or after fermentation. Their final alcohol content is 17–21%. Wine coolers that are usually diluted with juice contain an average of 6% alcohol (Matthews, 1995).

Distilled Spirits (liquor)

The alcoholic content of naturally fermented wine is limited to about 14% by volume. At higher levels the concentration of alcohol becomes too toxic and kills off the fermenting yeast thus halting the conversion of sugar into alcohol. In areas outside of Asia, drinks with greater than 14% alcohol weren't available until about **A.D. 800 when the Arabs discovered distillation.** This eventually led to the production of distilled spirits such as brandies, whiskies, vodka, and gin.

Brandy is distilled from wine, rum from sugar cane or molasses, vodka from potatoes, whiskey and gin from grains. Distilled spirits can be produced from many other plants including figs and dates in the Middle East or the agave plants in Mexico from which mescal and tequila are made.

One of the results of the invention of distilled beverages was that it became much easier to get drunk although this didn't start happening until centuries later. Initially the distilled alcohol was used more for medical reasons. **Alcoholism eventually exploded in Europe and other countries due to the increased manufacturing of distilled spirits and the desire for excise**

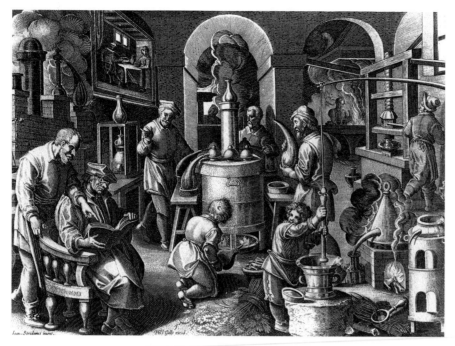

Distillatio by Philip Galle. Distillation in this sixteenth-century Dutch laboratory supplies alcohol for making medicines and for drinking. In distillation a liquid is boiled and the vapors are drawn off, cooled, and condensed into a clear, colorless, almost 100% pure grain alcohol distillate.

Courtesy of the National Library of Medicine, Bethesda, MD

tax revenues. Similarly alcoholism became a major social problem in Colonial America with the manufacture of increasing amounts of corn whiskey and rum that was easier and more profitable to transport and market than bushels of corn. Grains and other sugar-producing commodities could be reduced in volume into more potent and higher-priced commodities. Rum was so popular that the second publicly funded building in New Amsterdam (New York) was a rum distillery on Staten Island.

ABSORPTION, DISTRIBUTION, & METABOLISM

ABSORPTION & DISTRIBUTION

When someone drinks an alcoholic beverage, it is slightly broken down or metabolized by digestive juices in the mouth and stomach. Because alcohol is readily soluble in water and doesn't need to be digested, it immediately begins to be absorbed and distributed. **Absorption of alcohol into the bloodstream takes place at various sites along the gastrointestinal tract, including the stomach, the small intestines, and the colon.** In men about 10–20% of the alcohol is absorbed by the stomach while in women there is very little absorption there. **Most of the alcohol enters the capillaries in the walls of the small intestines** through passive diffusion.

Given the same body weight, women and men differ in their processing of alcohol. **Women have higher blood alcohol concentrations than men do from the same amount of alcohol.** A woman who weighs the same as a man and drinks the same number of drinks as a man absorbs about 30% more alcohol into the bloodstream and feels its psychoactive effects faster and more intensely (NIAAA, 1990).

This difference between women's

and men's reaction to alcohol results from three possible explanations.

◇ Women have a lower percentage of body water than men of comparable size, so there is less water to dilute the alcohol.

◇ Women have less alcohol dehydrogenase enzyme in the stomach to break down alcohol, so less alcohol is metabolized before getting into the blood.

◇ Finally, changes in gonadal hormone levels during menstruation affect the rate of alcohol metabolism (NIAAA, 1990).

Thus chronic **alcohol use causes greater physical damage to women than to men**—female alcoholics have death rates 50–100% higher than male alcoholics (NIAAA, 1990).

The alcohol is absorbed into the bloodstream and partially metabolized by the liver (first-pass metabolism) and then quickly distributed throughout the body. Since alcohol molecules are small, water- and lipid-soluble, and move easily through capillary walls by passive diffusion, they can enter any organ or tissue and in the case of pregnancy, can even cross the placental barrier into the fetal circulatory system (O'Brien & Chafetz, 1991). Once alcohol reaches the brain and passes through the blood-brain barrier, psychoactive effects gradually begin to occur.

The highest levels of blood alcohol concentration occur 30–90 minutes after alcohol is drunk. How quickly the effects are felt is determined by the rate of absorption. Absorption is influenced by an individual's weight, body chemistry, and factors such as emotional state (e.g., fear, stress, fatigue, or anger), state of health, body fat, food taken with the alcohol, and even the outside temperature. Women absorb more alcohol during the premenstrual period than at other times.

Other **factors that speed absorption** in both men and women are

◇ increasing the amount drunk or the drinking rate;

◇ drinking on an empty stomach;

TABLE 5–2   APPROXIMATE PERCENTAGE OF ALCOHOL IN CERTAIN BEVERAGES – BY VOLUME

WINE

Unfortified (red, white, rosé)	12–14%
Fortified (dessert, sherry, port)	17–21%
Champagne	12%
Vermouth	18%
Wine cooler	6%

BEER

Regular beer	4–5%
Light beer	3.4–4.2%
Malt liquor	6–9%
Ale	5–6%
Ice beer	5–6%
Low-alcohol beer	1.5%
Nonalcoholic beers (O'Doul's®)	0.5%

MALT BEVERAGES

Hard lemonade, Bacardi Silver®, Smirnoff Ice®, Stolichnaya Citrona®	5–6%

LIQUORS & WHISKEYS

Bourbon, whiskey, scotch, vodka, gin, brandy, rum	40–50%
Overproof rum	75%
Tequila, cognac, Drambui®	40%
Amaretto®, Kahlua®	26%
Everclear®	95%

(Note: To calculate the proof of a product, double the alcohol content: e.g., 40% alcohol = 80 proof, 100% alcohol = 200 proof.)

Metabolism of Alcohol

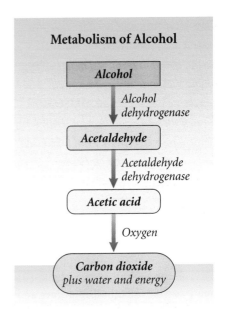

Figure 5-2 •

Metabolism is accomplished in several stages involving oxidation. First the enzyme alcohol dehydrogenase (ADH), found in the stomach and the liver, acts on the ethyl alcohol (C_2H_5OH) to form acetaldehyde (CH_3CHO), a highly toxic substance. Acetaldehyde is then quickly acted on by a second enzyme, acetaldehyde dehydrogenase (ALDH), that oxidizes it into acetic acid (CH_3COOH). Acetic acid is then further oxidized to carbon dioxide (CO_2) and water (H_2O).

◊ using high alcohol concentrations in drinks, up to a maximum of 95% with Everclear®;

◊ drinking carbonated drinks, such as champagne, sparkling wines, soft drinks, and tonic mixers;

◊ warming the alcohol (e.g., hot toddies, hot saké).

Factors that slow absorption are

◊ eating before or while drinking (especially eating meat, milk, cheese, and fatty foods);

◊ diluting drinks with ice, water, or fruit juice.

METABOLISM

Because the body treats alcohol as a toxin or poison, elimination begins as soon as it is ingested. Approximately 2–10% of the alcohol is eliminated directly without being metabolized—a small amount is exhaled via the lungs while additional amounts are excreted through sweat, saliva, and urine. The remaining **90–98% of alcohol is neutralized through metabolism (mainly oxidation) by the liver and then by excretion through the kidneys and lungs** (Jones & Pounder, 1998).

Alcohol is metabolized in the liver, first by alcohol dehydrogenase (ADH) into acetaldehyde, which is very toxic to the body and especially the liver, and then by acetaldehyde dehydrogenase (ALDH) into acetic acid that is finally oxidized into carbon dioxide (CO_2) and water (H_2O) (Fig. 5-2). **The varying availability and efficiency of ADH and ALDH, due in part to hereditary factors, account for some of the variation in people's reactions to alcohol** (Bosron, Ehrig, & Li, 1993).

For example, it is suspected that the high rate of alcoholism and the high rate of cirrhosis of the liver in Native Americans are due to disruptions in the ALDH and ADH systems as well as a tradition of binge-drinking patterns. Besides ALDH irregularities, drugs such as aspirin also inhibit metabolism of alcohol and lead to higher blood alcohol concentration in both men and women.

In many countries, alcoholic beverages are used primarily as a source of nutrition (especially beer) while in others they are used primarily for their mind-altering effects. Pure alcohol is a very concentrated energy source, almost as much as pure fat but they are empty calories, i.e., high caloric content with no real food value. **Alcoholics are much more susceptible to malnutrition** because, on average, they get half their energy intake from alcohol.

Blood Alcohol Concentration (BAC)

Though absorption of alcohol is quite variable, **metabolism occurs at a relatively defined continuous rate.** About 1 ounce (oz.) of pure alcohol (2 drinks) is eliminated from the body every 3 hours. Thus we can usually predict the amount of alcohol that will be circulating through the body and brain and how long it will take that amount to be metabolized and eliminated. However, each person's biochemical makeup due to heredity can have a strong effect on metabolism and elimination. In addition **the actual reaction and level of impairment can vary widely depending on drinking history, behavioral tolerance, mood, and a dozen other factors.** Physical impairment is greater in a rising BAC. From the moment of ingestion, it takes about 15–20 minutes for alcohol to reach the brain via the intestines and begin to cause impairment. **It takes 30–90 minutes after ingestion to reach maximum blood alcohol concentration** (NIAAA, 1997).

This **BAC table** (Table 5-3) measures the concentration of alcohol in an average drinker's blood. (Some other versions of BAC tables give slightly lower levels than this table. The differences are minimal.) In most states **legal intoxication is .08 or .10 whether the driver can function or not.** Some think it should be .05 for safety. For truck drivers the legal limit is .04 and for pilots it is .02 after 24 hours from the last drink. The unit of measurement for BAC is weight by volume, e.g., milligrams per deciliter, but can be expressed as a percentage, e.g., .10% alcohol by volume (Bailey, 1998).

For example, if a 200 lb. male has 5 drinks in 2 hours, his blood alcohol would be .108 minus the timetable factor of .030, so his BAC would be about .078 and he would be legally sober enough to drive in many states. If his 200 lb. female companion has 5 drinks in 2 hours, her blood alcohol level

TABLE 5–3 APPROXIMATE BLOOD ALCOHOL CONCENTRATION FOR DIFFERENT BODY WEIGHTS

No. of Drinks	1	2	3	4	5	6	7	8	9	10
Male										
100 lbs.	.043	.087	.130	.174	.217	.261	.304	.348	.391	.435
125 lbs.	.034	.069	.103	.139	.173	.209	.242	.287	.312	.346
150 lbs.	.029	.058	.087	.116	.145	.174	.203	.232	.261	.290
175 lbs.	.025	.050	.075	.100	.125	.150	.175	.200	.225	.250
200 lbs.	.022	.043	.065	.087	.108	.130	.152	.174	.195	.217
225 lbs.	.019	.039	.058	.078	.097	.117	.136	.156	.175	.195
250 lbs.	.017	.035	.052	.070	.087	.105	.122	.139	.156	.173
Female										
100 lbs.	.050	.101	.152	.203	.253	.304	.355	.406	.456	.507
125 lbs.	.040	.080	.120	.162	.202	.244	.282	.324	.364	.404
150 lbs.	.034	.068	.101	.135	.169	.203	.237	.271	.304	.338
175 lbs.	.029	.058	.087	.117	.146	.175	.204	.233	.262	.292
200 lbs.	.026	.050	.076	.101	.126	.152	.177	.203	.227	.253

If a person drinks over a period of time, the alcohol is metabolized at a rate of .015 per hour. Use the following table to factor in the time since the first drink.

TIMETABLE FACTORS

Hours since first drink	1	2	3	4	5
Subtract from BAC	.015	.030	.045	.060	.075

(O'Brien & Chafetz, 1991)

Drink Equivalency

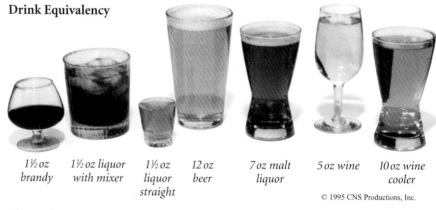

| 1½ oz brandy | 1½ oz liquor with mixer | 1½ oz liquor straight | 12 oz beer | 7 oz malt liquor | 5 oz wine | 10 oz wine cooler |

© 1995 CNS Productions, Inc.

Figure 5-3 •

One drink is defined as 1½ oz. brandy, 1½ oz. liquor w/wo mixer, 12 oz. lager beer, 7 oz. malt liquor, 5 oz. wine, 10 oz. wine cooler.

There is slightly more than ½ oz. of pure alcohol in the average alcoholic beverage.

would be .126 minus the timetable factor of .030, so her BAC would be .096 and not only would she be quite a bit more intoxicated than her companion even though they weighed the same and drank the same amount over the same period of time but she would also be legally impaired in many states.

DESIRED EFFECTS, SIDE EFFECTS, & HEALTH CONSEQUENCES

"I really enjoyed drinking. I really did. And I haven't found anything, actually I haven't looked very hard, but I just haven't found anything that I enjoy as much."
65-year-old man

"Escape, absolutely escape. It's all about running away, numbing your feelings because you can't, I can't, accept life on life's terms."
35-year-old woman

LEVELS OF USE

The effects of any drug depend on the dosage. The same substance can be a poison, a powerful prescription medicine, or an over-the-counter mild medication depending on the dose and frequency of use. Alcohol is no exception and, as with other psychoactive drugs, there are **escalating patterns of use.**

Abstention (nonuse)

"My brother experimented with Puerto Rican rum on New Year's Eve when he was 15. He threw up on me on the way to the toilet. That took care of his drinking for 5 years and mine forever."
54-year-old nondrinker

Experimentation (use for curiosity with no subsequent drug-seeking behavior)

"When you're a little boy, your dad says, 'Go get me a beer.' You pop it open

for him and they let you take a sip every once in a while as long as mom's not looking. It tasted good. When you're 10 or 12, you don't really know what alcohol is, you just experience it every once in a while."
33-year-old drinker

Social/Recreational Use (sporadic infrequent drug-seeking behavior with no established pattern)

"We know which dorm has the drinkers, so when we feel like a bit of a party and a few drinks, that's where we go. They're more serious about their drinking; they like '40s [40 oz. malt liquor bottles or cans] but I can take it with a grain of salt."
20-year-old college sophomore

Habituation (established pattern of use with no major negative consequences)

"I think the pleasure left. This was the only way I knew how to have fun. This was the only way I knew how to feel better. But it didn't work and it took me awhile to realize that it had become a habit."
36-year-old recovering alcoholic

Abuse (continued use despite negative consequences)

"I always got Bs, and then my grades dropped down to Ds, and then I started failing my classes, and I skipped school, and I got suspended all the time for that when I got caught. I'd skip school and I'd go get high or we'd just skip it because we were always high."
15-year-old high school dropout in treatment

Addiction (compulsion to use, inability to stop use, major life dysfunction with continued use)

"I would have the shakes, just really sick. I mean my body could not take

alcohol at all. I would be sick in the morning like for days. It was hard to go to work and hard to take care of my children, hard to do my daily chores. It took me a long time to get well in the morning until I realized there was a magical cure. I could start drinking Bloody Marys."
33-year-old recovering alcoholic

The effects of alcohol depend on the amount used, frequency of use, and duration of use:

◇ **low-to-moderate-dose use** (up to 1 drink a day for women and 2 drinks a day for men) can occur with experimentation, social/recreational use, and even habituation;

◇ **high-dose use** can occur at any level of drinking;

◇ **chronic high-dose use** occurs with abuse and addiction (alcoholism).

LOW-TO-MODERATE-DOSE EPISODES

Most studies show that

◇ **small amounts of alcohol generally do not have negative health consequences for men**, even over extended periods of time;

◇ **infrequent mild intoxication episodes generally do not have lasting adverse health consequences for most male drinkers**.

However **low-level alcohol use is generally not safe for** people who

◇ are **pregnant**;

◇ have certain **preexisting physical or mental health problems** that are aggravated by alcohol;

◇ are **allergic to alcohol, nitrosamines, or other congeners and additives**;

◇ have a high **genetic/environmental susceptibility** to addiction;

◇ have a **history of abuse and addiction problems** with alcohol or other drugs;

◇ are **at risk for breast cancer**.

Sometimes it is difficult to define moderate drinking because each person has a different definition. We will define moderate drinking as "drinking that doesn't cause problems for the drinker or for those around him or her" (Alcohol Alert, 1992). However, drinkers begin to have pathological consequences from alcohol when they have more than 2 drinks per day in men and up to 1 drink per day in women. Severe effects and long-term health and social consequences usually result from high-dose use episodes and frequent high-dose or chronic use.

Low-to-Moderate-Dose Use: Physical Effects

Therapeutic Uses. Alcohol is used as a solvent for other medications since it is water- and lipid-soluble. It is used as a **topical disinfectant, as a body rub to reduce fever** since it evaporates so quickly, and as a **pain reliever** for certain nerve-related pain; it is occasionally used to prevent premature labor (Woodward, 1998). Systemically ethanol is used to treat methanol and ethylene glycol poisoning.

Desired Effects. Some people who drink alcoholic beverages think that they **taste good, quench the thirst, and relax muscle tension.** Consumed in low doses before meals, alcoholic beverages activate gastric juices, improve stomach motility, and **stimulate the appetite.** They produce a feeling of warmth since vessels dilate and increase blood flow to subcutaneous tissues (Woodward, 1998).

Light-to-moderate use of alcohol has been shown to **reduce the incidence of heart disease** and plaque formation whether the cause is

◇ an increase in high-density lipoproteins, particularly HDL$_3$;

◇ a different interaction with lipoproteins;

◇ or simply the decrease in tension that a drink can induce.

The doses must be low enough not to cause liver damage, induce other adverse health effects, or trigger heavier

drinking (Mukamal & Rimm, 2001; NIAAA, 2000). Of course any beneficial effects may also be obtained through exercise, low-fat diets, stress-reduction techniques, and an aspirin a day. (On autopsy many end-stage alcoholics have clean blood vessels and badly damaged livers, hearts, and brains.)

One or 2 drinks decrease the chance of gallstones in men and women. In postmenopausal women, alcohol seems to slow bone loss because of its effect on estrogen. Women who drink in moderation seem to have a higher bone mass than women who don't drink (Turner & Sibonga, 2001).

Researchers at Columbia University found in a study of 677 stroke victims that those who have 1 or 2 drinks a day have a **lower risk of strokes** because alcohol keeps blood platelets from clumping (Sacco, Elkind, Boden-Albala, et al., 1999). But again, since heavy drinking actually increases the risk of stroke, and even moderate drinking has unwanted side effects, and since no benefit is shown in recommending moderate drinking to abstainers, using alcohol as a stroke-preventive measure should only be done in consultation with a physician.

Sleep. Alcohol is often used by people **to get to sleep** particularly if anxiety is causing insomnia. In fact alcohol does decrease the time it takes to fall asleep but it also seems to disturb the second half of the sleep period especially if consumed within an hour of bedtime (Landolt et al., 1996; Vitiello, 1997). It interferes with REM (rapid eye movement) and dreaming, both essential to feeling fully rested. Drinking also puts one at higher risk for experiencing obstructive sleep apnea, a disorder where the upper breathing passage (pharynx) narrows or closes during sleep causing the person to wake up, often a number of times during a sleep period, thus leading to severe fatigue, along with neurological and cardiac problems. Not only do those with alcoholism have an increased risk of sleep apnea, those with the condition seem to aggravate their disease by drinking (Miller et al, 1988; Dawson, Bigby, Poceta, & Mitler, 1993).

Low-to-Moderate-Dose Use: Psychological Effects

The mental and emotional effects depend more on the environment (setting) where the drug is used, along with the mood and general psychological makeup of the user (set) (Peele, 1995).

In general, alcohol affects people psychologically by **lowering inhibitions, increasing self-confidence, and promoting sociability.** It calms, relaxes, sedates, and reduces tension. But for someone who is already lonely, depressed, suicidal, or angry, **the depressant and disinhibiting effects of alcohol can deepen negative emotions** including verbal or physical aggressiveness and even violence.

"I started out drinking when I was about 15 out of peer pressure but it made me forget about everything. It felt like a whole new way of life. I was happy, I was gregarious, I was outgoing—more extroverted I guess. I love dancing and I thought I was Ginger Rogers in that I thought I could do anything."
42-year-old recovering alcoholic

Unfortunately alcohol's **disinhibiting effect at low-to-moderate doses** in both men and women can result in problems such as automobile crashes and legal problems. Disinhibition can also cause **high-risk sexual activity** leading to unwanted pregnancies and sexually transmitted diseases, including HIV/AIDS.

"When I used, my behavior was really dangerous. I'd do things that normal people wouldn't do. I was very promiscuous, I had a lot of unsafe sex. I contracted hepatitis C. I don't know if I'm HIV. I get tested periodically but I'm like, very high risk. I've also had numerous STDs."
37-year-old recovering female alcoholic

Neurotransmitters, Inhibition, & Other Effects

Alcohol's psychological effects are caused by its alteration of neuro-

chemistry in the higher centers of the cortex that control reasoning and judgment and the lower centers of the limbic system that rule mood and emotion. Most psychoactive drugs affect just a few types of receptors or neurotransmitters, e.g., anandamide for marijuana or norepinephrine, epinephrine, and dopamine for cocaine. Alcohol on the other hand interacts with receptors, neurotransmitters, cell membranes, intracellular signaling enzymes, and even genes to a greater extent.

◊ Alcohol initially elevates mood by causing the release of **serotonin** (a key mood neurotransmitter) then depletes it with excess use; scarcity causes depression.

◊ **Dopamine** release at multilevels of alcohol use gives a surge of pleasure in the mesolimbic dopaminergic reward pathway as does **norepinephrine** release.

◊ **Met-enkephalin** release by drinking reduces pain.

◊ **Glutamate** release causes stimulation thus reinforcing the drinking.

◊ The alcohol-induced release of **endorphins** and **anandamide** also enhances the reinforcing effect.

◊ In addition alcohol reduces excitatory neurotransmission at the **NMDA receptors** (a subtype of glutumate receptors) inhibiting their reactions and affecting memory and movement (Stahl, 2000).

◊ **Most importantly alcohol causes GABA (the major inhibitory neurotransmitter in the brain)** to enhance neurotransmission at the GABA-A receptor thus lowering psychological inhibitions and eventually slowing down all of the brain processes (Valenzuela & Harris, 1997).

"I always had to use alcohol to be able to socialize. If I go to the party and I'm not drinking, I wouldn't be able to function. I felt like I couldn't dance right or everybody was looking at me, just really uncomfortable. One or two drinks, that'd loosen me up and then I'd keep going 'til I got to a level that I wanted to be at. Where I thought that I was acceptable."
43-year-old recovering alcoholic

Low-to-Moderate-Dose Use: Sexual Effects

Alcohol's physical effects on sexual functioning are closely related to blood alcohol levels. **In low doses alcohol usually increases desire in males and females, often heightening the intensity of orgasm in females and slightly decreasing erectile ability and delaying ejaculation in males** (Blume, 1997).

"It's no mystery why guys in college fraternities, many of whom don't have all that much money, still come up with plenty of money to have outrageous amounts of alcohol and let any woman in for free. The whole point is they're setting up an environment whereby people are going to get more drunk. Women's inhibitions and a guy's inhibitions are going to get lowered."
23-year-old college peer counselor

More than any other psychoactive drug, alcohol has insinuated itself in the lore, culture, and mythology of sexual and romantic behavior: a beer "keg-ger" party to look for a date, a glass of wine before sex, or champagne to celebrate an anniversary. Almost half of a group of 90,000 college students at a number of 2- and 4-year institutions believed that alcohol facilitates sexual opportunities (Presley et al., 1997). Whether it does so because of actual psychological and physiological changes or because of expectations that it will is still open to question.

"When I drink, I wasn't drinking to have sex. I wasn't gonna say, okay, I'm gonna drink this beer and then sit here so a guy can uh, take me in the bedroom and have sex with me. No. In fact I never had sex when I was drunk because of the fact that you could end up having sex with a guy you don't even know that has AIDS or something."
20-year-old female college student

The acceptability of using alcohol in sexual situations extends to high school students. A survey done for the U. S. Surgeon General found that 18% of high school females and 39% of high school males say it is acceptable for a boy to force sex if the girl is stoned or drunk (U.S. Surgeon General, 1992).

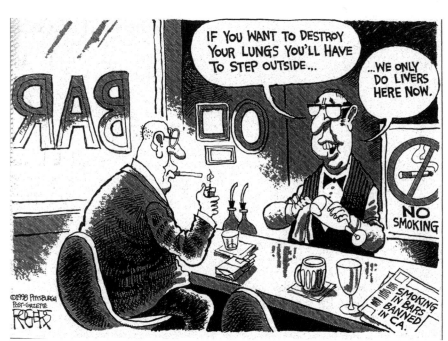

© 1998 Pittsburgh Post-Gazette, Rogers. Reprinted, by permission. All rights reserved

HIGH-DOSE EPISODES

High-Dose Use: Physical Effects of Intoxication

Intoxication is a combination of psychological mood, expectation, mental/physical tolerance, and past drinking experience as well as the physiological changes caused by elevated blood alcohol levels. However, the effects of intoxication can be partially masked by experienced drinkers (behavioral tolerance).

"When a man drinks wine he begins to be better pleased with himself, and the more he drinks the more he is filled full of brave hopes, and conceit of his power, and at last the string of his tongue is loosened, and fancying

---

Level of Impairment vs. Blood Alcohol Concentration

.00 Blood Alcohol Concentration

Lowered inhibitions, relaxation
Some loss of muscular coordination
Decreased alertness
Reduced social inhibitions
Impaired ability to drive
Further loss of coordination
Slowed reaction time
Clumsiness, exaggerated emotions
Unsteadiness standing or walking
Hostile behavior
Exaggerated emotions
Slurred speech
Severe intoxication
Inability to walk without help
Confused speech
Incapacitation, loss of feeling
Difficulty in rousing
Life-threatening unconsciousness
Coma
Death from lung and heart failure

.50 Blood Alcohol Concentration

Figure 5-4 •

As consumption increases, the amount of alcohol absorbed increases and therefore the effects increase but at different rates depending on the physical and mental makeup of the drinker.

---

himself wise, he is brimming over with lawlessness, and has no more fear or respect, and is ready to do or say anything."
Athenian Stranger in *The Laws* by Plato, 360 B.C.

Binge drinking is defined as consuming 5 or more drinks at one sitting for males and 4 or more for females. About 44% of college students say they are binge drinkers and 21% (of the total) say they binge frequently (Wechsler et al., 2002). Adults between 21 and 25 went on drinking binges an average of 18 times in the past year while those between 18 and 20 did it 15 times (Bellandi, 2003). Underage binge drinking increased almost 50% since 1993.

Heavy drinking is defined as 5 or more drinks in one sitting at least 5 times a month. Any person who binge drinks is more likely to have hangovers, experience injuries, aggravate medical conditions, damage property, and have trouble with authorities (Presely et al., 1997).

After enough drinks are consumed, the depressant effects of the alcohol take over. Expectation, setting, and the mood of the drinker cease to have a strong influence. Blood pressure is lowered, motor reflexes are slowed, digestion and absorption of nutrients become poor, body heat is lost as blood vessels dilate, and sexual performance is diminished. In fact every system in the body is strongly affected. Slurred speech, staggering, loss of balance and alertness, and mental confusion are all signs of an increased state of intoxication.

High-Dose Use: Alcohol Poisoning (overdose)

If truly large amounts of alcohol are drunk too quickly, severe alcohol poisoning occurs with **depression of the central nervous system (CNS) possibly leading to respiratory and cardiac failure then to unconsciousness (passing out), coma, and death**. Some clinicians use a BAC level of .40 as the threshold for alcohol poisoning. When other depressants, including

sedative-hypnotics or opiates, are used, the danger is greatly increased because metabolism of alcohol takes precedence over metabolism of other substances thus delaying neutralization and elimination of those other drugs. Symptoms also include reduced body temperature and low blood pressure.

However even blood alcohol concentration levels of .20 or greater, especially in individuals who have low tolerance, can result in severely depressed respiration and vomiting while semiconscious. The vomit can be aspirated or swallowed, blocking air passages to the lungs, resulting in asphyxiation and death. This can also cause infections in the lungs.

High-Dose Use: Blackouts

About one-third of drinkers report experiencing at least one blackout while the percentage doubles for alcohol-dependent individuals especially during heavy drinking bouts (Schuckit, 2000). **During blackouts, a person seems to be acting normally and is awake and conscious but afterwards cannot recall anything that was said or done.** Sometimes even a small amount of alcohol may trigger a blackout. Blackouts, which are caused by an alcohol-induced electrochemical disruption of the brain, are often early indications of alcoholism. They are different from passing out or loss of consciousness during a drinking episode since any drinker can pass out from too much alcohol. **A drinker can also have only partial recall of events, which is known as a "brownout."**

A possible indicator of susceptibility to blackouts and brownouts and therefore a marker for alcoholism can be seen on an electroencephalogram (EEG). The marker is a dampening of the P3 or P300 brain wave that affects cognition, decision-making, and processing of short-term memory. **This dampening is found in alcoholics and their young sons** but generally not in individuals without a drinking problem (Begleiter, 1980; Blum et al., 2000). Other researchers found that auditory P300 amplitude waves are reduced in alcoholics, particularly in those with anxiety disorders (Enoch, White, Harris, Rohrbaugh, & Goldman, 2001).

"With alcohol I was out of control because I would drink to the point where I didn't know what I was doing, which made it easier for the man to do whatever he wanted and my not realizing it until the next day or the next morning when I woke up and didn't have any recollection of what had happened."

32-year-old recovering female binge drinker

High-Dose Use: Hangover

A hangover is the body's response to excessive amounts of alcohol. The effects of **a hangover can be most severe many hours after alcohol has been completely eliminated** from the system. Typical effects include nausea, vomiting, headache, thirst, dizziness, mood disturbances, abbreviated sleep, sensitivity to light and noise, dry cottony mouth, inability to concentrate, and a general depressed feeling. Hangovers can occur with any stage of drinking from experimentation to addiction. More severe **withdrawal symptoms usually occur with chronic high-dose users**.

Some research shows that those with a high genetic susceptibility to alcoholism suffer more severe hangover and withdrawal symptoms and often continue drinking to find relief (NIAAA, 1998; Span & Earleywine, 1999).

The causes of hangover are not clearly understood. Additives (congeners) in alcoholic beverages are thought to be partly responsible although even pure alcohol can cause hangovers. Irritation of the stomach lining by alcohol may contribute to intestinal disorders. Low blood sugar, dehydration, and tissue degradation may also play their parts. Symptoms vary according to individuals but it is evident that the greater the quantity of alcohol consumed, the more severe the aftereffects (Swift & Davidson, 1998).

High-Dose Use: Sobering Up

A person can control the amount of alcohol in the blood by controlling the amount drunk and the rate at which it is drunk. But the **elimination of alcohol from the system is a constant**. As mentioned, the body metabolizes alcohol at the rate of $\frac{1}{4}$ oz. to $\frac{1}{3}$ oz. of pure alcohol per hour. Until the alcohol has been eliminated and until hormones, enzymes, body fluids, and bodily systems come into equilibrium, hangover symptoms will persist. An analgesic may lessen the headache pain while fruit juice can help hydrate the body and correct low blood sugar but **neither coffee, nor exercise, nor a cold shower cures a hangover. Feeling better comes only with rest and sufficient recovery time.** One danger of using acetaminophen (Tylenol®) to relieve a hangover-induced headache while alcohol is still in the system is the chance of liver damage.

High-Dose Use: Mental & Emotional Effects

"I remember being beat up physically and being emotionally abused and drinking a gallon of wine and feeling like I just wanted to be out of it. And for me, that was the way to deal with the pain. I think women tend to do those things; either they'll take drugs with the perpetrator to have some kind of relationship or after they've been beat up, use alcohol or drugs as a way not to deal with the pain."

39-year-old ex-wife of abuser

High-dose alcohol use depresses other functions of the central and peripheral nervous systems. Initial relaxation and lowered inhibitions at low doses often become **mental confusion, mood swings, loss of judgment, and emotional turbulence at higher doses**. At a BAC of .10, a drinker may demonstrate slurred speech and beyond that level, progressive mental confusion and loss of emotional control. Heavy alcohol consumption before sleep, as with light-to-moderate consumption, may also interfere with the REM or dreaming sleep essential to

feeling fully rested. Chronic alcoholics may suffer from fatigue during the day and insomnia at night as well as nightmares, bed wetting, and snoring.

CHRONIC HIGH-DOSE USE

"In the past year due to my alcoholism and drug addiction, I have had two overdoses. I have been in Two North, that is the mental ward of the hospital. I have set myself on fire, passed out with a cigarette in my hand, and I have fallen down all over the place, receiving various broken bones. The last time my husband saw me, I was near death."

43-year-old recovering alcoholic

The effect of long-term alcohol abuse not only on physical health but also on neurochemistry and cellular function is more wide-ranging and profound than most other psychoactive drugs.

Liver Disease

Since about 80% of the alcohol drunk passes through the liver and must be metabolized, high-dose and chronic drinking inevitably affect this crucial organ. In the United States approximately **10–35% of heavy drinkers develop alcoholic hepatitis and 10–20% develop cirrhosis** (NIAAA, 1993).

Alcoholic hepatitis causes inflammation of the liver, areas of fibrosis, necrosis (cell death), and damaged membranes. It can take months or years of heavy drinking to develop this condition that is manifested by jaundice, liver enlargement, tenderness, and pain. It is a serious condition that can only be arrested by abstinence from alcohol and even then the scarring of the liver and collateral damage remains (Moddrey, 1988).

Cirrhosis occurs when alcohol kills many liver cells and causes scarring. It is the most advanced form of liver disease caused by drinking and is the leading cause of death among alcoholics. Approximately 10,000 to

TABLE 5–4 RATES OF CIRRHOSIS OF THE LIVER IN THE UNITED STATES

Year	Rate of Cirrhosis per 100,000
1911	17.0
1932	8.0 (end of Prohibition)
1973	14.9
2000	9.6 (26,552 deaths)

(Grant, 1985; Saadatmand, Stinson, Grant, & Dufour, 2000; National Center for Health Statistics, 2002)

24,000 Americans die each year from cirrhosis due to alcohol consumption (DeBakey, Stinson, Grant, & Dufour, 1996). The damaging effects of alcohol to tissues occur not only because alcohol itself is toxic but because the metabolic process produces metabolites, such as free radicals and acetaldehyde, that are even more toxic than alcohol itself (Kurose, Higuchi, Kato, Miura, & Ishii, 1996). Cirrhosis is even less amenable to treatment and cannot be reversed although abstinence can often arrest the progression of the disease.

"I was sick to my stomach and I threw up and little did I know because it was dark that it was blood and I turned on the light and I had a little garbage can there by the bed and the damn thing filled up. There was an artery in my liver that had just exploded I guess and they said when that happens it's a gusher. And so after they put me out, they said you've got cirrhosis very bad. Well they put me on the transplant list. I didn't know it at the time but you have to be sober for a year before they'll even consider transplanting your liver."

65-year-old recovering alcoholic

Over the years liver cirrhosis rates have gone up and down with the rise and fall of alcohol consumption. With the increase in hepatitis C however, many more nonalcohol-related cases of cirrhosis will be altering the statistics.

It is estimated that alcoholic cirrhosis is a major contributing factor in 44–80% of all cases of cirrhosis in the United States (Nidus Information Services, 2002). The prevalence of cirrhosis in the United States also varies from ethnic group to ethnic group, from male to female, and by age. For example, in one study by the National Institute on Alcohol Abuse and Alcoholism (NIAAA), Hispanic men showed the highest cirrhosis mortality rates followed by Black men, White men, Hispanic women, Black women, and White women. A majority of the Hispanic men were of Mexican ancestry. About 2½ times more men than women of all races die from cirrhosis (mostly because more men drink than women).

The drinking habits of various cultures worldwide have a strong effect on the incidence of cirrhosis. **Heavy drinking countries such as France and Germany have rates of cirrhosis 2 to 3 times higher than the United States** (Table 5-5).

A problem with estimates about drinking rates is that in many countries, particularly poorer countries, there are large amounts of unreported alcohol production and consumption. The World Health Organization (WHO) reports that in a country such as Kenya 80–90% of alcohol consumption is not officially reported. In the Russian Federation about one-half of the consumption is unreported, while in Slovenia 40% is unreported (WHO, 2003). In comparing the increase in drinking, the WHO report found that the largest increases in consumption were among developing countries and those in transition, such as former Soviet bloc countries.

Fatty liver, the accumulation of fatty acids in the liver, can begin to occur after just a few days of heavy drinking. Abstention will eliminate much of the accumulated fat.

When the liver becomes damaged due to cirrhosis, fatty liver, or hepatitis, its ability to metabolize alcohol decreases thus allowing the alcohol to travel to other organs in its original toxic form. Even persistent moderate drinking can damage the liver.

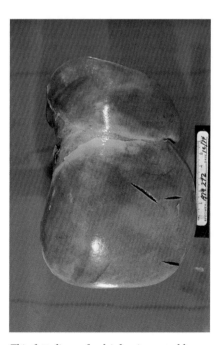

This fatty liver of a drinker is caused by accumulation of fatty acids. When drinking stops, the fat deposits usually disappear.
Courtesy of Boris Ruebner, M.D.

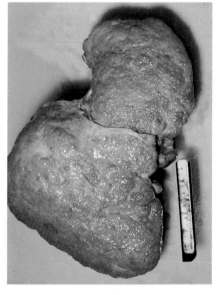

Cirrhosis of the liver usually takes 10 or more years of steady drinking. The toxic effects of alcohol cause scar tissue to replace healthy tissue. This condition remains permanent even when drinking stops.
Courtesy of Boris Ruebner, M.D.

TABLE 5–5   WORLDWIDE PER CAPITA USE OF ALCOHOL VS. INCIDENCE OF CHRONIC LIVER DISEASE

	Alcohol in Liters of Pure Ethanol			Cirrhosis Rate per 100,000		
	Total	Beer	Spirits	Wine	Total	Men	Women
Slovenia	24.19 (est.)	10.79	10.14	3.26	19.6	32.9	8.7
Kenya	17.29 (est.)	8.70	8.40	0.19	N/A	N/A	N/A
Russian Federation	14.49 (est.)	4.38	8.37	1.14	N/A	N/A	N/A
Republic of Korea	14.40	2.41	11.97	0.02	N/A	N/A	N/A
Denmark	14.36	8.15	1.85	4.84	10.4	14.7	6.3
Germany	13.77	8.01	2.50	3.26	15.4	22.6	9.0
France	13.74	2.45	3.01	8.91	12.1	17.8	7.2
Greece	12.51	2.43	4.23	5.88	3.4	5.4	1.6
Ireland	11.90	9.32	2.22	2.35	2.7	2.8	2.5
Spain	11.09	3.86	2.86	4.34	12.2	19.1	6.2
Italy	9.62	1.41	1.06	7.74	13.9	19.6	9.0
Argentina	9.59	2.05	0.42	7.11	8.3	14.3	3.3
Australia	9.55	6.07	1.72	2.78	4.6	7.0	2.4
United Kingdom	9.41	6.34	1.72	1.94	6.4	8.3	4.7
New Zealand	9.21 (est.)	5.11	1.51	2.59	2.6	3.5	1.8
United States	8.90	5.36	2.43	1.12	7.7	10.9	4.8
Japan	7.85	3.21	2.62	0.14	7.2	11.2	3.5
Kazakhstan	7.71	0.47	7.09	0.16	23.9	33.2	16.8
Canada	7.52	4.23	2.16	1.19	5.3	7.5	3.4
Costa Rica	5.72	0.92	4.67	0.12	17.4	25.3	9.9
China	5.39	0.95	4.38	0.06	N/A	N/A	N/A
Israel	1.75	0.81	0.42	0.52	4.9	7.3	2.9
India	0.99	0.04	0.95	0.00	N/A	N/A	N/A
Egypt	0.53	0.05	0.47	0.01	N/A	N/A	N/A
Indonesia	0.13	0.06	0.07	0.00	N/A	N/A	N/A

(WHO, 2003)

Digestive System

Alcohol's other effects on the digestive system are caused by its direct effects on organs and tissues. While lower doses of alcohol can aid digestion, moderate-to-higher doses stimulate the production of stomach acid and delay the emptying time of the stomach. Excessive amounts can cause acid stomach and diarrhea.

"One night I drank a bunch of hard A, and then beer, and then hard A again. And it will really mess up your stomach. So I was, oh, 6 hours into my drinking; I was in the bathroom by the toilet all night long. I couldn't leave.

Every minute I was throwing up and when I couldn't throw up, I was dry heaving. And at the end when I wasn't throwing up anymore, I wanted to drink again."
43-year-old recovering female alcoholic

Gastritis (stomach inflammation) is common among heavy drinkers as are inflammation and irritation of the esophagus, small intestine, and the pancreas (**pancreatitis**). Inflammation of the pancreas is often caused by blockage of pancreatic ducts and overproduction of digestive enzymes. Other serious disorders including **ulcers, stomach hemorrhage, and gastroin-**

testinal bleeding are also linked to heavy drinking. Damage to the liver also causes problems with digestion and proper metabolism.

"I have acid reflux so bad that I can't hold certain things down before it just comes back up—from throwing up alcohol constantly and making my stomach throw up. There are certain things I'm limited to eat; some foods can really make me sick, you know."
34-year-old recovering alcoholic

Alcohol contains calories (about 150 per drink) but almost no vitamins, minerals, or proteins. Heavy drinkers receive energy but little nutritional value from their drinking. As a result **alcoholics may suffer from primary malnutrition**, including vitamin B_1 deficiency leading to beriberi, heart disease, peripheral nerve degeneration, pellagra, scurvy, and anemia (caused by iron deficiency). In addition, because heavy drinking irritates and inflames the stomach and intestines, alcoholics may suffer from secondary malnutrition (especially from distilled alcohol drinks) as a result of faulty digestion and absorption of nutrients, even if they eat a well-balanced diet.

Another problem with alcohol is its effect on the body's sugar supply. **Alcohol can cause hypoglycemia (too little sugar [glucose]) in drinkers who are not getting sufficient nutrition** and have depleted their own stores of glucose. The liver is kept busy metabolizing the alcohol, so it cannot use other nutrients to manufacture more glucose. Blood sugar levels can drop precipitously causing symptoms of weakness, tremor, sweating, nervousness, and hunger. If the levels drop too low, coma is possible, particularly in those with liver damage or diabetics who are insulin dependent. **If there is sufficient nutrition, alcohol use can cause the opposite effect, hyperglycemia (too much sugar)**, in susceptible individuals. This condition is of particular danger to diabetics who have developed a problem controlling their blood sugar in the first place (Kinney, 2002).

Cardiovascular Disease

Though the headlines talk about the positive cardiovascular effect of light-to-moderate drinking, **chronic heavy drinking is related to a variety of heart diseases including hypertension** (high blood pressure) and cardiac arrhythmias (abnormal irregular heart rhythms) (Klatsky, 1988). Heavy drinking increases the risk of hypertension by a factor of 2 or 3 (He, 2001). Coronary diseases occur in alcohol-dependent people at a rate up to 6 times normal (Schuckit, 2000).

Since acetaldehyde, a metabolite of

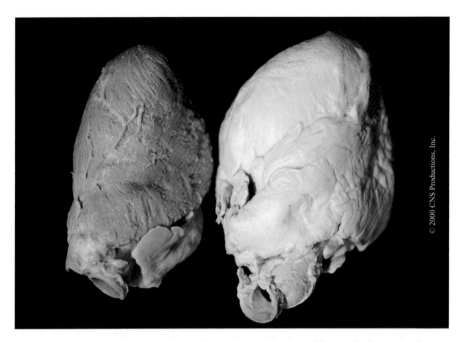

On the left is a normal heart. On the right is a fatty and enlarged heart of a heavy drinker.

alcohol, damages striated heart muscles directly, **cardiomyopathy, an enlarged, flabby, and inefficient heart**, is often found in chronic heavy drinkers. The heart of a heavy drinker can be twice the size of a normal heart. One form of irregular heart rhythm is called "holiday heart syndrome" because it appears in patients from Sundays through Tuesdays or around holidays after a large amount of alcohol has been consumed. Heavy drinking **increases the risk of stroke** and other intracranial bleeding within 24 hours of a drinking binge (Geller, 1997). The exact mechanism for many of the cardiovascular problems is not definitely known but the connection is clear.

Nervous System

Alcohol limits the brain's ability to use glucose and oxygen thus killing brain cells as well as inhibiting message transmission. Low-to-moderate use does not seem to cause permanent functional loss whereas **chronic high-dose use causes direct damage to nerve cells**. Alcohol-induced malnutrition can also injure brain cells and disrupt brain chemistry.

Both physical brain damage and impaired mental abilities have been linked to advanced alcoholism. Brain atrophy (loss of brain tissue) has been documented in 50–100% of alcoholics at autopsy. Breathing and heart rate irregularities caused by damage to the brain's autonomic nervous system have also been traced to brain atrophy. **Dementia (deterioration of intellectual ability, faulty memory, disorientation, and diminished problem-solving ability) is a further consequence of prolonged heavy drinking.**

One of the more serious diseases due to brain damage caused by chronic alcoholism and thiamin (vitamin B_1) deficiency is **Wernicke's encephalopathy** whose symptoms include delirium, visual problems, imbalance, and muscle tremors. The other serious condition that involves thiamin deficiency is **Korsakoff's psychosis**. Its symptoms include disorientation, memory failure, and repetition of false memories (confabulation) (Goodwin & Gabrielli, 1997).

Hippocrates wrote about the association between alcohol and seizures/epilepsy more than 2,000 years ago. The prevalence of epilepsy is up to 10 times greater in those with alcoholism (Devantag, Mandich, Zaiotti, & Toffolo, 1983). While the seizures could be caused by head trauma due to drunkenness or other causes, the direct damage to neurological systems as well as the adrenaline storm caused by withdrawal are strongly implicated.

Reproductive System

Female. While light drinking lowers inhibitions, prolonged use **decreases desire and the intensity of orgasm**. In one study of chronic female alcoholics, 36% said they had orgasms less than 5% of the time. Chronic alcohol abuse can inhibit ovulation, decrease the gonadal mass, delay menstruation, and cause sexual dysfunction (Blume, 1997). Heavy drinking also raises the chances of infertility and spontaneous abortion.

Male. Though low-to-moderate levels of alcohol can lower inhibitions and enhance the psychological aspects of sexual activity, the depressant effects soon take over. Chronic use causes effects beyond a temporary inability to perform. Long-term alcohol abuse **impairs gonadal functions and causes a decrease in testosterone** (male hormone) levels. Decreased testosterone causes an increase in estrogen (a female hormone) that can lead to male breast enlargement, testicular atrophy, low sperm count, loss of body hair, and loss of sexual desire. **About 8% of alcoholics are impotent and only half can recover sexual function during sobriety.** When returning to sexual activity, a recovering alcoholic may experience excessive anxiety; dysfunction can be intensified by one or two bad performances.

One of the most long-lasting effects of alcohol abuse is the resulting inability to experience normal sexual relationships because, before sobriety, meeting people of the opposite sex often occurred in bars or at parties where alcohol was readily available.

"I don't really remember making love with a woman when I was sober. It was usually when I had a couple of drinks in me or if I was that far gone, then I would probably go with the woman or bring the woman home, and I would go to bed with her, and I would probably fall asleep."
43-year-old recovering alcoholic

Cancer

Breast Cancer. The association between heavier drinking (3 or more drinks a day) and breast cancer is clear. The evidence is less compelling concerning the association between drinking small amounts of alcohol and the incidence of breast cancer. In one study of 1,200 women with breast cancer there was an association between moderate alcohol use and breast cancer—even amounts as low as 1 drink a day increased the risk by 50%. In fact 25% of all breast cancer was associated with even brief use of alcohol (Bowlin, 1997). However, other studies have found only small increases in the incidence of breast cancer (Ellison, Zhang, McLennan, & Rothman, 2001).

Other Cancers. The risk of mouth, throat, larynx, and esophageal cancer are 6 times greater for heavy alcohol users**, 7 times greater for smokers, and an astonishing **38 times greater for those who smoke and drink alcohol** (Blot, 1992). Some studies give different rates of cancer in heavy drinkers but the increase is there in all cases (Bagnardi, Blangiardo, Vecchia, & Corrao, 2001).

Systemic Problems

Musculoskeletal System. Alcohol leeches minerals from the body causing a **much greater risk of a fracture** of the femur, the wrist, vertebrae, and the ribs. The unbalancing of electrolytes by chronic or acute use, along with direct toxic effects, can cause myopathy (painful swollen muscles).

Dermatologic Complications. The reddish complexion of chronic alcoholics is caused by **acne rosacea, psoriasis, eczema, and facial edema**, all of which are potentiated by the toxic effects of alcohol. Skin problems also arise from nutritional deficiencies.

Immune System. Excessive drinking has been linked to infectious diseases such as respiratory infections, tuberculosis, pneumonia, and cancer. Heavy drinking may **disrupt white blood cells** and in other ways weaken the immune system, resulting in greater susceptibility to infections.

Other Susceptibilities. Alcohol can contribute to a host of other problems including atrophied muscle fibers resulting in flabby muscles and weight loss (more so for women than men).

Chronic High-Dose Use: Mental/Emotional Effects

With chronic high-dose use, almost **any mental, emotional, or psychiatric symptom is a possibility** including memory problems, hallucinations, paranoia, severe depression, insomnia, and intense anxiety. These symptoms, particularly amnesia and blackouts, become more common as alcohol abuse progresses. In addition to specific conditions one of the more general long-term mental/emotional effects is the inability to learn problem-solving techniques that help one cope with life.

"I think for the most part 16, 17, 18 year-olds are pretty comfortable with, you know, dealing with people of the opposite sex. When you're drunk and dealing with that whole part of your life at that age, you kinda sidestep the awkward part and you never get any confidence built up without having some kind of a social lubricant."
43-year-old recovering alcoholic

Alcohol and memory problems go hand-in-hand. Alcohol damages activity in frontal lobes making it difficult to concentrate and get information into the brain. Alcohol also damages the memory centers, so heavy drinkers have trouble retaining information not just getting it into the brain.

TABLE 5–6   SOME ALCOHOL-RELATED CAUSES OF DEATH

Diseases *(directly caused by alcohol)*	Diseases *(indirectly caused by alcohol)*	Injuries/Adverse Effects *(indirectly caused by alcohol)*
Alcoholic psychoses	Tuberculosis	Boating accidents
Alcoholism	Cancer of the lips, mouth,	Motor vehicle, bicycle, other road
Alcohol abuse	and pharynx	accidents
Nerve degeneration	Cancer of the larynx, esophagus,	Airplane accidents
Heart disease	stomach, and liver	Falls
Alcoholic gastritis	Diabetes	Fire accidents
Fatty liver	Hypertension	Drownings
Hepatitis	Stroke	Suicides, self-inflicted injuries
Cirrhosis	Pancreatitis	Homicides or shootings
Other liver damage	Diseases of stomach, esophagus, and	Choking on food
Excessive BAC	duodenum	Domestic violence
Accidental poisonings	Cirrhosis of bile tract	Rapes or date rapes
Seizure activity		

MORTALITY

Drinking can affect a person's lifespan since heavy drinking increases the chances of dying from disease or trauma. For instance, the average lifespan is shortened 4 years by cancer, 4 years by heart disease, and from 9–22 years for alcoholic liver disease. In one study a difference in lifespan was found even between abstainers (defined as 12 drinks or less per year) and light drinkers (1–2 drinks per day) (Vaillant, 1995; NIAAA, 2000). Overall **if people continue heavy drinking, they are likely to die 15 years earlier than the general population** (Moos, Brennan, & Mertens, 1994).

ADDICTION (alcohol dependence, alcoholism)

◇ About **10–12% of the 140 million adult drinkers in the United States have developed addiction**.

◇ The incidence of **alcoholism in men is approximately 2 to 3 times greater than in women** (14% of male drinkers vs. 6% of female drinkers).

◇ Onset of alcoholism usually occurs at a younger age in men than in women.

◇ In terms of consumption, **20% of drinkers consume 80% of all alcohol** (Greenfield & Rogers, 1999).

CLASSIFICATION

Early Classifications

Over the years there have been many attempts to classify different types of alcoholism. **The purpose of classification is to develop a framework by which an illness or condition can be studied systematically** rather than relying strictly on experience.

One of the earliest attempts at imposing scientific reasoning on drinking was by **Dr. Benjamin Rush**, physician, medical educator, patriot, reformer, and the first U.S. Surgeon General. He published the first American treatise on alcoholism in 1804—*An Inquiry into the Effects of Ardent Spirits on the Human Body and Mind*. It was a compendium of current attitudes towards abuse of alcohol.

At about the same time, **Dr. Thomas Trotter** in *An Essay, Medical, Philosophical and Chemical, on Drunkenness and Its Effects on the Human Body* expounded, in scientific terms, his thesis that drunkenness was a disease produced by a remote cause that disrupts health.

According to scientific literature from the nineteenth and early twentieth centuries, researchers developed dozens of classifications of alcoholics, e.g., acute, periodic, and chronic oenomania; habitual inebriate; continuous and explosive inebriate; and dipsomaniac among others.

It wasn't until the 1930s that scientific progress on the study of alcoholism really accelerated with the experiences of the newly created **Alcoholics Anonymous** and the founding of **Yale's Laboratory of Applied Psychology** (Trice, 1995). Researchers Yandell Henderson, Howard Haggard, Leon Greenberg, and later E. M. Jellinek made the study of alcoholism scientifically respectable, aided by their founding of the *Quarterly Journal of Studies on Alcoholism* and the Yale Center of Alcohol Studies.

E. M. Jellinek

In 1941 psychiatrist Karl Bowman and biometrist E. M. Jellinek presented an integration of 24 classifications of alcoholism that had appeared over the years in scientific literature, reducing alcoholics into four types:

◇ primary or true alcoholics: immediate liking for alcohol and rapid development of an uncontrollable need;

◇ steady endogenous symptomatic drinkers: alcoholism is secondary to a major psychiatric disorder;

◇ intermittent endogenous symptomatic drinkers: periodic binge drinking, again often with a psychiatric disorder;

◇ stammtisch drinkers: drinkers in whom alcoholism is precipitated by outside causes, often start as social drinkers.

Twenty years later Jellinek, in his landmark book *The Disease Concept of Alcoholism*, proposed five types of alcoholism: alpha, beta, gamma, delta, and epsilon. Gamma and delta alcoholics were considered true alcoholics (Jellinek, 1961).

◇ **Gamma alcoholics** mainly have a high psychological vulnerability but also a high physiological vulnerability; they develop tissue tolerance rapidly; they lose control quickly; and their progression to uncontrolled use is marked.

◇ **Delta alcoholics** mainly have strong sociocultural and economic influences, along with a high physiological vulnerability; they also acquire tissue dependence rapidly and it's hard for them to abstain; their progression to alcoholism is much slower than gamma alcoholics.

(Babor, 1996; Jellinek, 1961)

Modern Classifications

As valuable as Jellinek's classification was, the scientific basis for alcoholism wasn't as clear cut as with other illnesses and conditions. Four developments starting in the 1950s led to a deeper understanding of alcoholism as a biological phenomenon.

◇ First was the **discovery of the nucleus accumbens**, the area of the brain that gives a surge of pleasure and a desire to repeat the action when stimulated by an experience, by electricity, or by psychoactive drugs (Olds & Milner, 1954; Olds, 1956; Heath, 1995).

◇ Next was the **discovery of endogenous neurotransmitters**, starting in the '70s, that showed that drugs worked by influencing existing neurological pathways and receptor

sites in the central nervous system including the reward pathway that researchers had hinted at in the '50s and '60s (Goldstein, 2001).

◇ In the '80s and '90s **genetic research tools** developed insights into hereditary influences on addiction; in 1990 the first gene (DRD_2A_1 allele) that seemed to have an influence on vulnerability to alcoholism was discovered (Noble, Blum, Montgomery, & Sheridan, 1991; Blum et al., 2000).

◇ In the 1990s and 2000s **imaging techniques** visualized the actual reaction of the brain to drugs (Volkow, Wang, & Doria, 1995).

These developments moved classification of alcoholism and addiction away from qualitative classification towards a more quantifiable and empirical basis.

Type I & Type II Alcoholics. These studies were based on an extensive study of Swedish adoptees and their biological or adoptive parents by Dr. C. Robert Cloninger and colleagues. Type I alcoholism (also called "milieu-limited") was defined as a later-onset syndrome that can affect both men and women. It requires the presence of a genetic and environmental predisposition, it can be moderate or severe, and takes years of drinking to trigger it (much like Jellinek's delta alcoholic). Type II alcoholism (also called "male-limited") mostly affects sons of male alcoholics, is moderately severe, is primarily genetic, and is only mildly influenced by environmental factors (Bohman, Sigvardson, & Cloninger, 1981; Cloninger, Bohman, & Sigvardson, 1996).

Type A & Type B Alcoholics. Dr. T. F. Babor and his research colleagues at the University of Connecticut School of Medicine introduced the A/B typologies in 1992. They are similar to Dr. C. Robert Cloninger's type I/II typologies. Type A, like type I, is a later onset of alcoholism, less family history of alcoholism, and less severe dependence. Type B, like type II, refers to a more severe alcoholism with an earlier on-

set, more impulsive behavior and conduct problems or disorders, more co-occurring mental disorders, and more severe dependence (Babor et al., 1992).

The Disease Concept of Alcoholism

Much of the current research in the treatment of alcoholism is based on the disease concept. The idea of alcoholism as a disease goes back thousands of years but only recently has the concept become widely accepted.

◇ In 1972 the National Council on Alcoholism developed *Criteria for the Diagnosis of Alcoholism, Signs and Symptoms* and defined it as a "chronic progressive disease, incurable but treatable."

◇ In 1980 the American Psychiatric Association (APA) made Substance Use Disorders a separate major diagnostic category in their *Diagnostic and Statistical Manual of Mental Disorders (DSM-III)* (American Psychiatric Association, 2000).

◇ *The Natural History of Alcoholism* published in 1983 by Dr. George Vaillant, Professor of Psychiatry at Harvard Medical School, was based mostly on a long-term study of 2 groups of men (college students vs. inner-city young men). His major conclusions were that poverty and preexisting personality or psychological problems were not predictors of the development of alcoholism but rather the symptoms or consequences of alcohol dependence. The predictors of alcoholism were much more likely to be a family history of alcoholism and/or an environment with a high rate of alcoholism.

◇ In 1994 remission and substance-induced conditions were defined in *DSM-IV.*

◇ The latest edition of the APA manual, *DSM-IV-TR*, lists Alcohol Dependence and Alcohol Abuse under Alcohol Use Disorders. Under Alcohol-Induced Disorders they list Alcohol Intoxication, Alcohol Withdrawal, Delirium, and 10 other conditions.

Both the World Health Organization (WHO) and the American Medical Association (AMA) view alcoholism as a specific disease entity (O'Brien & Chafetz, 1991). In 1992 a medical panel from the American Society of Addiction Medicine (ASAM) and the National Council on Alcoholism and Drug Dependence (NCADD) defined alcoholism as follows:

"Alcoholism is a primary chronic disease with genetic, psychosocial, and environmental factors influencing its development and manifestation. The disease is often progressive and fatal. It is characterized by impaired control over drinking, preoccupation with the drug (alcohol), use of alcohol despite adverse consequences, and distortions in thinking, most notably denial. Each of these symptoms may be continuous or periodic" (Morse, Flavin, et al., 1992).

"I don't consider myself an alcoholic. I have five drinks a day—and that's an average. It's always three and sometimes it's a lot more but it's never interfered with my work. I haven't been to the doctor for 15 years. But since it's never interfered with my work, I see nothing wrong with sitting down and having a drink."
Avowed habitual drinker

HEREDITY, ENVIRONMENT, & PSYCHOACTIVE DRUGS

Instead of focusing on typologies, it is useful to look at alcoholism and addiction as continuums of severity that depend, to varying degrees, on genetic predisposition, environmental influences (family, workplace, school, community, or even diet), and from the action of alcohol and other psychoactive drugs themselves, which can alter the body's neurochemistry and instill craving (*see Chapter 2*).

Heredity

"... women who drink wine excessively give birth to children who drink excessively of wine."
Aristotle, 350 B.C.

As early as the fourth century B.C., the philosopher Aristotle wrote about the tendency of alcohol abuse to run in families but it hasn't been until the last 40 years that the scientific basis for this belief has been explored.

"I think that there are genes that impact a variety of different characteristics that increase or decrease your risk for alcoholism. We already know the genes related to the alcohol-metabolizing enzymes; some very good laboratories are closing in on some of the genes likely to contribute to disinhibition. Other laboratories are certainly actively searching for genes that might indirectly increase your risk for alcoholism through psychiatric disorders, such as schizophrenia and bipolar disorder. And our group and others are searching for the genes that are contributing to the low response to alcohol, which indirectly increases your risk for alcoholism in a heavy drinking society (Schuckit, Edenberg, Kalmijn, et al., 2001). Obviously there are going to be a whole slew of genes that contribute to the alcoholism risk but altogether they're explaining a very important part of the picture, probably 60% of the risk."
Marc Schuckit, M.D., Professor of Psychiatry, University of California Medical School, San Diego, CA

Family studies, twin studies, animal studies, and adoption studies show strong genetic influences particularly in severe alcoholism (Nutt, 1998; Anthenelli & Schuckit, 1998; Knop, Goodwin, Teasdale, Mikkelsen, & Schulsinger, 1984; Blum, Cull, Braverman, & Comings, 1996; Li, Lumeng, McBride, & Chao, 1986; Goodwin & Gabrielli, 1997). A twin study that assessed alcohol-related disorders among 3,516 twins in Virginia concluded that the genetic influence was 48–58% of the various influences, a rate much higher than postulated in the past (Prescott & Kendler, 1999). It is theorized that **several genes have an influence**

on one's susceptibility to alcoholism and other drug addictions. A person could have one, several, or all of the genes that make someone susceptible to addiction not just a single gene such as the dopamine DRD_2 A_1 allele receptor gene (Blum et al., 2000). The drinker could have a defective $ALDH_2$ gene that encodes aldehyde dehydrogenase, a key liver enzyme that helps metabolize alcohol. The gene is more prevalent in Asians. Because the defective gene means less enzyme to rid the body of alcohol, its presence acts as a preventive to alcoholism because the person becomes uncomfortable or ill after even a few drinks. In addition about half of all Japanese, along with some other Asian populations (e.g., Chinese), are born with a more efficient ADH (alcohol dehydrogenase), called "atypical ADH," and a less efficient form of ALDH, known as "KM $ALDH_1$." Thus when they drink even small amounts of alcohol, the toxic acetaldehyde builds up (up to 10 times the normal amount) and causes a flushing reaction due to vasodilation. Tachycardia and headaches also occur. At higher doses, edema (water retention), hypotension, and vomiting ensue (Goedde, Harada, & Agarwal, 1979; Teng, 1981; Woodward, 1998). Though Asians have a higher rate of abstention and lower rate of alcoholism, Asian Americans' rate of alcoholism is higher, showing that environmental and cultural influences can overcome biological propensities (Lee, 1987).

Other markers for a strong genetic influence are a tendency to have blackouts, a greater initial tolerance to alcohol, an impaired decision-making area of the brain, a major shift in personality while drinking, an impaired ability to learn from mistakes, and retrograde amnesia.

"When I was younger I was always surrounded by alcohol and drugs. My mom became an alcoholic, my sister used, and so did my two stepbrothers and stepsister. My stepdad also used to grow [marijuana]. So I was kind of around it a lot."
19-year-old recovering alcoholic

There also seems to be a hereditary link to the physical consequences of alcoholism, especially cirrhosis and alcoholic psychosis; concordance (agreement) rates were 0.47 for cirrhosis and 0.61 for alcoholic psychosis (Reed, Pagte, Viken, & Christian, 1996).

Environment

For other people the **environmental factors** are the overwhelming influences: child abuse, poor nutrition, alcohol/other drug-abusing friends and relations, and extreme stress.

"I remember holidays, it being pretty disgusting; my father would be pretty intoxicated. And I remember the Tooth Fairy, the Easter Bunny and Santa Claus all smelling the same way."
23-year-old recovering alcoholic

Alcohol & Other Drugs

For some the toxic effects of **alcohol and other drugs that change neurochemistry** are most important.

"After a while it got to the point where I didn't care what it tasted like. You just wanted that buzz to keep going. The brain was craving alcohol. It was the hard liquor and the higher volume of alcohol involved with it, I think. To this day I still like the taste of Jack Daniels® and I watch myself real close."
Recovering 32-year-old alcoholic

In the end what is important varies with the point of view of the person involved.

◇ To a researcher or scientist, classification and a systematic view of the science of alcoholism is important.

◇ To a psychiatrist, counselor, or social worker, the environmental factors and neurochemical effects of addiction are important because they lead to strategies to counteract craving and lack of control.

◇ To the problem drinker or alcoholic, any help, knowledge, or methods that will keep them sober and lessen the craving are important.

◇ To all involved, understanding the harm that chronic use can cause is important.

"Most alcohol-dependent people or drug-dependent people, when terrible crises occur, they can stop. Their trouble however is staying stopped. So when they go back to use, whether it's the first or the thirtieth time they use, you can bet money that one of those times, they won't be able to stop and problems are going to develop dramatically."
Marc Schuckit, M.D., Professor of Psychiatry, University of California Medical School, San Diego, CA

TOLERANCE, TISSUE DEPENDENCE, & WITHDRAWAL

"Exposure of the brain to alcohol initiates a process of adaptation that works to counteract the altered brain function resulting from initial exposure to alcohol. This adaptation or change in brain function is responsible for the processes called 'alcohol tolerance,' 'alcohol dependence,' and 'alcohol withdrawal syndrome' (NIAAA, 2000, p. 69)."

Tolerance

Tolerance is a process through which the brain defends itself against the effects of alcohol. The rate at which tolerance develops varies widely among drinkers. Dispositional (metabolic) tolerance, pharmacodynamic tolerance, behavioral tolerance, and acute tolerance are four ways the body tries to adapt to the effects of alcohol and protect itself. The result of tolerance is that the chronic drinker is able to handle larger and larger amounts of alcohol. It also indicates the body's growing dependence (tissue dependence) as it attempts to maintain its normal physiological balance in the face of alcohol's toxic effects.

"Well I started drinking one beer and then I went on to two. A week later I went on to a six-pack, and then through the years I went on to two six-packs, and then I ended up drinking tequila. I used to drink a fifth of tequila 2 years after I got addicted to the alcohol. So I drank tequila most of the day and I used to numb myself."
38-year-old recovering female alcoholic

Dispositional (metabolic) tolerance means the body changes so that it metabolizes alcohol more efficiently. As a person drinks over a period of time, the liver adapts to create more enzymes to process the alcohol and its metabolite acetaldehyde (Tabakoff, Cornell, & Hoffman, 1992; Lieber, 1998). This accelerated process eliminates alcohol more quickly from the body. It also accelerates the elimination of other prescription drugs lessening their effectiveness. In addition since liver cells are also being destroyed by drinking and by the natural aging process, **the liver eventually becomes less able to metabolize the alcohol, a process called "reverse tolerance."** A heavy

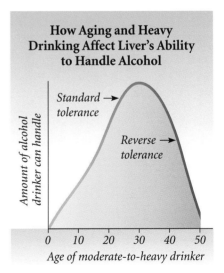

How Aging and Heavy Drinking Affect Liver's Ability to Handle Alcohol

Figure 5-5 •

This graph shows the decrease in liver capacity to process alcohol as a person ages. As the liver is taxed and poisoned by the alcohol, its capacity is diminished to the point where an older chronic drinker can get tipsy on just one drink.

drinker who could handle a fifth of whiskey at the age of 30 can become totally incapacitated by half a pint of wine or less at the age of 50.

Pharmacodynamic tolerance means brain neurons and other **cells become more resistant to the effects of alcohol** by increasing the number of receptor sites needed to produce an effect or by creating other cellular changes that make tissues less responsive to alcohol. When GABA receptors are activated by ethanol, they change over time to become less sensitive not only to ethanol but to GABA, benzodiazepines, and other GABA agonists as well (Valenzuela & Harris, 1997).

Behavioral tolerance means **drinkers learn how to "handle their liquor"** by modifying their behavior or by trying to act in such a way that they hope others won't notice they are inebriated. If they practice acting normally while under the influence, they learn behavioral tolerance more quickly (Vogel-Sprott, Rawana, & Webster, 1984).

Acute tolerance also develops from high-dose alcohol use. **This rapid tolerance starts to develop with the first drink** and is the body's method of providing instant protection to the poisonous effects of ethanol.

Select tolerance means that **tolerance does not develop equally to all the effects of alcohol**, so while a person may learn how to walk steadily with a .14 BAC, they might have trouble performing a task that requires manual dexterity.

Withdrawal

"Your body is going through so many changes, you can't hardly breathe; you're shaking. A hangover, yeah, you might be sick for a couple of hours. That's different than withdrawals but with withdrawals, it will kill you."
32-year-old recovering female alcoholic

As mentioned, hangovers can occur with any level of drinking from experimentation to addiction. More severe withdrawal symptoms occur with chronic high-dose use.

"I hurt so much when I sobered up that I said the heck with this. I said if that's going to kill the pain, I'll go back to drinking and I really thought about it several times and it was a war within myself whether to drink or not drink."
65-year-old recovering alcoholic

In 1 year, more than ½ million drinkers with alcoholism suffered withdrawal symptoms severe enough to require pharmacologic treatment (Griffin, Gross, & Teitelbaum, 1993). A majority of patients develop significant symptoms of withdrawal when they come in for detoxification and treatment for their alcoholism (Saitz & O'Malley, 1997). However, **85–95% of those experiencing withdrawal will only have the more minor symptoms**, not the life-threatening ones (Schuckit, 1996). To the inexperienced eye, minor withdrawal symptoms will look like hangover symptoms. The presence of true withdrawal symptoms is one important indication that the drinker has developed dependence on alcohol. However, the alcoholic coming into treatment will often try to explain away what he/she is feeling as a hangover instead of accepting it as true withdrawal.

Various classic experiments have shown that **minor withdrawal symptoms will develop for people who drink heavily for 7–34 days while major withdrawal symptoms will probably develop after 48–87 consecutive days of heavy drinking** (Isbell, Fraser, Wikler, et al., 1955). Many withdrawal symptoms involve the autonomic nervous system.

Minor symptoms of withdrawal include

◇ rapid pulse,
◇ sweating,
◇ increased body temperature,
◇ hand tremors,
◇ anxiety and/or depression,
◇ insomnia,
◇ nausea or vomiting.

Major symptoms of withdrawal include

◇ tachycardia,
◇ transient visual, tactile, or auditory hallucinations and illusions,
◇ psychomotor agitation,
◇ grand mal seizures,
◇ delirium tremens.

"I was very sick, very nauseous, pains in my stomach, headaches, shaking,

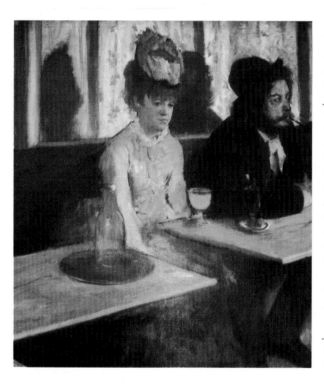

The Absinthe Drinkers *by Edgar Degas, 1876. Absinthe, a distilled liquor that is 68% alcohol, was first produced commercially in 1797. It proved so powerful and dangerous due to a toxin in the wormwood that could cause delirium and death that it was banned in France in 1915 and subsequently by many other countries. Many bohemian artists overindulged in absinthe during the nineteenth century. Currently it is making somewhat of a comeback in the United States and a few European countries. Musée D'Orsay.*

filled with sheer terror. I've never known fear like that in my life. This has been the hardest thing I've had to do but the alternative is worse."
34-year-old recovering alcoholic

Since the main symptoms of severe withdrawal can combine with medical complications, such as malnutrition, pneumonia, depressed respiration, liver problems, or physical damage, medical care for a chronic alcohol abuser or alcoholic needs to be a consideration in any course of treatment.

In less than 1% of serious cases of alcohol withdrawal, full-blown **delirium tremens, called "the DTs,"** occurs. The DTs usually begins 48–96 hours after the last drink in a period of long heavy drinking and can last for 3 to 5 sometimes up to 10 days although some cases have been reported to last up to 50 days (Mayo-Smith, 1998). The dramatic symptoms can include trembling over the whole body, grand mal seizures, severe auditory, visual, and tactile hallucinations, disorientation, insomnia, and delirium. The DTs is **a serious condition requiring hospitalization**. Untreated, the mortality rate ranges from 10–20%.

Neurotransmitters & Withdrawal. Alcohol at first increases the effectiveness of GABA thus blocking the actions of the brain's energy chemicals, making the person drowsy and depressing other body functions. Over time **the brain compensates by creating an excess of energy chemicals and decreasing (down regulating) the number of GABA receptors, resulting in hyperarousal**. During withdrawal the rebound excess of energy chemicals causes anxiety, increased muscular activity, tachycardia, hypertension, and occasionally seizures. The brain becomes less able to control the hyperactivity (Blum & Payne, 1991). Current research also explores the role of serotonin in the alcohol withdrawal process. A 30% reduction in the availability of brainstem serotonin transporters was found in chronic alcoholics, which correlate with their self-reported ratings of depression and anxiety during withdrawal (Heinz, Ragan, Jones, et al., 1998).

Kindling. With many long-term heavy drinkers, a process called "kindling" occurs. What happens is that **repeated bouts of drinking and withdrawal actually intensify subsequent withdrawal symptoms and can cause seizures**. The theory is that the repeated presence of alcohol actually alters brain chemistry, impairing the body's natural defenses against damage from alcohol (Becker, 1998). Kindling is also known as "inverse tolerance."

DIRECTIONS IN RESEARCH

As it becomes more evident that the cause of alcoholism is a combination of heredity, environment, and the toxic effects of alcohol, research has divided itself along those lines. **Research into heredity has focused on identifying the genes that make a user more susceptible to addiction** (e.g., DRD_2A_1 allele, $ALDH_2$).

"If you are going to have a way to intervene therapeutically, what you want to know is which are the most important genes and which are the most important proteins and enzymes that are carrying out the mission of those genes because those are the ideal targets for new medications. Those genes are also changed by our thoughts, by our pleasures, by our experiences and so there's a complicated mixture of the changes of molecules in the brain. I can imagine a day in the future when we will be able to sort out the different kinds of alcoholic subjects and we'll learn that some of them have problems with one transmitter system, others have a problem with a different transmitter system, the end result will still be alcoholism but the treatment designed for those patients will be designed to meet their specific needs."
Ivan Diamond, M.D., Director, Ernest Gallo Clinic and Research Center

Research into environmental causes of alcoholism has focused on **identifying which changes in the addict's surroundings will decrease the use of alcohol and other drugs**. Studies on raising the drinking age, reducing child abuse in the home, limiting sales of alcohol, and lowering stress in everyday life are reported every month in dozens of professional medical and sociological journals worldwide.

Research into **physiological and psychological changes that occur with chronic and high-dose drinking** also keep many researchers occupied. Studying the impact on the immune system, on the development of dispositional and pharmacodynamic tolerance, on the beneficial cardiovascular effects, and on the learning disabilities in drug-affected infants all show promise in identifying risk factors and treatment for alcoholism.

OTHER PROBLEMS WITH ALCOHOL

These groups of problems with alcohol, including polydrug abuse, mental health involvement, violence, suicide, drunk driving, and alcohol use during pregnancy, can occur at almost any level of use although high-dose chronic use and alcoholism are involved most often.

POLYDRUG ABUSE

Most illicit drug users also drink alcohol and most alcohol abusers use other drugs. The reasons vary.

◇ Alcohol taken before using cocaine will prolong and intensify the cocaine's effects by creating the metabolite cocaethylene, which also seems to trigger violence.

◇ Alcohol can be used to come down off a 3-day speed run.

◇ Some drink alcohol to get loaded if the desired shot of heroin or sedative-hypnotic capsule is unavailable.

◊ Drinking alcohol and shooting cocaine together will provide a speedball effect.

◊ Users will switch from alcohol to another addiction when the effects of the alcohol have become too damaging.

"I used downers just to come down off the alcohol because I was so shaky. And then I would try using amphetamines just to lift me up so I wouldn't drink so much. But what I would do was stay awake longer and drink more, so that didn't work."
40-year-old recovering polydrug abuser

As mentioned in Chapter 4, when alcohol is used with another drug, the liver becomes busy metabolizing the alcohol and so the other drug passes through unmetabolized and signifi-

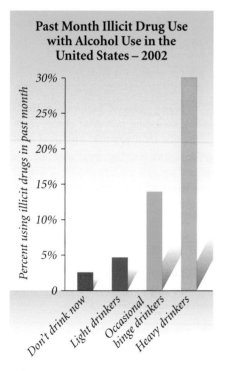

Past Month Illicit Drug Use with Alcohol Use in the United States – 2002

Figure 5-6 •
This chart shows that excessive drinking is associated with the use of other illicit drugs. Whether it's the association with other people who drink and use drugs, the lowering of inhibitions that makes other drug use acceptable, or the desire for stronger and stronger experiences, the association is quite clear.

cantly stronger; thus the chance of overdose becomes much greater.

Polydrug abuse has become so common that treatment centers have had to learn how to treat simultaneous addictions. Although the emotional roots of addiction are similar no matter what drug is used, the physiological and psychological changes that each drug causes, particularly during withdrawal, often have to be treated differently. For example, if a client of the Haight Ashbury Detox Clinic has a serious alcohol and benzodiazepine problem, the Clinic has to be extremely careful detoxifying the client since it can't use a benzodiazepine to control any alcohol withdrawal symptoms.

There is a strong association between smoking and drinking. Approximately **70% of alcoholics are heavy smokers** (more than one pack a day) compared to 10% of the general population. The converse is not as dramatic—smokers are only slightly more likely to drink alcohol compared to nonsmokers. There is also a strong link between early use of tobacco and alcohol. Adolescents who smoke are 3 times more likely to begin using alcohol (Shiffman & Balabanis, 1995).

ALCOHOL & MENTAL PROBLEMS

Alcohol is often used to change one's mood or mental state. The mood could be sadness, boredom, or depression. The mental state could be as mild as confusion or as major as symptoms of an existing mental illness such as major depression, schizophrenia, bipolar illness, panic disorder, or a personality disorder (Petrakis, Gonzalez, Rosenheck, & Krystal, 2002).

The person could **use alcohol (or other drugs) to try to control the symptoms of his/her mental state** or to avoid asking for psychiatric help. For example, a study of adults with panic disorder showed that the subjects reported significantly less anxiety and fewer panic attacks when drinking. Unfortunately the use of alcohol to control the symptoms resulted in a higher rate of alcohol-use disorders

among those with panic disorder (Kushner, Mackenzie, Flazdon, et al., 1996).

An association has been found between drinking and certain mental illnesses. In a study of alcohol-dependent men and women, 4% also had an independent bipolar disorder, 4 times the rate for the general public (Schuckit, Tipp, Bucholz, et al., 1997). Whether the relationship is causal or associative, it is the subject of much debate among professionals in the mental health community and those in the chemical dependency treatment community. In another study alcoholics were

◊ 3.9 times more likely to have another drug abuse disorder,

◊ 6.2 times more likely to have manic-depressive disorder,

◊ 4 times more likely to have schizophrenia (Helzer & Pryzbeck, 1988).

"I would pick up some beer to put me out of it. I didn't like the effect that regular psychiatric drugs, such as antidepressants, had on my brain and I'd rather just put myself out with the booze."
Patient with major depression and an alcohol problem

On the other hand, if alcohol is used to excess, **drinking or withdrawal from drinking can induce symptoms of a mental illness.** For example, a person may use alcohol to escape sadness although chronic alcohol abuse may actually contribute to depression (Miller, Klamen, Hoffman, & Flaherty, 1995).

"The problems did get worse when I was drinking. That was one reason that I never figured out I was a manic-depressive. I figured I was depressed because I was drunk all the time."
Alcoholic who has bipolar illness

For the above reasons, **any psychiatric diagnosis must always take into account the possibility of drug-induced symptoms** and the professional must wait, often weeks or months, for the user's brain chemistry and cognition to rebalance before making an accurate diagnosis (Shivani, Goldsmith, & Anthenelli, 2002). **The majority of alcoholics who come into treatment at the Haight Ashbury Clinic are initially diagnosed as suffering from depression**. The depression can last for as long as a month after abstinence begins but then the number of depressed clients drops dramatically once the drinker is abstinent.

"The alcohol, that came later on. It intensified my depression and intensified everything. I already felt bad about myself and the alcohol just made it worse. It definitely made it worse."
Recovering 16-year-old alcoholic with major depression

Researchers from the Scripps Institute found that heavy drinking disrupts the brain's natural chemicals (opioid peptides, dopamine, serotonin, and GABA) that trigger feelings of wellbeing in the mesolimbic/dopaminergic reward pathway. **Heavy drinking also raises the levels of chemicals that cause tension and depression** (Koob, 1999). The brain tries to compensate for the depletion of neurotransmitters by releasing corticotropin-releasing factor, a stress chemical that unfortunately can induce depression.

On the other end of the spectrum, a diagnosis of alcohol dependence can attribute all of the erratic behavior to the effects of the drug and miss the psychiatric diagnosis. The client keeps relapsing because the more serious and overwhelming psychiatric problems have not been addressed. Experience has shown that if indeed there is a true dual diagnosis or co-occurring disorders, both conditions must be treated in order to achieve an effective recovery.

These problems are especially confusing with psychiatric diagnoses of antisocial personality disorder and borderline personality disorder (BPD). The symptoms of these two illnesses are very common in those who come in for alcohol and other drug abuse treatment. One evaluation of public and private inpatient alcoholic programs

measured the incidence of the antisocial personality disorder at 15% for male alcoholics and 5% for female alcoholics. Conversely **80% of those with antisocial personality disorder develop substance dependence** (Schuckit et al., 1997; Schuckit, 2000). The symptoms of high impulsivity, no remorse for causing harm to others, and inability to learn from mistakes are found in this illness and among drug abusers. In order to diagnosis borderline personality disorder or antisocial personality disorder, the symptoms should exist outside of the drug-seeking/using behavior and should have existed prior to use of the drugs.

In one older study of alcohol treatment admissions, the incidence of BPD was 13% (Nace, Saxon, & Shore, 1983). Among admissions for any drug abuse, the incidence of BPD was 17% (Nace, Saxon, Davis, & Gaspari, 1991). This illness is characterized by intense negative emotions such as depression, self-hatred, anger, and hopelessness and these individuals often use impulsive maladaptive behaviors such as suicidal actions and substance abuse to deal with their feelings. **There is much debate as to the actual incidence of this disease** since it's symptoms often shift from moment to moment and can be drug induced. Some treatment personnel refer to the diagnosis as a "catchall diagnosis" when the real problems aren't clear. However, patients who seem to have these problems are difficult to treat and take up a disproportionate amount of the staff's time.

ALCOHOL & PREGNANCY

Maternal Drinking

"I had been using for years before I got pregnant and when I got pregnant, I tried to stop but I just couldn't do it. I wanted the drug more than I wanted the baby."
27-year-old recovering alcoholic

Alcohol use during pregnancy is the **leading cause of mental retardation in the United States** (Abel & Sokol, 1986; May & Gossage, 2001). Alcohol over-

use during pregnancy also increases the number of miscarriages and infant deaths; there are more problem pregnancies and the newborns are smaller and weaker (NIAAA, 2000).

A survey of pregnant women in the United States found that 12.4% drank some alcohol during several months of pregnancy, 3.9% used in a binge pattern, while 0.7% were heavy drinkers. In addition 5.5% used illicit drugs at least once (SAMHSA, 2002; Morbidity and Mortality Weekly Report, 2002).

Dr. Sarajini Budden, an expert on FAS at Legacy Emmanuel Children's Hospital in Portland, Oregon, did a survey of the mothers of 293 infants born with fetal alcohol syndrome (FAS) or alcohol-related neurodevelopmental disorder (ARND), both caused by heavy drinking. **During their pregnancy about 89% of the women were using alcohol with at least 2 other drugs** and 49% were using just 2 drugs, usually alcohol and cocaine. Interestingly all of them were smoking, so nicotine was included as one of the toxins. Most were single moms, most were school dropouts, most had been or were being physically or sexually abused, and often there was a history of alcohol or drug abuse in the family. There is also a suspicion that a number of the mothers also had learning problems in school and possibly were alcohol or drug affected themselves.

Through the University of Washington in Seattle, 2 groups of children with fetal alcohol syndrome were studied. By the time that the first group was 5 years old, 38% of the biological mothers had died as a direct result of their alcoholism. By the time the second group was in early adolescence, 69% of the biological mothers died as a direct result of their alcoholism.

"Wally's birth mom was a severe alcoholic. I never got to really meet her, to sit down and talk to her but I know that when she went into labor she was in a bar and had fallen off a barstool. And she was so intoxicated that they said that when Wally was born he reeked of alcohol. That's how much she

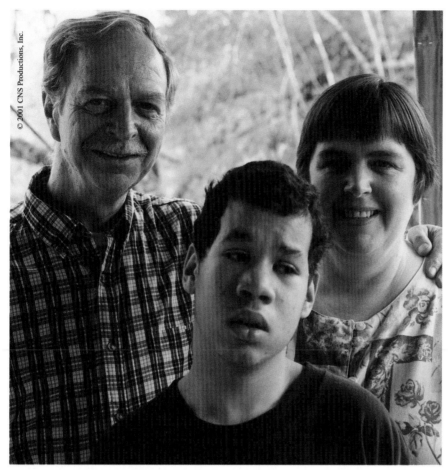

Wally, who was adopted at birth, is seen with his foster parents. The physical abnormalities of fetal alcohol syndrome (FAS) are readily apparent.

● ●

drank. And now she's deceased. She was murdered. It was very sad. He's our little boy but that was who gave life to him. And it was very very hard."
Foster mother of Wally, a 14-year-old with severe FAS and autism

Fetal Alcohol Syndrome (FAS), Alcohol-Related Neurodevelopmental Disorder (ARND), & Alcohol-Related Birth Defects (ARBD)

Certain specific toxic effects of alcohol on the developing fetus are known as "fetal alcohol syndrome" or FAS, a term first coined in 1973 although the diagnosis was first written about in France in 1968 (Jones & Smith, 1973). Initially it was thought that the defects were the result of malnutrition but the **toxicity of alcohol was eventually recognized as the cause**. The de-

fects can range from obvious gross physical defects, to mental deficits, to behavioral problems. In 1996 the Institute of Medicine of the National Academy of Sciences reclassified the effects of prenatal alcohol exposure into five categories. Three categories refer to the facial features and two categories are for alcohol-affected infants without the specific facial features. The last two categories are ARND, in which there's evidence of CNS abnormality, and alcohol-related birth defects (ARBD), in which there are any number of physical anomalies (Stratton, Howe, & Battaglia, 1996). ARND and ARBD used to be referred to as "FAE" (fetal alcohol effects) or "PFAE" (possible fetal alcohol effects) but the complexity of the diagnosis in regard to mental and emotional functioning made it necessary to expand the definitions.

Not all women who drink heavily

during pregnancy bear children with FAS. There is as yet no definitive test for confirming FAS at birth and only the most severe cases are diagnosable at birth. The minimal standards for a diagnosis of FAS are

◇ **retarded growth** before and after birth including height, weight, head circumference, brain growth, and brain size;

◇ **facial deformities** including shortened eye openings, thin upper lip, flattened midface, missing groove (filtrum) in the upper lip;

◇ occasional **problems with heart and limbs**;

◇ **central nervous system involvement** such as delayed intellectual development, neurological abnormalities, behavioral problems, visual problems, hearing loss, and balance or gait problems (Sokol & Clarren, 1989).

In tests of 178 individuals with **FAS, IQ test scores ranged from 20 to 120 with a mean of 79**; in 295 individuals who were FAE, PFAE, or ARND, IQ scores ranged from 49 to 142 with a mean score of 90 (Streissguth, Barr, Kogn, & Bookstein, 1996). (Mental retardation is defined as an IQ of less than 70.)

Alcohol kills cells and changes the wiring of the fetus's brain. Huge gaps in brain development destroy natural connections that can never be regained. Specific neurological problems associated with FAS as well as ARND in terms of a neurocognitive profile include

◇ difficulty with short-term memory,

◇ problems storing and retrieving information,

◇ impaired ability to form links and make associations,

◇ difficulty making good judgments and forming relationships,

◇ problems controlling temper tantrums and aggression,

◇ oversensitivity to stimuli where they can't tolerate a bright light, loud sounds, smells, or certain kinds of textures or tastes in their mouths.

Children of mothers who drank but who do not have a diagnosis of FAS have many of the same neurological abnormalities as children who have been diagnosed with full FAS.

Worldwide studies estimate that **FAS births occur anywhere from 0.33 to 2.9 cases per 1,000 live births**. The incidence can vary greatly, e.g. the rate in one survey in South Africa where alcoholism is rampant was 40 cases per 1,000. The worldwide incidence of ARBD and ARND (which are difficult to diagnose) is probably 5–10 times greater than the incidence of FAS and FAE (May, 1996; Hans, 1998).

In the United States rates of 0.5 to 2.0 per 1,000 are the accepted figures. African Americans have about 6 FAS births per 1,000; Asians, Hispanics, and Whites about 1 to 2; and Native Americans about 30 although rates from 10–120 per 1,000 have been reported in various specific Native American and Canadian Indian communities (May, Brooke, Gossage, et al., 2000).

Alcohol exposure appears to damage some parts of the brain while leaving other parts unaffected. Some children exposed to alcohol in utero will have neurological problems in just a few brain areas. Other exposed children may have problems in many areas of the brain. The majority of children who are exposed to alcohol and other psychoactive drugs prenatally aren't going to have the physical symptoms that are associated with the diagnosis of full FAS. They will have a subtle neurobehavioral disorder.

These cognitive/behavioral deficits are not unique to alcohol exposure. Many other substances and physiological problems can cause similar conditions in children. For that reason the concept that alcohol might be the cause of this problem is often missed in the absence of those unique facial features. Many of the symptoms are not obvious until several years after birth. For example, children with any prenatal alcohol exposure were 3.2 times as likely to have delinquent-behavior scores in the clinical range compared with nonexposed children (Sood & Delaney-Black, 2001).

"What you're seeing at birth is a disorder of the brain's ability to regulate itself and its emotions and later on, especially in the toddler years and preschool years, what you're seeing are problems with sleep and problems with behavior; they're sitting and playing and they're pretty happy and then suddenly out of the blue they become aggressive. They throw temper tantrums and you really don't know what's going on. But that's the up-and-down emotional instability that these children demonstrate."
Sarajini Budden, M.D., FAS specialist, Legacy Emmanuel Children's Hospital, Portland, OR

In addition children with FAS are liable for **increased risks of other common birth defects** including heart disease, cleft lip and palate, and spina bifida. A weak and irregular sucking response, jitteriness, trembling, and sleep disturbances have been reported in babies exposed to large doses of alcohol (NIAAA, 1997).

"He was very inconsolable. He would take 10 cc of feed, he wouldn't sleep. He slept for maybe 15, 20 minutes at a time, 24 hours a day. That's what we went through. And it was like that for a couple of years. He was a very hard baby to parent but we loved him."
Foster mother of child with FAS

Critical Period. Because the brain is among the first organs to develop and the last to finish, it appears to be vulnerable throughout pregnancy; however **weeks 3 through 8, at the onset of embryogenesis (formation of the embryo), are crucial**. For example, the corpus callosum, a crucial structure that connects the cerebral hemispheres, is extremely vulnerable to alcohol use during the 6th to 8th gestational weeks; damage to the basal ganglia affects fine motor coordination and cognitive ability (Rosenberg, 1996). Generally

◇ during the 1st trimester alcohol interferes with the migration and organization of brain cells;

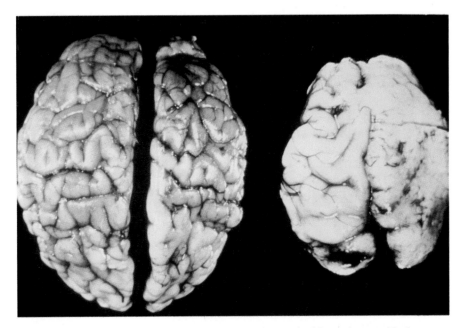

The greatest danger of alcohol use by a pregnant woman is fetal brain damage. The larger brain on the left is the normal brain of a human newborn (that died in an accident). The smaller brain on the right is of a child born with FAS. The FAS brain is obviously small and malformed.

Courtesy of Sterling K. Clarren, M.D., Children's Hospital, Seattle, WA

◇ in the 2nd trimester, especially the 10th to 20th week, facial features are greatly affected;

◇ during the 3rd trimester the hippocampus is strongly affected, which leads to difficulties encoding visual and auditory information (Miller, 1995; Goodlett & Johnson, 1999; Coles, 1994; Streissguth, 1997).

"It wasn't like they were meaning to do this to their child. At the time that they were drinking or using drugs, they didn't even know they were pregnant. And, in fact, we've had women who were almost into their 6th and 7th month of pregnancy who didn't know they were pregnant."
Sarajini Budden, M.D., FAS specialist, Legacy Emmanuel Children's Hospital, Portland, OR

Critical Dose. Animal models suggest that peak blood alcohol concentration rather than the total amount of alcohol drunk determines the critical level above which adverse effects are seen. A pattern of rapid drinking and the resulting high BAC seems to be the most dangerous style of drinking.

How many drinks are safe during pregnancy? One study concludes that **7 standard drinks per week by pregnant mothers are a threshold level below which most neurobehavioral effects are not seen.** This might lead some health care professionals to feel that they need not recommend total abstinence. However 7 drinks per week are an average and if a pregnant woman consumes a large number of those drinks at one sitting, the fetus may be much more at risk. Also some neurobehavioral tests are so sensitive that effects on the fetus can be found even with extremely low levels of exposure to alcohol.

"What they've tried to understand is how much alcohol does it take during what period of gestation to cause problems. And I think the message really is that if you know you're pregnant, don't drink because you don't know whether

an ounce is going to cause a problem or whether 12 ounces is going to cause a problem because it may have a different effect on people. But it's fairly clear that if you are using alcohol throughout pregnancy, every day, even a glass of wine every day is going to have some impact on the growing child."
Sarajini Budden, M.D., FAS specialist, Legacy Emmanuel Children's Hospital, Portland, OR

A new animal study showed that even one high-dose use episode of alcohol in rats when the developing brain is creating neurons and neuronal connections at a furious pace will also kill brain cells at a furious pace. In the experiment they showed that normally 1.5% of brain cells die during a certain period in a rat's growth but in rats exposed to alcohol during that critical period, 5–30% of neurons will die. When extrapolating these results to humans, the blood alcohol concentration would be .20, about twice the legal allowable limit for drivers and the crucial period would be 6 months into the pregnancy until the baby is born. During the brain growth spurt, a single prolonged contact with alcohol lasting 4 hours or more is enough to **kill vast numbers of brain cells** (Ikonomidou, Bitigau, Ishimaru, et al., 2000).

The U.S. Surgeon General advises that women should not drink at all while pregnant since **there is no way to determine which babies might be at risk from even very low levels of alcohol exposure** (NIAAA, 1997; Hans, 1998; Maier & West, 2001).

"I think like anybody that has a child with FAS or FAE, we have a tendency to take a closer look at people who are not acting quite right. The behaviors are a little bit different and you start to wonder if there isn't some alcohol in their past."
Foster father of 13-year-old with FAS

Paternal Drinking

As we have seen in Chapter 2, genetic transmission of alcoholism by fa-

thers is strongly suspected. There is now some evidence that the **detrimental effects of alcohol on the fetus may also be transmitted by paternal alcohol consumption**. Researchers are unable to say definitively whether paternal exposure to alcohol results in FAS or in some other damage. In laboratory tests alcoholic-sired rats of nonalcohol-using mothers produced male offspring with disturbed hormonal functions and spatial learning impairments. Adolescent male rats subjected to high alcohol intake produced both male and female offspring suffering from abnormal development including decreased body weight (Bielawski, Zaher, Svinarich, & Abel, 2002).

Observations of male children of alcoholic fathers indicate no gross physical deficits but do show an association with intellectual and functional deficits in these offspring. In addition to the deficits in verbal, thinking, and planning skills of children of alcoholics (COAs), sons of male alcoholics (SOMAs) exhibit further deficiencies in visual/spatial skills, motor skills, memory, and learning (NIAAA, 2000).

Some explanations of the causes of these abnormalities suggest that alcohol may mutate genes in sperm, kill off certain kinds of sperm, or biochemically and nutritionally alter semen and influence sperm (Little & Sing, 1986).

AGGRESSION & VIOLENCE

In a situation involving violence there are usually three people involved: the **victim**, the **perpetrator**, and one or more **bystanders**. Most often the bystanders are the children that witness violence in their homes or their neighborhoods. The victims can be the recipients of sexual assault or a beating (by a spouse). The perpetrator can be of any age; the common denominator being anger with perhaps a psychoactive drug thrown into the mix.

"I've always just been an angry child, growing up with a lot of anger that's been stuffed. And then it's like on the fifth drink I'm a party girl but on the seventh drink, I'd kick in your car door,

you know. I'd just totally change to that Dr. Jekyll and Mr. Hyde syndrome. There's no end of my anger when I drink. Mine comes from a lot of past abuse as a kid and it comes from just not fitting in."

28-year-old recovering female alcoholic

Most research suggests that a tendency to violence already resides in some people and is due to a combination of factors (heredity, environment, and alcohol or other drugs) working together to biochemically and emotionally put them at risk.

"He was a pretty mean guy when he wasn't drunk when I think about it, so it is really hard for me to tell. But we know that when people are addicted and are alcoholics, they can be dry drunks, which makes them just as mean when they're not using as when they are."

38-year-old victim of domestic violence

Among many neurochemical effects, alcohol has been shown to increase aggression by interfering with **GABA** (the main inhibitory neurotransmitter) in ways that **provoke intoxicated people with preexisting aggressive tendencies**. In addition alcohol decreases the action and levels of serotonin thus lowering impulse control. Lowered impulse control can cause drinkers to act out their aggressive impulses but also makes them less able to stop drinking once it has started (Gustafson, 1994; Javors, Tiouririne, & Prihoda, 2000).

Other causes of alcohol-related violence involve personality, setting, sociocultural factors, and economic conditions. Experiments have shown that even the expectation that alcohol will make one braver leads people to be more aggressive even if they are drinking a nonalcoholic beverage that they believe contains alcohol (Bushman, 1997; Higley, 2001).

"On a typical Friday night at least 50% of our calls will be some kind of alcohol

and drug violent behavior situation whether it be a shooting, stabbing, or a beating. A lot of those involve significant others, a spouse, or cohabitants."

Emergency medical technician, San Francisco Fire Department

Based on victim reports, 15% of robberies, 26% of aggravated assaults, and 50% of all homicides involved alcohol use. **About one-fourth of the 11.1 million victims of violent crime report that the offender had been drinking alcohol prior to committing the crime.** Not only had the offenders been drinking but their blood alcohol concentrations (BAC) were 2 or 3 times the drunk-driving threshold: levels of .18 for probationers, .20 for local jail inmates, and an incredible .28 for state prisoners at the time of their offense. In domestic violence situations, the association is particularly important—alcohol is involved at least three-fourths of the time (Roizen, 1997; Greenfield, 1998; NIAAA, 2000).

In a 1995 study in Memphis, Tennessee that examined police calls for domestic violence in that city, 92% of the perpetrators had used alcohol and 67% had used cocaine on the day of the assault. Almost half the perpetrators had often been loaded on alcohol and/or cocaine during the past 30 days. Other studies (Fig. 5-7) showed similar results.

"The use of alcohol would really bring out the hit man in me. I mean, I could talk to my partner or whoever fairly good if I was sober but after I started drinking, the deep emotions really would come out."

28-year-old male in an anger management class

Alcohol encourages the release of pent-up anger, hatred, and desires forbidden by society, especially in people prone to violence. Alcohol can also undermine moral judgment and reasoning, so when someone drinks, the common sense that would keep that person out of trouble is often suppressed (Collins & Messerschmidt, 1993).

"Seems like alcohol is always referred to as this 'liquid courage,' you know. And I guess it depends where you're at—courage to do what? Courage to ask a girl on a date that you hadn't had the courage to do before, or courage to dance like a fool on the floor, or is it courage to beat your wife or to beat your girlfriend cause you didn't have the guts to do it before?"

College peer counselor

There are three major kinds of interpersonal violence and one can escalate into another: **emotional violence, physical violence, and sexual violence.** The most common form of violence as well as the most underreported is emotional violence, which includes verbal abuse often caused by alcohol's freeing effect on the tongue.

Any type of violence can cause

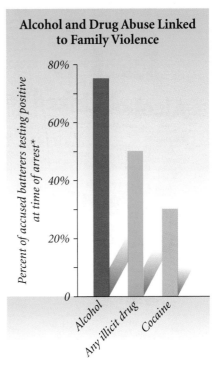

Figure 5-7 •

Three out of four of those arrested for family violence tested positive for alcohol. Half had used some illicit drug and more than one in four tested positive for cocaine.

The National Research Council, 1993

permanent biochemical changes in the victim that then can make them more susceptible to drug abuse and other emotional problems. MRI studies in 1997 at Yale and Harvard Universities showed that severely abused children had permanent changes to the brain. These changes often led to more behavioral problems including hyperactivity, impulsive behavior, increased aggression, exaggerated fears and nightmares, trouble keeping a job, and difficulty with relationships. The studies showed that the changes could also be caused just by severe emotional abuse.

"It doesn't matter if alcohol was involved in the situation. He raped me. There's more attention paid to the fact that there was alcohol involved than the fact that a woman was assaulted and that her life changed and that all of these things happened as a result of that. Alcohol's involved in almost every social situation but it doesn't mean that we recognize it or validate it."

22-year-old female college senior (rape victim)

Depending on the study, **34–74% of sexual assault perpetrators had been drinking as had 30–79% of the victims**. In most cases the perpetrator and victim are drinking simultaneously; rarely is the victim drinking alone (Abbey, Zawacki, Buck, Clinton, & Auslan, 2001).

Another mechanism that connects alcohol and violence is that alcohol can cause a drinker to misjudge social cues causing a person to perceive a threat where none exists. What occurs is that alcohol disrupts the judgment and rea-

soning center of the brain (Miczek et al., 1997).

DRIVING UNDER THE INFLUENCE

"An officer can pull up to a traffic light and the person is staring straight ahead and their face is up against the windshield of the car. Those are all indicators that that person might be under the influence of intoxicants. The people that we arrest try to stall as much as they can. They'll ask for a lawyer, they'll ask all kinds of questions, they'll try to let enough time go by. But it's been our experience that it doesn't help. The alcohol's gonna be in the system."

Lt. Rich Walsh, Ashland, OR, Police Department

Drink began day that ended in murder

By MARK FREEMAN
of the Mail Tribune

Ruben Landeros awoke at 10:30 a.m. Saturday and, as was his custom, poured a smidgeon of orange juice into a glass that he then filled with whiskey poured from a half-gallon plastic bottle.

The whiskey and orange juice flowed

more money than him. How she was leaving him for good.

Ten hours and a half-bottle of whiskey later, Ruben Landeros ended his marital dilemmas, but this time with the family pistol, family members say.

He shot Bobbi Jo dead inside her North Columbus

"She (Bobbi Jo) loved Ruben with all her heart," said Brenda Landeros, Ruben's sister-in-law and the dead woman's cousin, as she poured the last swig of whiskey from Ruben's bottle onto the ground Monday outside their Tripp Street apartment.

"The bottle took the best of

Office.

Prosecutors on Monday planned to issue formal arrest warrants for Ruben on charges of murder and attempted murder, and on Jose, 32, for hindering prosecution, said Doug McGeary, an assistant district attorney, Jackson County.

pair won't be charged until prosecuter esent the case to a Jackson County McGeary said. No grand jury

Alcohol Linked to 40 Percent of Violent Crimes

Associated Press Writer

Washington

Although declining as a cause of death, alcohol remains a factor in nearly 40 percent of violent crimes, the Justice Department reported yesterday.

Alcohol is an even bigger factor in violence by a

Of the 5.3 million convicted adult offenders in prison, jail or on parole or probation in 1996, 36 percent reported they had been drinking at the time of the offense for which they were convicted, the report estimated.

The report also said

victims of
'inancial
age out-

'inancial
'iolence,
million,

since 1990. In the past decade, highway fatalities blamed on alcohol sank from 24,000 in 1986 to 17,126 in 1996.

Nevertheless, local police made 1,467 arrests nationwide in 1996, for driving un the influence of alcohol. That was down the peak of 1.9 million arrests in 1983 33 states permitted alcohol consumptic fore age 21. Since then, responding to f highway funding requirements, ever has gone to a minimum drinking age

The most common state laws defin ication as 0.10 grams of alcohol per

Domestic Abuse Linked To Alcohol, Job Stability

Male ethnicity is not a factor, study says

LOS ANGELES TIMES

Men's alcohol abuse and shaky nployment status rank among the ost important precipitating factors domestic violence against womwhile ethnicity plays virtually no at all, according to one of the st comprehensive studies to date ssailants and their victims.

Student Barflies Take to Streets In Daylight-Saving Time Protest

Associated Press

Athens, Ohio

For the second year in a row, a rowdy crowd confronted police in this college town yesterday as bars closed early for the switch to daylight-saving time.

An estimated 2,000 people gathered outside downtown bars that cater to Ohio University students before the bars started closing at 2 a.m., half an hour earlier than usual because of the time change, authorities said.

No civilia
Sheriff Dave
dispersed the

Five offic
juries, and a
arrested, aut
rests were p
photograph
lice said.

One yea
change sen
to the stre
were arres

Those

Teenage Beer Party Leads to Rape Arrests

By Sandy Kleffman
Chronicle Correspondent

Two Union City teenagers were in custody yesterday for allegedly raping a 15-year-old girl during an afternoon gathering at one boy's apartment.

Police arrested the boys, ages 16 and 14, on Thursday and took them to Alameda County Juvenile Hall in San Leandro.

The girl told police the rape oc-

on the bed she was undressed and raped by at least two of the boys who were present," Packard said.

The girl told police she drifted in and out of consciousness during the attack.

Later, the boys helped her get dressed and leave the apartment. She then went to a friend's house and called police at 10:45 p.m.

Of the estimated 700,000 rapes committed yearly in the United States, around 80% of them are committed by acquaintances, intimate partners, and other family members.

Approximately 40% of motor vehicle fatalities (16,652) in 2001 involved alcohol use, an increase of 5.2% from 1999 but the same as in 2000. However over the last 10 years there has actually been a 13% drop in fatalities despite a 28% increase in miles driven. In addition, of the 3 million traffic-related accidents, 1 million were alcohol related (National Highway Traffic Safety Administration [NHTSA], 2001). According to the National Highway Traffic Safety Administration (NHTSA),

◇ more than 1 in 4 drivers gets behind the wheel within 2 hours of drinking;

◇ on any weekday night between 10 p.m. and 1 a.m., 1 in 13 drivers is legally drunk; on weekend mornings between 1 a.m. and 6 a.m., 1 in 7 drivers is drunk (Miller, Lestina, & Spicer, 1996);

◇ **of those convicted of DUI, 61% drank beer only**, 2% drank wine only, 18% drank liquor only, and 20% drank more than one type of alcoholic beverage;

◇ **alcohol-related crashes cost an estimated $148 billion in the United States every year** (NHTSA, 2001, NIAAA, 2000).

Since alcohol is a depressant, susceptibility to traffic accidents and fatalities is usually directly related to the blood alcohol level: coordination is decreased, judgment is impaired. There are some skills that are even impaired at .02 BAC such as the ability to divide attention between two or more visual inputs. At .05 BAC, eye movement,

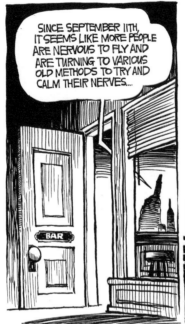
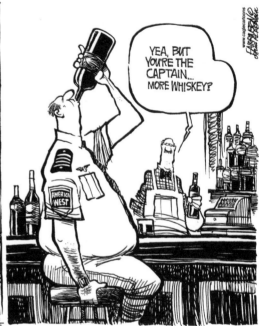

© 2002, Farrington. Printed with permission of Cagle Cartoons

glare resistance, visual perception, and reaction time are affected (Moskowitz, Burns, Fiorentino, Smiley, & Zador, 2000; Moskowitz & Fiorentino, 2000). Impairment for other forms of transportation also begins at relatively low BAC levels. Flight simulators show impaired pilot performance at .04 BAC and for up to 14 hours after reaching BACs between .10 and .12 (Yesavage & Leirer, 1986).

"A number of years ago I did a test in which I brought a number of individuals down to the police department, had them drink various amounts of alcohol and then drive a short obstacle course.

Some were social drinkers and some didn't drink at all except on very rare occasions. What I found was this:

◇ *one of the social drinkers felt he did the driving test fairly well and that he felt 'absolutely fine to drive.' I told him I would have arrested him for driving under the influence. When I put him on the breathalyzer machine, his was the highest blood alcohol of everybody there. This overconfidence in drinkers is fairly common;*

TABLE 5–7	BAC VS. CHANCES OF BEING KILLED IN A SINGLE-VEHICLE CRASH
Blood Alcohol Concentration	**Chances of Being Killed**
0.02–0.04	1.4 times normal
0.05–0.09	11.0 times normal
0.10–0.14	48.0 times normal
0.15 and above	380.0 times normal

(Zador, 1991)

TABLE 5–8	PERMISSIBLE BAC LIMITS IN OTHER COUNTRIES
Country	**Permissible BAC**
United States	.08–.10
Canada, Austria, Switzerland, United Kingdom, Germany	.08
Australia	.05–.08
Netherlands, Finland, France, Belgium	.05
Israel	.05
Japan	.03
Sweden, Poland	.02

◇ *the people who didn't drink very often and actually had much less to drink than this individual were saying when they took the driving test, 'There's no way in the world that I'd drive.' Their breathalyzer results were way under the limit."*
Traffic Safety Officer

The laws in the United States do not make exceptions. **When the BAC is over the legal limit (.08 or .10), the officer does not have to prove the person is impaired; the driver is guilty per se.** Usually though, an officer will observe the driver and if telltale signs are observed, the officer will pull the driver over and test coordination and other physical abilities to see if there is physical or mental impairment before requiring a breath or blood test. One of the most effective tests given on the spot is the eye nystagmus test.

"For some reason alcohol affects the eyeballs and the eyeball will start jerking if it tries to follow a moving finger or object. It's amazing, you can watch people's eyes just twitching away when they're under the influence. They can't follow the finger to the side, they're turning their whole head back and forth."
Lt. Rich Walsh, Ashland Police Department

Among those arrested for DUI, two-thirds have never been arrested before, so laws and programs have to be aimed at all segments of the population. In fact a majority of drivers in fatal alcohol-related crashes did not have a DUI conviction on their record and many did not have a history of problem drinking (NHTSA, 2001; Baker, Braver, Chen, Li, & Williams, 2002). More importantly, **only 1 driver is arrested for every 300 to 1,000 drunk-driving trips,** so effective enforcement can be a daunting task (Voas, Wells, Lestina, Williams, & Greene, 1997).

There are a quite a few **prevention strategies** that have reduced the number of alcohol-related traffic fatalities and injuries over the years:

◇ lowering the BAC limit from .10 to .08;

◇ imposing administrative license revocation (ALR) in which a police officer or other official can immediately confiscate the license of a driver whose BAC exceeds the legal limit. Some ALR laws also permit other penalties to be imposed immediately (making punishment more swift and certain);

◇ increasing the minimum legal drinking age to 21 years;

◇ having zero tolerance laws for those under 21 (i.e., prohibiting driving with any alcohol or a minimum of alcohol in the system [.01 or .02 BAC for those under 21]). These laws have reduced alcohol-related crashes involving youth by 17% to 50%;

◇ passing specific laws to deter repeat offenders, e.g., lowering the allowable BAC for repeat offenders;

◇ impounding or towing vehicles of drunk drivers;

◇ requiring mandatory treatment for DUI arrestees;

◇ increasing taxes on alcohol;

◇ training alcohol servers and mandating sanctions and liability. Legally servers have to stop serving drinkers who seem intoxicated;

◇ promoting designated-driver ideas;

◇ enacting mandatory seat belt laws, air bag laws, and child restraint laws;

◇ requiring licensing where driving privileges are granted gradually, not all at once.

"A DUI would definitely curb my drinking, like if I got a DUI right now, I would be hating life. You know that's like a year you don't drive or maybe like 6 months or whatever. I'm over 21, so it's like if I get a DUI, it's on me, you know"
22-year-old college student

There is no single prevention strategy that is most effective. The best results seem to occur with community-wide efforts when a combination of the above suggestions, along with media campaigns, police training, high school and college prevention programs, and better control of liquor sales, are implemented.

Injuries & Suicide

"I was medicating myself, covering it up, and I would take a sports bottle of wine with me to work in the morning, and I was operating heavy machinery, I would go home for lunch, and refill it, and come back, and drive a forklift, and operate this thing with spinning blades, and it's just insanity."
40-year-old recovering female alcoholic

Medical examiner reports indicate that alcohol dramatically increases the risk of injury.

◇ Emergency room studies confirm that **15–25% of emergency room patients tested positive for alcohol** or reported alcohol use, with relatively high rates among those involved in fights, assaults, and falls.

◇ Alcoholics are 16 times more likely to die in falls and 10 times more likely to become burn or fire victims.

◇ The U. S. Coast Guard reported that **31% of boating fatalities had a BAC of .10 or more**.

◇ In the workplace up to **40% of industrial fatalities** and 47% of injuries involved alcohol.

(Bernstein & Mahoney, 1989; NCADI, 2003)

"Putting a guy in the ground did nothing for our feeling indestructible, you know, kids that we were. That age of, 'God we're young and strong and there's nothing we can't do. There are no consequences to this behavior.' And even seeing it, going to the funeral, watching the hearse drive by, it was like, 'Duh, didn't make the connection.'"
40-year-old recovering alcoholic

Among adult alcoholics, **suicide rates are twice as high** as for the general population and even greater than the nonmentally ill population and rates increase with age. There seems to be a 3–10% suicide rate for those with alcoholism (Schuckit, 2000). One reason given for the increase in suicide with age is that the longer the alcoholism, the greater the social, health, and interpersonal problems. The alcoholic suicide victim is typically White, middle-aged, male, and unmarried with a long history of drinking. Additional risk factors for suicide include depression, loss of job, living alone, poor social support, and other illnesses.

"I just didn't want to live. I mean, my family and people that I love so much, I feel like they hated to see me coming and it's something that I wouldn't wish on anybody to go through. I was drinking on a day-to-day basis, just drinking and then I wound up at the hospital. I had tried to commit suicide and they put me in the psych ward."

38-year-old recovering female alcoholic

EPIDEMIOLOGY

PATTERNS OF ALCOHOL CONSUMPTION

It is difficult to get accurate, comparable, and consistent alcohol use data in other countries but as Table 5-5 (earlier in the chapter) points out, most European countries have higher per capita alcohol consumption rates than the United States while most Asian countries have lower per capita consumption. These differences result from a combination of physiological, cultural, social, religious, and legal factors.

Culture is one of the main determinants of how a person drinks. Different drinking patterns are found in the so-called wet and dry drinking cultures in Europe and North America.

Wet drinking cultures (e.g., Austria, Belgium, France, Italy, Switzerland) sanction daily or almost daily use and **integrate social drinking into everyday life**. In France children are served watered-down wine at the dinner table (Vaillant, 1995). Wet cultures consume more wine and beer—5 times the amount of wine drunk in dry cultures.

Dry drinking cultures (e.g., Denmark, Finland, Norway, Sweden) **restrict the availability of alcohol** and tax it more heavily. Dry cultures consume more distilled spirits, almost 1.5 times the amount in wet cultures, and are characterized by binge-style drinking particularly by males on weekends (Eurocare, 2003).

Canada, England, Ireland, the United States, Wales, and Germany exhibit combinations of wet and dry or **mixed drinking cultures** where patterns such as binge drinking in social situations are common. A relatively higher incidence of violence against women is found in mixed drinking cultures than in dry or wet cultures, probably because binge drinking often occurs in social situations.

Chinese families generally don't drink much, often because of cultural pressures. However in Japan and South Korea, social pressures to drink are very strong. **In Japan most of the men and half the women drink**, yet their alcoholism rate is half of that in the United States.

In Russia vodka is traditionally drunk between meals in large quantities. Alcoholism had become so rampant in Russia that in 1985 Premier Mikhail Gorbachev severely restricted the availability of alcohol almost to the point of prohibition. Illegal stills and the consumption of anything with alcohol in it, such as shoe polish and insecticides, soared. In just 1 year 11,000 died of alcohol and related poisonings. Many of those restrictions have since been lifted. When the restrictions were in place, Russian male life expectancy started to increase. Once the restrictions were lifted, male life expectancy dropped 6 years. Currently 9% of Russian men and 35% of Russian women abstain from alcohol (Bobak, 1999; Segal, 1990; Davis, 1994; Courtwright, 2001).

In England a trip to the pub for warm beer and darts is a tradition, so **70% of Britons drink regularly**. About two-thirds of the alcohol consumption in England is beer. In a recent campaign to stem alcoholism, Britons were urged to reduce their average daily consumption to three drinks a day.

In the United States much drinking is done in social settings away from lunch and dinner tables. In a land of many different cultures and lifestyles, a variety of culturally influenced drinking customs are present.

POPULATION SUBGROUPS

Men

In all age groups **men drink more per drinking episode than women** do,

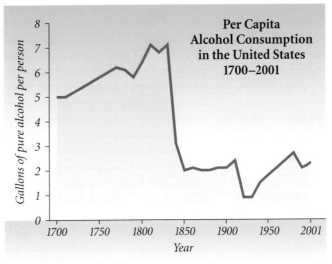

Figure 5-8 •
In the United States the per capita consumption of pure alcohol at present is 2.2 gallons but as this chart shows, the rate has varied wildly with the rise and fall of prohibition movements, health concerns, and the availability of a good water supply.
Adapted from David F. Musto's Alcohol in American History, *Scientific American*, April, 1996

TABLE 5–9   ALCOHOL ABUSE OR DEPENDENCE WITHIN THE PAST YEAR

	Males	Females	
Abstainers	28.0%	38.0%	
Light drinkers	58.7%	45.1%	(at least once a month)
Moderate drinkers	25.4%	9.6%	(at least once a week)
Binge drinkers	23.2%	8.6%	(5 or more drinks on the same occasion at least once in the last 30 days)
Heavy drinkers	9.7%	2.4%	(5 or more drinks per day at least 5 or more days in the last 30 days)

(SAMSHA, 2002)

TABLE 5–10   WOMEN & ALCOHOL PROBLEMS

More Likely to Have Drinking Problems	Less Likely to Have Drinking Problems
Younger women	Older women (60+)
Loss of role (mother, job)	Multiple roles (married, stable, work outside the home)
Never married	Married
Divorced, separated	Widowed
Unmarried and living with a partner	Children in the home
White women	Black women
Using other drugs	Hispanic women
Experiencing sexual dysfunction	Nondrinking spouse
Victim of childhood sexual abuse	

(National Institute on Drug Abuse, 1994)

regardless of country. Much of this difference has to do with the cultural acceptability of male drinking and the disapproval of female drinking. The other reason for the difference reflects the ability of men to more efficiently metabolize higher amounts of alcohol. As expected, **men also have more adverse social and legal consequences** and develop problems with alcohol abuse or alcohol dependence (alcoholism) at a higher rate than women.

Women

Women's alcohol problems become greater in their 30s not in their 20s as for men (Blume, 1997). Alcohol-dependent women as a group drink about one-third less alcohol than alcohol-dependent men (York, 1990).

Several studies demonstrate that **even low levels of drinking in women with a certain genetic susceptibility can result in major health consequences** such as an increase in breast cancer (Thun et al., 1997; Zhang et al., 1999). Proportionally **more women than men die from cirrhosis of the liver, circulatory disorders, suicide, and accidents**. As mentioned, female alcoholics have a 50–100% higher death rate than male alcoholics. But just as health problems develop after sustained heavy drinking, some health disorders, especially depression, may precede heavy drinking and even contribute to it. Also since women get higher BACs from the same amount of alcohol drunk than men, negative health consequences develop faster for women than for men (NIAAA, 1997; Maher, 1997).

Since **society more readily accepts the alcoholic male but disdains the alcoholic female**, women are less likely to seek treatment for alcoholism than men but are quicker to utilize mental health services when, in fact, their primary problem is alcohol or other drugs. Women are also more likely to enter treatment when their physical or mental health is suffering whereas men are more likely to seek treatment when they have problems with their employment or with the law (Gomberg, 1991; Ross, 1989).

Alcohol, Students, & Learning

It used to be that only college students, away from the control of their parents, began heavy drinking. But in the late 1980s and 1990s the age of first use and heavy use dropped to where many students had "done it all" by the time they finished their senior year in high school. The problem is that since so much maturing and developing takes place during high school and college years, **drinking can negatively affect learning and maturation**.

"Often it's the style of drinking, not experimentation, that gets college students (as well as high school kids and young adults) in trouble. Many think the name of the game is to get drunk. They drink too fast, they drink without eating, they play drinking games or contests, or they binge drink. They drink heavily and hard on 'hump day' [Wednesday] or over the weekend. But because they drink heavily only once or twice a week, they think that there is no problem. But there usually is a problem: lower grades, disciplinary action, or behavior they regret, which usually means sexual behavior. And both males and females talk to me about having been drunk and regretting the person they were with or their conduct with that person."

Shauna Quinn, drug and alcohol counselor, California State University - Chico

Doonesbury

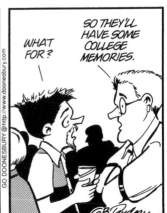

DOONESBURY © 1998 G. B. Trudeau. Reprinted, by permission, Universal Press Syndicate. All rights reserved.

Forty-four percent of college students admit to binge drinking at least once every 2 weeks (Wechsler et al., 2002). Binge drinking is defined as having 5 or more drinks at one sitting for males, 4 for females. About half the students in one study who admitted to binge drinking also admitted that their grades fell in the C to F range. Many binge drinkers missed classes on a regular basis. In a national study there was a startling, dramatic, and direct correlation between the number of drinks consumed per week and the grade point average.

Notice that women's grades start to deteriorate at slightly less than half the drinking level it takes for men's grades to go down. The *National Household Survey on Drug Abuse* (Fig. 5-9) indi-

cates that the higher the level of educational attainment, the more likely was the current use (not necessarily abuse) of alcohol. This seems a contradiction with the statistics about grade performance; however, the rate of heavy alcohol use in the 18–34 age group among those who had not completed high school was twice that of those who had completed college. In general, college students learn to moderate their drinking before they graduate.

"Secondhand drinking is a large problem on a college campus and it is a problem on our campus. We have a lot of students complain about their roommate or their boyfriend or girlfriend you know, being drunk, violence occurring, vandalism occurring, being unable to study, having to stay up all night with that person who may have had too much to drink and they need to stay with them to make sure they make it through the night and they don't die from alcohol poisoning."

Shauna Quinn, drug and alcohol counselor, California State University - Chico

Older Americans

"I visited my granddad in the retirement center/nursing home when he was 93 years old. He showed me the medicine cabinet. It was a small closet

that, when opened by a nurse, revealed dozens of bottles of alcohol—whiskey, rum, scotch, vodka, and a variety of wines—each one with the name of one of the elderly residents. Depending on the health of the patient, they could

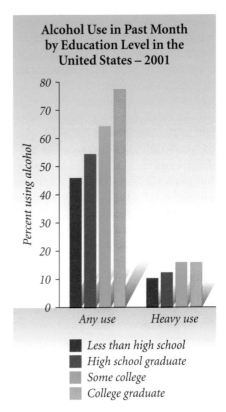

Alcohol Use in Past Month by Education Level in the United States – 2001

Figure 5-9 •

This chart compares the use and abuse of alcohol vs. the level of education.
(SAMHSA, 2002).

TABLE 5–11   AVERAGE NUMBER OF DRINKS PER WEEK, LISTED BY GRADE AVERAGE

Grade Average	Drinks Per Week		
	Males	Females	Overall
A	5.4	2.3	3.3
B	7.4	3.4	5.0
C	9.2	4.1	6.6
D or F	14.6	5.2	10.1

(College Core Study of 56 four-year and 22 two-year colleges by Southern Illinois University - Carbondale, 1993)

have one or two drinks a day for their health. He was still healthy at 96 when a fall killed him."

42-year-old grandson

People who are 65 years or older constitute the fastest growing segment of the U.S. population. About 6–21% of elderly hospital patients, 20% of elderly psychiatric patients, and 14% of elderly emergency room patients exhibit symptoms of alcoholism (American Medical Association, 1996). One study indicates that approximately **2.5 million older adults have alcohol-related problems.**

Research indicates that **patterns of drinking persist into old age** and that the amount and frequency of drinking are a result of general trends in society rather than the aging process. Hip fractures, one of the most debilitating injuries that occurs to the elderly, increase with alcohol consumption mainly due to **decreases in bone density caused by the deleterious effects of alcohol** (Adams, Yuan, Barboriak, et al., 1993). In nursing homes as many as 49% of the patients have drinking problems although some nursing homes are used as a place to hospitalize problem drinkers, so the rate may seem higher than the general population (Joseph, 1997). Another problem is that the average American over 65 years old takes two to seven prescription medications daily and so **alcohol/prescription drug interactions among older people are quite common** (Korrapati & Vestal, 1995).

About one-third of elderly alcohol abusers are of the late-onset variety. Some older people may increase their drinking because of isolation, retirement, more leisure time, financial pressures, depression over health, loss of friends or a spouse, lack of a day-to-day structure, or simply the availability and access to alcohol in the home or at friends' homes. The elderly alcohol abuser is less likely to be in contact with a workplace, the criminal justice system, or drug abuse treatment providers. Thus it may be **more difficult to identify elderly abusers and get them help.** This is also because of a more tolerant attitude towards drinking by the elderly. The common reaction is, "So what, if they are heavy drinkers? At their age, they deserve it. They've contributed to society and what harm could it do now anyway?"

One of the reasons diagnosis of drug or alcohol problems is difficult in the elderly is the **coexistence of other physical or mental problems** that become much more prevalent due to the aging process. Dementia, depression, hypertension, arrhythmia, psychosis, and panic disorder are just some of the conditions whose symptoms are mimicked by either the use of or withdrawal from alcohol and other drugs (Gambert, 1997).

However even with all the reasons and pressures to drink, people 65 and older have the lowest prevalence of problem drinking and alcoholism. There are several reasons for the lower rates.

◇ People who become alcohol abusers or alcoholics usually do so before the age of 65, suggesting a high degree of self-correction or spontaneous remission with age.

◇ Cutting down on drinking or giving up drinking may be related to the relatively high cost of alcohol for those on a fixed income.

◇ The body is less able to handle alcohol since liver function declines with age. The general aging process also decreases tolerance and slows metabolism, so the older drinker often has to limit intake.

◇ Side effects are increased if someone is ill or is taking medications thus encouraging temperance.

Homeless

For various reasons, some obvious, some not, it is hard to estimate the number of homeless in the United States. Varied sources suggest figures from **500,000 to 2 million with the average length of homelessness to be 6 months**. The breakdown of the homeless population is

◇ 46% are single males,

◇ 14% are single women,

◇ 36.5% are female heads of household with children,

◇ 25% are children.

Underrepresented ethnic groups are overrepresented:

◇ **56% are African American,**

◇ 12% are Hispanics,

◇ 29% are Caucasian,

◇ 2% are Native Americans,

◇ 1% are Asians.

Finally it is estimated that

◇ 8% have HIV or AIDS,

◇ **23% could be considered mentally ill,**

◇ and a staggering **45% have serious substance abuse problems.**

Street young adult: "We wake up and we drink."

Street teenager #1: "Drink a beer."

Street teenager #2: "And we go to sleep right after we're done drinking at night. But we drink all day long, every day, all the time, constantly."

Street teenager #3: "Except for right now 'cause we don't have enough money for a beer."

Counselor: "How long have you been doing that?"

Street young adult: "All my life, pretty much since I was a teenager."

Counselor: "How old are you now?"

Street young adult: "Twenty eight. And I've been living like this since I was 13. I take breaks. I'll get a job and shit but I still drink then too. Don't get me wrong. I have money for beer even if I have to pawn stuff."

Interview with street people by a counselor from the Haight Ashbury Clinic Youth Outreach Program

The reasons for homelessness vary widely. There are

◇ the situationally homeless who, because of job loss, spousal abuse, poverty, or eviction, find themselves on the street;

◇ the street people who have made the streets their home and have made an adjustment to living outside;

◇ the chronic mentally ill who have been squeezed out of inpatient mental facilities in the last 3 decades in favor of less costly outpatient health facilities;

◇ the homeless substance abusers, particularly alcohol abusers, whose lives center around their addiction that has made them incapable of living within the boundaries of normal society.

Within the last two groups are the mentally ill person who has begun to use drugs (often to self-medicate) and the drug abuser who has developed mental/emotional problems as a result of drug use. One of the keys to all these groups is to understand their **lack of affiliation with any kind of support system**. Services that identify and treat substance abuse or mental health problems are hard to come by or, if available, are shunned by the homeless person (Joseph & Paone, 1997).

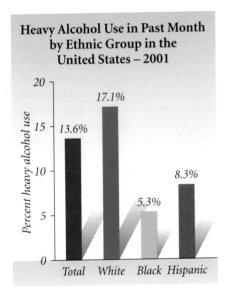

Heavy Alcohol Use in Past Month by Ethnic Group in the United States – 2001

Figure 5-10 •

In the United States during 2001, Caucasians continued to have a high rate of heavy alcohol use (5 or more drinks 5 or more times in the past month) at 6.4%. The rate for Hispanics was 4.4% and for African Americans, 4.1%.
SAMHSA, 2002

A comprehensive program to alleviate the drug and mental problems of the homeless usually involves outreach that will bring some basic services to the clients and which encourages them to eventually come into treatment facilities. Many cities try to locate services at shelters and gathering places for the homeless but since a wide variety of services are needed to meet the wide variety of problems, budget constraints often become the deciding factor.

UNDERREPRESENTED POPULATIONS

Biological and neurochemical differences between different ethnic groups account for some of the different patterns of alcohol and drug use in different communities. However, **diverse cultural traditions seem to make a greater contribution to alcohol use and abuse patterns** as does the degree of assimilation into the drinking patterns of the dominant culture. Sensitivity to ethnic traditions and degrees of assimilation can help us understand how alcohol use affects the health, family life, and social interactions of various cultures and in turn can contribute to more effective treatment and prevention.

African Americans

In the *2001 National Household Survey on Drug Abuse*, **heavy use of alcohol was lower among African Americans (4.1%) than among Caucasians (6.4%) or Hispanics (4.4%)** as in previous years. Use on a monthly basis by Black men (35.1%) is also less than by White men (52.7%) (SAMHSA, 2002). On the other hand even though more Black women abstain than White women, there is greater heavy drinking among those Black women who do drink. **Peak drinking for Blacks occurred after the age of 30** whereas drinking among Whites peaked at a younger age. Two reasons for the higher rate of abstention and the lower rate of heavy drinking among African Americans is their long history of spirituality, along with a strong matriarchal family structure, both of which look down upon heavy drinking.

TABLE 5–12   HISTORY OF ALCOHOLISM IN FAMILIES IN THE UNITED STATES

Native Americans and Alaskan natives	48%
Caucasians	23%
African Americans	22%
Hispanics	25%

(NCADI, 2003)

One disturbing fact is that **medical problems brought on by heavy drinking among African Americans are more severe** (Caetano & Clark, 1998). This is probably due to less access to health care facilities, insurance programs, and prevention programs as well as a delayed entrance into treatment for alcoholism as compared to Whites (John, Brown, & Primm, 1997).

Hispanics

In 2002 there were **32 million Hispanics in the United States or about 12.5% of the total population** (U.S. Bureau of the Census, 2003). One of the problems with examining Hispanic alcohol or drug use is the diversity of cultures involved: Mexican American, Cuban American, Puerto Rican, Colombian American, and individuals from dozens of other Spanish-speaking countries. In addition a single culture consists of anywhere from first- to tenth-generation immigrant Americans. **About 60% of all Hispanics in the United States are of Mexican origin**, 9.5% of the total are of Puerto Rican origin, and 3.2% are of Cuban origin (U.S. Bureau of the Census, 2003). In a survey done in the early '80s, heavy alcohol use was highest in the Mexican American community, somewhat lower in the Puerto Rican community, and very low in the Cuban American community. Alcohol use in Hispanic communities in 2001 were: past-month use, 39.5%; binge use, 21.3%; heavy drinking, 4.4%; and those reporting dependence in the past year, 6.2% (SAMHSA, 2002).

Unlike the general population,

drinking in the Hispanic community increases with both sexes as education and income increase. One of the problems with alcohol abuse and addiction in the Hispanic community is a **lack of culturally relevant treatment facilities and personnel**. Part of the severity of the problem has to do with the disruption of the family unit and the degree of assimilation.

"I think the cultural differences are crucial. To give you an example, I was in detox once and this woman came in, an Hispanic woman, and she was being interviewed by another counselor, and she was in an abusive relationship, and the other counselor told her that she would have to leave her relationship if she wanted to stay clean. And I thought, 'This woman's going to bolt. She's not going to leave her family.' And I had to intervene in a delicate way because otherwise I felt we were going to lose her."

35-year-old female Hispanic drug counselor

The rate of alcohol use among female Hispanics has grown over the last 20 years possibly due to the different attitude towards women's rights, more female heads of household, or because of different cultural traditions. Generally Hispanic women still drink considerably less than Hispanic men. In treatment a strong involvement of the family is necessary plus an appreciation of the values of **dignidad, respeto, y cariño** (dignity, respect, and love) (Ruiz & Langrod, 1997).

Asian & Pacific Islanders (APIs)

Asian and Pacific Islanders (APIs) are the **fastest growing ethnic group in the United States** though currently they only make up about 4% of the total population, approximately 11 million people. However because the label API encompasses dozens of distinct ethnicities throughout the Pacific Basin, including Japanese, Chinese, Filipino, Korean, Vietnamese, Thai, Indonesian, Burmese, and Pacific Islanders, mak-

TABLE 5–13	DRINKING PATTERNS OF 1,100 LOS ANGELES ASIAN AMERICANS		
Group Drinking	**Heavy Drinking**	**Moderate Drinking**	**Abstaining**
Japanese Americans	25%	42%	33%
Chinese Americans	11%	48%	41%
Korean Americans	14%	24%	62%
Filipino Americans	20%	29%	51%

(NIAAA, 1991)

ing generalized statements about APIs can lead to inaccuracies regarding the extent of their drug use and the reasons for that use. However a few general statements can be made.

Asian and Pacific Islanders are reported to have the **lowest rate of drinking and drug problems in the United States**. However as the APIs became more highly acculterated (more generations in America and increased ease with English), drinking increased (Sue, 1987; Zane & Kim, 1994). There are genetic factors that may help deter heavy drinking among APIs. The other major influence seems to be cultural (i.e., heavy drinking is strongly disapproved of in most API cultures). Surveys confirm that there are significant differences in drinking patterns among different national API groups (Johnson & Nagoshi, 1990). Note that there are sometimes large differences between Asian and Asian American drinking patterns for the same country—the foreign-born vs. American-born Asians of the same ethnic origin and even among the same generation of Asian Americans with identical ethnicities (Westermeyer, 1997).

In one study in Los Angeles (Table 5-13), **Filipino Americans and Japanese Americans were twice as likely to be heavy drinkers as Chinese Americans**. The Korean Americans have the highest number of abstainers. In general, Asian American males under 45 who are educated and in the middle class are most likely to drink but there is relatively little problem drinking even among this group (Makimoto, 1998).

As with other ethnic groups, treatment is much more effective when it is culturally relevant. For example, in San Francisco at the Haight Ashbury Clinic, relatively few APIs came in for treatment often because of the **stigma involved in admitting that there was a problem**. When research was done on the drug use patterns of the API communities in San Francisco, **when more API counselors were hired, and when a specific treatment facility for Asian Americans was created, the API population in treatment vastly increased**.

Native Americans & Alaskan Natives

There are approximately 2.4 million Native Americans and Alaskan Natives in the United States (U.S. Bureau of the Census, 2003). They **are divided into more than 300 tribal or language groups. In general, drinking patterns vary widely among these tribes** who make up about 1% of the population of the United States. Some tribes are mostly abstinent; some drink moderately with few problems; and some have high rates of heavy drinking and alcoholism. Stereotypes and old western movies seem to have influenced much of the thinking about Native Americans and drinking. The picture of the "Indian who can't hold his liquor" has been perpetuated for generations. One explanation is that although the rate of abstinence is quite high in many tribes, it is the pattern of heavy binge drinking among males in various tribes, especially on reservations, that accounts for the highly visible Native American alcoholic. (However in a survey of Sioux tribes, the women drank as much as the men.) The fact that many surveys are done on reservations where only one-third of the total Native American population lives, coupled with the grinding poverty found on many of those tribal reservations, may explain the rates of heavy drinking reported for this population (Beauvais, 1998).

Historically Native Americans only drank weak beers or other fermented beverages and usually just for ceremonial purposes. When distilled alcoholic beverages were introduced, most Native American cultures did not have time to develop ethical, legal, and social customs to handle the stronger drinks.

A study of a group of Native Americans (Mission Indians) looked at the inherited sensitivity to alcohol and found that they were not more sensitive to the effects of alcohol. Rather they were less sensitive and so had to drink more to get drunk (a sign of susceptibility to developing alcoholism) (Garcia-Andrade, Wall, & Ehlers, 1997).

Generally the abuse of alcohol accounts for 5 of the 10 leading causes of death in most Native American tribes. Alcohol-related motor vehicle deaths are 5.5 times higher than for the rest of the U.S. population. Cirrhosis of the liver is 4.5 times higher; alcoholism, 3.8 times higher; homicide, 2.8 times higher; and suicide, 2.3 times higher. Although Native American women drink less than men, they are especially vulnerable to cirrhosis and account for almost half of the deaths from cirrhosis (Manson, Shore, Baron, et al., 1992).

One study in Oklahoma found alcohol-related causes of death varied from less than 1% up to 24% among the 11 tribes surveyed, compared with 2% for Blacks and 3% for Whites (Manson et al., 1992).

CONCLUSIONS

Because alcohol causes many serious health and societal problems, its use has often been restricted or banned by almost every country. However most restrictions ultimately have been overturned because of demand and the lure of tax revenues by governments.

The road to alcoholism can take 3 months, 30 years, or it may never occur. One has to recognize that alcohol is a psychoactive drug and can cause irreversible physiological changes that make one more susceptible to alcoholism with continued use.

CHAPTER SUMMARY

Overview

1. Except for Islamic countries and a few others, drinking alcoholic beverages is a worldwide phenomenon.

2. One hundred and nine million Americans drank some alcoholic beverages last month.

3. About 25–30% of all U.S. hospital admissions were due to alcohol.

4. Two million people worldwide died last year due to alcohol.

5. Since the process of fermentation occurs naturally, alcohol was initially discovered by accident and then purposefully cultivated and manufactured.

6. Over the centuries alcohol, a central nervous system depressant, has been used as a reward, as food, as a medicine, as a sacrament, as a water substitute, as a social lubricant, as a source of taxes, and as a tranquilizer (to cover emotional and mental problems).

7. Because alcohol (a legal drug) also causes the most health and societal problems, its use has often been restricted or banned by almost every country but because of consumer demand and tax revenues, most severe restrictions were eventually overturned.

Alcoholic Beverages

8. Though there are hundreds of different alcohols, ethyl alcohol (ethanol) is the main psychoactive ingredient in all alcoholic beverages, along with nonpsychoactive fermentation products called "congeners" that add tastes, colors, and aromas.

9. When yeast is added to certain fruits, vegetables, or grains, they ferment into alcoholic beverages.

10. When fruits, particularly grapes, ferment, wine is the result. When grains ferment, beer is the result (e.g., ale, stout, lager, malt beverages). More highly concentrated spirits are distilled from the original fermentation of grains or vegetables such as potatoes (vodka) and from wine.

11. Most wines are 12–14% alcohol; most beers are 4–7% alcohol; and most liquors and whiskeys are about 35–45% alcohol. Higher-proof alcoholic beverages increase the incidence of alcoholism.

Absorption, Distribution, & Metabolism

12. When alcohol is drunk, it is absorbed (mostly through the capillaries in the small intestine), metabolized (mostly in the liver), and then excreted.

13. The rate of absorption depends on body weight, sex, health, and a dozen other factors including what additives are in the drink. The effects on women of a given amount of alcohol are generally more damaging.

14. Alcohol dehydrogenase (ADH) and acetaldehyde (ALDH) are central to the liver's metabolism of alcohol.

15. About 2–10% of alcohol is excreted directly through the urine

and lungs. The rest is metabolized by the liver and then excreted as carbon dioxide and water through the kidneys and lungs.

16. Alcohol is metabolized at a defined continuous rate, so it is possible to roughly approximate what level of drinking will produce a certain blood alcohol concentration (BAC). A BAC of .08 to .10 defines legal intoxication in all 50 states. However, behavioral reactions vary widely. It takes 30–40 minutes after taking a drink to reach maximum alcohol concentration.

Desired Effects, Side Effects, & Health Consequences

Levels of Use

17. The six levels of alcohol use are abstention, experimentation, social/recreational use, habituation, abuse, and addiction (alcohol dependence, alcoholism).

Low-to-Moderate-Dose Episodes

18. Small amounts of alcohol or occasional episodes of intoxication are usually not harmful and have some positive health benefits.

19. The negative side effects of low-to-moderate drinking are accidents, legal problems, and high-risk sexual activities leading to unwanted pregnancies, sexually transmitted diseases, and relationship problems.

20. People who are pregnant or who have preexisting physical or mental health problems, allergies to alcoholic beverages, high genetic/environmental susceptibility to addiction, and preexisting abuse problems should avoid any use of alcohol.

21. Low-dose use can help digestion, promote relaxation and sleep, and slightly lower the risk of heart attacks or other coronary diseases.

22. Psychological effects depend on the mood of the drinker (set) and where the alcohol is consumed (setting) as well as how much was drunk. Negative emotions can be exaggerated by drinking alcohol.

23. Since alcohol is a disinhibitor, low-dose use can increase self-confidence, sociability, and sexual desire. The disinhibition is mostly due to alcohol's effects on GABA, an inhibitory neurotransmitter, and NMDA, a glutamate receptor.

24. Alcohol's influence on the brain's neurotransmitters (serotonin, dopamine, met-enkephalin, and especially GABA) cause the effects.

25. In low doses, alcohol often increases sexual desire but eventually decreases sexual performance.

High-Dose Episodes

26. Intoxication is a combination of blood alcohol concentration, psychological mood, expectation, and drinking history. Binge drinking (5 or more drinks for men at one sitting and 4 or more for women) and heavy drinking (bingeing 5 or more times a month) cause the most problems.

27. As the blood alcohol concentration rises, depressant effects go from lowered inhibitions and relaxation, to decreased alertness and clumsiness, to slurred speech and inability to walk, to alcohol poisoning that can result in unconsciousness and death (respiratory and cardiac failure).

28. Blackouts are caused by heavy drinking in susceptible individuals and are marked by loss of memory even though the drinker is awake and conscious. Partial blackouts are known as "brownouts."

29. Hangovers usually disappear within hours on their own while withdrawal symptoms that occur with chronic high-dose use can last for days.

30. Mental confusion, mood swings, loss of judgment, and emotional turbulence replace desired effects at high doses.

Chronic High-Dose Use

31. The liver is the organ most severely affected. Problems include a fatty liver, alcoholic hepatitis, and cirrhosis (a scarring of the liver

that is often eventually fatal). Usually the higher a country's drinking rate, the higher the cirrhosis rate.

32. Digestive effects of chronic drinking include gastritis, ulcers, pancreatitis, internal bleeding, and malnutrition. Low blood sugar and high blood sugar are often the result of chronic drinking.

33. Though beneficial to the cardiovascular system at low doses, with chronic high-dose drinking, enlarged heart, high blood pressure, intracranial bleeding, and stroke are seen.

34. Heavy drinking kills neurons since alcohol is toxic to all cells. Alcohol-caused vitamin B_1 deficiency can cause brain damage and dementia.

35. With chronic use, alcohol can decrease desire and orgasm in females and impair gonadal functions and decrease testosterone in males.

36. In moderate-to-heavy drinkers, the chance of breast cancer in women as well as the chance of mouth, throat, and esophageal cancer in both men and women increases especially if they also smoke.

37. Mental and emotional problems, especially depression and anxiety, increase with chronic use. Chronic use also impairs concentration and memory.

Mortality

38. The average lifespan of the chronic heavy drinker is shortened by 15 years.

Addiction (alcohol dependence, alcoholism)

39. About 10–12% of drinkers progress to frequent, high-dose use (alcoholism); 2 to 3 times more men than women have a major problem with alcohol.

40. Just 20% of drinkers consume 80% of all alcohol.

41. There have been numerous attempts to classify alcoholism so

that the condition can be studied more systematically and strategies for treatment can be more effective.

42. Classifications have progressed from E. M. Jellinek's gamma and delta alcoholics, to type I and II alcoholics, to type A and B alcoholics, and finally to the disease concept of alcoholism.

43. The discovery of the nucleus accumbens (reward/reinforcement center), the identification of endogenous neurotransmitters, the use of genetic research tools, and the development of imaging techniques has increased the understanding of alcoholism.

44. Most current concepts look at addiction as a progressive disease that is caused by a combination of hereditary and environmental influences that are triggered and aggravated by the use of alcohol or other drugs.

45. Tolerance and tissue dependence occur as the body, especially the liver, attempts to adapt to the increasing levels of use and the cumulative toxic effects of alcohol.

46. Withdrawal after cessation of frequent high-dose use can be painful and even life threatening. Symptoms (e.g., rapid pulse, breathing, and heart rate, tremors, anxiety) will occur after cessation of 7–34 days of heavy drinking. Delirium tremens (DTs) is a life-threatening form of severe withdrawal that includes hallucinations and convulsions.

47. Research is focusing on identifying marker genes that make one more susceptible to alcoholism; learning which environmental changes will lessen risk; studying specific physical and mental changes caused by chronic use.

Other Problems with Alcohol

48. Most drug abuse involves more than one substance, one of them usually being alcohol. The problems of polydrug abuse can be synergistic not just additive.

Simultaneous addictions must be treated simultaneously. Tobacco is heavily used by drinkers.

49. Drinkers can have preexisting mental health problems and try to self-medicate symptoms or the alcohol and other drugs can induce symptoms of mental illness, particularly depression, and lead to misdiagnosis of mental problems.

50. Personality disorders, especially antisocial and borderline personality disorders (BPDs), seem overrepresented among alcoholics and addicts.

51. Heavy drinking during pregnancy can cause birth defects, most notably fetal alcohol syndrome (FAS), that involve abnormal growth and mental problems. It is not known what level of drinking and drug use, if any, is safe during pregnancy. Mental deficits, particularly memory problems, without facial abnormalities are more likely to affect the infant. Drinking during weeks 3 through 8 of pregnancy is the most dangerous to the fetus. Paternal drinking can also affect the fetus. Heavy drinking is also the leading cause of all mental retardation in the United States.

52. Alcohol is heavily involved in emotional/physical/sexual violence, mostly from the lowering of inhibitions in people with a predisposition to violence. Alcohol and violence affect victim, perpetrator, and bystanders. The mood of the drinkers and the setting also affect violence. From 34–74% of sexual assault perpetrators had been drinking, about the same percentages as the victim.

53. Approximately 40% of motor vehicle fatalities involve alcohol. A .08 to .10 BAC means legal guilt even though the level of impairment can vary greatly. An intoxicated driver is arrested for every 300 to 1,000 drunk-driving trips.

54. About 15–25% of emergency room patients tested positive for alcohol. Large percentages of ho-

micides, suicides, and accidents involve alcohol.

Epidemiology

55. Culture is one of the main determinants of how a person drinks. Wet cultures (e.g., France) integrate social drinking into every day life while dry drinking cultures (e.g., Denmark) place numerous limitations on its use. The United States has a mixed drinking culture and does much social drinking away from lunch and dinner tables.

56. Men drink more per episode than women and have a higher level of addiction and of sociolegal consequences while women suffer more health consequences. This is because of a combination of hereditary, physiological and psychological differences, and social expectations.

57. The amount and frequency of binge alcohol consumption are high in both high school and colleges. About 44% of college students have 5 or more drinks at one sitting. The greater the amount of alcohol used, the lower the grade point average.

58. About 2.5 million older Americans have alcohol-related problems. As the drinker ages, the liver is less able to handle alcohol but even so, the elderly have the lowest prevalence of problem drinking and alcoholism.

59. About 45% of the homeless have serious substance abuse problems and 23% have a mental illness. Treatment must first be brought to the homeless rather than expecting they will come to an agency for treatment.

60. Each ethnic group in the United States has unique drinking patterns and problems due to physiological and cultural variances.

61. Heavy drinking is lower in the African American community than in Caucasian or Hispanic communities. The Asian & Pacific Islander community has so many

components that it is hard to make generalizations. There is also a wide variation in the Native American communities although in some tribes 5 of the 10 leading causes of death are due to alcohol. In all groups a lack of culturally

relevant treatment facilities is a major barrier to recovery.

Conclusions

62. The road to alcoholism can take 3 months, 30 years, or it may never occur. One has to recognize that al-

cohol is a psychoactive drug and can cause irreversible physiological changes that make one more susceptible to alcoholism with continued use.

REFERENCES

Abbey, A., Zawacki, M. A., Buck, M. A., Clinton, A. M., & Auslan, P. (2001). Alcohol and sexual assault. *Alcohol Research & Health, 25*(1), 43–51.

Abel, E. L., & Sokol, R. J. (1986). Fetal alcohol syndrome is now leading cause of mental retardation. *Lancet, 2*, 1222.

Adams, W. L., Yuan, Z., Barboriak, J. J., et al. (1993). Alcohol-related hospitalizations of elderly people. *Journal of the American Medical Association, 270*(10), 1222–1225.

Alcohol Alert. (1992). Moderate drinking: Benefits and risks. *Alcohol Alert, 16.*

Alcoholics Anonymous. (1934, 1976). *Alcoholics Anonymous.* New York: Alcoholics Anonymous World Services, Inc.

American Medical Association. (1996). Alcoholism in the elderly. AMA Council on Scientific Affairs. *Journal of the American Medical Association, 275*(10), 797–801.

American Psychiatric Association. (2000). *Diagnostic and Statistical Manual of Mental Disorders* (4th ed., text revision [DSM-IV-TR]). Washington, DC: Author.

Anthenelli, R. M., & Schuckit, M. A. (1998). Genetic influences in addiction. In A. W. Graham & T. K. Schultz (Eds.), *Principles of Addiction Medicine* (2nd ed., pp. 41–51). Chevy Chase, MD: American Society of Addiction Medicine, Inc.

Babor, T. F. (1996). The classification of alcoholics. *Alcohol Health & Research World, 20*(1), 6–18.

Babor, T. F., Dolinsky, Z. S., Meyer, R. E., Brock, M., Hofmann, M., & Tennen, H. (1992). Types of alcoholics: Concurrent and predictive validity of some common classification schemes. *British Journal of Addiction, 87,* 1415–1431.

Bagnardi, V., Blangiardo, M., Vecchia, C. L., & Corrao, G. (2001). Alcohol consumption and the risk of cancer. *Alcohol Research & Health, 25*(4).

Bailey, W. J. (1998). Indiana Prevention Resource Center FactLine on high potency alcoholic beverages [Online]. Available: *http://www.drugs.indiana. edu/publications/iprc/factline/high_ potency.html*

Baker, S. P., Braver, E. R., Chen, L-H., Li, G., & Williams, A. F. (2002) Drinking histories of fatally injured drivers. *Injury Prevention, 8,* 221–226.

Beauvais, F. (1998). American Indians. *Alcohol Health & Research World, 22*(4).

Becker, H. C. (1998). Kindling in alcohol withdrawal. *Alcohol Health & Research World, 22*(1), 25–33.

Begleiter, H. (1980). *Biological Effects of Alcohol.* New York: Plenum Press.

Bellandi, D. (2003, January 1). Underage binge drinking climbs by 56 percent. *Medford Mail Tribune,* p. 1.

Bernstein, M., & Mahoney, J. J. (1989). Management perspectives on alcoholism: The employer's stake in alcoholism treatment. *Occupational Medicine, 4*(2), 223–232.

Bielawski, D. M., Zaher, F. M., Svinarich, D. M., & Abel, E. L. (2002). Paternal alcohol exposure affects sperm cytosine methyltransferase messenger RNA levels. *Alcoholism: Clinical and Experimental Research, 26,* 347–351.

Blot, W. J. (1992). Alcohol and cancer. *Cancer Research Supplement, 52,* 2119s–2121s.

Blum, K., Braverman, E. R., Cull, J. G., Holder, J. M., Luck, R., Lubar, J., Miller, D., & Comings, D. E. (2000). Reward deficiency syndrome (RDS): A biogenetic model for the diagnosis and treatment of impulsive, addictive, and compulsive behaviors. *Journal of Psychoactive Drugs, 32*(1).

Blum, K., Cull, J. G., Braverman, E. R., & Comings, D. E. (1996). Reward deficiency syndrome. *American Scientist, 84,* 132–145.

Blum, K., & Payne, J. E. (1991). *Alcohol and the Addicted Brain* (p. 165). New York: The Free Press.

Blume, S. (1997). Women: Clinical aspects. In J. H. Lowinson, P. Ruiz, R. B. Millman, & J. G. Langrod (Eds.), *Substance Abuse: A Comprehensive Textbook* (3rd ed., pp. 645–654). Baltimore: Williams & Wilkins.

Bobak, M. (1999). Alcohol consumption in a national sample of the Russian population. *Addiction, 94*(6), 857–866.

Bohman, M., Sigvardson, S., & Cloninger, C. G. (1981). Maternal inheritance of alcohol abuse: Cross-fostering analysis of adopted women. *Archives of General Psychiatry, 38,* 965–969.

Bosron, W. F., Ehrig, T., & Li, T. K. (1993). Genetic factors in alcohol metabolism and alcoholism. *Seminars in Liver Disease, 13*(2), 126–135.

Bowlin, S. J. (1997). Alcohol intake and breast cancer. *International Journal of Epidemiology, 26,* 915–923.

Bushman, B. J. (1997). Effects of alcohol on human aggression. In M. Galanter (Ed.), *Recent Developments in Alcoholism* (Vol. 13, pp. 227–243). New York: Plenum Press.

Caetano, R., & Clark, C. L. (1998). Trends in alcohol-related problems among Whites, African Americans, and Hispanics: 1984–1995. *Alcoholism: Clinical and Experimental Research, 22*(2), 534–538.

Cloninger, C. R., Bohman, M., & Sigvardson, S. (1996). Type I and type II alcoholism: An update. *Alcohol Health & Research World, 20*(1), 18–23.

Coles, C. (1994). Critical periods for prenatal alcohol exposure: Evidence from animal and human studies. *Alcohol Health & Research World, 18,* 22–29.

Collins, J. J., & Messerschmidt, P. M. (1993). Epidemiology of alcohol-related violence. *Alcohol Health & Research World, 17*(2), 93–100.

Courtwright, D. T. (2001). *Forces of Habit.* Cambridge, MA: Harvard University Press.

Davis, R. (1994). Drug and alcohol use in

the former Soviet Union: Selected factors and future considerations. *International Journal of Addictions,* 29(3), 88–89.

Dawson, A., Bigby, B. G., Poceta, J. S., & Mitler, M. M. (1993). Effect of bedtime ethanol on total inspiratory resistance and respiratory drive in normal nonsnoring men. *Alcoholism: Clinical and Experimental Research,* 17(2), 256–262.

Dawson, D. A., & Grant, B. F. (1998). Family history of alcoholism and gender. *Journal of Studies on Alcohol,* 59(1), 97–106.

DeBakey, S. F., Stinson, F. S., Grant, B. F., & Dufour, M. C. (1996). Liver cirrhosis mortality in the United States, 1970–1993. *Surveillance Report #41.* Bethesda, MD: National Institute on Alcohol Abuse and Alcoholism.

Devantag, F., Mandich, G., Zaiotti, G., & Toffolo, G. G. (1983). Alcoholic epilepsy: Review of a series and proposed classification and etiopathogenesis. *Harvard Journal of Neurologic Science, 4,* 275–284.

Ellison, R. C., Zhang, Y., McLennan, C. E., & Rothman, K. J. (2001). Exploring the relation of alcohol consumption to risk of breast cancer. *American Journal of Epidemiology, 154,* 740–747.

Enoch, M., White, K. V., Harris, C. R., Rohrbaugh, J. W., & Goldman, D. (2001). Alcohol use disorders and anxiety disorders: Relation to the P300 event-related potential. *Alcohol Clinical Experimental Research,* 25(9), 1293–1300.

Eurocare. (2003). Report on European alcohol use [Online]. Available: *http://www. eurocare.org/profiles*

Gambert, S. R. (1997). The elderly. In J. H. Lowinson, P. Ruiz, R. B. Millman, & J. G. Langrod (Eds.), *Substance Abuse: A Comprehensive Textbook* (3rd ed., pp. 693–699). Baltimore: Williams & Wilkins.

Garcia-Andrade, C., Wall, T. L., & Ehlers, C. L. (1997). The firewater myth and response to alcohol in Mission Indians. *American Journal of Psychiatry, 154,* 983–988.

Geller, A. (1997). Neurological effects. In A. W. Graham & T. K. Schultz (Eds.), *Principles of Addiction Medicine* (2nd ed., pp. 775–784). Chevy Chase, MD: American Society of Addiction Medicine, Inc.

Goedde, H. W., Harada, S., & Agarwal, D. P. (1979). Racial differences in alcohol sensitivity: A new hypothesis. *Human Genetics, 51,* 331–334.

Goldstein, A. (2001). *Addiction: From Biology to Drug Policy* (2nd ed.). New York: W.H. Freeman and Company.

Gomberg, E. A. L. (1991). Alcoholic women in treatment: New research. *Substance Abuse, 12*(1), 6–12.

Goodlett, C. R., & Johnson, T. B. (1999). Temporal windows of vulnerability to alcohol during the third trimester equivalent. In: J. H. Hannigan, L. P. Spear, N. E. Spear, & C. R. Goodlett (Eds.), *Alcohol and Alcoholism: Effects on Brain and Development* (pp. 59–91). Hillsdale, NJ: Lawrence Erlbaum Associates.

Goodwin, D. W., & Gabrielli, W. F. (1997). Alcohol: Clinical aspects. In J. H. Lowinson, P. Ruiz, R. B. Millman, & J. G. Langrod (Eds.), *Substance Abuse: A Comprehensive Textbook* (3rd ed., pp. 142–147). Baltimore: Williams & Wilkins.

Grant, B. F. (1985). Liver cirrhosis mortality in the United States. *Alcohol Epidemiologic Data Reference Manual* (2nd ed., Vol. 2). Washington, DC: Department of Health and Human Services.

Greenfield, L. A. (1998). *Alcohol and crime: An analysis of national data on the prevalence of alcohol involvement in crime.* Report prepared for National Symposium on Alcohol Abuse and Crime. Washington, DC: U.S. Department of Justice.

Greenfield, T. K., & Rogers, J. D. (1999). Who drinks most of the alcohol in the U.S.? The policy implications. *Journal of Studies on Alcohol.*

Griffin, R. E., Gross, G. A., & Teitelbaum, R. (1993). Delirium tremens: A review. *Journal of the American Osteopath Association, 93,* 929.

Gustafson, R. (1994). Alcohol and aggression. *Juvenile Offender Rehabilitation, 21*(3/4), 41–80.

Hans, S. L. (1998). Developmental outcomes of prenatal exposure to alcohol and other drugs. In A. W. Graham & T. K. Schultz (Eds.), *Principles of Addiction Medicine* (2nd ed., pp. 1223–1237). Chevy Chase, MD: American Society of Addiction Medicine, Inc.

Harwood, H., et al. (2000). *Updating Estimates of the Economic Costs of Alcohol Abuse in the United States.* Report prepared by the Lexin Group for the National Institute on Alcohol Abuse and Alcoholism.

He, J. (2001). Alcohol reduction advised for heavy drinkers with hypertension. *Hypertension, 38,* 1112–1117.

Heath, D. B. (1995). Alcohol: History. *Encyclopedia of Drugs and Alcohol* (Vol.1, pp. 70–78). New York: Simon & Schuster Macmillan.

Heinz, A., Ragan, P., Jones, D. W., et al. (1998). Reduced central serotonin transporters in alcoholism. *The American Journal of Psychiatry, 155,* 1544–1549.

Helzer, J. E., & Pryzbeck, T. R. (1988). The co-occurrence of alcoholism with other psychiatric disorders in the general population and its impact on treatment. *Journal of Studies on Alcohol, 49*(3), 219–224.

Higley, J. D. (2001). Individual differences in alcohol-induced aggression. *Alcohol Research & Health, 25*(1), 12–19.

Ikonomidou, C., Bitigau, P., Ishimaru, M. J., et al. (2000). Ethanol-induced apoptotic neurodegeneration and fetal alcohol syndrome. *Science, 287,* 1056–1060.

Internal Revenue Service. (2002). Federal excise taxes [Online]. Available: *http:// www.irs.gov/pub/irs-soi/02ex21te.xls*

Isbell, H., Fraser, H. F., Wikler, A., et al. (1955). An experimental study of the etiology of "rum fits" and delirium tremens. *Quarterly Journal on Alcohol, 16*(1).

Javors, M., Tiouririne, M., & Prihoda, T. (2000). Platelet serotonin uptake is higher in early-onset than in late-onset alcoholics. *Alcohol and Alcoholism, 35,* 390–393.

Jellinek, E. M. (1961). *The Disease Concept of Alcoholism.* New Haven, CT: College & University Press.

John, S., Brown, L. S. Jr., & Primm, B. J. (1997). African Americans: Epidemiologic, prevention, and treatment issues. In J. H. Lowinson, P. Ruiz, R. B. Millman, & J. G. Langrod (Eds.), *Substance Abuse: A Comprehensive Textbook* (3rd ed., pp. 699–705). Baltimore: Williams & Wilkins.

Johnson, R. C., & Nagoshi, C. T. (1990). Asians, Asian Americans and alcohol. *Journal of Psychoactive Drugs, 22*(1), 45–52.

Jones, A. W., & Pounder, D. J. (1998). Measuring blood alcohol concentration for clinical and forensic purposes. In S. B. Karch (Ed.), *Drug Abuse Handbook* (pp. 327–355). Boca Raton, FL: CRC Press.

Jones, K. L., & Smith, D. W. (1973). Recognition of the fetal alcohol syndrome in early infancy. *Lancet, 2,* 999–1001.

Joseph, C. L. (1997). Misuse of alcohol and drugs in the nursing home. In A. M.

Gumack (Ed.), *Older Adults' Misuse of Alcohol, Medicines, and Other Drugs: Research and Practice Issues.* New York: Springer Science.

Joseph, H., & Paone, D. (1997). The homeless. In J. H. Lowinson, P. Ruiz, R. B. Millman, & J. G. Langrod (Eds.), *Substance Abuse: A Comprehensive Textbook* (3rd ed., pp. 733–743). Baltimore: Williams & Wilkins.

Keller, M. (1984). Alcohol consumption. *Encyclopaedia Britannica* (Vol. 1, pp. 437–450). Chicago: Encyclopaedia Britannica.

Kinney, J. (2002). *Loosening the Grip* (7th ed.). Boston: McGraw-Hill.

Klatsky, A. L. (1988). The cardiovascular effects of alcohol. *Alcohol, 22* (1), 1178–124.

Knop, J., Goodwin, D. W., Teasdale, T.W., Mikkelsen, U., & Schulsinger, F.A. (1984). A Danish prospective study of young males at high risk for alcoholism. In D. W. Goodwin, K. Van Dusen, & S. A. Mednick (Eds.), *Longitudinal Research in Alcoholism.* Boston: Kluwer-Nijhoff.

Koob, G. (1999, August 23). *Alcohol stimulates release of stress chemicals.* Speech presented at a meeting of the American Chemical Society, New Orleans, LA.

Korrapati, M. R., & Vestal, R. E. (1995). Alcohol and medications in the elderly: Complex interactions. In T. Beresford & E. Gomberg (Eds.), *Alcohol and Aging* (pp. 42–55). New York: Oxford University Press.

Kurose, I., Higuchi, H., Kato, S., Miura, S., & Ishii, H. (1996). Ethanol-induced oxidative stress in the liver. *Alcoholism: Clinical and Experimental Research, 20*(1), 77A–85A.

Kushner, M. G., Mackenzie, T. B., Flazdon, J., et al. (1996). The effects of alcohol consumption on laboratory-induced panic and state anxiety. *Archives of General Psychiatry, 53,* 264–270.

Landolt, H. P., et al. (1996). Late-afternoon ethanol intake affects nocturnal sleep and the sleep EEG in middle-aged men. *Journal of Clinical Psychopharmacology, 16*(6), 428–436.

Langton, P. A. (1995). Temperance movement. *Encyclopedia of Drugs and Alcohol* (Vol. 3, pp. 1019–1023). New York: Simon & Schuster Macmillan.

Lee, J. A. (1987). Chinese, alcohol and flushing: Sociohistorical and biobehavioral considerations. *Journal of Psychoactive Drugs, 19*(4), 319–327.

Li, T. K., Lumeng, L., McBride, W. J., Waller, M. B., & Murphy, J. M. (1986). Studies on an animal model of alcoholism. In M. C. Braude & J. M. Chao (Eds.), *Genetic and Biological Markers in Drug Abuse and Alcoholism. NIDA Research Monograph 66.* Rockville, MD: Department of Health and Human Services.

Lichine, A. (1990). Distilled spirits. *Encyclopedia Americana* (pp. 188–190). Danbury, CT: Grollier, Inc.

Little, R. E., & Sing, C. F. (1986). Association of father's drinking and infant's birth weight. *New England Journal of Medicine, 314,* 1644–1645.

Lukas, S. E. (1995). Beer. *Encyclopedia of Drugs and Alcohol* (Vol.1, pp. 146–149). New York: Simon & Schuster Macmillan.

Maher, J. (1997). Exploring alcohol's effects on liver function. *Alcohol Health & Research World, 21*(1), 10.

Maier, S. E., & West, J. R. (2001). Drinking patterns and alcohol-related birth defects. *Alcohol Research & Health,* 25(3), 168–174.

Makimoto, K. (1998). Drinking patterns and drinking problems among Asian Americans and Pacific Islanders. *Alcohol Health & Research World,* 22(4), 265–269.

Manson, S. M., Shore, J. H., Baron, A.E., et al. (1992). Alcohol abuse and dependence among American Indians. In J. E. Helzer & G. J. Canino (Eds.), *Alcoholism in North America, Europe, and Asia* (pp. 113–130). New York: Oxford University Press.

Matthews, J. (1995). *Beer, Booze and Books: A Sober Look at Higher Education.* Peterborough, NH: Viaticum Press.

May, P. A. (1996). Research issues in the prevention of fetal alcohol syndrome and alcohol-related birth defects. *Research Monograph 32, Women and Alcohol: Issues for Prevention Research.* Bethesda, MD: National Institute on Alcohol Abuse and Alcoholism.

May, P. A., Brooke, L., Gossage, J. P., et al. (2000). Epidemiology of FAS in a South African community. *American Journal of Public Health, 90*(12), 1905–1912.

May, P. A., & Gossage, J. P. (2001). Estimating the prevalence of fetal alcohol syndrome. A summary. *Alcohol Research & Health,* 25, 159–167.

Mayo-Smith, M. (1998). Management of alcohol intoxication and withdrawal. In A. W. Graham & T. K. Schultz (Eds.), *Principles of Addiction Medicine* (2nd

ed.). Chevy Chase, MD: American Society of Addiction Medicine, Inc.

Miczek, K. A., et al. (1997). Alcohol, GABA-benzodiazepine receptor complex and aggression. In M. Galanter (Ed.), *Recent Developments in Alcoholism* (Vol. 13, pp. 139–171). New York: Plenum Press.

Miller, M. M., et al. (1988). Bedtime ethanol increases resistance of upper airways and produces sleep apneas in asymptomatic snorers. *Alcohol Clinical Experimental Research, 12*(6), 801–805.

Miller, M. M. (1998). Traditional approaches to the treatment of Addiction. In A. W. Graham & T. K. Schultz (Eds.), *Principles of Addiction Medicine* (2nd ed., pp. 315–326). Chevy Chase, MD: American Society of Addiction Medicine, Inc.

Miller, M. W. (1995). Effect of pre- or postnatal exposure to ethanol. Cell proliferation and neuronal death. *Alcohol Clinical Experimental Research, 19*(5), 1359–1363.

Miller, N. S., Klamen, D., Hoffman, N. G., & Flaherty, J. A. (1995). Prevalence of depression and alcohol and other drug dependence in addictions treatment populations. *Journal of Psychoactive Drugs, 28*(2), 111–124.

Miller, T. R., Lestina, D. C., & Spicer, R. S. (1996). Highway crash costs in the United States by driver age, blood alcohol level, victim age, and restraint use. In *40th Annual Proceedings of the Association for the Advancement of Automotive Medicine* (pp. 495–517).

Moddrey, W. C. (1988). Alcoholic hepatitis: Clinicopathologic features and therapy. *Seminars in Liver Disease, 8*(1), 91–102.

Moos, R. H., Brennan, P. L., & Mertens, J. R. (1994). Mortality rates and predictors of mortality among late, middle-aged and older substance abuse patients. *Alcoholism: Clinical and Experimental Research, 18,* 187–195.

Morbidity and Mortality Weekly Report. (2002). Alcohol use among women of childbearing age – United States, 1991–1999. Centers for Disease Control and Prevention. *Morbidity and Mortality Weekly Report, 51*(3).

Morse, R. M., Flavin, D. K., et al. (1992). The definition of alcoholism. *Journal of the American Medical Association (JAMA), 268,* 1012–1014.

Moskowitz, H., Burns, M., Fiorentino, D., Smiley, A., and Zador, P. (2000). *Driver Characteristics and Impairment at*

Various BACs. Washington, DC: National Highway Traffic Safety Administration.

Moskowitz, H., & Fiorentino, D. (2000). *A Review of the Literature on the Effects of Low Doses of Alcohol on Driving-Related Skills.* Washington, DC: National Highway Traffic Safety Administration.

Mukamal, K. J., & Rimm, E. B. (2001). Alcohol's effects on the risk for coronary heart disease. *Alcohol Research & Health, 25*(4), 255–261.

Nace, E. P. (1997). Alcoholics Anonymous. In J.H. Lowinson, P. Ruiz, R.B. Millman, & J. G. Langrod (Eds.), *Substance Abuse: A Comprehensive Textbook* (3rd ed., pp. 383–390). Baltimore: Williams & Wilkins.

Nace, E. P., Saxon, J. J., Davis, C. W., & Gaspari, J. P. (1991). Axis II comorbidity in substance abusers. *American Journal of Psychiatry, 148*, 118–120.

Nace, E. P., Saxon, J. J., & Shore, N. (1983). A comparison of borderline and nonborderline alcoholic patients. *Archives of General Psychiatry, 40*, 56–58.

National Center for Health Statistics. (2002). National vital statistics report (Vol. 50, No. 15) [Online]. Available: *http://www.cdc.gov/nchs/fastats/liverdis.htm*

National Clearinghouse on Alcohol and Drug Information. (2003). Alcohol [Online]. Available: *http://store.health.org/catalog/facts.aspx?topic=3&h=Publications*

National Highway Traffic Safety Administration. (2001). *Alcohol and Highway Safety, 2001.* Springfield, VA: National Technical Information Service.

National Institute on Alcohol Abuse and Alcoholism. (1990). Alcohol and women. *Alcohol Alert No. 10.*

National Institute on Alcohol Abuse and Alcoholism. (1991). Alcohol & Asian Americans. *Alcohol Health & Research World, 2*(2), 41.

National Institute on Alcohol Abuse and Alcoholism. (1993). Alcohol and the liver. *Alcohol Alert No. 19.*

National Institute on Alcohol Abuse and Alcoholism. (1997). Alcohol metabolism. *Alcohol Alert No. 35.*

National Institute on Alcohol Abuse and Alcoholism. (1998). Alcohol and tobacco. *Alcohol Alert No. 39.*

National Institute on Alcohol Abuse and Alcoholism. (2000). *Tenth Special Report to U.S. Congress on Alcohol and Health.* Bethesda, MD: U.S. Department of Health and Human Services.

National Institute on Drug Abuse. (1994). *Women and Drug Abuse: You and Your Community Can Help.* Bethesda, MD: Substance Abuse and Mental Health Services Administration.

Nidus Information Services. (2002). What is cirrhosis? [Online]. Available: *http://www.reutershealth.com/wellconnected/doc75.html*

Noble, E. P., Blum, K., Montgomery, A., & Sheridan, P. J. (1991). Allelic association of the D2 dopamine receptor gene with receptor-binding characteristics in alcoholism. *Archives of General Psychiatry, 48*, 648–654.

Nutt, D. J. (1998). The neurochemistry of Addiction. In A. W. Graham & T. K. Schultz (Eds.), *Principles of Addiction Medicine* (2nd ed.). Chevy Chase, MD: American Society of Addiction Medicine, Inc.

O'Brien, R., & Chafetz, M. (1991). *The Encyclopedia of Alcoholism,* (2nd ed.). New York: Facts on File.

Olds, J. (1956). Pleasure centers in the brain. *Scientific American, 195*(4), 105–116.

Olds, J., & Milner, P. (1954). Positive reinforcement produced by electrical stimulation of septal area and other regions of rat brain. *Journal of Comprehensive Physiology and Psychology, 47*, 419–427.

Peele, S. (1995). Controlled drinking versus abstinence. *Encyclopedia of Drugs and Alcohol* (Vol. 1, pp. 92–97). New York: Simon & Schuster Macmillan.

Petrakis, I. L., Gonzalez, G., Rosenheck, R., & Krystal, J. H. (2002). Comorbidity of alcoholism and psychiatric disorders: An overview. *Alcohol Research & Health, 26*(2), 81–89.

Prescott, C. A., & Kendler, K. S. (1999). Genetic and environmental contributions to alcohol abuse and dependence in a population-based sample of male twins. *The American Journal of Psychiatry, 156*, 34–40.

Presley, C. A., et al. (1997). *Alcohol and Drugs on American College Campuses: Issues of Violence and Harassment.* Carbondale IL: Southern Illinois University at Carbondale.

Reed, T., Pagte, W. F., Viken, R. J., & Christian, J. C. (1996). Genetic predisposition to organ-specific endpoints of alcoholism. *Alcohol Clinical Experimental Research, 20*(9), 1528–1533.

Roizen, J. (1997). Epidemiological issues in alcohol-related violence. In M. Galanter (Ed.), *Recent Developments in Alcoholism* (Vol. 13). New York: Plenum Press.

Rosenberg, A. (1996). Brain damage caused by prenatal alcohol exposure. *Science & Medicine, 3*(4), 43–51.

Ross, H. E. (1989). Alcohol and drug abuse in treated alcoholics: A comparison of men and women. *Alcohol Clinical & Experimental Research, 13*, 810–816.

Ruiz, P., & Langrod, J. G. (1997). Hispanic Americans. In J. H. Lowinson, P. Ruiz, R. B. Millman, & J. G. Langrod (Eds.), *Substance Abuse: A Comprehensive Textbook* (3rd ed., pp. 705–711). Baltimore: Williams & Wilkins.

Saadatmand, F., Stinson, F. S., Grant, B. F., & Dufour, M. C. (2000). *Surveillance Report #54. Liver Cirrhosis Mortality in the United States, 1970–1997.* Bethesda, MD: National Institute on Alcohol Abuse and Alcoholism.

Sacco, R. L., Elkind, M., Boden-Albala, B., et al. (1999). The protective effects of moderate alcohol consumption on ischemic stroke. *Journal of the American Medical Association (JAMA), 281*(1).

Saitz, R., & O'Malley, S. S. (1997). Pharmacotherapies for alcohol abuse. Withdrawal and treatment. *Medical Clinics of North America, 81*, 881.

Schuckit, M. A. (1996). Hangovers: A rarely studied but important phenomenon. *Vista Hill Foundation Drug Abuse & Alcoholism Newsletter, 23*(1).

Schuckit, M. A. (2000). *Drug and Alcohol Abuse* (5th ed.). New York: Kluwer Academic/Plenum Publishers.

Schuckit, M. A., Edenberg, J. J., Kalmijn, J., et al. (2001). A genome-wide search for genes that relate to a low level of response to alcohol. *Alcohol Clinical Experimental Research, 25*(3), 323–329.

Schuckit, M. A., Tipp, J. E., Bucholz, K. K., et al. (1997). The lifetime rates of three major mood disorders and four major anxiety disorders in alcoholics and controls. *Addiction, 92*, 1289–1304.

Segal, B. (1990). *The Drunken Society: Alcohol Abuse and Alcoholism in the Soviet Union.* New York: Hippocrene Books.

Shiffman, S., & Balabanis, M. (1995). Associations between alcohol and tobacco. In J. B. Fertig & J. P. Allen (Eds.), *Alcohol and Tobacco: From Basic Science to Clinical Practice, NIAAA Research Monograph No. 30* (pp. 17–36). Washington, DC: U.S. Government Printing Office.

Shivani, R., Goldsmith, J., & Anthenelli, R. M. (2002). Alcoholism & psychiatric disorders. *Alcohol Research & Health, 26*(2), 90–98.

Sokol, R. J., & Clarren, S. K. (1989). Guidelines for use of terminology describing the impact of prenatal alcohol on the offspring. *Alcoholism: Clinical and Experimental Research, 13*(4), 597–509.

Sood, B., Delaney-Black, V., et al. (2001). Prenatal alcohol exposure and childhood behavior at age 6 to 7 years. Dose response effect. *Pediatrics, 108*(2).

Span, S. A., & Earleywine, M. (1999). Familial risk for alcoholism and hangover symptoms. *Addictive Behaviors, 24*(1), 121–125.

Stahl, S. M. (2000). *Essential Psychopharmacology* (pp. 522–523). Cambridge, England: Cambridge University Press.

Stratton, K., Howe, C., & Battaglia, F. (Eds.). (1996). *Fetal Alcohol Syndrome: Diagnosis, Epidemiology, Prevention, and Treatment.* Washington, DC: National Academy Press.

Streissguth, A. P. (1997). *Fetal Alcohol Syndrome.* Baltimore: Paul H. Brookes Publishing Co.

Streissguth, A. P., Barr, H. M., Kogn, J., & Bookstein, F. L. (1996). *Understanding the occurrence of secondary disabilities in clients with FAS and FAE* (Tech. Rep. No. 96-06). Atlanta, GA: Centers for Disease Control and Prevention.

Substance Abuse and Mental Health Services Administration. (2002). *Summary of Findings from the 2001 National Household Survey on Drug Abuse.* Rockville, MD: SAMHSA, Office of Applied Studies.

Sue, D. (1987). Use and abuse of alcohol by Asian Americans. *Journal of Psychoactive Drugs, 19*(1), 57–66.

Swift, R., & Davidson, D. (1998). Alcohol hangover: Mechanisms and mediators. *Alcohol Health & Research World, 22*(1), 54–60.

Tabakoff, B., Cornell, N., & Hoffman, P. L. (1992). Alcohol tolerance. *Annals of Emergency Medicine, 15*(9), 1005–1012.

Teng, Y. S. (1981). Human liver aldehyde dehydrogenase in Chinese and Asiatic Indians: Gene deletion and its possible implications in alcohol metabolism. *Biochemical Genetics, 19,* 107–114.

Thun, M. J., Peto, R., Lopez, A. D., Monaco, J. H., Henley, S. J., Heath, C. W., & Doll, R. (1997). Alcohol consumption and mortality among middle-aged and elderly U.S. adults. *New England Journal of Medicine, 337*(24), 1711.

Trice, H. M. (1995). Alcohol: History. In D. B. Heath (Ed.), *Encyclopedia of Drugs and Alcohol* (Vol.1, pp. 85–92). New York: Simon & Schuster Macmillan.

Turner, R. T., & Sibonga, J. D. (2001). Effects of alcohol use and estrogen on bone. *Alcohol Research & Health, 25*(4), 276–281.

University of Michigan. (2002). Monitoring the Future Study [Online]. Available: *http://www.MonitoringTheFuture.org*

U. S. Bureau of the Census. (2003). Resident population of the United States by sex, race, and Hispanic origin [Online]. Available: *http://www.census.gov/population/estimates/nation/intfile3-1.txt*

U.S. Department of Justice. (1998). Alcohol and crime: An analysis of national data on the prevalence of alcohol involvement in crime [Online]. Available: *http://www.ojp.gov/bjs/pub/pdf/ac.pdf*

U.S. Surgeon General. (1992). *Youth and Alcohol: Dangerous and Deadly Consequences: Report to the Surgeon General.* Bethesda, MD: Substance Abuse and Mental Health Services Administration.

Vaillant, G. E. (1995). *The Natural History of Alcoholism Revisited.* Cambridge, MA: Harvard University Press.

Valenzuela, C. F., & Harris, F. A. (1997). Alcohol: Neurobiology. In J. H. Lowinson, P. Ruiz, R. B. Millman, & J. G. Langrod (Eds.), *Substance Abuse: A Comprehensive Textbook* (3rd ed., pp. 119–141). Baltimore: Williams & Wilkins.

Vitiello, M. V. (1997). Sleep, alcohol, and alcohol abuse. *Addiction Biology, 2,* 151–158.

Voas, R. B., Wells, J. K., Lestina, D. C., Williams, A. F., & Greene, M. A. (1997). *Drinking and Driving in the U. S.: The 1996 National Roadside Survey.* NHTSA Traffic Task No. 152. Arlington, VA: Insurance Institute for Highway Safety.

Vogel-Sprott, M., Rawana, E., & Webster, R. (1984). Mental rehearsal of a task under ethanol facilitates tolerance. *Pharmacology, Biochemistry & Behavior, 21*(3), 329–331.

Volkow, N., Wang, G. J., & Doria, J. J. (1995). Monitoring the brain's response to alcohol with positron emission tomography. *Alcohol World: Health and Research: Imaging in Alcohol Research, 19*(4).

Waugh, A. (1968). *Wines and Spirits.* New York: Time-Life Books.

Wechsler, H., Lee, J. E., Kuo, M., Seibring, M., Nelson, T. F., & Lee, H. (2002) Trends in college binge drinking during a period of increased prevention efforts. *Journal of American College Health, 50*(5).

Westermeyer, J. (1997). Native Americans, Asians, and new immigrants. In J. H. Lowinson, P. Ruiz, R. B. Millman, & J. G. Langrod (Eds.), *Substance Abuse: A Comprehensive Textbook* (3rd ed., pp. 712–716). Baltimore: Williams & Wilkins.

Woodward, J. J. (1998). The pharmacology of alcohol. In A. W. Graham & T. K. Schultz (Eds.), *Principles of Addiction Medicine* (2nd ed., 103–116). Chevy Chase, MD: American Society of Addiction Medicine, Inc.

World Health Organization. (1999). Health and development in the twentieth century. *The World Health Report.* Geneva: WHO.

World Health Organization. (2003). Alcohol consumption [Online]. Available: *http://www.who.int/substance_abuse/PDFfiles/global_alcohol_status_report/4Alcoholconsumption.pdf*

Yesavage, J. A., & Leirer, V. O. (1986). Hangover effects on aircraft pilots 14 hours after alcohol ingestion. *American Journal of Psychiatry, 143*(12).

York, J. L. (1990). High blood alcohol levels in women. *New England Journal of Medicine, 323*(1), 59–60.

Zador, P. L. (1991). Alcohol-related relative risk of fatal driver injuries in relation to driver age and sex. *Journal of Studies of Alcohol, 52*(4), 302–310.

Zane, N. W., & Kim, J. C. (1994). In N. W. Zane, D. T. Takeuchi, & K. N. J. Young (Eds.), *Confronting Critical Health Issues of Asian and Pacific Islander Americans* (pp. 316–346). Thousand Oaks, CA: Sage Publications.

Zhang, Y., Schatzkin, A., Kreger, B. E., Dorgan, J. F., Splansky, G. L., Cupples, L. A., & Ellison, R. C. (1999). Alcohol consumption and risk of breast cancer: The Framingham study revisited. *American Journal of Epidemiology, 149.*

All Arounders

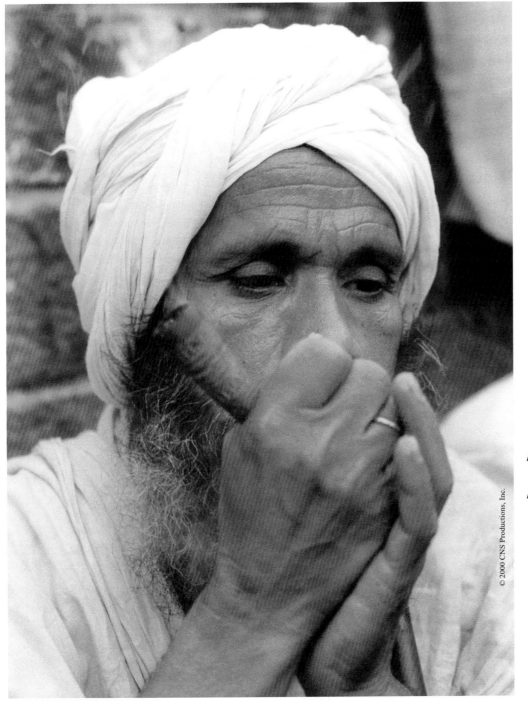

In India, ganja, the more potent leaves and flowering tops of the Cannabis plant, are smoked in chillums, hollow cone-shaped pipes. The smoker cups his hands over the opening at the bottom of the pipe and draws the smoke in through his hands. Charas, the concentrated resin of the marijuana plant, is also called "hashish." Bhang, the less-potent stems and leaves of the Cannabis plant, can also be smoked in a chillum.

- **History:** All arounders (psychedelics) have been available since the origin of man. They were originally found in plants and fungi.
- **Classification:** LSD, MDMA, ketamine, psilocybin mushrooms, DMT, PCP, peyote, and especially marijuana are the most commonly used all arounders (also called "hallucinogens" and occasionally "intactogens" or "empathogens").
- **General Effects:** Psychedelics cause intensified sensations, crossed sensations (e.g., visual input becomes sound), illusions, delusions, hallucinations, stimulation, impaired judgment, and distorted reasoning.
- **LSD, Psilocybin Mushrooms, & Other Indole Psychedelics:** LSD, an ergot alkaloid, is very potent; it causes stimulation and can induce hallucinations and illusions. Psilocybin mushrooms cause nausea and induce hallucinations. Ibogaine and yage, two other indole psychedelics, are much less common.
- **Peyote, MDMA, & Other Phenylalkylamine Psychedelics:** Peyote cacti (mescaline), used in sacred rituals and ceremonies, cause more hallucinations than LSD. Psycho-stimulants like MDMA (ecstasy) are pharmacologically similar to amphetamines but also have calming and psychedelic effects.
- **Belladonna & Other Anticholinergic Psychedelics:** Plants such as belladonna, jimsonweed, and henbane have been used in the rituals of ancient cultures for more than 3,000 years mostly to induce visions.
- **Ketamine, PCP, & Other Psychedelics:** Ketamine is an anesthetic used on animals and humans. It causes mind-body disassociation, a sensory-deprived state, and hallucinations. PCP is similar to ketamine and produces many of the same effects. It predates ketamine in street popularity. PCP and ketamine are also known as "dissociative anesthetics." *Amanita* mushrooms, nutmeg, and mace are also psychedelics but rarely used in Europe and the United States. *Salvia divinorum* (diviner's sage) has become somewhat popular in the 2000s.
- **Marijuana & Other Cannabinols:** Marijuana is the most popular illicit psychoactive drug. It magnifies the existing personality traits of users. Effects often depend on the mind-set of the user and the setting. Recently there has been an intense social and legal battle over the use of marijuana for medical purposes. Marijuana can cause relaxation, sedation, increased appetite, giddiness, bloodshot eyes, short-term memory impairment, impaired tracking ability, and mental confusion.

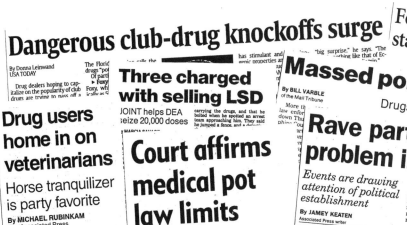

HISTORY

Psychedelic plants and fungi have probably been used since the origin of man and were around for 250 million years before then (Schultes & Hofmann, 1992). In an evolutionary pattern plants and fungi mutated and developed chemical defenses against animals, insects, and disease. Often those defenses were alkaloids such as cocaine and nicotine that could induce psychedelic effects. **More than 4,000 plants have psychedelic (hallucinogenic) or psychoactive properties** but only a few hundred have continued to be used over the ages. Primitive people stumbled across these plants and fungi, probably tried them as food, and had hallucinogenic experiences (Siegel, 1985).

Neanderthal men and women and eventually shamans, witches, and healers experimented with different methods of ingestion: boiling and drinking, smoking, eating, or absorbing (through the nasal passages, the gums, or the skin). Even after the hypodermic needle was invented 150 years ago, hallucinogens were rarely injected since the **object of using them was to alter**

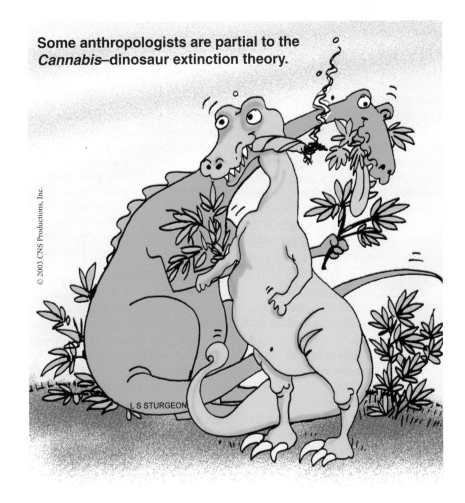

Some anthropologists are partial to the *Cannabis*–dinosaur extinction theory.

one's consciousness and perception of reality rather than to induce a **rush** (Escohotado, 1999).

"When the mushrooms took effect on them, then they danced, then they wept. But some, while still in command of their senses, entered and sat there by the house; they danced no more, but only sat there nodding. . . . And when the effects of the mushrooms had left them, they consulted among themselves and told one another what they had seen in vision."
Bernardo de Sahagun, 1542 (Sahagun, 1985)

Historically *Amanita* mushrooms were eaten in India and pre-Columbian Mexico, belladonna was drunk in ancient Greece and medieval Europe, marijuana was inhaled and eaten in ancient China and Egypt, and poisonous ergot, found in rye mold (a natural form of LSD), was accidentally consumed in renaissance Europe. No matter where explorers and anthropologists ventured, they found that every culture had discovered and was using a psychoactive substance from some natural source (Goldstein, 2001).

In the twenty-first century, even though psychedelics can still be found in every country, **the majority of these drugs are grown and used in the Americas, Europe, and Africa** (the major exception is marijuana, which is grown in most countries). Hundreds of primitive tribes in the Americas, such as the Aztecs and Toltecs in the past and the Kiowas and Huichols in the present, have used peyote, psilocybin mushrooms, yage, marijuana, and morning glory seeds among others **for religious, social, ceremonial, and medical rites** (Diaz, 1979; Efferink, 1988).

Recently there has been an upsurge of interest in psychedelics—MDMA (ecstasy), LSD, and psilocybin mushrooms ("'shrooms")—among students in colleges, high schools, and even middle schools throughout the United States. The percentage of high school seniors who used LSD at least once per month surged in 1994 and 1995 and has

leveled off since then (2.3% per month used LSD in 2001). It is about the same percentage that used cocaine in the past month (2.1% in 2001). Use of marijuana, the most preferred psychedelic, declined from a high of 37.4% past month use in 1979 to a low of 11.9% in 1992 but since then it has risen again (22.4% in 2001) (University of Michigan, 2003). Other than marijuana, **psychedelics, as in the '60s and '70s, were and still are most popular among young White users**, then Hispanics, and finally, the lowest per capita use, the Black community (Substance Abuse and Mental Health Services Administration [SAMHSA], 2002).

"I got into marijuana and particularly LSD in the university setting in the late 1960s where we all felt it was a spiritual thing. We went to Dead concerts, Grateful Dead that is. We traveled around to wherever they were playing. Also I went to about 20 Santana concerts. Later on we got out of it because everybody started doing it and doing it just to get loaded—no spirituality there. Some could maintain while they were taking LSD, some just became idiots. I started just after my 17th birthday. Nowadays kids get into it when they're 12."
48-year-old former psychedelic abuser

CLASSIFICATION

Uppers stimulate the body and downers depress it. All arounders usually act as stimulants and occasionally as depressants but mostly **psychedelics dramatically alter a user's perception and create a world in which reason takes a back seat to intensified sensations by creating illusions, delusions, or hallucinations**. From alphabet soup psychedelics (MDMA, LSD, PMA) to naturally occurring plants used socially or in religious ceremonies (marijuana, peyote, mushrooms, belladonna), all arounders represent a diverse group of substances.

The five main classes of psychedelics are

◊ the indole psychedelics (e.g., **LSD, psilocybin mushrooms**);

◊ the phenylalkylamines (e.g., **peyote, MDMA [ecstasy]**);

◊ the anticholinergics (e.g., **belladonna, datura**);

◊ those in a class by themselves (e.g., **ketamine, PCP, *Salvia divinorum*, dextromethorphan [DXM]**);

◊ the cannabinols found in **marijuana** (*Cannabis*) plants.

GENERAL EFFECTS

ASSESSING THE EFFECTS

Even though many psychedelics predate more modern stimulants and depressants such as methamphetamines and benzodiazepines, the research has been minimal since most psychedelics are grown illegally or manufactured by street chemists. For this reason, **much of the information about the effects of psychedelics has been anecdotal rather than the result of extended scientific testing**. In addition most plant-based psychedelics contain more than one active ingredient, so it is hard to say which chemical is causing which effect. Also many drugs that are sold as one psychedelic may actually be another cheaper psychedelic, so even the anecdotal information can be incorrect. Some common examples of misrepresentation are ketamine sold as THC (the active ingredient in marijuana) or regular mushrooms dosed with LSD and sold as psilocybin mushrooms (Weil & Rosen, 1998).

Besides the toxicity, the effects of many psychedelics are dependent on the amount of drug ingested. A drug like LSD is thousands of times more powerful by weight than a similar amount of peyote.

Besides the toxicity of the psychedelic and the amount used,

◊ **experience with the drug,**

◊ **the basic emotional makeup of the user,**

TABLE 6–1   ALL AROUNDERS (PSYCHEDELICS)

Common Names	Active Ingredients	Street Names
INDOLE PSYCHEDELICS		
LSD (LSD-25 & -49) (Schedule I)	Lysergic acid diethylamide	Acid, sugar cube, window pane, blotter, illusion, boomers, yellow sunshine
Mushrooms (Schedule I)	Psilocybin	'Shrooms, magic mushrooms
Tabernanthe iboga (Schedule I)	Ibogaine	African LSD
Morning glory seeds or Hawaiian woodrose	Lysergic acid amide	Heavenly blue, pearly gates, wedding bells, ololiuqui
DMT (synthetic or from yopo beans, epena, or Sonoran Desert toad) (Schedule I)	Dimethyltryptamine	Businessman's special, cohoba snuff
Yage, ayahuasca, caapi	Harmaline (also mixed with DMT)	Visionary vine, vine of the soul, vine of death, mihi, kahi
Foxy	5-Me-DIPT	
AMT	Alphamethyltryptamine	
PHENYLALKYLAMINE PSYCHEDELICS		
Peyote cactus (Schedule I)	Mescaline	Mesc, peyote, buttons
Designer psychedelics, e.g., MDA, MDMA (MDM), MMDA, MDE (Schedule I)	Variations of methylenedioxy-amphetamines	Ecstasy, rave, love drug, XTC, Adam, Eve
2C-B or CBR (Schedule I)	4-bromo-2,5-dimethoxy-phenethylamine	Nexus
2C-T-2 (Schedule I)	2,5-dimethoxy-4-ethyl-thiophenethylamine	
2C-T-7 (Schedule I)	2,5-dimethoxy-4-propyl-thiophenethylamine	
STP (DOM) (synthetic) (Schedule I)	4 methyl 2,5 dimethoxy-amphetamine	Serenity, tranquility, peace pill
STP-LSD combo	Dimethoxy-amphetamine with LSD	Wedge series, orange and pink wedges, Harvey Wallbanger
PMA(Schedule I)	Paramethoxyamphetamine	Death, Mitsubishi Double-Stack
U4Euh (Schedule I)	4-methylpemoline	Euphoria
ANTICHOLINERGICS		
Belladonna, mandrake, henbane, datura (jimson weed, thornapple), wolfbane (Schedule I)	Atropine, scopolamine, hyoscyamine	Deadly nightshade
Artane®	Trihexyphenidyl	
Cogentin®	Benztropine	
Asmador® cigarettes	Belladonna alkaloids	
OTHER PSYCHEDELICS		
Ketamine (Schedule III)	Ketajet®, Ketalar®	Special K, K, vitamin K, super-K
PCP (Schedule II)	Phencyclidine	Angel dust, hog, peace pill, krystal joint, ozone, Sherms, Shermans
Nutmeg and mace	Myristicin	
Amanita mushrooms (fly agaric) (Schedule I)	Ibotenic acid, muscimole	Soma
Salvia divinorum	Salvinorin A	Diviner's sage, sage
DM in Romilar®, Coricidin®	Dextromethorphan	DXM, robo, red devils, dex, skittles
CANNABINOLS		
Marijuana (Schedule I) (Marinol® is legal prescription THC)	Δ-9-tetrahydro-cannabinol (THC)	Grass, pot, weed, Mary Jane, joint, reefer, honey blunt, chronic, sens, stink weed, herb, charas, ganja, grifa, the kind, bhang, ditch weed, Colombian, BC bud
Sinsemilla (Schedule I)	High-potency THC	Sens, skunk weed, ganja
Hashish, hash oil (Schedule I)	High-potency THC	Hash

◇ **the mood and mental state at the time of use,**

◇ **any preexisting mental illnesses,**

◇ **and the surroundings in which the drug is taken**

are also crucial to the kind, duration, and intensity of the effects. For instance, a first- or second-time psychedelic user may become nauseous, extremely anxious, depressed, and totally disoriented whereas an experienced user may only experience euphoric feelings or some mild illusions. A user with schizophrenia or major depression could get a severe reaction from LSD because it might trigger any unstable tendencies. Someone who is basically aggressive might become violent when using PCP whereas a young and immature user of marijuana could become more docile (Schuckit, 2000).

Physical & Mental Effects

LSD and most other **hallucinogens stimulate the sympathetic nervous system**. This stimulation results in a rise in pulse rate and blood pressure. Many psychedelics can trigger sweating, palpitations, or nausea. Generally psychedelics interfere with neurotransmitters such as dopamine, norepinephrine, acetylcholine, anandamide, alpha psychosin, and especially serotonin. Serotonin affects sensory perception, behavior control, hunger, body temperature, sexual behavior, and muscle control. Because serotonin neurons are amply represented in the limbic system, the emotional center of the brain, most psychedelics greatly affect mood. Serotonin $5HT_2A$ receptors are especially affected by the indole psychedelics, e.g., LSD. The strength of most psychedelics is related directly to their influence on the $5HT_2A$ receptors (Snyder, 1996; National Institute on Drug Abuse [NIDA], 2001).

The stimulation of the brainstem, and specifically the reticular formation, can **overload the sensory pathways making the user acutely aware of all sensation**. Disruption of visual and auditory centers can confuse perception. An auditory stimulation such as music might jump to a visual pathway causing the music to be "seen" as shifting light patterns; visual impulses might shift to auditory neurons resulting in strange sounds. **This crossover or mixing of the senses is known as "synesthesia."** Some practitioners of certain forms of religion or mysticism say that many psychedelic experiences are similar to the transcendental state of mind achieved through deep meditation.

Illusions, Delusions, & Hallucinations

It is important to note the differences between an illusion, a delusion, and a hallucination. **An illusion is a mistaken perception of an external stimulus.** For example, a rope can be misinterpreted as a snake or smooth skin as silk.

"All the trees were caving in on me and the bus was melting. I couldn't think. I couldn't comprehend what the teacher was telling everybody and here I am walking around dumbfounded. The rocks are moving and I can't pay attention to anything."
18-year-old psychedelic mushroom user

A delusion is a mistaken idea that is not swayed by reason or other powerful evidence. An example is someone who thinks he can fly or thinks he has become deformed or ugly.

"I have strange thoughts. I have a tunnel vision effect. I feel unified; I feel very asexual, like sex would be beside the point because I feel unified with everything."
38-year-old psychedelic user

A hallucination is a sensory experience that doesn't come from external stimuli, such as seeing a creature or object that doesn't exist.

"You go to places that you could never reach before to where you were never coming back and then out of a dream and you step up back into your body

and come back to your senses and come back to reality."
16-year-old psychedelic user

With LSD and most psychedelics, illusions and delusions are the primary experiences. With mescaline, psilocybin, and PCP, hallucinations are the primary experience.

LSD, PSILOCYBIN MUSHROOMS, & OTHER INDOLE PSYCHEDELICS

LSD (lysergic acid diethylamide)

"LSD was very colorful, a super rush, magical, trippy, giggly, sometimes scary. I was called the 'King of Acid' because I always had a very good trip unlike some friends who took it every day. I waited at least 3 or 4 days in between trips because your body needs some time to recover. My friends who used it daily, they got pretty burnt out with insomnia, grinding teeth, and exhaustion because of the total nerve action."
48-year-old accountant, former "Deadhead"

History (also see Chapter 1)

"Acid," "blotter," "barrels," "sunshine," "illusion," and "window panes" are just some of the street names for **LSD (lysergic acid diethylamide), a semisynthetic form of an ergot fungus toxin that infects rye and other cereal grasses**. The brownish-purple fungus, *Claviceps purpura*, was responsible for many outbreaks of ergot poisoning (ergotism) and thousands of deaths over the centuries when people accidentally ate the infected grain, particularly in parts of Europe and Russia. There are two types of ergotism, gangrenous and convulsive. **Gangrenous ergotism, also known as "St. Anthony's Fire," is marked by feverish hallucinations** and rotting away of gangrenous extremities of the body. The gangrene is caused by the extreme vasoconstriction of small blood vessels that causes the unnourished tissues to die. **Convulsive ergotism is marked by visual and auditory hallucinations**, painful muscular contractions, vomiting, diarrhea, headaches, disturbances in sensation, mania, psychosis, delirium, and convulsions (Siegel, 1985).

LSD was first extracted in 1938 by Dr. Albert Hoffman at Sandoz Pharmaceuticals when he and Dr. Arthur Stoll were investigating the alkaloids of *Claviceps purpurea* looking for a circulatory stimulant (analeptic). LSD (technically LSD-25) was the 25th derivative the doctors tried. Five years later Dr. Hoffman discovered the hallucinogenic properties of the new drug when he accidentally ingested a dose of LSD while developing a new way to chemically synthesize it in his laboratory.

"I suddenly became strangely inebriated. The external world became changed as in a dream. Objects appeared to gain in relief, they assumed unusual dimensions and colors became more glowing. Even self-perception and the sense of time were changed. [Another time] I lost all control of time; space and time became more and more disorganized and I was overcome with fears that I was going crazy."

Dr. Albert Hoffman in 1943 describing one of his experiences with LSD (Stafford, 1992)

LSD was investigated as a therapy for mental illnesses and alcoholism and as a key to investigating thought processes (Marnell, 1997). In the 1950s it was sold as Delysid® (the trade name for LSD) and prescribed to enhance psychological insight in psychotherapy. In the early 1950s the CIA conducted a number of experiments with LSD as a truth drug or mind-control drug in a program code-named "MK-ULTRA." The drug did not do what was expected and the program

was discontinued in the mid-1960s (Stafford, 1985).

LSD-25 was popularized by Harvard psychologists Drs. Timothy Leary and Richard Alpert (among others) who did psilocybin and LSD research in the 1960s as a way to explore consciousness and feelings. Dr. Leary's first experience with a large amount of LSD kept him "unable to speak for five days." He wrote that he never recovered from that mind-shattering experience. He even started a religion called the "League for Spiritual Discovery" (Stafford, 1992). Dr. Leary's slogan **"Turn on, tune in, and drop out"** was used in endless newspaper articles and TV news shows as the rallying cry for the youth of the '60s and '70s. (It led to the suspicion that the media was as much responsible for the rise and fall of LSD as was its identification and subsequent vilification as the drug of the hippie generation.)

Ken Kesey, who wrote *One Flew Over the Cuckoo's Nest,* was one of the subjects of early LSD experiments. He went on to become one of the founders of the Merry Pranksters, a group of counter-culture advocates who popu-

larized psychedelics, particularly LSD, through a series of concerts often involving the Grateful Dead. They held happenings called the "Kool Aid Acid Test," where diluted vats of LSD were distributed freely to all partygoers.

LSD was made illegal on February 1, 1966, under provisions of the Federal Drug Abuse Control Amendments. LSD was classified as a Schedule I drug in 1970. In 1974 the National Institute of Mental Health concluded that LSD had no therapeutic use (Henderson & Glass, 1994). Scientific research virtually ceased in the early '70s and it wasn't until recently that any research on LSD or psychedelics in general was renewed. LSD use continued to decline in the '80s but in the '90s there was a resurgence in its popularity.

Epidemiology

Younger and younger Americans were using LSD in the early 1990s but those numbers dropped by the early 2000s possibly due to the increasing popularity of the psycho-stimulant ecstasy. Anecdotal reports at the Haight Ashbury Clinic in San Francisco indi-

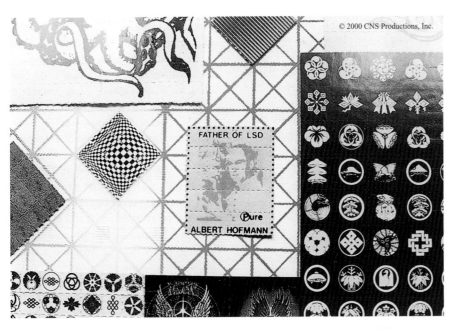

© 2000 CNS Productions, Inc.

FATHER OF LSD

Pure
ALBERT HOFMANN

The hallucinogen LSD is manufactured as a liquid and dropped onto perforated blotter paper. A small square is swallowed for the effect. The designs varied from cartoon characters to a picture of Dr. Albert Hoffman, the Sandoz Pharmaceuticals chemist who first synthesized the drug.

TABLE 6–2   30-DAY PREVALENCE OF LSD USE AMONG 8th, 10th, & 12th GRADE STUDENTS

	1975	1985	1991	1993	1995	1997	1999	2002
8th Grade	—	—	0.6%	1.0%	1.4%	1.5%	1.1%	0.7%
10th Grade	—	—	1.5%	1.6%	3.0%	2.8%	2.3%	0.7%
12th Grade	2.3%	1.6%	1.9%	2.4%	4.0%	3.1%	2.7%	0.7%

The use of LSD by high school students started climbing in 1991 after years of decline. The use of LSD for those who have been arrested is double the above figures (University of Michigan, 2003).

cate that low doses of LSD are abused on occasion by junior high and high school students while they are sitting in class. This is because low-dose use results in less detectable physical symptoms (e.g., stimulation) than alcohol or marijuana and only mild psychedelic effects. In the '60s, "acidheads" were usually in their early 20s and many were searching for a quasi religious experience. In the 1990s and 2000s most younger teenagers said they just wanted to get high or augment the effects of ecstasy and other drugs.

Besides the normal reasons for using a drug like LSD (experimentation, peer pressure, availability, and curiosity), there are three other factors that have spurred current popularity. One is the proliferation of what used to be called "rave" clubs and parties where MDMA, LSD, ketamine, GHB, and amphetamines are used (Pechnick & Ungerleider, 1997). Another reason is that **standard drug testing usually does not test for LSD** and even when tested for, the effective dose is so small that it is almost impossible to detect.

Manufacture of LSD

"We had Palo Alto Owsley stuff— Augustus Stanley Owsley. He ran the sound for the Grateful Dead for years. Supposedly he made pure LSD with no additives or bad chemistry. I started with 200 mics then up to 400. The best dose was 100 to 150. If we were out of doors, we would only take 50, so we'd still be able to navi-

gate. Back in 1969 and the early '70s, it cost about $1 to $3 a hit."
48-year-old former LSD user

The majority of LSD has been and still is manufactured in northern California, mostly in the San Francisco Bay area, although there is some secondary manufacture in the Pacific Northwest and recently the Midwest (Drug Enforcement Administration [DEA], 2003a). The labs are hard to find since the quantities of raw material needed to make the drug are very small. Indeed the entire U.S. supply for 1 year could be carried by one person. For example, 60 lbs. of ergotamine tartrate, the basic synthetic raw ingredient for LSD, could produce 11 lbs. of LSD, the nation's annual consumption (Marnell, 1997). One pound of LSD is sufficient to make up to 9 million hits of the drug. LSD can also be synthesized from morning glory plants that contain lysergic acid amide. The production of LSD is tedious and involves volatile and dangerous chemicals. The end product of the initial synthesis, **crystalline LSD, is dissolved in alcohol and drops of the solution are put on blotter paper and chewed or swallowed**. It has also been put into microdots or tiny squares of gelatin and eaten or dropped onto a moist body tissue and absorbed (NIDA, 2001). Each dose on the blotter is 1 cm square and has been impregnated with 10–50 micrograms (mics) of liquid LSD. To reach the younger group of potential users, illegal manufacturers even printed images of Mickey Mouse, Donald Duck, a teddy bear, and other characters on the blotter paper.

Pharmacology

LSD ($C_{20}H_{25}N_3O$) is remarkable for its potency. Doses as low as 25 micrograms, or **25 millionths of a gram, can cause mental changes** (spaciness, decreased perception of time, mild euphoria) and mild stimulatory effects.

Effects appear 15 minutes to 1 hour after ingestion and last 6–8 hours. The usual psychedelic dose of LSD is 150–300 micrograms. The Drug Enforcement Administration (DEA) reports that the current strength of LSD street samples ranges from 20–80 micrograms and each dose costs \$.50 to \$5.00 or more. In the late '60s and '70s, samples ranged from 100–200 micrograms or more (DEA, 2003a). **Tolerance develops very rapidly** to the psychedelic effects of LSD. Within a few days of daily use, a person can tolerate a 300-microgram dose without experiencing any major psychedelic effects. The tolerance is lost rapidly after cessation of use—usually within a few days. Some cross-tolerance can also develop to the effects of mescaline and psilocybin but there is little cross-tolerance between LSD and DMT, another indole psychedelic (Pechnick & Ungerleider, 1997).

"When we took it every day, we got off less 'cause we depleted our brain chemistry, and you just get burned out, and you have to take twice as much. Some had to take five times as much, about 2,000 mics to get any reaction, like a depleted speed freak, like in a cloud."
28-year-old former LSD user

Withdrawal after LSD use is usually more mental and emotional than physical—a psychedelic hangover.

"Withdrawal was like the next day; the Germans call it 'Katzenjammer,' which is like a chemical depletion of mind and body, similar to a really bad hangover. You're still psychedelically spaced the next day and you're dealing with all the revelations. Dependence

was more of a social urge to do it rather than a private urge."
24-year-old former LSD user

Physical Effects

LSD can cause a **rise in heart rate and blood pressure, a higher body temperature, dizziness, dilated pupils, and some sweating**, much like amphetamines. Users see many light trails, like afterimages in cheap televisions where there is always an afterimage of whatever is happening on camera (this aftereffect is known as the "trailing phenomena").

Mental Effects

"In a real strong acid you'll see the walls melting like candles and water running down the wall. That kind of distortion is not a complete hallucination or anything real solid like a bottle where you wonder whether it's there or not. The thing that got me really crazy was hearing a dog or airplane or passenger car miles away and you didn't know whether that was real or an illusion. There was also what we called the psychedelic hummmmmm that we thought we heard."
Recovering 38-year-old LSD and marijuana user

Mentally LSD overloads the brainstem, the sensory switchboard for the mind, causing **sensory distortions (seeing sounds, feeling smells, or hearing colors [synesthesia]), dreaminess, depersonalization, altered mood, and impaired concentration and motivation**. The locus coeruleus is activated to release extra amounts of norepinephrine, which greatly enhances alertness. This heightened awareness of the senses is possibly responsible for the introspection and awareness of the inner self that is common with LSD users (Snyder, 1996).

It becomes difficult to express oneself verbally while on LSD. Single word answers and seemingly nonassociated comments (nonsequiturs) are common. A user might experience intense sensations and emotions but find it difficult to tell others what he or she is feeling.

"It is fake, ersatz. Instant mysticism. . . . There's no wisdom there. I solved the secret of the universe last night, but this morning I forgot what it was."
Arthur Koestler, writer, LSD user

One of the **greatest dangers of LSD is the loss of judgment and impaired reasoning**. This, coupled with slowed reaction time and visual distortions, can make even the driving of a car risky at best.

"I stuck my hand in this flame and then I went, 'Uh-oh, my hand is in the flame,' and I pulled it out and I thought it didn't burn but later that night, my hand started blistering and I'm going, 'Oh no, I got burned.'"
43-year-old male former LSD user

Bad Trips (acute anxiety reactions)

Because LSD affects the emotional center in the brain and distorts reality, some users, particularly **first-time users who take it without supportive experienced users around them, are subject to the extremes of euphoria and panic**. Depersonalization and lack of a stable environment can trigger acute anxiety, paranoia, fear over loss of control, and delusions of persecution or feelings of grandeur leading to dangerous behaviors. One survivor of a jump from the Golden Gate Bridge claimed he was jumping through the "golden hoop." (*See Chapter 9 concerning treatment for bad trips.*)

"I've done acid one time. I took a couple of hits, you know, little tabs, and walls started melting and everything like that. Everybody started looking like monsters and just weird crazy shit, man. I was freaking out. I had a real bad trip that time, worse than the

"shrooms.' I was too scared to do that ever again."
15-year-old polydrug abuser in recovery

Mental Illness & LSD

Much of the research as well as enthusiasm for LSD as an adjunct to psychotherapy has decreased over the years. Proponents of psychotherapeutic use claim that **drug-stimulated insights afford some users a shortcut to the extended process of psychotherapy** in which uncovering traumas and conflicts from the subconscious helps to heal the patient. Opponents of this kind of therapy say that the dangerous side effects of LSD more than outweigh any benefit.

The popular picture of someone using LSD just one time and becoming permanently psychotic or schizophrenic is incorrect. It is a very unusual occurrence. What usually happens is that in people **with a preexisting mental illness or instability, LSD use can aggravate those conditions into more severe mental disturbances**. Use can also cause some people to experience their mental illness at an earlier age or it may provoke a relapse in someone who has previously suffered a psychotic disorder or a major depression.

"The whole thing started with my schizophrenia. That always plays a part. And any time I get too involved in the music scene, the acid starts to trigger the schizophrenia, like flashbacks, and sometimes it makes me want to use. But I'm drawn to it like a moth drawn to a light."
Recovering LSD user with schizophrenia

Also some otherwise normal users can be thrown into a temporary but prolonged psychotic reaction or severe depression that requires extended treatment. Prolonged trips (extended LSD effects) devoid of other psychiatric symptoms have also occurred. Though very rare, these reactions can be emotionally crippling and may last for years (NIDA, 2001).

Hallucinogen Persisting Perception Disorder (HPPD). **A number of users experience mental flashbacks of sensations or of a bad trip** they had while under the influence of LSD even when they have not used any drugs in several months or even years. The flashbacks, which can be triggered by stress, the use of another psychoactive drug, or even exercise, recreate the original experience. This sensation can also cause anxiety and even panic since it is unexpected and the user seems to have little control over its recurrence. Most flashbacks are provoked by some sensory stimulus: sight, sound, odor, or touch. Seeing trails of moving objects seems fairly common (American Psychiatric Association, 2000). It is thought that HPPD has a strong hereditary component.

A number of hallucinogens have the capacity to cause HPPD, e.g., LSD, MDMA, MDA, mescaline, DMT, marijuana, and psilocybin, though it is most common with LSD. It has been estimated that flashbacks occur in about 23% to 64% of regular LSD users (Hollister, 1984; Carroll & Comer, 1998; Jaffe, 1989). Although the **LSD flashback appears to be similar to a posttraumatic stress disorder**, recent case reports suggest that medications like sertraline, clonidine, and naltrexone may be useful in treating this problem (Lerner et al., 2000; Wilkins, Gorelick, & Conner, 1998; Young, 1997; Lerner, Oyffe, Issacs, & Sigal, 1997). A number of other medications have been tried on HPPD with limited success.

Dependence

Since LSD does not generally produce compulsive drug-seeking behavior, it is not considered addictive though some use it frequently. Five hundred LSD trips or more are reported by a number of users probably due to **a psychological dependence rather than a physical dependence** even though tolerance does develop rapidly. Frequent and repeated use of low-dose LSD for its stimulant not its psychedelic effects is an example of this psychological dependence.

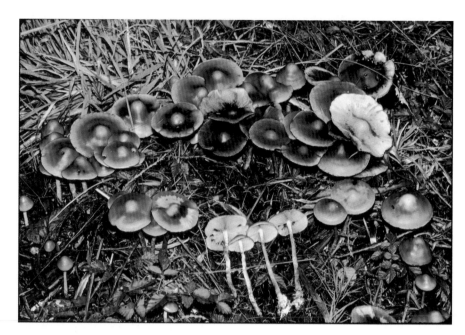

One of the 75 species of mushrooms containing psilocybin or psilocin. The "'shrooms" can be used fresh or dried although fresh psilocybin mushrooms are more potent than dried ones.
© 2000 Paul Stamets. Reprinted by permission.

"MAGIC MUSHROOMS" (psilocybin & psilocin)

"In 2002 Japan banned the sale of hallucinogenic mushrooms in stores. Up until then only the hallucinogenic chemical, psilocybin, had been illegal not the mushrooms themselves. 'Cases of young people doing harm to their health have been on the rise,' said a Health Ministry official."
Reuters News Service, 2002

Psilocybin and psilocin are the active ingredients in a number of psychedelic mushrooms found in Mexico, the United States, South America, Southeast Asia, and Europe. These mushrooms, originally called "*Teonanacatl*" (divine flesh) by the Aztecs, were especially important to Indian cultures in Mexico and some other areas in the pre-Columbian Americas and were **used in ceremonies dating as far back as 1000 B.C.** More than 200 stone sculptures of mushrooms have been found in El Salvador, Guatemala, and parts of Mexico (Furst, 1976). The existence of a mushroom cult that

flourished from 100 B.C. to A.D. 400 has been found in northwestern Mexico (Schultes & Hofmann, 1992). They are still used today although persecution by the Spaniards, who conquered much of Central and South America in the sixteenth and seventeenth centuries, drove the ceremonial use of mushrooms underground for hundreds of years. It wasn't until the 1950s that much was known about the ceremonies conducted by Mazatec, Chol, and Lacandon Mayan shamans or curanderas (medicine women or men). The ceremonies include eating or drinking the extracted psychedelic substances in order to get intoxicated, along with hours of chanting, all to **induce visions that will help treat illnesses, solve problems, or get in contact with the spirit world**.

The famous Mazatec shaman María Sabina wrote,

"The sacred mushroom takes me by the hand and brings me to the world where everything is known. It is they, the sacred mushrooms, that speak in a way I can understand. When I return from the trip that I have taken with

them, I tell what they have told me and what they have shown me."
María Sabina (Schultes & Hofmann, 1992)

In 1957, when mushroom researcher R. Gorden Wasson's article "Seeking the Magic Mushroom" appeared in *Life Magazine*, millions of Americans were introduced to the concept of psychedelic fungi and over the next 10 years experimentation began (Stamets, 1996).

"We tried strawberry psilocybin or rather psilocin, a synthetic version of psilocybin. The second batch we got was pink and we called that 'pink silly.' Then we tried 'Czechoslovakian microdot.' The psilocybin was very similar to LSD. There was a lot of romantic adventure. I remember eating rhododendron flowers in the park. All the flowers were smiling. After concerts the music would continue in my head for hours. There wasn't much difference but you didn't know if the psilocin was really LSD."
48-year-old ex-psychedelic user

Pharmacology

In 1956 the active psychedelic ingredients psilocybin and psilocin were isolated by mycologist (mushroom expert) Roger Heim and researcher Dr. Albert Hoffman, the same scientist at Sandoz Pharmaceutical who had discovered LSD-25. **Psilocybin and psilocin are found in about 75 different species of mushroom** from 4 genera: *Psilocybe, Panaeolus, Stropharia,* and *Conocybe* (Stamets, 1996). Fifteen species have been identified in the U.S. Pacific Northwest. Psychic effects are obtained from doses of 10 mg to 60 mg and generally last for 3 to 6 hours.

Both wild and cultivated **mushrooms vary greatly in strength, so a single potent mushroom might have as much psilocybin as 10 weak ones.** When the caps and stems are ingested, either fresh or dried, the psilocybin is converted to psilocin. However psilocy-bin is more plentiful and is almost twice as potent as psilocin. It also crosses the blood-brain barrier more readily. **The chemical structure of psilocybin is similar to that of LSD.**

Effects

"We were living in an Indian village in the mountains of central Mexico where the 'hongos' [mushrooms] grow. One night when it rained, the locals were shouting, 'Hongos mañana,' and they were right. We got some and it made all the colors seem softer and more pastel. My body felt like there was a river running through it and all sorts of visceral feelings were let loose. The environment was fortunately non-threatening."
Former psychedelic user

Most mushrooms containing psilocybin cause nausea and other physical symptoms before the psychedelic effects take over. The psychedelic effects include **visceral sensations, changes in sight, hearing, taste, and touch, and altered states of consciousness.** There seems to be less disassociation and panic than with LSD. Prolonged psychotic reactions are rare. However these effects are not consistent with every user and depend on the setting in which the drug is taken. As with LSD and other indole psychedelics, many of the effects are caused by disruption of the neurotransmitters serotonin and dopamine, along with the sudden release of norepinephrine, a stimulatory neurotransmitter that overheightens the senses (Pechnick & Ungerleider, 1997).

"With 'shrooms' sometimes you catch yourself just like, not out of your body but out of your mind kind of. You're not controlling your actions. You're not controlling what you're saying or what you're feeling. You know, the drug just takes hold of you."
23-year-old psilocybin mushroom user

There is a small market for mail order kits containing spores for growing mushrooms in a closet or basement. Some users also tramp the countryside looking for a certain species. **The major danger in "'shroom" harvesting is mistaking poisonous mushrooms for those containing psilocybin.** Some poisonous mushrooms (e.g., *Amanita phalloides*) can cause death or permanent liver damage within hours of ingestion. Further, grocery-bought mushrooms can be laced with LSD or PCP and often sold to those seeking the "magic mushroom" experience.

OTHER INDOLE PSYCHEDELICS

Ibogaine

Produced by the African *Tabernanthe iboga* shrub and some other plants, ibogaine in low doses acts as a stimulant. In higher doses it produces long-acting psychedelic effects and a self-determined catatonic reaction that can be maintained up to 2 days. It is rarely found in the United States although it has been synthesized in laboratories. Its use is generally limited to native cultures in western and central Africa, such as the Bwiti tribe of Gabon. They use it to help stay alert and motionless while hunting. They also claim to experience ancestral visions while using it (O'Brien, Cohen, Evans, & Fine, 1992).

There has been **research into the use of ibogaine to treat heroin or cocaine addiction.** Anecdotal reports as well as some limited studies claim that just a few treatments eliminated withdrawal symptoms and craving for opioids. However several deaths have been associated with ibogaine administration. Animal studies indicate cerebellum neurotoxicity results from ibogaine use. These concerns have effectively limited further research into ibogaine as a medical treatment for heroin dependence (Wilkins, Gorelick, & Conner, 1998).

Morning Glory Seeds (ololiuqui)

Seeds from the morning glory plant (*Ipomoea tricolor*) or the Hawaiian woodrose (*Argyreia nervosa*) contain several LSD-like substances, particularly **lysergic acid amide, which is about one-tenth as potent as LSD**. The lysergic acid amide can be used to make lysergic acid diethylamide (LSD). Used by Indians in Mexico before the Spanish arrived, several hundred seeds have to be taken to get high, so the nauseating properties of the drug are magnified. In sufficient quantities the seeds cause LSD-like effects but they are not particularly popular among those who use psychedelics. Along with sensory disturbances and mood changes come the nausea, vomiting, drowsiness, headaches, and chills. Effects last up to 6 hours and LSD-like flashbacks are somewhat common. **Morning glory seeds are sold commercially** but to prevent misuse, many of these seeds are dipped in a toxic substance that induces vomiting (O'Brien et al., 1992). The seeds have street names such as "heavenly blue" and "pearly gates."

DMT (dimethyltryptamine)

Dimethyltryptamine is found in South American trees, vines, shrubs, and mushrooms or it is synthesized by street chemists. DMT is a psychedelic substance similar in structure to psilocin. Since digestive juices destroy the active ingredients, the drug, which is usually a white, yellow, or brown powder, can be snorted or injected but usually smoked. South American tribes have used it for at least 400 years. They **prepare it from several different plants as a snuff** called "yopo," "cohoba," "vilca," "cebil," or "epena." They blow it into each other's noses through a hollow reed and then dance, hallucinate, and sing. The synthetic form can be made in basement laboratories (Schultes & Hofmann, 1992).

DMT causes intense visual rather than auditory hallucinations, intoxication, and often a loss of awareness of surroundings lasting about 30–60 minutes or less. The **short duration of action** gave rise to the nickname "businessman's special" because the white-collar worker can get high and almost sober during lunch.

Newspaper reports have sensationalized a variant of DMT, 5-MeO-DMT, the venom of the Sonoran Desert toad. Contrary to anecdotes about people licking the toad to get high, the substance is milked onto cigarettes, dried, and smoked (Lyttle, Goldstein, & Gartz, 1996; Chilton, Bigwood, & Jensen, 1979).

Foxy (5-methoxy-N, N-diisopropyltryptamine [5-Me-DIPT]) & AMT (alphamethyltryptamine)

These two psychedelic tryptamines appeared in the early 2000s while they were still not listed as scheduled drugs under the Controlled Substances Act. However they have been prosecuted under the federal drug analogue statute. Law enforcement agencies have seized samples in a number of states but the drugs have been only occasionally used at raves in Arizona, California, Florida, and New York (DEA, 2002).

Effects include hallucinations, euphoria, empathy, visual and auditory disturbances (illusions), and emotional distress. They also can cause nausea, vomiting, and diarrhea. The effects from 20 mg of either of the drugs can last 12–24 hours while smaller doses will last only 3–6 hours. The powder is prepared in capsules or tablets in a variety of colors.

Yage

Yage or ayahuasca is a psychedelic drink made from the leaves, bark, and vines of *Banisteriopsis caapi* and *Banisteriopsis inebrians*, Amazon Jungle vines. Drinking this preparation **causes intense vomiting, diarrhea, and then a dreamlike condition that usually lasts up to 10 hours**. The Chama, Tukanoan, and Zaparo Indians of Peru, Brazil, and Ecuador use it for prophecy, divination, sorcery, and medical purposes. They believe that yage frees the soul to wander at will and return at will and communicate with ancestors (Schultes & Hofmann, 1992).

The active ingredient is harmaline, an indole alkaloid found in several other psychedelic plants, such as the Syrian rue herb from China. Native cultures often mix yage with DMT plant extracts in order to intensify the effects. It has been recently discovered that harmaline protects the DMT from being deactivated by gastric enzymes thus allowing DMT to be effective when taken orally.

In the last few years cults using ayahuasca as the focus of their beliefs have sprung up in Brazil. The use has spread to the United States and other countries.

PEYOTE, MDMA, & OTHER PHENYLALKYLAMINE PSYCHEDELICS

This class of psychedelics is **chemically related to adrenaline and amphetamine** although many of the effects are quite different. Whereas the effects of amphetamines will peak within half an hour, much sooner if smoked, many of the **phenylalkylamines take several hours to reach their peak**, much longer than indole psychedelics like LSD.

PEYOTE (mescaline)

The search for connections to the inner self and the outer spiritual worlds led many cultures to experiment with hallucinogenic plants. In the late nineteenth and early twentieth centuries, the interest in the inner workings of the mind, as delineated in the writings of Drs. Sigmund Freud, Alfred Adler, and Carl Jung among others, led many to search for the philosopher's stone (plant) that would chemically help them to understand themselves. Aldous Huxley, one of the earliest writers/philosophers to examine this connection, used mescaline from the peyote cactus for his exploration.

"The urge to transcend self-conscious selfhood is, as I have said, a principal appetite of the soul. When, for whatever reason, men and women fail to

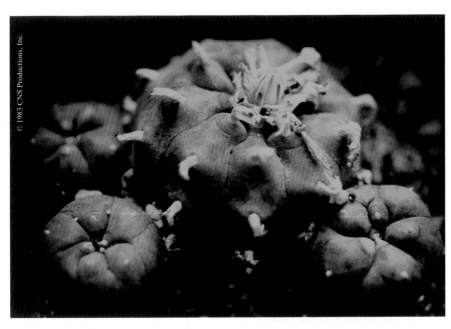

A mature peyote cactus (Lophophora williamsii) *is ripe for harvesting. Each button (the top of the cactus) contains about 50 mg of mescaline. It can take from 2–10 buttons to get high.*

transcend themselves by means of worship, good works, and spiritual exercises, they are apt to resort to religion's chemical surrogates— alcohol and 'goof pills' in the modern West, alcohol and opium in the East, hashish in the Mohammedan world, alcohol and marijuana in Central America, alcohol and coca in the Andes."
Aldous Huxley, The Doors of Perception, 1954

Mescaline is the active component of the peyote cactus (*Lophophora williamsii***) and the San Pedro cactus (***Trichocereus pachanoi***).** San Pedro cacti have been depicted in 3,000-year-old Chavin art from coastal Peru. The use of the peyote cacti stretches back to 300 B.C. Over the centuries the Aztecs, Toltecs, Chichimecas, and several Meso-American cultures included it in their rituals. When they invaded the New World, the Spanish Conquistadores regarded peyote as evil and the hallucinations as an invitation from the devil. They tried to abolish it but never succeeded. In the 1800s its use spread north to the United States where about 50 North American tribes were still taking it by the early 1900s

(Furst, 1976). Many challenges have been made concerning the legality of using a psychedelic substance for a religious ceremony. **In 1990 the U.S. Supreme Court ruled that the use of peyote during religious ceremonies is not protected by the Constitution and that states can ban it.** For this reason many ceremonies are held in secret.

Peyote cacti are still eaten in ritual ceremonies by the northern Mexican tribes (e.g., Huichol, Tarahumara, Cora Indians), and by the Southwest Plains Indian tribes (e.g., Comanche, Kiowa, Ute). In addition **peyote is used by the Native American Church of North America**, with a claimed membership of 250,000, as part of their ceremonies. Their stated reason for using peyote is to build spirituality and community. In 2002 in an appeal of a divorce suit in which a Native American got custody of his son on the proviso that he not give him peyote, he claimed the ruling interfered with his practice of religion. The litigation continues.

In the '50s and '60s peyote cacti (called "buttons") were available by mail order. Presently they are still available by mail but one has to file documentation of membership in the Native

American Church. About 2 million buttons are harvested in Texas each year. Heavy active users might consume up to 1,000 buttons a year. There are nine licensed distributors of peyote in the United States (Marnell, 1997; DEA, 2003c).

Effects

The gray-green crowns of the peyote cactus are cut at ground level or uprooted and can be **used fresh or dried**. The bitter nauseating substance is either eaten (seven to eight buttons is an average dose) or boiled and drunk as a tea. They can also be ground and eaten as a powder (Schultes & Hofmann, 1992). Synthetic mescaline, which was isolated in 1890, consists of thin needle-like crystals that are sold in capsules. **The effects of mescaline last approximately 12 hours and are very similar to LSD with an emphasis on colorful visions.** Users term it the "mellow LSD" but actual hallucinations are more common with mescaline than with LSD. Each use of peyote is usually accompanied by a severe episode of nausea and vomiting although some users can develop a tolerance to these effects. As with most psychedelics, tolerance to the psychedelic effects can also develop rapidly (La Barre & Weston, 1979).

A peyote ceremony might consist of ingesting the peyote buttons, then singing, drumming, chanting hymns, and trying to understand the psychedelic visions in order to have spiritual experiences. Many participants also have hallucinatory visions of a deity or spiritual leader whom they are able to converse with for guidance and understanding (Furst, 1976).

"When you get fresh buttons, they go down easier. No doubt about it, peyote is the worst taste I've ever experienced. Whenever I took it I got into projectile vomiting. It would happen as I was coming on to it. My reaction was intensely visual but it was different than LSD in that I could have a conversation despite the hallucinations."
Former psychedelic user

Since the reaction to many psychedelics depends on the mind-set and setting almost as much as on the actual properties of the drug, use of a mind-altering substance in a structured ceremonial setting can induce more spiritual feelings than if it's used at a rock concert.

PSYCHO-STIMULANTS (MDA, MDMA, 2C-B, PMA, 2C-T-7, 2C-T-2, et al.) & CLUB DRUGS

"There is a wealth of information built into us. . . tucked away in the genetic material in every one of our cells. Without some means of access, there is no way even to begin to guess at the extent and quality of what is there. The psychedelic drugs allow exploration of this interior world and insights into its nature."

Dr. Alexander Shulgin, psychopharmacologist and chemist

One of the first groups of synthetic drugs used for mental exploration and later for so-called recreational purposes were designer psychedelics or psycho-stimulants, chemically defined as **phenylethylamine derivatives similar to mescaline**. Phenylethylamines are naturally occurring compounds found in the human brain (Shulgin & Shulgin, 2000).

The first of these **laboratory variations of the amphetamine molecule** was synthesized in 1910 (MDA) and 1914 (MDMA) although the psychic effects weren't explored until a generation later. The drugs can **cause feelings of well-being and euphoria, some psychedelic effects, and stimulatory effects** as well as side effects and toxicity similar to amphetamines. The differences among the more than 150 compounds of these psycho-stimulants in current limited use have to do with duration of action, extent of delusional, illusional, or hallucinogenic effects, and degree of euphoria. Hundreds of other compounds have been created but strictly for experimental purposes.

MDA was the first of these compounds to be widely used and abused (in the late '60s, '70s, and early '80s), often on college campuses. Though originally designed as a medication to stop bleeding, when the psychic effects were discovered it became the "love drug" as it was touted to increase libido. When research showed damage to serotonin-producing neurons in the brain, a few overdose deaths, and increased legal scrutiny, its popularity waned and by the mid-1980s, MDMA had taken over as the psycho-stimulant of choice.

MDMA (ecstasy, rave, "XTC," "X," "Adam," "E," et al.)

The compound **MDMA, chemical name 3,4-methylenedioxymethamphetamine**, is shorter acting than MDA (4–6 hrs. vs. 10–12 hrs.). MDMA can be swallowed, snorted, or injected, much like methamphetamine, though it is **usually sold as a capsule, tablet, or powder**. MDMA is often taken at parties, raves, and music clubs because users claim it creates a strong desire to move about, dance, and interact with other people (Morgan, 1997).

"We'd have 'E' parties; a bunch of people would go and take 'E' and like it's really like a friendly drug. Like you take it and then you feel happy, so you talk to your friends a lot. You talk to strangers and you find things in common and everyone is like your best friend but when you come down off of the drug, it's like a totally different experience, it's like a downer."

17-year-old ecstasy user

History. MDMA was first discovered in 1914 by Merck Pharmaceuticals in Germany as an intermediate chemical step in its synthesis of MDA. It wasn't until 1953 that it surfaced again when the U.S. Army experimented on animals with a number of psychedelic compounds. The psychological warfare/brainwashing experimental compounds included MDPEA, MDA, BDB, DMA, TMA, and MDMA. It took another 16 years before the **first published human study of MDMA appeared, written by Dr. Alexander Shulgin** (a chemist and psychopharmacologist) and Dave Nichols, another chemist. They described the insight that the drug seemed to give and **recommended it to a number of therapists to help their patients see into their emotions and repressed memories**. Dr. Ann Shulgin, a psychotherapist, who along with her husband Alexander developed over 150 amphetamine analogues (many for the DEA), estimated that as many as 4,000 therapists were introduced to MDMA in the late '70s and '80s (Holland, 2001; Pentney, 2001).

As with any drug that develops a reputation, entrepreneurs started making it available (legally) for recreational use. After a series of hearings starting in 1985 and continuing for several years, MDMA was finally **banned as a Schedule I drug in 1988 in the United States** making it impossible to continue psychotherapeutic experimentation legally. Of course all the publicity made the drug more desirable among drug experimenters. The name "ecstasy" was supposedly chosen by a street chemist as a marketing tool possibly because the name "empathy," which is closer to the true initial effects of the drug, wasn't sexy enough for the young crowd.

"I had no inhibitions. I mean it was like whatever sexual compromise or you know, touching or conversation that I would have normally had boundaries for, I didn't when I took ecstasy."

28-year-old ecstasy user

When ecstasy was legal, the main manufacturer sold up to 50,000 tablets a week. After it was made illegal, just one bust in Holland in 2000 netted 1.25 million tablets. It was a sign that the traffic in this psycho-stimulant had reached unprecedented proportions. Most of the MDMA used in the United States has been smuggled in from

Europe. Recently however a significant amount of "E" tabs have been manufactured by clandestine laboratories across the United States that use a variety of safrole compounds extracted from sassafras oil to synthesize MDMA (DEA, 2003a).

In 2002 about **7.4% of high school seniors had used MDMA but only 2.4% used on a monthly basis**, about the same amount that tried LSD (University of Michigan, 2003). By comparison, 21.5% used marijuana on a monthly basis, 26.7% smoked cigarettes, and 48.6% drank alcohol. Recent reports indicate that the use of ecstasy has leveled off.

Use & Cost.   Ecstasy use is often called "rolling," the Generation X term coming from the practice of concealing an "E" tablet in the middle of a Tootsie Roll® that is then rewrapped. Vicks® inhalants and other pungent substances that are said to be pleasingly enhanced by the use of "E" are also found at rave clubs, along with Tiger Balm® and certain oils used while massaging the muscle tightness that occurs with the onset of MDMA effects.

A capsule, tablet, or equivalent powder packet (75–125 mg) costs anywhere from $10 to $35. The cost of producing each tablet ranges from $0.50 to $2.00 each, so there is a huge profit margin. Wholesale prices in the United States for large quantities range from $8 to $12 per pill. Tablets come in almost every color with off-white to a light tan being the most common. They also have a variety of logos stamped on them. The Mitsubishi® emblem, the butterfly, and various heart renditions have been some of the hundreds of "E" tab logos.

A DEA report found that **30–50% of the tablets sold as MDMA at rave parties actually contain no MDMA** but do contain other illicit drugs like PCP, methamphetamine, PMA, or MDA. Of those with MDMA, only 24% had only MDMA and no other psychoactive drug. In addition 57% of "rolling ravers" were knowingly under the influence of other illicit drugs besides "E" (DEA, 2001; DEA; 2003a).

"The first time I did 'E,' I chewed the bottom of my lip open because there was so much speed in it. I woke up the next morning and my stomach was like completely hollow. I felt like there was nothing in my stomach at all. My legs were going, I was bouncing my legs and they were vibrating; they were going so fast. It was so weird. My eyes were popping out of their sockets."
17-year-old ecstasy user

At a number of raves and concerts, a private organization (DanceSafe®) does testing of ecstasy samples, so people who buy pills can find out if there is actually any MDMA in them. The main problem is that the tests are fairly basic and cannot test for what is actually in the pills. Some users can get a false sense of security and take the drug anyway. The testing group does give out information about ecstasy and other drugs, so they do function as a method of harm reduction that minimizes some of the damage "rollers" can do to themselves (DanceSafe, 2003).

Physical Effects.   MDMA has many stimulant effects similar to amphetamines, such as increased heart rate, faster respiration, excess energy, fainting, sweating, chills, and hyperactivity. The more that is used, the greater the physical effects. The effects of "E" start to appear about 30 minutes after ingestion (the usual route of administration). **The onset of action usually consists of tightness in muscles with generalized muscle spasms, trismus (jaw muscle spasm), and bruxism (clenching of the teeth) just before most of the psychic effects begin to appear.** Because of the clenched jaw and other effects, a variety of paraphernalia is associated with MDMA including baby pacifiers and lollipops to avoid tooth damage. Though some report more heightened sensations, prolonged use decreases orgasm in men and sexual arousal in women (DuPont, 2000). Since MDMA releases less adrenaline than most methamphetamines, a user doesn't receive quite as much

sympathetic nervous system stimulation of heart rate and blood pressure. However, **tolerance to its mental effects develops rapidly**, so users increase doses often causing greater physical harm.

When the Rock Medicine Program of the Haight Ashbury Free Clinics provides medical care at concerts, the more serious MDMA effects they see include

◇ water toxicity and electrolyte imbalances as well as dehydration;

◇ pupil dilatation, blurred vision, and twitches of the eyelid;

◇ headaches, agitation, nausea, and anorexia;

◇ serotonergic axon apoptosis (cell death) resulting in thought and memory impairment;

◇ rapid and potentially dangerous heart rhythm problems;

◇ seizure activity, stroke, cardiovascular failure, and coma;

◇ malignant hyperthermia (**high body temperature**) that can also result in rhabdomyolysis (muscle damage)

◇ and renal (kidney) failure; the extreme heat can even coagulate the blood.

"At raves ecstasy causes the natural thermostat in your body to go haywire, so there's a lot of heat because people are very active. It's a stimulant, so people are dancing, forget to drink water, forget to hydrate, and these places are mostly hot and we've seen people with extended body temperatures. So those are the things to spot, cool down, and then in the extreme states, medicate and transport."
Glen Razwick, Director, Rock Medicine Program, Haight Ashbury Free Clinics

High-dose use can result in **high blood pressure and seizure activity** much like that seen in amphetamine overdose. In recent animal experiments (rats and monkeys), it was found that MDMA damaged serotonin-producing neurons in the brain similar to the way that MDA was proven to do in humans. Much of the damage remained even 12–18 months after use (Fischer, Hatzidimitriou, Wlos, Katz, & Ricaurte, 1995).

Mental/Emotional Effects. Twenty minutes to 1 hour after ingestion and continuing for 3 to 4 more hours, MDMA induces feelings of happiness, clarity, peace, pleasure, and altered sensory perceptions without causing any depersonalization or detachments of the users from the realities of their environment. Users also claim to experience increased **nonsexual empathy for others**, heightened self-esteem, more self-awareness, open mindedness, acceptance, and intimacy in their interactions. For these reasons it is also called a "hug drug" rather than a "love drug" like MDA.

Many of the psychic effects are probably due to serotonergic activity though it doesn't give the visual illusions most often associated with psychedelics (Snyder, 1996). For the first few hours of use, **ecstasy continues to overwhelm the vesicles and forces them to discharge their reservoirs of serotonin** into the synaptic gap thus continuing to dramatically amplify the brain's response to its internal and external environment.

After about 3 hours into the trip, ecstasy is still trying to force the vesicles to release more serotonin but the supplies have been depleted. More ecstasy is usually taken at this point but it results in smaller effects. Because of this reaction, ecstasy is often combined with other drugs like LSD and amphetamines to prolong the feelings. **It can take up to a week or more to produce a sufficient amount of serotonin to reexperience similar feelings.**

Due to this excessive stimulation, serotonin receptors also retreat into the cell membrane to avoid damage. This process, called "down regulation," leads to more long-lasting mood changes since there are now fewer receptors to respond to the serotonin.

"The next day you wake up and it's what you call 'E-tarded.' You feel

retarded but you're coming off of 'E' so you're 'E-tarded' and you're just, you know, totally tired and just, you know, just, 'Duh, what's going on?' You are really slow in your thinking."
17-year-old ecstasy user

Following an ecstasy experience, users have also been known to become extremely depressed and suicidal. **High-dose use has resulted in an acute anxiety reaction** ("bum trip"), prolonged reaction, and even flashbacks after cessation of use (Carroll & Comer, 1998).

Physical dependency is generally not a problem but, as with amphetamines and cocaine, psychological dependence can cause compulsive use. If used daily, tolerance develops rather quickly, as with amphetamines (Markert & Roberts, 1991).

MDMA Polydrug Combinations. Ecstasy is currently being ingested simultaneously with a number of other prescription and illicit drugs.

◇ **LSD with ecstasy**, known as "candy flipping," "flip flopping," "X&Ls," "candy snaps," is said to intensify the effects of both drugs and increase the duration of action of MDMA.

◇ **Hydrocodone/OxyContin®/ codeine/heroin with ecstasy** is a Generation X **speedball combination** that can enhance the euphoric feelings of both drugs.

◇ **GHB with ecstasy** is another type of modern day speedball.

◇ **Nitrous oxide with ecstasy** is used to intensify the inhalant rush sometimes resulting in traumatic injuries from passing out.

◇ **Prozac® (fluoxetine) with ecstasy** is thought to protect serotonin brain cells from the neurotoxic effects of ecstasy. Recent animal studies indicate that Prozac® may actually neutralize all effects of MDMA.

◇ **MDMA with Viagra®** when used to enhance sexuality is called "sextacy."

Lichtbild der Vorderseite: Bezeichnung: Rückseite:								
ADAM	EVA 130 mg	Amor Bruchrille	Love Herz	Herz Bruchrille	Drops Bruchrille	Sonne Bruchrille	Halbmond Bruchrille	Herzpfeil Bruchrille
Käfer	Mercedes	Triple Five	V.I.P.	CAL Bruchrille	PT Bruchrille	Schlitzauge Bruchrille	ANADIN	Boomerang	Bulls Bruchrille
Elephant Bruchrille	Hund Bruchrille	Pigs Ringelschwanz	Pelikan Bruchrille	Taube Bruchrille	Friedenstaube	Spatz Bruchrille	Vogel	Kermit Bruchrille	Feuerstein Bruchrille
Superman	Popeye Bruchrille	Chiemsee Bruchrille	Fido Bruchrille	Häuptling Bruchrille	Sonic Sonic/Bruchrille	Smiley SMILE	Playboy Bruchrille	Schwalbe	Dino Bruchrille
Pilz Bruchrille	Olympics	Hammer & Sichel	Gorbys CCCP	Kleeblatt Kleeblatt	Kleeblatt Bruchrille	Liebessymbol Bruchrille	Yellow Shunshine	Pink Panther	Snowball

(Fotomaterial: Bundeskriminalamt Wiesbaden)

These are some MDMA (ecstasy) tablets confiscated in Europe by various police agencies and Interpol. Seizures by the U.S. Customs Service have soared from 400,000 pills in 1997 to 7.2 million in 2001. About 90% of ecstasy comes from Northern Europe, mainly the Netherlands and Belgium, although in recent years Canada has manufactured more and more of the drug (DEA, 2003a).

Courtesy of the Bundeskriminalant Wiesbaden, U.S. Customs Service, and Trinka Porrata

"I smoked a 'blunt' that had about a gram of coke in it and five pills of ecstasy. And the ecstasy, I had gotten, I had about a thousand pills, I was doing it a lot. It was bad, it was a bad dose. And it put me in the hospital for about a month; attacked my heart and gave me a heart problem."

32-year-old recovering addict

Parties, Raves, & Music Clubs

A rave is a social or dance party gathering where very loud computer-generated **techno or electronic trace beat music is played, light shows and laser light effects are performed, and at many, both club drugs and drug paraphernalia are promoted or condoned.** These are convened in actual dance clubs (with no alcoholic drinks for sale), or at rented warehouses and abandoned buildings, or even at desolate outdoor locations (outlaw or underground raves and desert raves). Some of the clubs are legal and some are nomadic. The stars of many of the raves are disc jockeys with names such as Nahah, Fat Boy Slim, and Moby. A well-known DJ will help attract larger crowds.

When a rave is going to occur, flyers are handed out during the week for a party that weekend while the exact time and date are available on the Internet only a few hours before the party to avoid police involvement. These gatherings are so popular that they have become a big business enterprise often charging as much as $20 to $50 per admission (DuPont, 2000). The drugs that have become popular at these gatherings are **primarily ecstasy, nitrous oxide (laughing gas), GHB or GBL, and occasionally dextromethorphan, ketamine, PCP, and nexus (2C-B). The more traditional street drugs are also available** especially methamphetamine, marijuana, cocaine, LSD, psilocybin mushrooms, alcohol, and various sedative-hypnotics (e.g., Rohypnol®).

"I did a lot of ecstasy when I went to raves, and 'special K,' and coke, and even meth every now and then. It intensifies it. When you're on ecstasy like you take a hit of nitrous, you don't even need like a balloon, you just need like a whippet can and you're, like it intensifies it like a hundred times more for just those 30 seconds and I remember doing that like all the time but, um, I never thought of whip cream cans as a drug."

17-year-old ecstasy "roller"

Generation X butterfly emblems or references to "E" or "X" on clothing and jewelry, along with use of glow sticks or light wands to create a light show by exaggerated movements in front of a "rolling raver," are common at raves. Glow sticks, strobes, laser and light shows are all said to be more mesmerizing with fascinating light trails and visual distortions experienced while "rolling on X."

The problems that occur at these gatherings include **bad reactions to drugs, overheating, falling injuries, passing out, and bad psychedelic trips.** Most of the trips to emergency rooms are due to, in order of frequency, alcohol, then methamphetamines, LSD, GHB, MDMA, and ketamine abuse (Drug Abuse Warning Network [DAWN], 2002a).

Nexus (2C-B or 4-bromo-2,5-dimethoxy phenylethylamine)

"I found only mild visual and emotional effects at the 20 mg dose, so I took the remaining 44 mg. I was propelled into something not of my choosing. Everything that was alive was completely fearsome. My gaze moved to the right and caught a bush growing outside the window and I was petrified. It was a life form I could not understand."

40-year-old physician (Shulgin & Shulgin, 2000)

This amphetamine analogue was synthesized by Dr. Alexander Shulgin. Like many of the psycho-stimulants, the effects of 2C-B are **very dependent on the amount taken: mild stimulation at low doses and intense psychedelic experiences at high doses**.

A number of users combine 2C-B and MDMA to intensify the experience. Experienced psychedelic users have generally learned to control their reactions to various substances and can report on the subtleties between one psycho-stimulant and another but most experiment with whatever drug is available.

STP (DOM) (2,5-dimethoxy-4-methylamphetamine)

STP, also called the "serenity," "tranquility," or "peace" pill, is similar to MDA. It causes a 12-hour intoxication characterized by intense stimulation and several mild psychedelic reactions. There are, however, reports that it is a thicker duller trip than those experienced from mescaline or LSD. DOM is 80 times more active than mescaline (Smith, 1981). Low doses of 2–3 mg cause perceptual distortion while 4–9 mg cause hallucinations and severe sympathetic nervous system stimulation. The combination of STP and LSD, called "pinks" and "purple (or "orange") wedges," was briefly popular in the late 1960s but is rarely seen today because of the high incidence of bad trips (Stafford, 1992).

PMA (4-MA or paramethoxyamphetamine)

Recently PMA has been found in pills purporting to be ecstasy that were smuggled in from Europe. After 1 hour this short-acting drug causes a sudden rise in blood pressure, distinct afterimages, and a pins-and-needles tingly feeling like a chill or hair standing on end.

This hallucinogen can negatively surprise the unaware user causing severe sympathetic nervous system stimulation (seizures), hyperthermia, coagulation of blood, and muscle damage. PMA became popular because street lore said it was close to LSD in its effects (which was not really true). Most of the reported deaths were caused by overdosage. At one time it was sold in the United States and Canada as "Chicken Power" and "Chicken Yellow."

2C-T-7 & 2C-T-2

Two other phenethylamines, originally developed and then later introduced to the general public by Dr. Alexander Shulgin in his 1991 book *PiHKAL, A Chemical Love Story* have also found their way into the recent psychedelic drug-taking subculture. The common effects of these two phenethylamine psycho-stimulant drugs are their ability to **induce delirium, heighten sensitivity, and increase awareness** in the user. They can also cause dangerous cardiovascular effects and even death when taken in high doses.

2C-T-7 (2,5 dimethoxy-4-propylthiophenethyamine), known by its Netherlands trade name Blue Mystic®, was first synthesized in January of 1986 by Dr. Shulgin. By 2000, "smart shops" were selling the psycho-stimulant under the brand names "Tripstacy," "7th Heaven," "7-Up," "Lucky 7," and "Beautiful" (The Vaults of Erowid, 2001). These shops, the current equivalent of "head shops," are boutiques that promote and sell New Age psychedelic substances, paraphernalia, literature, and fashion accessories that promote drug use. There are over 200 of these "smart shops" in Holland and most sell fresh and dried varieties of magic mushrooms, herbal ecstasy, ephedra, guarana, other herbal stimulants, psychoactive herbs, cannabis seeds, and grow kits.

2C-T-2 (2,5-dimethoxy-4-ethylthiophenethyamine) was synthesized by Dr. Shulgin 5 years before he created 2C-T-7. The rapidly spreading abuse of this drug through "smart shops" in the Netherlands, Sweden, Germany, and even in Japan led to it being banned in the Netherlands on April 12, 1999.

BELLADONNA & OTHER ANTICHOLINERGIC PSYCHEDELICS

BELLADONNA, HENBANE, MANDRAKE, & DATURA (jimsonweed, thornapple)

From ancient Greek times through the Middle Ages and the Renaissance, these plants, which contain scopolamine, hyoscyamine, and atropine, have been used in magic ceremonies, sorcery, witchcraft (black mass), and religious rituals. They've also been used as a poison, to mimic insanity, and even as a beauty aid by ancient Greek, Roman, and Egyptian women because they dilate pupils and make the eyes more striking (Ott, 1976). In fact *belladonna* in Latin means "beautiful woman." Datura is more widely grown and references to it are found in Chinese, Indian, Greek, and Aztec history.

One of the effects of these plants is to block acetylcholine receptors in the central nervous system. Acetylcholine helps regulate reflexes, aggression, sleep, blood pressure, heart rate, sexual behavior, mental acuity, and attention. This disruptive effect can cause a form of delirium and make it hard to focus vision. It can also **speed up the heart, create an intense thirst, and raise the body temperature to dangerous levels. Anticholinergics also create some hallucinations, a separation from reality, and a deep sleep for up to 48 hours** (Schultes & Hofmann, 1980). They are still used today by some native tribes in Mexico and Africa. Synthetic anticholinergic prescription drugs like Cogentin® and Artane® that are used to treat the side effects of antipsychotic drugs and Parkinson's disease symptoms are diverted from legal sources and abused for their psychedelic effects. Further, even belladonna cigarettes (Asmador®) used to treat asthma have been abused in the past by youth in search of a cheap high (Smith, 1981).

Jimson weed, also known as "thornapple," "angel's trumpet," "Jamestown weed," "mad apple," and "stinkweed," is a bristly looking plant with coarse green leaves and white flowers found growing naturally in many parts of the United States. The drug induces severe hallucinations such as imaginary snakes, spiders, and lizards. Not too many users try the drug twice since it is often described as a horrible experience. Over 140 jimson weed poisonings were reported in the United States in 1999.

KETAMINE, PCP, & OTHER PSYCHEDELICS

KETAMINE

The effects of ketamine, a dissociative general anesthetic used in human and veterinary medical procedures, are very similar to those of **PCP** (phencyclidine), its close chemical relative and predecessor. Both share the same receptor sites in the brain although they each have a different duration of action—PCP lasts longer than ketamine. Ketamine was the most used anesthetic in the Vietnam War. As an abused club drug, the IV solution of ketamine is diverted from medical and dental supplies to be crystallized by a microwave oven heating process. **The crystals are then smoked in a cocaine freebase pipe or they are ground up and snorted**, the most common method of use. Occasionally the drug is taken orally or injected. Ketamine is sold under the trade names Ketalar® and Ketajet® and is known on the streets as "special K," "vitamin K," and "kit kat."

In 2002, raids in the United States, Mexico, and Panama by the DEA and local authorities dismantled North America's largest illegal producer and distributor of ketamine. The group allegedly handled 60–70% of the illegal ketamine sold in the United States. About 200,000 vials of the drug were confiscated in a veterinary office in Tijuana, Mexico. The drug had been advertised on the Internet and smuggled into the United States (Fox, 2002). A number of veterinary offices in the United States have been broken into in order to steal ketamine.

"K-heads" (ketamine abusers) usually use a level coke spoon, about 20 mg of powder (also piled up as a "line" or a "bump" on a mirror), snorted into each nostril repeatedly for two to five times until the desired effects are achieved. A total dose of 200 mg or less results in a mellow, colorful, mild, dreamlike intoxication known as "being

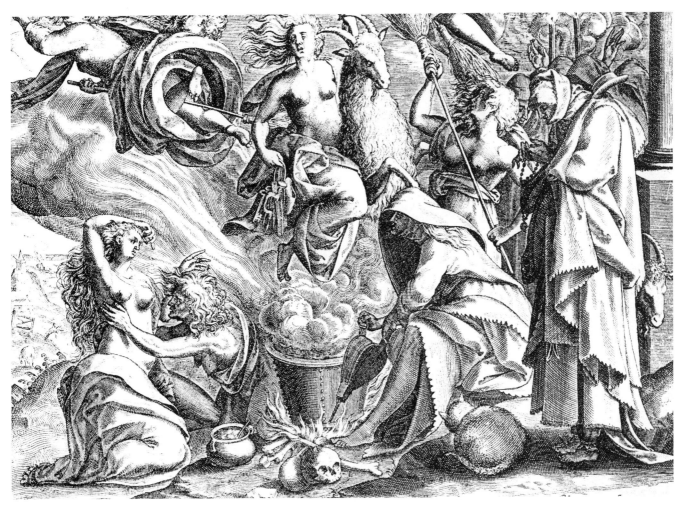

This etching on leather by Adrien Hubertus from medieval Europe gives the artist's impression of hallucinations caused by the hexing herbs, along with visions of sexual activity and death.

Reprinted, by permission, EMB Service for Publishers.

in the K-land." The "K-land" experience is also characterized by a sensation of a mind/body separation, dizziness, slurred speech, and impaired muscular coordination.

"You don't care about anything whatsoever. You are a distance from whatever it is. Whether someone is talking to you, whether there is an argument going on right next to you, you don't know it. You are in your own little place. Nothing around you is connected to you."
43-year-old recovering psychedelic user

A 300–500 mg dose of ketamine is usually needed to produce the full psy-

chedelic experience known as **"being in a K-hole,"** described as an **out-of-body near-death encounter with depersonalization, hallucinations, delirium**, and occasionally bizarre or mystical experiences. Users are also anesthetized against pain, including injuries sustained by rough activities such as fighting or dancing in a "mosh pit" at a rock concert where people bang against each other.

"I walked into a cactus garden during a party. I just walked right through, walked right out. The next day my feet were all bloody and I was pulling stickers out and stuff but at the time there wasn't anything to it."
43-year-old recovering psychedelic user

Ketamine's toxic side effects include respiratory depression, increased heart rate and blood pressure, combative or belligerent behavior, convulsions, and in a few cases, coma.

The retail price of ketamine for veterinarians is about $7 per vial. Middle-level street dealers pay $30 to $45 per vial and the users may pay $100 to $200 per vial. A vial contains about 1 gram of powder (5 to 10 doses) (DEA, 2003c). A single 100–200 mg dose of illicit ketamine usually costs about $20 to $40.

Several researchers have used ketamine to treat alcoholism in a technique known as "ketamine-assisted psychotherapy." The ketamine is injected intramuscularly supposedly to make the

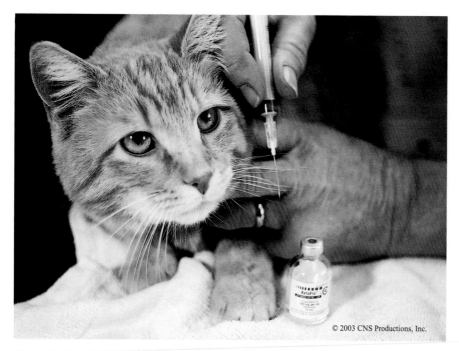

Ketamine is most often used as an animal tranquilizer.

brain more accessible to emotions and dialogue. The researchers reported that about two-thirds of their clients treated this way stayed abstinent for more than a year compared to one-fourth of a control group that tried conventional treatment (Krupitsky & Grinenko, 1997).

Rapid and dramatic development of tolerance, along with a profound psychic dependence, occurs with regular daily use of ketamine (Jansen & Darracot-Cankovic, 2001). It was classified as a Schedule III drug in August 1999. **Major ketamine effects last for only about an hour or less while PCP effects last for several hours.** However, coordination, judgment and sensory perceptions may be affected for 18–24 hours after ketamine use.

PCP

PCP (phencyclidine hydrochloride) was originally created during the 1950s by Parke-Davis Pharmaceuticals (under the trade name Sernyl®) as a new type of disassociative general anesthetic for humans. However, the frequency and severity of toxic and hallucinogenic effects soon limited its use to veterinary medicine starting in 1965 (Petersen, 1980; Zukin, Sloboda, & Javitt, 1997). Eventually

use of PCP was even discontinued in veterinary medicine. **Now the only supplies are illegal ones.** The drug is fairly easy to manufacture in a home laboratory although the pungent odor is easily detectable. **PCP can be smoked in a joint, snorted, swallowed, or injected.** As with ketamine, it appears to distort sensory messages sent to the central nervous system, stifling inhibitions, deadening pain, and resulting in the same mind-body separation as ketamine. In one study almost three-fourths of the users reported forgetfulness, difficulty concentrating, aggressive and violent behavior, depersonalization, and/or estrangement while **a smaller percentage (about 40%) reported hallucinations (tactile, visual, or auditory)** (Siegel, 1989).

PCP, also called "angel dust," "peep," "KJ," "Shermans," or "ozone," is **often misrepresented as THC, mescaline, or psilocybin.** PCP comes in liquid, crystal, or powdered form. It is often smoked in a Nat Sherman® cigarette or sprinkled onto marijuana in a joint. It can also be snorted, swallowed, or injected.

"When I smoke PCP, I feel just like on top of the world, you know. You don't

feel pain. You don't think about your past. It's a good drug if you want to cover up your feelings, you know? You feel like Superman. It's like acid without the mind trip. A couple of times I got scared on it though 'cause I smoked too much. And it was just like a scary experience, like a nightmare, you know? Weird."
Recovering PCP user

Since PCP is so strong, particularly for first-time users, the range between a dose that produces a pleasant sensory deprivation effect and one that induces catatonia, coma, or convulsions is very small. Low dosages (2–5 mg) first produce mild depression then stimulation. Moderate doses (10–15 mg) can produce a more intense sensory-deprived state. Dosages just a little higher, above 20 mg, can cause catatonia, coma, and convulsions. Large PCP doses have also produced seizures, respiratory depression, rigidity of muscles, cardiovascular instability, and even kidney failure (Jaffe, 1989).

"I've had seizures before on it and banged my head really hard—continually on hard objects—and got lots of bumps and everything and felt them the next few days but never realized I was doing it and never felt hurt from it."
Recovering PCP user

A low dose of PCP will last 1–2 hours, a moderate dose 4–6 hours but the effects of a large dose can last up to 48 hours, much longer than the effects produced by an equivalent dose of LSD. PCP is not widely used by the general drug-using population because **there is a high frequency of bad trips associated with it.** When the psychedelic effects kick in, first-time or surprised users can have a bad trip and often do not even remember what happened during the trip. This type of amnesia, which occurs after the use of PCP, is called "anterograde amnesia" and is frequently seen with date rape drugs like Rohypnol® or GHB and with alcohol (blackouts).

In 2002 a number of researchers found that a certain monoclonal antibody called "Fab," developed by NIDA-supported scientists, is a PCP antagonist and can reduce PCP concentrations in the brains of rats and possibly human beings. It is being studied as a possible treatment for PCP overdose and even to treat babies born with PCP in their systems (Proksch, Gentry, & Owens, 2000).

SALVIA DIVINORUM (salvinorin A)

"Me and my friends, when we did it there wasn't very much communication. We were just pretty much all trapped in our little trip. We weren't very talkative. It's not a party drug at all.

18-year-old psychedelic user

Recently *Salvia divinorum*, commonly referred to as "sage" or "diviner's sage" **a psychedelic plant whose effects have been likened to PCP**, has started showing up in some high schools and colleges. *Salvia divinorum* has been used for centuries by Mazatac shamans and curanderas (medicine men and women) in the Sierra Madre Oriental Mountains in northeastern Mexico. It is used to induce a trance-like state in order to search for the cause of the patient's illness.

Dried leaves and live cuttings of this member of the mint family can be chewed and absorbed through the buccal membranes or smoked and absorbed through the lungs **causing dreamlike hallucinations, occasional delirium, and out-of-body sensations**. When smoked, the major effects last for only a few minutes, taper off after 7–10 minutes, and disappear within 30 minutes, much like DMT. As with most psychedelics, the experience is very dependent on the mind-set of the user and the surroundings when taken. An ounce of *Salvia divinorum* contains 100–200 leaves, enough for 4–12 doses although the strength of the plant and suscepti-

bility of the user vary widely. **Salvinorin A is thought to be the key psychoactive extract** responsible for *Salvia divinorum's* major psychoactive effects. When smoked, doses of 200–500 micrograms of salvinorin A are said to produce similar yet more intense psychedelic effects than 100–200 micrograms of LSD.

"And then there's the extract of Salvia, which is a whole other ball game. It's similar to a DMT experience but without such a hard edge thing going on. You definitely get removed from whatever situation you are in at the moment."

24-year-old Salvia divinorum user

It takes 3 lbs. of leaves to make 1 oz. of extract. Using salvinorin A extract can also produce hallucinations, delirium, and out-of-body sensations, along with an inability to function physically or even communicate. It is not understood how the extract works in the brain and no receptor sites have yet been identified as its site of action. *Salvia divinorum* **is currently legal** and is considered to be an herb though there are some indications that the authorities are reviewing the substance for scheduling as a controlled substance. Live cuttings of the plant can even be obtained on the Internet.

AMANITA MUSHROOMS

Although many members of this family of mushrooms are deadly, the *Amanita muscaria* (fly agaric) and the *Amanita pantherina* (panther mushroom) have been used as psychedelics for many centuries. The *Amanita muscaria*, a large mushroom that has an orange, tan, red, or yellow cap with white spots, **can cause dreamy intoxication, hallucinations, delirious excitement, and deadly physical toxic effects as well**. The effects start one-half hour after ingestion and can last for 4–8 hours (Schultes & Hofmann, 1992). The active ingredients are ibotenic acid and the alkaloid muscimole, substances that resemble the inhibitory neurotransmitter GABA. The *Amanita pantherina* contains more of the active ingredients and taking too much of the mushroom can make the user sick for up to 12 hours (Weil & Rosen, 1998).

The *Amanita* mushroom is mentioned in sacred writings in India dating back to 1500 B.C. where it is referred to as the god Soma. *Amanita* has also been used by native tribes in Siberia but its use is limited in the modern age because of the unpredictability of its effects and because many even more deadly mushrooms can be mistaken for it. The use of *Amanita muscaria* in ancient ritual ceremonies is still practiced today by some Ojibway Indians in Michigan (Ott, 1976).

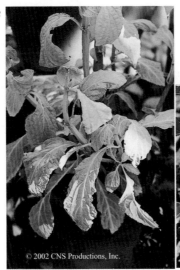

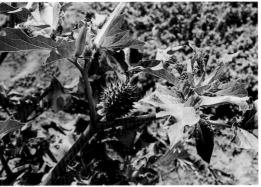

a. Salvia divinorum, *a member of the sage family, is cultivated in many parts of the United States.*
b. Jimsonweed (datura), an anticholinergic psychedelic, is also found throughout the United States.

DEXTROMETHORPHAN
(Robitussin DM®, Romilar®, & other cough syrups)

Dextromethorphan is a **nonprescription opioid cough suppressant** that has been available in several cold and cough medications, such as Coricidin®, Romilar®, Robitussin DM®, and over 140 other liquids, tablets, and capsules since the 1960s. **The effects of an excess dose can be euphoria, dissociation of mind and body, auditory and visual hallucinations, and a loss of coordination.** Those who participate in the club drug scene say that a **very high dose is somewhat similar to LSD or "magic mushrooms."** Alcohol is found in many of these cough medications, so **the effects are of a drunken deliriant.**

"I only took a capful and it was kind of a bluish tint. It kinda reminded me of acid sort of where like wherever I'd walk, I'd feel like the world was kinda rushing towards me. Wherever I looked, it was just like the visuals, almost like tracers, coming at me. I smoked a lot of weed with those."
Recovering club drug user

Occasional yet persistent reports of dextromethorphan abuse have continued since the early 1960s resulting in the evolution of many street names for the drug like "CCC," "robo," "dex," "DXM," and even "red devils" (a street name used for Seconal® in the '60s).

A normal therapeutic dose is 10–50 mg or up to 120 mg in a 24-hour period. **A strong dose by a drug abuser who wants the psychedelic effects is 300–600 mg and the effects will last 6–8 hours.** Some will take a heavy dose, 600–1,500 mg, in the search for more mental effects. Those who get totally carried away might use a dose of 2,500–20,000 mg and at that level death can occur particularly if used in conjunction with alcohol.

The drug can also dilate pupils, decrease orgasm, upset the stomach, and induce nausea. Additional negative results are itching, rashes, fever, and tachycardia. Tolerance does develop to dextromethorphan and when used in excess can be mildly addicting.

In addition to toxic side effects resulting in acute anxiety and panic reactions ("bad trips"), DXM is also an opioid and an overdose can result in coma and respiratory depression that is somewhat treatable with naloxone, an opioid antagonist (Elora, 2001). Dextromethorphan has also been studied as a treatment for heroin and opioid addiction both by addicts themselves and by researchers (*see Chapter 9*).

NUTMEG & MACE

At the low end of the psychedelic drug spectrum, nutmeg and mace—both from the nutmeg tree (*myristica fragrans*)—**can cause varied effects from a mild floating sensation to a full-blown delirium.** So much has to be consumed (about 20 grams) that the user is left with a bad hangover and a severely upset stomach. The active chemicals in nutmeg and mace are variants of MDA (methylenedioxyamphetamine) (Marnell, 1997). Since this dose exposes a user to the nauseating and toxic effects of other chemicals in nutmeg, its **abuse is extremely rare outside of prisons** where convicts are driven to use it since they have limited access to other psychedelics.

MARIJUANA & OTHER CANNABINOLS

"A federal jury in San Francisco found Ed Rosenthal, one of the nation's most prominent marijuana advocates, guilty Friday of felony conspiracy and cultivation charges — a triumph for federal prosecutors seeking to override California's endorsement of pot as medicine."
San Francisco Chronicle, Feb 1, 2003

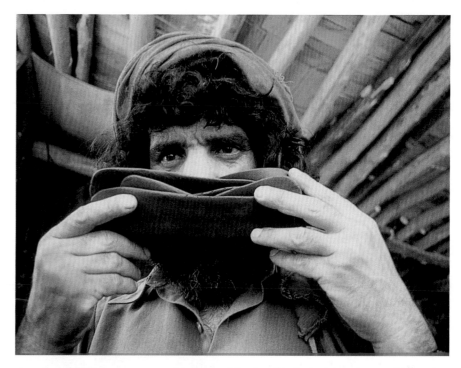

A smuggler in Afghanistan covers his face with bricks of hashish, the concentrated form of marijuana that has been around for over 1,000 years. Hashish is the Arab word for "dry herb." The word is also associated with an eleventh-century Persian cult of terrorists called "The Hashishi" (hashish eaters). "Assassin" is a derivative of the word "Hashishi." The Middle East, north Africa, Pakistan, and Afghanistan are the main sources of hashish.
© 1990 Alain Labrousse.

Growers

According to the DEA, **the majority of the marijuana used in the United States comes from Mexico and Colombia**. In addition **tens of thousands of Americans grow their own marijuana**, either a few plants for their own use or hundreds, even thousands for large-scale dealing. Because of stiffer penalties and greater surveillance by law enforcement agencies, more growers have moved their operations indoors. A disturbing recent change has been noted in California where three-fourths of the marijuana seized in the state during the fall of 2002 was grown by Mexican cartels running growing operations in the richer soils of remote forests. The plantings contained anywhere from 2,000 to 10,000 plants ("Cartels," 2002). Estimates of the percentage of marijuana that is homegrown vary nationwide from 10% to 50% of total consumption.

The indoor growing of marijuana has led to very high-potency plants grown all over the United States and the world. Some marijuana is even grown hydroponically (in water). Other major growing countries in the western hemisphere besides Mexico, Colombia, Canada, and the United States are Jamaica, Brazil, Belize, Guatemala, Trinidad, and Tobago. In the Far East, Thailand, Laos, Cambodia, and the Philippines are big growers. The African and the Middle Eastern countries Morocco, Lebanon (greatly reduced in recent years), Nigeria, and South Africa produce mostly *Cannabis indica*. In southwest and central Asia, Pakistan and Afghanistan are the big producers (DEA, 2003a).

The average street price of marijuana in the United States rose steadily from 1981 to a peak in 1991. Retail prices fell over the next decade but began to level off to about $10 per gram from 1996 to 1998. Since the common unit of sale for marijuana is 1 oz. (called a "lid"), the average street price by the beginning of the 2000s ranged from $100 up to $400 per "lid" (Office of National Drug Control Policy, 2002; Marnell, 1997). Prices for commercial-

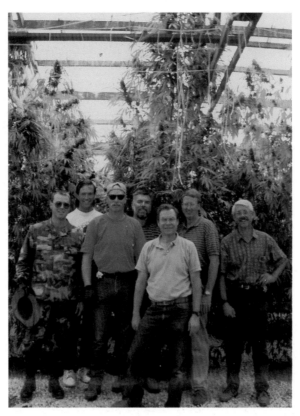

This indoor marijuana-growing operation was busted by JACNET, a drug task force run by the Sheriff's Department in Jackson County, Oregon. Growers can use grow lights or filtered sunlight to avoid detection by law enforcement agencies or passers-by.
© 1996 JACNET

grade marijuana when bought in larger quantities have remained relatively stable ranging from $400 to $1,000 per pound in U.S. southwest border areas to between $700 to $2,000 per pound in the Midwest and northeastern United States. The national price range for sinsemilla, a higher quality marijuana usually grown domestically, is between $900 and $6,000 per pound. In Vancouver, British Columbia, "BC bud" sells for between $1,500 and $2,000 per pound but when smuggled into the United States and sold in smaller quantities, the dealer can make between $5,000 and $8,000 per pound in major metropolitan areas.

PHARMACOLOGY

At last count researchers had discovered some 420 chemicals in a single *Cannabis* plant. Interestingly adolescents use the number 420 as their phone-beeper code to signal the availability of marijuana. At least 30 of these chemicals, called "cannabinoids," have been studied for their psychoactive effects. **The most potent psychoactive chemical is called "Δ-9-tetrahydro-cannabinol" or "THC."** When smoked or ingested, this potent psychoactive chemical is converted by the liver into over 60 other metabolites, some of which are also psychoactive. In addition the widespread use of the sinsemilla-growing technique has increased the average concentration of THC from 1–3% in the '60s to 4–15% since then (DEA, 2003a). **High-concentration THC marijuana has been around for many years—it just hasn't been so readily available.** What this means is that a user would have to smoke 3 to 5 of the weak joints from the '60s and '70s to equal just 1 of the stronger joints available in the 2000s. Unfortunately many of the early studies on marijuana and many of the attitudes of the counterculture about the effects of the drug were based on the weaker plants. Fortunately there has been a great increase in research over the last few years using the higher-potency marijuana.

Marijuana Receptors & Neurotransmitters

At Johns Hopkins University **in 1990, receptor sites in the brain that** were specifically reactive to the THC in marijuana were discovered (Howlett, Evans, & Houston, 1992). This discovery implied that the brain has its own natural neurotransmitters that fit into these receptor sites and that they affect the same areas of the brain as marijuana.

Two years later researchers at the National Institute on Drug Abuse announced the **discovery of anandamide, the natural neurotransmitter that fits into the receptor sites** (Devane et al., 1992). Receptors for anandamide were found in several areas of the limbic system including the reward/reinforcement center. Other parts of the brain with anandamide receptor sites are those regulating the integration of sensory experiences with emotions as well as those controlling functions of learning, motor coordination, and some automatic body functions. The presence of anandamide receptors means that these are the areas of the brain most affected by marijuana. It is important that there are fewer anandamide receptors in the brainstem for marijuana, compared to endorphin receptors for opioids and norepinephrine receptors for cocaine since this area of the brain controls heart rate, respiration, and other body functions. It is the reason why dangerous overdoses can occur with cocaine and opioids due to depression or overstimulation of these functions and why it is so **difficult to physically overdose with marijuana** (Smith et al., 1994; Huestis et al., 2001).

SHORT-TERM EFFECTS

Physical Effects

The immediate physical effects of marijuana often include **physical relaxation or sedation, some pain control, bloodshot eyes, coughing from lung irritation, an increase in appetite, and a loss in muscular coordination**. Other physical effects include an increased heart rate, decreased blood pressure, decreased eye pressure (Marinol® capsules or marijuana joints are used as a treatment for glaucoma), increased blood flow through the mucous membranes of the eye resulting in

conjunctivitis or red eye, and decreased nausea (capsules and joints are also used for cancer patients undergoing chemotherapy).

Marijuana impairs tracking ability (the ability to follow a moving object, such as a baseball) and causes a trailing phenomenon where one sees an afterimage of a moving object. Impaired tracking ability, the trailing phenomenon, and sedating effects make it more difficult to perform tasks that require depth perception and good hand-eye coordination, such as flying an airplane, catching a football, or driving a car.

Marijuana can act as a stimulant as well as a depressant depending on the variety and amount of chemical that is absorbed in the brain, the setting in which it is used, and the personality of the user.

"Marijuana is not a downer for me, it's a speed thing. I have plenty of friends who smoke marijuana and become quiet. They can't speak. They become immobile. They're total veggies, you know, sitting around and cannot move whereas I become more active."
48-year-old marijuana smoker

Marijuana also causes a small temporary disruption of the secretion of the male hormone testosterone. That might be important to a user with hormonal imbalance or somebody in the throes of puberty and sexual maturation. The testosterone effect also results in a slight decrease in both sperm count and sperm motility in chronic pot users (Wilkins, Conner, et al., 1998; Joy, Watson, & Benson, 1999; Marnell, 1997).

Mental Effects

Within a few minutes of smoking marijuana, the user becomes a bit confused and **mentally separated from the environment**. Marijuana produces a feeling of deja vu where everything seems familiar but really isn't. Additional effects include **an aloof feeling, drowsiness, and difficulty concentrating**.

"It's kind of like life without a coherent thought. It's kind of like an escape. It's like when you go to sleep, you forget about things. It's like everything's dreamlike and there are no restraints on anything. You can have freedom to say what you want to say."
16-year-old marijuana smoker

Stronger varieties of marijuana can produce giddiness, increased alertness, and major distortions of time, color, and sound. Very strong doses can even produce a sensation of movement under one's feet, visual illusions, and sometimes hallucinations. Two of the most frequently mentioned psychological problems with smoking marijuana are paranoia and a deeper depersonification (detachment from one's sense of self).

"I'd keep smoking, and keep smoking, and keep smoking, and I'd get paranoid. If you're not relaxed and having fun, it seems really insane to keep doing it. And I did keep doing it for a long time after I had started developing fear."
35-year-old marijuana user

Marijuana acts somewhat as a mild hypnotic. Charles Baudelaire, the nineteenth-century French poet, referred to it as "the mirror that magnifies." **It exaggerates mood and personality and makes smokers more empathetic** to others' feelings but also makes them more suggestible.

Marijuana disrupts short-term memory but not long-term memory. This effect occurs because of marijuana's impact on the hippocampus, that part of the brain responsible for memory formation. The hippocampus normally loses neurons due to aging. Chronic marijuana use seems to increase that loss (NIDA, 2002).

"I'd be doing the job and all of a sudden I'd look up and freeze and not know what to do. I would have a handful of checks in my hand and just

look at the machine for a while and just think to myself, 'What is this and what do I do with it?'"
38-year-old recovering marijuana addict

The distortion of a sense of time (temporal disintegration) is responsible for several of the perceived effects of marijuana. Dull repetitive jobs seem to go by faster. In Jamaica some cane field workers smoke "ganja" (marijuana) to make their hard monotonous work pass by more quickly. On the other hand students who smoke marijuana while studying get easily bored and often abandon their books. There is also a spatial disintegration that is a loss of the ability to appropriately discern distances and depth.

The effects of mental confusion, distortion of the passage of time, impaired judgment, and short-term memory loss result in a user's inability to perform multiple and interactive tasks, like programming a VCR, while under the influence (Wilkins, Conner, et al., 1998; Joy et al., 1999; Marnell, 1997; Stafford, 1992). A study of present and former marijuana users tested the smokers at 1, 7, and 28 days after stopping various levels of use. Significant impairment was found at days 1 and 7 for heavy users but by day 28 the difference in impairment had mostly disappeared (Pope, Gruber, Hudson, Huestis, & Yurgelun-Todd, 2001).

LONG-TERM EFFECTS

Respiratory Problems

THC is a bronchodilator; it opens up the airways, at least initially. As smoking becomes chronic, so does irritation to the breathing passages. Because marijuana is grown under a wide variety of conditions and is unrefined, the joints made from the buds and/or leaves are harsh, unfiltered, irregular in quality, and composed of many different chemicals. Therefore, when it is inhaled and held in the lungs, smoking four to five joints gives the same harmful exposure to the lungs and mucous membranes as smoking a full pack of cigarettes according to studies by Dr. Donald Tashkin at UCLA (Tashkin,

Simmons, & Clark, 1988; Tashkin et al., 1997). For these and other reasons, a major concern of health professionals is the damaging effect that marijuana smoking has on the respiratory system. **Marijuana smoking on a regular basis leads to symptoms of increased coughing with acute and chronic bronchitis.** In microscopic studies of these mucous membranes, Dr. Tashkin has found that **most damage occurs in the lungs of those who smoke both cigarettes and marijuana.** This is significant because most marijuana smokers also smoke cigarettes.

"It's just like cigarettes. I started smoking cigarettes at the age of 13 right behind the marijuana. Now as soon as I got done with a joint or two, I'd smoke a cigarette to get rid of the smell. Then I'd hide it from my wife and go outside and smoke outside on the porch or outside in my woodshed."
32-year-old recovering compulsive marijuana smoker

In the series of slides, the normal ciliated surface epithelial cells in the mucous membranes of a nonsmoker of either cigarettes or marijuana (Fig. 6-3a) show healthy densely packed cilia that clear the breathing passages of mucous, dust, and debris.

The breathing passage of a chronic smoker of only marijuana (Fig. 6-3b) shows increased numbers of mucous-secreting surface epithelial cells that do not have cilia, so **phlegm production is increased but is not cleared as readily from the breathing passages.** Some of the changes involve the cell nucleus, suggesting that malignancy may be a consequence of regular marijuana smoking since some of these changes are precursors of cancer.

"I'm sure I've done some damage to my lungs. I mean, you can't put that kind of tar down in your system, heated tar going into your system constantly for 23 years and sit here and say there's nothing wrong and nothing

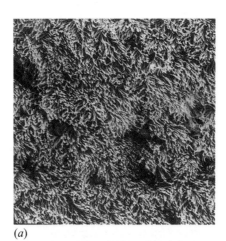
(a)

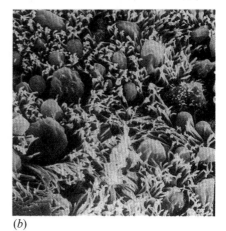
(b)

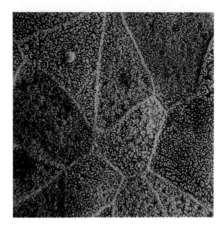
(c)

Figure 6-3 •

a. Healthy mucous membrane of nonsmoker.

b. Mucous membrane of a marijuana smoker.

c. Mucous membrane of a marijuana and cigarette smoker.

Courtesy of Dr. Donald Tashkin, Chief, Pulmonary Research Department, UCLA Medical Center, Los Angeles, CA

has happened. Surely something has happened."
48-year-old marijuana smoker

Finally the breathing passage of a chronic marijuana and cigarette smoker (Fig. 6-3c) shows that the normal surface cells have been completely replaced by nonciliated cells resembling skin, so the **smoker has to cough to clear any mucous from the lungs since the ciliated cells are gone**. Marijuana and cigarette smokers also have a greatly increased risk for developing cancer of the tongue, larynx, or lungs (Joy et al., 1999; Tashkin, 1999; Tashkin et al., 1988; Wilkins, Conner, et al., 1998).

Immune System

Some evidence suggests that heavy use of marijuana can depress the immune system making users more susceptible to a cold, the flu, and other viral infections. If such were the case, it could be somewhat counterproductive for people who are already immune depressed, either as a result of AIDS or as a result of chemotherapy for cancer, to smoke marijuana for therapeutic (pain relief or antinausea) purposes. The user is further exposing the lungs to pathogens, such as fungi and bacteria, found in marijuana smoke. However, the health impact of marijuana on the immune system remains unclear from lack of definitive research (Joy et al., 1999; Hollister, 1992).

Learning & Emotional Maturation

"If you go home and have homework to do that night and you say, 'O.K. I'm going to get stoned before I do my homework,' you're never going to get your homework done."
High school student

Marijuana use has been shown to slow learning and disrupt concentration by its influence on short-term memory. Short-term memory, in contrast to long-term memory, is a processing of information to be retained for only a short period of time, such as a grocery list, a proper assortment of tools for a certain job, or facts crammed into the brain for an upcoming exam. Marijuana greatly impairs a person's ability to retain this information. However, it has a much smaller effect on long-term memory, which is the processing and storing of information for a long period of time, e.g., remembering a theory in physics that has been studied for several weeks. This explains why some students have been able to maintain good grades while using marijuana on a regular basis while others end up flunking out. A recent study of 150 heavy marijuana users in treatment found that not only memory but attention span and cognitive functioning were impaired and as expected, the heavier the use, the greater the impairment (Solowij, Stephens, Roffman, et al., 2002). Overall in one study, those who averaged a D in school were 4 times more likely to have used marijuana than those who got A's (SAMHSA, 2001).

Although more research is needed into what some researchers call an "amotivational syndrome," a number of patients treated at the Haight Ashbury Clinic for marijuana addiction do show a lack of motivation. They have a tendency to avoid problems and evade meaningful work.

"You know how they tell you go to school to get an education so you can get a good job? They did tell me how to get a job, so that's 8 hours a day. I knew how to sleep, that's 8 hours a day. I had another 8 hours a day that I didn't know how to fill and I used marijuana to fill those 8 hours. Period."
38-year-old recovering compulsive marijuana smoker

The way this mechanism operates is similar to the effects of other psychoactive drugs. What happens is that if users come to depend on this drug to gain pleasure or avoid pain rather than learn how to receive satisfaction naturally or deal with painful situations directly, they will habituate their minds and bodies to this chemical solution.

"I liked to do it so much that, it's like, why not do it? I couldn't find a reason for not doing it. It was too enjoyable. It was like going and looking in your refrigerator and seeing a thing of ice cream and a thing of Hershey's" chocolate syrup and going, 'No, I'm going to have a bran muffin instead.' Why? You can have ice cream and the chocolate syrup, man. That's what you want. Why don't you have it?"
17-year-old marijuana smoker

Since marijuana is "the mirror that magnifies," smoking it often exaggerates natural tendencies in the user. Thus if a person really isn't interested in working, studying, having a relationship, or reading a book and smokes marijuana, his or her primitive brain is given the edge over the new brain and says, "You don't have to do those things." So rather than the new brain, the neocortex, giving guidance and saying, "These are necessary things that you're going to have to do," the primitive brain takes over and says, "Forget it, let's not do this."

"When I got high I thought I was the smartest person in the world. I knew I had the answer to everything and one day I sat down with the tape recorder and I started rattling off all this brilliance that I had and the next day when I woke up in the morning and I played it back, it was almost like I wasn't even speaking English."
38-year-old recovering compulsive marijuana smoker

With marijuana many thoughts and feelings are internalized. Long-term marijuana smokers feel that they're thinking, feeling, and communicating better but often they're not.

"When I have worked with couples where one of the principal partners in the relationship has been using marijuana for a long period of time, the biggest complaint is, 'He never says

anything,' or 'She never says anything. We don't talk. We don't communicate.' For the marijuana user, that person feels when they're under the influence that they are trying to communicate. So the intentions are there, the feelings are there, and the emotions are there but it's all internal. It never gets out to the other person."

John DeDomenico, counselor, Haight Ashbury Detox Clinic

Acute Mental Effects

Lasting mental problems from short-term use are unusual but in someone with preexisting mental problems or with latent emotional problems, particularly **if marijuana with high THC levels is smoked, acute anxiety or temporary psychotic reactions can occur** (National Institutes of Health, 1997; Os et al., 2002). Individuals believe that they have lost control of their mental state. Besides paranoia there is often a belief that they have severely damaged themselves or that their underlying insecurities are insurmountable. These acute problems are usually treatable but what is problematic is when the symptoms persist. Counselors at the Haight Ashbury Clinic have seen a number of cases where people who, after experiencing a bad trip, don't come all the way back and may have problems going on with their lives. They experience continued confusion, concentration difficulty, memory problems, and feel as if their mind is always in a fog.

"I'm working with a 13-year-old client who had no premorbid symptoms that could be identified prior to his 13th birthday when his friends turned him on to a 'honey blunt,' which is a cigar packed with marijuana soaked in honey and dried. It happened to be very strong sinsemilla and he experienced an acute anxiety reaction followed by a post-hallucinogenic drug perceptual disorder including a profound depression and an inability to concentrate.

We don't know how long these problems will last."

Counselor, Haight Ashbury Detox Clinic

Even seasoned veteran smokers who've been smoking some low-grade pot and then get some strong "Buddha Thai" sinsemilla may feel that somebody has slipped them a psychedelic like PCP or LSD. They begin to experience anxiety and paranoia that then create even more anxiety.

There is also an increase in the practice of mixing marijuana with other drugs like cocaine, amphetamine, and PCP that can cause exaggerated reactions. Some users even smoke joints that have been soaked in formaldehyde and embalming fluid ("clickems," "fry") for a bigger kick. "Clickems" give a PCP-like effect when smoked.

TOLERANCE, WITHDRAWAL, & ADDICTION

Tolerance

Tolerance to marijuana occurs in a rapid and dramatic fashion. Although high-dose chronic users can recognize the effects of low levels of

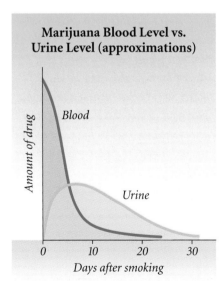

Marijuana Blood Level vs. Urine Level (approximations)

Figure 6-4 •

This chart shows the blood and urine levels of marijuana over time. The marijuana persists in the urine longer. The majority of drug testing only measures marijuana in the urine.

THC in their systems, they are able to tolerate much higher levels without some of the more severe emotional and psychic effects experienced by a first-time user.

One great concern is that marijuana **persists in the body of a chronic user for up to 3 months** though the major effects last only 4 to 6 hours after smoking. These residual amounts in the body can disrupt some physiological, mental, and emotional functions.

Withdrawal

Because there is not the rapid onset of withdrawal from marijuana as with alcohol or heroin, many people deny that withdrawal occurs. The withdrawal from marijuana is more drawn out because much of the THC has been retained in the brain and **only after a relatively long period of abstinence will the withdrawal effects appear**.

"Sometimes people who've been smoking for 5 years decide to quit. They stop 1, 2, 3 days, even a week, and they say [especially those who think marijuana is benign], 'Wow, I feel great. Marijuana's no problem. I have no withdrawal. It's nothing at all.' Then they start up again. They never experience withdrawal. We see that withdrawal symptoms to marijuana are delayed sometimes for several weeks to a month after a person stops."

Counselor, Haight Ashbury Detox Clinic

Withdrawal effects of marijuana include

◊ **anger** or irritability and aggression;
◊ **aches**, pains, chills;
◊ **depression**;
◊ **inability to concentrate;**
◊ slight tremors;
◊ sleep disturbances;
◊ decreased appetite;
◊ sweating;
◊ **craving**.

Not everyone will experience all of these effects but **everyone will experi-**

ence some of them, especially crav-ing. Recent human research demon-strated that irritability, anxiety, aggres-sion, and even stomach pain caused by marijuana withdrawal occurred within 3 to 7 days of abstinence (Kouri et al., 1999; Haney et al., 1999; Budney, Hughes, Moore, & Novy, 2001).

"I would break into a sweat in the shower. I could not maintain my con-centration for the first month or two. To really treasure my sobriety, it took me about 3 or 4 months before I really came out of the fog and really started getting a grasp of what was going on around me."
38-year-old recovering marijuana addict

The discovery by French scientists in 1994 of an antagonist that instantly blocks the effects of marijuana en-abled researchers to search for true signs of tolerance, tissue dependence, and withdrawal symptoms in long-term users. Experiments demonstrated that cessation of marijuana use could cause true physical withdrawal symptoms. Dr. Billy Martin of the Medical College of Virginia gave the THC antagonist SR14176A to rats who had been ex-posed to marijuana 4 days in a row. The antagonist negated the influence of the marijuana. Within 10 minutes the rats exhibited immediate physical with-drawal behaviors that included "wet dog shakes" and facial rubbing, which is the rat equivalent of withdrawal. These ex-periments indicated that **marijuana de-pendence occurs more rapidly than previously suspected.** This experiment, which compressed the withdrawal to minutes instead of weeks, allowed the addictive potential of cannabinoids to be more clearly understood. (Aceto, Scates, Lowe, & Martin, 1995; Rinaldi-Carmona et al., 1994; Tsou, Patrick, & Walker, 1995; Huestis et al., 2001).

Further, human studies have de-monstrated rapid eye movement (REM) sleep changes similar to those seen in other drug addictions. They include de-creased REM while smoking marijuana and increased REM during withdrawal.

Addiction

Just as the refinement of coca leaves into cocaine and opium into heroin led to greater abuse of those drugs, so have better sinsemilla cultiva-tion techniques increased the compul-sive liability of marijuana use.

"I thought I could control it because when I woke up in the morning, I didn't get high for the first hour and a half. I figured an hour and a half, that proves that I'm not hooked on this stuff because I don't really need it."
Recovering user in Marijuana Anonymous, a 12-step program

The research of the 1990s and 2000s has provided a different view of the addiction potential of this sub-stance. **Today many people smoke the drug in a chronic compulsive way and have difficulty discontinuing their use.** Like cocaine, heroin, alco-hol, nicotine, and other addictive drugs, marijuana does have the ability to in-duce compulsive use in spite of the negative consequences it may be caus-ing in the user's life.

"'Why am I doing this? What's wrong with me? Why do I have to keep doing this?' And I did this for a good 8–10 years. I used to buy it by the pound and then I found after a while that I wanted to make it harder on myself to smoke. So I started buying dime bags, figuring it would cost a lot more, and then eventually I got to the point where [the technique] didn't work. I just kept on buying."
38-year-old recovering marijuana addict

Finally, all earlier available research on marijuana was based on a THC cal-culation of 20 mg per marijuana ciga-rette (considered in the 1960s to be a high-dose exposure). Current marijuana joints used for research contain 40 mg of THC, still below most good quality street joints but closer than in the past. (The marijuana for these experimental joints is grown at a government farm in Mississippi.)

"The main problem we're dealing with is that today's potent form of mari-juana is causing a lot more problems than we saw in the 1960s. I never treated a single marijuana self-admitted addict in the Clinic through-out the '60s nor the '70s and pretty much through the '80s. But by the late '80s we started seeing people coming in. Every one of them came in on their own volition, saying, 'Help me. I want to stop smoking pot. It is causing me these problems, causing me to have memory problems, causing me to be too spaced out, not to function in my work. I can't complete tasks. It's causing me to be sick in the morning and cough. I have withdrawal symptoms. I want to stop and I can't stop.' At our program in San Francisco, we have about 100 patients who are in treatment at any given time specifically for marijuana addiction. So people who claim that marijuana is harmless have to sit down and listen to those people who are the walking wounded. For them marijuana has caused major problems—not propaganda or other people telling them it's causing problems but they themselves saying it's so."
Darryl Inaba, Pharm.D., CEO, Haight Ashbury Free Clinics

Is Marijuana a Gateway Drug?

In antidrug movies from the '30s like *Reefer Madness* and *Marijuana, Assassin of Youth,* the claim was that marijuana physically and mentally changed users, so they started using heroin and cocaine and became help-less addicts. The exaggeration of this idea undermined drug education be-cause people who smoked marijuana didn't become raving lunatics or de-praved dope fiends. The experimenters who had tried marijuana said, "I tried marijuana and that didn't happen, so I guess they're lying about all the drugs."

This exaggeration and resultant ridicule of propagandistic or scare films and books probably caused **more drug abuse than it prevented.** It also obscured an important idea, that is, the real role marijuana use plays in future drug use and abuse.

"I've been in a 12-step program [Narcotics Anonymous] for a little over 6 years and I'm not going to say like one and one equal two but just about everybody I meet in the 12-step program started out with either marijuana or alcohol."
Recovering marijuana addict

Marijuana is a gateway drug in the sense that **if people smoke it, they will probably hang around others who smoke it or use other drugs, so the opportunities to experiment with other drugs are greater**. Viewed from this perspective, it is not surprising that **most users of other illicit drugs have used marijuana first but only after they began using alcohol and or nicotine** (Joy et al., 1999; Kandel & Yamaguchi, 1993; Kandel, Yamaguchi, & Chen, 1992).

No two people will have the exact same reaction to marijuana but what has been observed is that those who continue to use it regularly establish a pattern of use and begin to find opportunities where drugs other than marijuana are available.

"The majority of people that I know, that I hang around with, if they ain't smoking weed, they're smoking crack, or drinking. I'm not saying that they are bad people but that's just how it is."
30-year-old polydrug user who started smoking marijuana at the age of 13

A recent study of 311 young adults in Australia who were identical or fraternal twins found that **those who smoked cannabis by age 17 had a 2.1 to 5.2 times higher chance of other drug use, alcohol dependence, and drug abuse/dependence** than those who didn't smoke it. There was no significant difference in drug/alcohol use

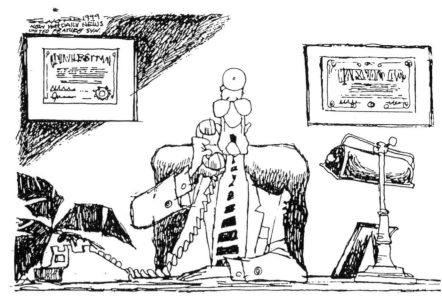

" SMOKE TWO JOINTS AND CALL ME IN THE MORNING..."

BILL SCHORR Reprinted, by permission of United Feature Syndicate, Inc.

or dependence between fraternal or identical twins emphasizing the effect of marijuana and environmental influences (Lynskey et al., 2003).

MARIJUANA (*Cannabis*) & THE LAW

Marijuana is one of the drugs that has never been out of favor over the last 40 years in the United States and is still popular at the start of the twenty-first century. Internationally, marijuana is the most widely used illicit drug in countries such as Canada, Mexico, Costa Rica, El Salvador, Panama, Australia, and South Africa (DEA, 2003a). In the United States the penalties for marijuana use or possession vary from federal laws to state laws and from state to state. Federal laws focus more on heavy trafficking although there are penalties for simple possession and personal use.

Marijuana, Driving, & Drug Testing

In more and more arrests for reckless driving or in investigations at the scene of an accident, the driver is tested for marijuana and other drugs. Four problems of marijuana testing are that

◇ the drug persists for a number of days in the body and can sometimes still be detected weeks after use;

◇ the elimination rate varies radically compared to alcohol that has a defined rate of metabolism;

◇ there is a scarcity of good data about the level of marijuana in the blood vs. the level of impairment;

◇ and most important (and most often), there is another drug besides marijuana in the system, especially alcohol, so even if marijuana has a relatively small effect, it is magnified by polydrug use and abuse. Added to the fact that 65% of heavy drinkers also use marijuana, it's no wonder that positive polydrug test results are the rule and not the exception in drivers arrested for DUI or DWI (SAMHSA, 2002; Gieringer, 1988).

As with alcohol, **driving impairment is directly related to the amount of THC in the brain.** One study found that 60% of smokers failed a field sobriety test $2\frac{1}{2}$ hours after smoking moderate amounts, while other tests have shown some impairment 3–7 hours after smoking. Some tests even showed minimal impairment

TABLE 6–3 PENALTIES FOR MARIJUANA POSSESSION

FEDERAL

2,000 lbs. or 1,000 or more plants	First offense: Not less than 10 yrs., not more than life
200 lbs. to 2,000 lbs. or 100–999 plants	First offense: Not less than 5 yrs., not more than 40 yrs.
More than 22 lbs. hashish; 100–200 lbs.; 50–99 plants	First offense: Not more than 20 yrs.
Less than 100 lbs.; 1–49 plants	First offense: Not more than 5 yrs.

STATE

Texas

2 oz. or less	Up to 180 days in prison and a fine up to $2,000
Greater than 4 oz.	Up to 2 yrs. in prison and a fine up to $10,000
Greater than 5 lbs.	2–10 yrs. in prison and a fine up to $10,000
Greater than 50 lbs.	2–20 yrs. in prison and a fine up to $10,000
Any amount greater than 2,000 lbs.	5–99 yrs. in prison and a fine up to $50,000

New York

1 oz. or less	$100 for the first offense and up to 15 days in prison
Greater than 2 oz.	Up to 1 yr. in jail and a fine up to $1,000
8 oz. to 16 oz.	Up to 4 yrs. in prison and a fine up to $5,000
Greater than 16 oz.	Up to 7 yrs. in prison and a fine up to $5,000
Any amount greater than 10 lbs.	Up to 15 yrs. in prison and a fine up to $5,000

(National Organization for the Reform of Marijuana Laws, 2003; DEA, 2003b; Robert Wood Johnson Foundation, 2003)

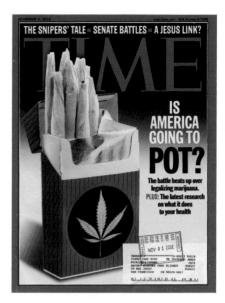

up to 8 hours later (Reeve et al., 1983; Smiley, 1986; Hollister, 1986).

Testing machines can measure minute amounts of the THC metabolite but are generally calibrated to start registering at 50 nanograms per milliliter (ng/mL) in urine samples. The 50-nanogram level doesn't necessarily measure impairment but only the fact that marijuana was used. Generally for long-term smokers it would take about 3 weeks before they wouldn't register on a test with a 50 ng/mL cutoff and another 3 weeks to be completely negative. In a few instances it has taken 10 weeks for the drug to clear completely. For someone who smoked a joint at a party but is not a long-time user, he or she usually tests negative 24–48 hours after use. The Olympic Committee uses just 15 nanograms as their cutoff level.

In drivers, marijuana generally

◇ **induces drowsiness and impairs judgment** (Mathias, 1996);

◇ **makes it difficult to complete complex tasks**;

◇ appears in the blood and urine 3–5 times more frequently in driver fatalities than in the general population (Gieringer, 1988).

Medical Use of Marijuana

Over the centuries the medical profession has examined the use of *Cannabis* **and its extracts for medicinal purposes.** Since there were a limited number of medications available in the past, substances that had a real effect were prized. In a report to the Ohio State Medical Society in 1860, Dr. R. R. McMeens said he was convinced of its immense value because of the immediate action of the drug in appeasing the appetite for chloral hydrate or opium and restoring the ability to appreciate food. He also recommended it as a treatment for disordered bowels, as a diuretic, and as a sleeping tonic (McMeens, 1860). The concentration of THC was probably fairly high, approaching that of hashish. As in the present day, there were also warnings about its dangers.

For example, in 1890 Dr. J. Russel Reynolds in writing about his 30 years of experience using *Cannabis* medicinally said the problems included a wide variation in the strength of any *Cannabis indica* preparation, that people vary widely in their reaction to the same dose, and that if high concentrations are taken, severe reactions are quite possible (Reynolds, 1890).

Historically marijuana has been used

◇ to treat insomnia,

◇ to calm anxiety,

◇ to cure venereal disease,

◇ to relieve coughs (antitussive),

◇ to calm whooping cough,

◇ to control headaches,

◇ as a childbirth analgesic,

◇ as a topical anesthetic,

◇ to control asthma,

◇ to treat nerve pains (neuralgias) and migraine headaches,

◇ to treat withdrawal from opiates and alcohol,

◇ as an antibiotic,

◇ to control spasms and convulsions,

◇ and to induce childbirth.

(Mikuriya, 1973; Aldrich, 1997; Gurley, Aranow, & Katz, 1998)

Recently marijuana has been recommended for some types of glaucoma, nausea control, pain control, and to help a patient who has lost too much weight (wasting disease) to gain it back by stimulating appetite.

There is evidence that marijuana does reduce intraocular pressure, does calm nausea, does reduce some pain, and does encourage people to eat, though there are other drugs that are as effective or in some cases better. Many people smoke marijuana therapeutically for their glaucoma, cancer, AIDS, or other illness even though it is illegal. A recent report by the U.S. General Accounting Office found that the average medical marijuana user in Hawaii, Oregon, and Alaska, states where medical marijuana is legal, is male and in his 40s. More than 70% of those registered were 40 or older and about 70% were male ("Medical marijuana," 2002).

There are also people and places such as **marijuana buyers clubs that supply marijuana for those who are ill**. The problem is that marijuana is still a Schedule I drug, so growing it is illegal in most states although some states allow growing by authorized users of medical marijuana. However growing by nonauthorized users was just declared illegal even if they are supplying their drug to medical marijuana buyers clubs (Egelko, 2002). Another ruling by a federal appeals panel stated that doctors can recommend marijuana in those states where its medical use is legal and that their licenses cannot be revoked (Kravets, 2002). The presence of medical marijuana laws have only had a limited effect on the jobs of law enforcement officers according to recent reports from California, Arizona, Oregon, and Hawaii (Freedman, 2002).

Synthetic Marinol®, a form of THC, is theoretically available for treatment of these health problems but in practice is rarely prescribed. People say they prefer marijuana in its smokable form because it works faster than Marinol®. If they smoke, they can smoke just as much or as little as they need to relieve symptoms whereas if they take a premeasured Marinol® capsule, it may not be enough or may be too much for their condition. **A major obstacle with smoking or ingesting marijuana for medical purposes is the great variation in the amount of active ingredients** in any given marijuana plant. Variations in Δ-9-THC potency, the relative concentration of other active cannabinoids, and the inconsistency of botanical factors make it difficult to rely on this substance to treat medical problems. For example, some forms of marijuana have been shown to increase intraocular pressure, making someone's glaucoma worse, although normally most forms of marijuana will lower intraocular pressure.

Beyond the physiological effects, there are the mental effects of marijuana. Like opium cure-alls, such as theriac and laudanum, it is the mental effects of calming, anxiety relief, or mild euphoria that make people feel good and think they are getting better even if the drug isn't actually helping the illness.

There is however reluctance in the medical community to prescribe or even approve of marijuana for medical use for several reasons, including those already stated.

◇ There are a number of drugs on the market that physiologically have the same or even better therapeutic effects than marijuana or Marinol®.

◇ Marijuana smoke contains a number of irritants, carcinogens, pathogens, fungi, insecticides, and other chemicals, most of which have not been studied. If marijuana is baked in brownies or otherwise eaten, the respiratory effects are avoided but the 420 or more compounds contained in marijuana remain, along with all their side effects.

◇ Marijuana is a psychoactive drug with abuse and addictive potential, which is particularly dangerous for those who are recovering from abuse or addiction. It can cause its own addiction or relapse to other addictions.

Contrary to popular belief, medical research about marijuana continues in many countries. Since the 1970s there have been more than 12,500 scientific studies conducted. Yet results continue to be conflicting, making it difficult to substantiate appropriate medical use of marijuana.

1999 Report From the Institute of Medicine to the Office of National Drug Control Policy

In 1999 a study entitled *Marijuana and Medicine: Assessing the Science Base* was released. It was commissioned in August 1996 by the Office of National Drug Control Policy. The Office asked the Institute of Medicine of the National Academy of Sciences to conduct a review of the scientific evidence and do field research concerning the health benefits and risks of marijuana. We present their major conclusions and recommendations. We do this because when the report was originally released in 1999, both sides of the argument (pro- and antimarijuana forces) went in front of the media and translated the report colored by what they thought it said. The result was that unless one read the original report, it was extremely difficult to know what was actually written.

Conclusions of the Report

Cannabinoid Biology

• Cannabinoids likely have a natural role in pain modulation, control of movement, and memory.

• The natural role of cannabinoids in immune systems is likely multifaceted and remains unclear.

• The brain develops a tolerance to cannabinoids.

• Animal research demonstrates the potential for dependence but this potential is observed under a narrower range of conditions than with benzodiazepines, opiates, cocaine, or nicotine.

• Withdrawal symptoms can be observed in animals but appear to be mild compared to opiates or benzodiazepines, such as diazepam (Valium®).

Efficacy of Cannabinoid Drugs

• Scientific data indicate the potential therapeutic value of cannabinoid drugs, primarily THC, for pain relief, control of nausea and vomiting, and appetite stimulation; smoked marijuana however is a crude THC delivery system that also delivers harmful substances.

Influence of Psychological Effects on Therapeutic Effects

- The psychological effects of cannabinoids, such as anxiety reduction, sedation, and euphoria, can influence the potential therapeutic value. Those effects are potentially undesirable for certain patients and situations and beneficial for others. In addition psychological effects can complicate the interpretation of other aspects of the drug's effect.

Physiological Risks

- Numerous studies suggest that marijuana smoke is an important risk factor in the development of respiratory disease.

Marijuana Dependence and Withdrawal

- A distinctive marijuana withdrawal syndrome has been identified but it is mild and short-lived. The syndrome includes restlessness, irritability, mild agitation, insomnia, sleep EEG disturbance, nausea, and cramping.

Marijuana as a "Gateway" Drug

- Present data on drug use progression neither support nor refute the suggestion that medical availability would increase drug abuse. However, this question is beyond issues normally considered for medical uses of drugs and should not be a factor in evaluating the therapeutic potential of marijuana or cannabinoids.

Use of Smoked Marijuana

- Because of the health risks associated with smoking, smoked marijuana should generally not be recommended for long-term medical use. Nonetheless for certain patients, such as the terminally ill or those with debilitating symptoms, the long-term risks are not of great concern. Further, despite the legal, social, and health problems associated with smoking marijuana, it is widely used by certain patient groups.

Recommendations of the Report

1. **Research should continue into the physiological effects of synthetic and plant-derived cannabinoids and the natural function of cannabinoids found in the body.** Because different cannabinoids appear to have different effects, cannabinoid research should include, but not be restricted to, effects attributable to THC alone.

2. Clinical trials of cannabinoid drugs for symptom management should be conducted with the goal of developing rapid-onset, reliable, and safe delivery systems.

3. Psychological effects of cannabinoids such as anxiety reduction and sedation, which can influence medical benefits, should be evaluated in clinical trials.

4. Studies to define the individual health risks of smoking marijuana should be conducted particularly among populations in which marijuana use is prevalent.

5. **Clinical trials of marijuana use for medical purposes should be conducted** under the following limited circumstances: be conducted in patients with conditions for which there is reasonable expectation of efficacy; be approved by institutional review boards; and collect data about efficacy.

6. Short-term use of smoked marijuana (less than 6 months) for patients with debilitating symptoms (such as intractable pain or vomiting) must meet the following conditions:
   - failure of all approved medications to provide relief has been documented;
   - the symptoms can reasonably be expected to be relieved by rapid-onset cannabinoid drugs;
   - such treatment is administered under medical supervision in a manner that allows for assessment of treatment effectiveness;
   - and involves an oversight strategy comparable to an institutional review board process that could provide guidance within 24 hours of a submission by a physician to provide marijuana to a patient for a specified use.

(Institute of Medicine, 1999) (The full report is available from the National Academy Press, Tel: (800) 624-6242.)

CHAPTER SUMMARY

History

1. All arounders, also known as "psychedelics," "hallucinogens," and "psycho-stimulants," have been around since before the origin of man. Virtually all of the early psychedelics were derived from some of the more than 4,000 plants and fungi.

2. Instead of a rush or high, psychedelics were most often used to alter one's reality and consciousness and for religious, social, ceremonial, and medical reasons.

3. Recently the most popular psychedelics besides marijuana (e.g., LSD, MDMA) have been synthetic, mostly among young White users.

Classification

4. The most commonly used psychedelics are marijuana, LSD, MDMA (or other variations of the amphetamine molecule), psilocybin ("magic mushrooms"), peyote, ketamine, and PCP.

General Effects

5. The effects of all arounders are particularly dependent on the size of the dose, the emotional makeup of the user, the mood, the surroundings, previous psychedelic experiences, and preexisting mental illness.

6. A major physical effect of some psychedelics, (e.g., LSD, psilocybin, peyote, MDMA), is stimulation.

7. The most frequent mental effects of psychedelics are mixed up sen-

sations (synesthesia), along with illusions, delusions, and hallucinations.

LSD, Psilocybin Mushrooms, & Other Indole Psychedelics

8. LSD (derived from an ergot fungus) is extremely potent. Doses as low as 25 micrograms (25 millionths of a gram) can cause stimulant effects and some psychic effects.

9. LSD has been tried as a therapy for mental illnesses, as a truth/mind control drug (by the CIA), and as a mind-expanding experience (Dr. Timothy Leary, Ken Kesey, et al.). It was made illegal in 1966 and classified as a Schedule I drug in 1970.

10. In the 1990s younger students tried LSD but in the late 1990s and early 2000s the number shrank, possibly due to the popularity of MDMA (ecstasy).

11. Blotter acid is the most popular dosage form of LSD.

12. LSD also acts like a stimulant and like many other psychedelics, it overloads the reticular formation in the brainstem, the sensory switchboard for the mind, and creates illusions, delusions, and hallucinations that can last 6 to 8 hours.

13. A first-time user or someone with a preexisting mental condition is more likely to have a bad trip and later experience hallucinogen persisting perception disorder (flashbacks).

14. Psilocybin and psilocin (chemically similar to LSD) are the active ingredients in more than 75 species of "magic mushrooms"; they have been used for spiritual rites for 3,000 years by many Native American and Mexican Indian tribes.

15. After initial nausea or vomiting, visceral sensations, visual illusions, other sensory distortions, and a certain altered state of consciousness are the most common effects of mushrooms.

16. Many mushrooms are poisonous while store-bought mushrooms spiked with LSD or other psyche-

delics are often misrepresented as being psilocybin mushrooms.

17. Other indole psychedelics include ibogaine, which is also a stimulant; morning glory seeds; DMT, a naturally occurring short-acting psychedelic snuff that can be extracted from several plants or synthesized; and yage (ayahuasca) a longer-acting psychedelic that induces a dreamlike condition.

Peyote, MDMA, & Other Phenylalkylamine Psychedelics

18. These drugs, chemically related to adrenaline and amphetamines, take several hours to reach their peak effects.

19. Mescaline is the active ingredient of the peyote cactus.

20. Eating peyote buttons or drinking them in a prepared tea causes visual distortions and vivid hallucinations after an initial nausea and physical stimulation.

21. Designer psychedelics, variations of the amphetamine molecule, include psycho-stimulants such as MDMA, MDA, 2C-B, and PMA. Their chemical structures are similar to mescaline.

22. MDMA (ecstasy), usually sold as a capsule or tablet for anywhere from $5 to $35, came to public attention in 1978 and was used widely by therapists to help patients see into their emotions and repressed memories.

23. Ecstasy use, called "rolling," is popular at rave and other music parties, along with other psychedelics, stimulants, and depressants, e.g., LSD, cocaine, methamphetamine, GHB, and alcohol.

24. Physically MDMA stimulates heart and respiration, tightens muscles, and causes teeth clenching and a dangerous rise in body temperature.

Belladonna & Other Anticholinergic Psychedelics

25. Belladonna and other nightshade plants contain scopolamine, hyoscyamine, and atropine. In low

doses these substances cause a mild stupor but as the dose increases, delirium, hallucinations, and a separation from reality are common.

Ketamine, PCP, & Other Psychedelics

26. Ketamine and PCP ("angel dust") are anesthetics that besides deadening sensations, disassociate users from their surroundings and senses.

27. Effects of the drugs include amnesia, extremely high blood pressure, and combativeness. Higher doses can produce tremors, seizures, catatonia, coma, and even kidney failure.

28. Ketamine ("special-K") has become a popular drug in the rave club scene.

29. *Salvia divinorum* ("designer sage") has become popular recently as a legal, New Age, short-acting psychedelic.

30. DXM, or dextromethorphan, in many cough or cold preparations continues to be abused since it acts as a powerful psychedelic when ingested in high doses.

Marijuana & Other Cannabinols

31. Historically the *Cannabis* plant has been grown to produce fibers for rope and cloth, seeds for food, various chemicals for medicinal effects, and a psychoactive resin for psychedelic effects.

32. Marijuana is the most widely used illicit psychoactive drug. Use has increased since 1992, particularly in high school students, after a decade of decline in the 1980s.

33. Discoveries in the 1990s of a marijuana receptor site, a neurotransmitter (anandamide) that fits into that receptor site, and a marijuana antagonist (that precipitates withdrawal) have accelerated research into the effects of marijuana.

34. The two most widely used marijuana species are *Cannabis sativa* and *Cannabis indica*. *Cannabis sativa* can be used for hemp or

psychedelic effects. *Cannabis indica* is used only for its psychedelic effects.

35. The sinsemilla technique of growing *Cannabis sativa* or *Cannabis indica* greatly increases the concentration of Δ-9-THC, the main psychoactive ingredient in marijuana. There are at least 420 other ingredients.

36. Street marijuana that is readily available in the 2000s is 5–14 times stronger than the marijuana of the '60s and '70s. Much growing is done indoors to avoid detection.

37. Short-term effects of smoking marijuana include a dreamlike sensation, sedation, and a mild self-hypnosis, making users more likely to exaggerate their mood and react to the surroundings.

38. Some of the negative effects of short-term marijuana use are a decrease in the ability to do complicated tasks, a temporary disruption of short-term memory, decreased tracking ability (an impairment of hand-eye coordination), a trailing phenomenon, a distorted sense of time, and lowered testosterone levels.

39. Large amounts of marijuana or prolonged use can cause anxiety reactions, paranoia, and some illusions.

40. Respiratory effects include a decrease in the cilia lining the mucous membranes in the breathing passages that makes the smoker more susceptible to coughs, chronic bronchitis, emphysema, and possibly cancer. Smokers of both marijuana and cigarettes do much more damage to their air passages and lungs than a smoker of only marijuana.

41. Chronic marijuana use can make some smokers less likely to do anything they don't want to do, leading to a tendency to neglect life's problems or to think about problems rather than do something about them.

42. Tolerance develops fairly rapidly with chronic marijuana use.

43. When stopping chronic marijuana use, a person can suffer delayed withdrawal symptoms that include headache, anxiety, depression, irritability, aggression, restlessness, tremors, sleep disturbances, decreased appetite, and continued craving for the drug.

44. Medical use of marijuana is the controversial new battleground. Although marijuana has been employed as a medicine for more than 5,000 years, it is used very sparingly today. Proponents say it should be available as a medicine whereas opponents say there are better medicines that are more reliable and don't have all the other chemicals with unresearched side effects. Several states have passed laws allowing the medical use of marijuana but federal law that prohibits this use still takes precedence.

REFERENCES

Aceto, M. D, Scates, S. M., Lowe, J. A., & Martin, B. R. (1995). Cannabinoid-precipitated withdrawal by a selective antagonist: SR 141716A. *European Journal of Pharmacology, 282*(1–3), R1–R2.

Aldrich, M. R. (1997). History of therapeutic *Cannabis*. In M. L. Mathre (Ed.), Cannabis *in Medical Practice*. Jefferson, NC: McFarland & Company, Inc.

American Psychiatric Association. (2000). *Diagnostic and Statistical Manual of Mental Disorders* (4th ed., text revisions [DSM-IV-TR]). Washington, DC: Author.

Arrestee Drug Abuse Monitoring Program. (2003).The rise of marijuana as the drug of choice among youthful adult arrestees. National Institute of Justice Research in Brief June 2001 [Online]. Available: *http://www.adam-nij.net/files/golub_ and_johnson_pub.pdf*

Bibra, B. E. (1855/1995). *Plant Intoxicants.* Rochester, VT: Healing Arts Press.

Blum, K. (1984). Marijuana: Heaven or hell. In K. Blum (Ed.), *Handbook of Abusable Drugs.* New York: Garner Press.

Brunner, T. F. (1977). Marijuana in ancient Greece and Rome? The literary evidence. *Journal of Psychoactive Drugs, 9*(3).

Budney, A. J., Hughes, J. R., Moore, B. A., & Novy, P. L. (2001). Marijuana abstinence effects in marijuana smokers maintained in their home environment. *Archives of General Psychiatry, 58*(10), 917–924.

Carroll, M., & Comer, S. (1998). The pharmacology of phencyclidine and the hallucinogens. In A. W. Graham & T. K. Schultz (Eds.), *Principles of Addiction Medicine* (2nd ed., pp. 153–162). Chevy Chase, MD: American Society of Addiction Medicine, Inc.

Cartels replace hippies in California's market for marijuana growers (2002, September 26). *Medford Mail Tribune,* p. A2.

Chilton, W. S., Bigwood, J., & Jensen, R. E. (1979). Psilocin, bufotenine and serotonin: Historical and biosynthetic observations. *Journal of Psychoactive Drugs, 11*(1–2), 61–69.

Courtwright, D. T. (2001). *Forces of Habit.* Cambridge, MA: Harvard University Press.

DanceSafe. (2003). Party drug web site [Online]. Available: *http://www.dance-safe.org/about.html*

Devane, W. A., Hanus, L., Breuer, A., Pertwee, R. G., Stevenson, L. A., Griffin, G., Gibson, D., Mandelbaum, A., Etinger, A.,

& Mechoulam, R. (1992). Isolation and structure of a brain constituent that bonds to the cannabinoid receptor. *Science, 258*(5090), 1882–1884, 1946–1949.

Diaz, J. L. (1979). Ethnopharmacology and taxonomy of Mexican psychodysleptic plants. *Journal of Psychoactive Drugs, 11*(1–2), 71–101.

Drug Abuse Warning Network. (2002a). Club drugs, 2001 update. The DAWN Report [Online]. Available: *http://www.samhsa. gov/oas/2k2/DAWN/clubdrugs2k1.pdf*

Drug Abuse Warning Network. (2002b). *Mid-Year 2002 Preliminary Emergency Department Data from DAWN.* Rockville, MD: Substance Abuse and Mental Health Services Administration (SAMHSA).

Drug Enforcement Administration. (2001). Ecstasy: Rolling across Europe [Online]. Available: *http://www.usdoj.gov/dea/ pubs/intel/01008/index.html*

Drug Enforcement Administration. (2002). Trippin' on tryptamines. The emergence of Foxy and AMT as drugs of abuse [Online]. Available: *http://www.usdoj.gov/dea/ pubs/intel/02052/02052.html*

Drug Enforcement Administration. (2003a). Drug trafficking in the United States

[Online]. Available: *http://www.usdoj.gov/dea/concern/drug_trafficking.html*

Drug Enforcement Administration. (2003b). Federal trafficking penalties [Online]. Available: *http://www.usdoj.gov/dea/agency/penalties.htm*

Drug Enforcement Administration. (2003c). Ketamine [Online]. Available: *http://www.usdoj.gov/dea/concern/ketamine.html*

DuPont, R. L. (2000). *The Selfish Brain.* Washington, DC: American Psychiatric Press, Inc.

DuToit, B. M. (1980). *Cannabis in Africa.* Rotterdam: Balkema.

Efferink, J. G. R. (1988). Some little-known hallucinogenic plants of the Aztecs. *Journal of Psychoactive Drugs, 20*(4), 427–434.

Egelko, B. (2002, October 15). Court affirms medical pot law limits. *San Francisco Chronicle,* p. 1.

Elora, H. (2001). Adolescent dextromethorphan abuse. *Toxalert, 18*(1), 1–3.

Emboden, W. A. (1981). The genus *Cannabis* and the correct use of taxonomic categories. *Journal of Psychoactive Drugs, 13*(1), 15–22.

Escohotado, A. (1999). *A Brief History of Drugs.* Rochester, VT: Park Street Press.

Fischer, C., Hatzidimitriou, G., Wlos, J., Katz, J., & Ricaurte, G. (1995). Reorganization of ascending 5-HT axon projections in animals previously exposed to recreational drug 3,4-methelenedioxymethamphetamine (MDMA, ecstasy). *Journal of Neuroscience, 15,* 5476–5485.

Fox, B. (2002, October 3). Authorities break up big club-drug ring. *Medford Mail Tribune,* p. 11.

Freedman, D. (2002, November 30). Report says medical marijuana laws have limited effect on crime fighting. *The Oregonian.*

Furst, P. T. (1976). *Hallucinogens and Culture.* San Francisco: Chandler & Sharp Publishers, Inc.

Gieringer, D. H. (1988). Marijuana, driving, and accident safety. *Journal of Psychoactive Drugs, 20*(1), 93–100.

Goldstein, A. (2001). *Addiction: From Biology to Drug Policy* (2nd ed.). New York: W. H. Freeman and Company.

Gurley, R. J., Aranow, R., & Katz, M. (1998). Medicinal marijuana: A comprehensive review. *Journal of Psychoactive Drugs, 30*(2), 137–148.

Haney, M., et al. (1999). Abstinence symptoms following smoked marijuana in humans. *Psychopharmacology, 141,* 395–404.

Henderson, L., & Glass, W. (Eds.). (1994). *LSD Report.* Lexington, MA: Lexington Books.

Holland, J. (2001). *Ecstasy: The Complete Guide.* Rochester, VT: Park Street Press.

Hollister, L. E. (1984). Effects of hallucinogens in humans. In B. L. Jacobs (Ed.), *Hallucinogens: Neurochemical, Behavioral, and Clinical Perspectives* (pp.19–34). New York: The Raven Press.

Hollister, L. E. (1986). Health aspects of cannabis. *Pharmacological Revues, 38*(1), 1–20.

Hollister, L. E. (1992). Marijuana and immunity. *Journal of Psychoactive Drugs, 24*(2), 159–164.

Howlett, A. C., Evans, D. M., & Houston, D. B. (1992). The cannabinoid receptor. In L. Murphy & A. Bartke (Eds.), *Marijuana/Cannabinoids: Neurobiology and Neurophysiology* (pp. 35–72). Boca Raton, FL: CRC Press.

Huestis, M. A., et al. (2001). Blockade of effects of smoked marijuana by the CBI-selective cannabinoid receptor antagonist SR141716. *Archives of General Psychiatry, 58*(4), 322–328.

Institute of Medicine. (1999). *Marijuana and Medicine: Assessing the Science Base.* Washington, DC: National Academy Press.

Jaffe, J. H. (1989). Psychoactive substance abuse disorder. In H. Kaplan & B. J. Sadock (Eds.), *Comprehensive Textbook of Psychiatry* (5th ed., pp. 642–686). Baltimore: Williams & Wilkins.

Jansen, K. L. R., & Darracot-Cankovic, R. (2001). The nonmedical use of ketamine, Part Two: A review of problem use and dependence. *Journal of Psychoactive Drugs, 33*(2), 151–158.

Joy, J. E., Watson, S. J., Jr., & Benson, J. A. (Eds.). (1999). *Marijuana and Medicine: Assessing the Science Base.* Washington, DC: National Academy Press.

Kandel, D. B., & Yamaguchi, K. (1993). From beer to crack: Developmental patterns of drug involvement. *American Journal of Public Health, 83,* 851–855.

Kandel, D. B., Yamaguchi, K., & Chen, K. (1992). Stages of progression in drug involvement from adolescence to adulthood: Further evidence for the gateway theory. *Journal of Alcohol Studies, 53,* 447–457.

Kouri, E. M., et al. (1999). Changes in aggressive behavior during withdrawal from long-term marijuana use. *Psychopharmacology, 143,* 302–308.

Kravets, D. (2002). Court: Doctors can recommend marijuana. *Medford Mail Tribune,* p. 1.

Krupitsky, E. M., & Grinenko, A. Y. (1997). Ketamine psychedelic therapy (KPT). A review of the results of ten years of research. *Journal of Psychoactive Drugs, 29*(2), 165–183.

La Barre, J., & Weston, D. (1979). Peyotl and mescaline. *Journal of Psychoactive Drugs, 11*(1–2), 33–39.

Lee, M. A., & Shlain, B. (1985). *Acid Dreams: The Complete Social History of LSD.* New York: Grove Weidenfeld.

Lerner, A. G., Gelkopf, M., Oyffe, I., Finkel, B., Katz, S., Sigal, M., & Weizman, A. (2000). LSD-induced hallucinogen persisting perception disorder treatment with clonidine: An open pilot study. *International Clinical Psychopharmacology, 15*(1), 35–37.

Lerner, A. G., Oyffe, I., Isaacs, G., & Sigal, M. (1997). Naltrexone treatment of hallucinogen persisting perception disorder. *American Journal of Psychiatry, 154,* 437.

Lynskey, M. T., Heath, A. C., Bucholz, K. K., Slutske, W. S., Madden, P. A. F., Nelson, E. C., Statham, D. J., & Martin, N. G. (2003). Escalation of drug use in early-onset *Cannabis* users vs. co-twin controls. *Journal of the American Medical Association, 289*(4), 427-433.

Lyttle, T., Goldstein, D., & Gartz, J. (1996). Bufo toads and bufotenine: Fact and fiction surrounding an alleged psychedelic. *Journal of Psychoactive Drugs, 28*(3), 267–270.

Markert, L. E., & Roberts, D. C. (1991). 3,4 methylenedioxyamphetamine (MDA) self-administration and neurotoxicity. *Pharmacology, Biochemistry and Behavior, 39,* 569–574.

Marnell, T. (Ed.). (1997). *Drug Identification Bible* (3rd ed.). Denver: Drug Identification Bible.

Mathias, R. (1996). Marijuana impairs driving-related skills and workplace performance. *NIDA Notes, 11*(3).

McMeens, R. R. (1860). Report to the Ohio State Medical Committee on *Cannabis indica.* In T. H. Mikuriya (Ed.), *Marijuana: Medical Papers 1839–1972.* Oakland, CA: Medi-Comp Press.

Medical marijuana users are male, 40ish. (2002, December 2). *Medford Mail Tribune,* p. 6A.

Mikuriya, T. H. (Ed.). (1973). *Marijuana: Medical Papers 1839–1972.* Oakland, CA: Medi-Comp Press.

Morgan, J. P. (1997). Designer drugs. In J. H. Lowinson, P. Ruiz, R. B. Millman, & J. G. Langrod (Eds.), *Substance Abuse: A Comprehensive Textbook* (3rd ed., pp. 142–147). Baltimore: Williams & Wilkins.

National Institute on Drug Abuse. (2001). Research report series: Hallucinogens and dissociative drugs [Online]. Available: *http://165.112.78.61/ResearchReports/hallucinogens/halluc2.html*

National Institute on Drug Abuse. (2002). Research report series: Marijuana abuse [Online]. Available: *http://www.nida.nih.gov/ResearchReports/Marijuana*

National Institute on Drug Abuse. (2003). InfoFacts: LSD [Online]. Available: *http://www.nida.nih.gov/Infofax/lsd.html*

National Institutes of Health. (1997). Workshop on the medical utility of marijuana [Online]. Available: *http:www.nih.gov/news/ medmarijuana/MedicalMarijuana.htm*

National Organization for the Reform of Marijuana Laws. (2003). State by state laws [Online]. Available: *http://www. norml.org/index.cfm?Group_ID=4516*

O'Brien, R., Cohen, S., Evans, G., & Fine, J. (1992). *The Encyclopedia of Drug Abuse* (2nd ed.). New York: Facts on File.

Office of National Drug Control Policy. (2002). *National Drug Control Strategy, 2002*. Bethesda, MD: National Drug Clearinghouse.

Os, J., Bak, M., Hanssen, R. V., Bijl, R. V., Graaf, R., & Verdous, H. (2002). *Cannabis use and psychosis: A longitudinal population-based study. American Journal of Epidemiology, 156*, 319–327.

Ott, J. (1976). *Hallucinogenic Plants of North America*. Berkeley, CA: Wingbow Press.

Pechnick, R. N., & Ungerleider, J. T. (1997). Hallucinogens. In J. H. Lowinson, P. Ruiz, R. B. Millman, & J. G. Langrod (Eds.), *Substance Abuse: A Comprehensive Textbook* (3rd ed., pp. 142–147). Baltimore: Williams & Wilkins.

Pentney, A. R. (2001). As exploration of the history and controversies surrounding MDMA and MDA. *Journal of Psychoactive Drugs, 33*(3), 213–221.

Petersen, R. C. (1980). *Phencyclidine: a Review* (NIDA Publication No. 1980-0-341-166/614). Washington, DC: U.S. Government Printing Office.

Pope, H. G., Gruber, A. J., Hudson, J. I., Huestis, M. A., & Yurgelun-Todd, D. (2001). Neuropsychological performance in long-term *Cannabis* users. *Archives of General Psychiatry, 58*(10).

Proksch, J. W., Gentry, W. B., & Owens, S. M. (2000). Anti-phencyclidine monoclonal antibodies provide long-term reductions in brain phencyclidine concentrations during chronic phencyclidine administration in rats. *Journal of Pharmacology and Experimental Therapeutics, 292*(3), 83–837.

Reeve, V. C., et al. (1983). Hemolyzed blood and serum levels of delta-9-THC: Effects on the performance of roadside sobriety tests. *Journal of Forensic Sciences, 28*(4), 963–971.

Reynolds, J. R. (1890). Therapeutical uses and toxic effects of *Cannabis indica. Lancet, 1*, 637–638. In T. H. Mikuriya (Ed.), *Marijuana: Medical Papers 1839–1972*. Oakland, CA: Medi-Comp Press.

Rinaldi-Carmona, M., et al. (1994). SR141716, a potent and selective antagonist of the brain cannabinoid receptor. *Federation of European Biochemical Sciences Letters, 350*(2–3), 240–244.

Robert Wood Johnson Foundation. (2003). State drug laws. Medical marijuana [On-line]. Available: *http://www.rwjf.org/ news/special/drugLawsMarijuana.jhtml*

Sahagun, B. (1985). *The Florentine Codex, General History of the Things of New Spain*. Santa Fe, NM: The School of American Research.

Schuckit, M. A. (2000). *Drug and Alcohol Abuse*. New York: Kluwer Academic/ Plenum Publishers.

Schultes, R. E., & Hofmann, A. (1980). *The Botany and Chemistry of Hallucinogens*. Springfield, IL: Charles C. Thomas.

Schultes, R. E., & Hofmann, A. (1992). *Plants of the Gods*. Rochester, VT: Healing Arts Press.

Shulgin, A., & Shulgin, A., (2000). *PiHKAL, A Chemical Love Story*. Berkeley, CA: Transform Press.

Siegel, R. K. (1985). LSD hallucinations: From ergot to electric Kool-Aid. *Journal of Psychoactive Drugs, 17*(4), 247–256.

Siegel, R. K., (1989). *Life in Pursuit of Artificial Paradise*. New York: E. P. Hutton Publishing.

Smiley, A. (1986). Marijuana: On-road and driving simulator studies. *Alcohol, Drugs, and Driving: Abstracts and Reviews, 2*(3–4), 121–134.

Smith, M. V. (1981). *Psychedelic Chemistry.* Port Townsend, WA: Loompanics Unlimited.

Smith, P. B., et al. (1994). The pharmacological activity of anandamide, a putative endogenous cannabinoid in mice. *Journal of Pharmacology and Experimental Therapeutics, 270*, 219–227.

Snyder, S. (1996). *Drugs and the Brain.* New York: W.H. Freeman and Company.

Solowij, N., Stephens, R. S., Roffman, R. A., et al. (2002). Cognitive functioning of long-term heavy *Cannabis* users seeking treatment. *Journal of the American Medical Association, 287*(9).

Stafford, P. (1985). Recreational uses of LSD. *Journal of Psychoactive Drugs, 17*(4), 219–228.

Stafford, P. (1992). *Psychedelics Encyclopedia* (Vol. 1, p. 157). Berkeley, CA: Ronin Publishing.

Stamets, P. (1996). *Psilocybin Mushrooms of the World*. Berkeley, CA: Ten Speed Press.

Substance Abuse and Mental Health Services Administration. (2001). *Summary of Findings from the 2000 National Household Survey on Drug Abuse*. Rockville, MD: SAMHSA, Office of Applied Studies.

Substance Abuse and Mental Health Services Administration. (2002). *Summary of Findings from the 2001 National Household Survey on Drug Abuse*. Rockville, MD: SAMHSA, Office of Applied Studies.

Tashkin, D P., et al. (1997). Respiratory symptoms and lung function in habitual heavy smokers of tobacco alone and nonsmokers.

American Review of Respiratory Disease, 135, 209–216.

Tashkin, D. P., Simmons, M., & Clark, V. (1988). Acute and chronic effects of marijuana smoking compared with tobacco smoking on blood carboxyhemoglobin levels. *Journal of Psychoactive Drugs, 20*(1), 27–32.

Tashkin, E. (1999). Effects of marijuana on the lung and its defenses against infection and cancer. *School Psychology International, 20*, 23–37.

The Vaults of Erowid. (2001). Sulfurous Samadhi: An investigation of 2C-T-2 & 2C-T-7 [Online]. Available: *http://www. erowid.org/chemicals/2ct7/article1/ article1.shtml*

Touw, M. (1981). The religious and medicinal uses of *Cannabis* in China, India, and Tibet. *Journal of Psychoactive Drugs, 13*(1), 23–33.

Tsou, K., Patrick, S., & Walker, M. J. (1995). Physical withdrawal in rats tolerant to delta-9-tetrahydrocannabinol precipitated by a cannabinoid receptor antagonist. *European Journal of Pharmacology, 280*, R13–R15.

University of Michigan. (2003). Monitoring the Future Study. 2002 data from in-school surveys of 8th, 10th, and 12th grade students [Online]. Available: *http://monitoringthefuture.org/data/02data.html#2002d ata-drugs*

Walton, R. P. (1938). *Marijuana: America's New Drug Problem*. Philadelphia: Lippincott.

Weil, A., & Rosen, W. (1998). *From Chocolate to Morphine*. Boston: Houghton Mifflin Company.

Wilkins, J. N., Conner, B. T., & Gorelick, D. A. (1998). Management of stimulant, hallucinogen, marijuana, and phencyclidine intoxication and withdrawal. In A. W. Graham & T. K. Schultz (Eds.), *Principles of Addiction Medicine* (2nd ed., pp. 583–592). Chevy Chase, MD: American Society of Addiction Medicine, Inc.

Wilkins, J. N., Gorelick, D. A., & Conner, B. T. (1998). Pharmacological therapies for other drug and multiple drug addiction. In A. W. Graham & T. K. Schultz (Eds.), *Principles of Addiction Medicine* (2nd ed., pp. 465–485). Chevy Chase, MD: American Society of Addiction Medicine, Inc.

Young, C. R. (1997). Sertraline treatment of hallucinogen persisting perception disorder. *Journal of Clinical Psychiatry, 58*, 85.

Zukin, S. R., Sloboda, Z., & Javitt, D. C. (1997). Phencyclidine (PCP). In J. H. Lowinson, P. Ruiz, R. B. Millman, & J. G. Langrod (Eds.), *Substance Abuse: A Comprehensive Textbook* (3rd ed., pp. 142–147). Baltimore: Williams & Wilkins.

Other Drugs, Other Addictions

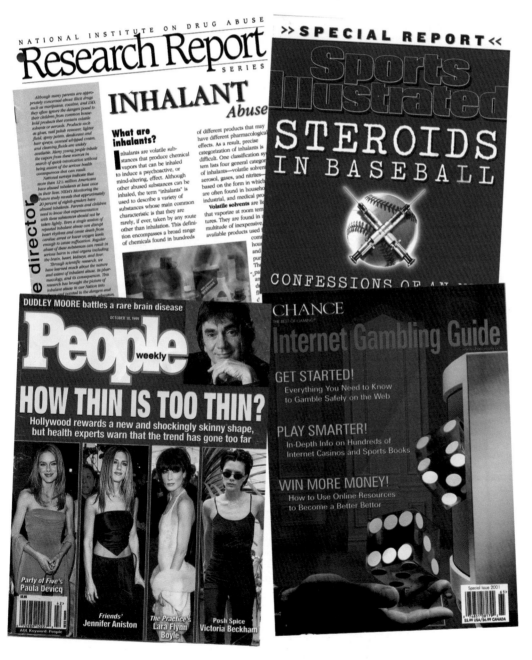

R esearchers, the media, and the general public have come to realize that addiction isn't limited only to hard drugs, alcohol, and tobacco. Compulsive eating, gambling, and Internet addiction are just some of the behavioral addictions that are part of people's lives.

- **Introduction:** It is unusual for a person to have only one addiction and this includes compulsive behaviors as well as drug addictions.

OTHER DRUGS

- **Inhalants:** The major inhalants (volatile solvents, volatile nitrites, and anesthetics) can cause mood elevation, central nervous system depression, disorientation, inebriation, and delirium. Dangerous effects include nerve damage, memory impairment, lack of coordination, and hypoxia (lack of oxygen leading to passing out or occasionally death).

- **Sports & Drugs:** Athletes have used therapeutic drugs, performance-enhancing drugs (especially steroids), and recreational/mood-altering drugs (legal and illegal). Steroids can build muscles and increase weight but they can also cause aggression, physical problems, abuse, and addiction. The safety of some performance-enhancing stimulants (e.g., ephedra) has been disputed.

- **Miscellaneous Drugs:** Toad secretions, embalming fluid, kava kava, and even cough medicine have been used to get high. In attempts to change mood and improve health, herbal medicines and supplements, amino acids, vitamins, and nutrients have been taken.

OTHER ADDICTIONS

- **Compulsive Behaviors:** People use compulsive behaviors to change their mood, get a rush, or self-medicate much as they do with psychoactive drugs. Compulsive behaviors include compulsive gambling, eating disorders, sexual addiction, compulsive shopping, and Internet addiction.

- **Heredity, Environment, & Compulsive Behaviors:** These factors can change brain chemistry and make someone more susceptible to turn a behavior into an addiction, just like substance addictions.

- **Compulsive Gambling:** Gambling has grown dramatically over the past 25 years. Almost 9 million adults are problem or pathological gamblers and another 15 million are at risk.

- **Compulsive Shopping:** In an era of easy credit and shopping networks, the debt load of the average American has exploded; many of those debtors are compulsive shoppers.

- **Eating Disorders:** There are three basic eating disorders.

  ◇ **Anorexia Nervosa:** Starving oneself by extreme measures including diet in order to look thin and feel in control of one's life.

  ◇ **Bulimia Nervosa:** Uncontrolled overeating followed by risky behaviors to avoid weight gain, such as vomiting, excessive exercise, and taking laxatives.

  ◇ **Binge-Eating Disorder (including compulsive overeating):** Uncontrolled eating, often involving large weight gains—usually a lifetime problem.

  All three eating disorders combine behavior and a substance (food) to create compulsive behaviors.

- **Sexual Addiction:** Sexual compulsivity, particularly pornography and masturbation, is often used to cope with personal problems and childhood traumas or stress.

- **Internet Addiction:** There are several Internet compulsions involving online services such as chat rooms, list servers, and even e-mail.

  ◇ **Cybersexual Addiction:** This includes online pornography along with X-rated chat rooms.

  ◇ **Computer Relationship Addiction:** This involves having relationships online in an obsessive manner.

  ◇ **Net Compulsions:** These consist of online gambling, shopping, auctions, stock day trading, and other Internet activities.

  ◇ **Information Addiction:** Endless surfing of the Internet for information and data is part of this compulsion.

  ◇ **Computer Games Addiction:** Online games, along with Sega® and Sony PlayStation® games, have become as popular and as compulsive as any drug.

- **Conclusions:** Although the roots of many compulsions are similar, one still has to be aware of differences, e.g., abstinence is necessary for recovery from some addictions while a return to normal levels of activity is a possibility with others.

INTRODUCTION

"Addiction is a state of mind. I was thinking of what addictions I have or have had. Well eating, that's my addiction. Well, no, I gamble, I got that. I watch TV too much—4 hours a day. Smoking, I smoked for 10 years—three packs a day. Drinking—I was drunk for 6 straight months in the Air Force and on a binge basis after that. It's not the substance. It's not the gambling. It's not the specific thing I do. It's all these behaviors. Instead of solving a problem to change how I feel in the long term, I take something or do something to change how I feel right now."

43-year-old male in recovery

It is unusual that a person will have only one addiction. Many sedative-hypnotic abusers are also alcoholics. Most marijuana smokers smoke cigarettes. It is the rare cocaine abuser who hasn't used methamphetamines. The addictions aren't limited to just psychoactive drugs. Behavioral addictions that include compulsive gambling, eating disorders, sexual addiction, compulsive shopping, and Internet addiction are also extremely common among substance abusers. For example, more than half of all compulsive gamblers are alcoholics. A 2003 study of 18–22 year-old women found that those who diet, even moderately, smoke significantly more than those who don't diet and if they are prone to binge eating and purging, they are more likely to drink alcohol as well as smoke (National Center on Addiction and Substance Abuse [NCASA], 2003). This chapter examines drugs (other than the ones covered in Chapters 3, 4, 5, and 6) and behaviors that are used compulsively and can cause harm to the user.

OTHER DRUGS

In addition to stimulants, depressants, and psychedelics, three classes of drugs that are used for the way they change physical or mental states are

◇ **inhalants** that have been around for thousands of years but whose use has expanded dramatically in the last 200 years;

◇ **sports drugs** that are used to heal injuries, increase performance, or to reward athletic prowess;

◇ miscellaneous drugs that include unusual substances that are difficult to classify: **herbal preparations, smart drugs/drinks, and nootropics**, some of which have been used as substitutes for the usual psychoactive drugs or as substances that will improve one's physical and mental health.

INHALANTS

"'Huffing'? I 'huffed' gas when I was like 9 years old. And then when I was 11 or 12, I 'huffed' for a year. I'd inhale 12 cans of air freshener a day. My mom would buy the big packs at Costco®— she didn't know I was 'huffing' them 'cause I'd throw them away and then when she found out, I had to stop. I'm surprised I'm not dead from it because I did it for a long time. I'd just sit there and use until I passed out."

17-year-old recovering inhalant and alcohol abuser

Inhalants, sometimes classified as deliriants, comprise a wide variety of volatile liquids that give off fumes or are found in certain gases and aerosol sprays. The volatile substances are often present in commercial products. **Inhalants are used for their stupefying, intoxicating, and less often slight psychedelic effects.** Inhalants, which are inhaled through the nose and/or mouth and occasionally sprayed directly in the mouth or nose, are classified differently from those substances like tobacco and heroin that are heated or burned and then smoked. They are also different than powders like cocaine hydrochloride that are sniffed.

There is some disagreement as to how to classify inhalants. This chapter uses three groupings (Table 7-1).

◇ **Volatile solvents (and aerosols):** Most of these substances are synthesized from petroleum and combined with other chemicals. Volatile solvents (hydrocarbons) are found in glues, gasoline, and nail polish remover among others. Some aero-

Solvent causes numb feeling

The Associated Press
ATLANTA — Repeated exposure to a chemical found in some car maintenance products

Youth trying to get high dies sniffing ScotchGard

14-year-old friend arrested on charge of manslaughter

System in Sacramento. "We are not talking about smoking and then dying 40 years down the road. We are talking about you are 14 — and then you...

breathe. He fell down and friend struggled to help.
Paramedics...

Swedes Say Laughing Gas Can Be Trouble

Reuters

Millions of U.S. kids have tried huffing

dangerous for regular users as well

First-time inhalant users

to 17 who reported an average grade of D in school were three times more likely to have huffed

Stockholm

Newest dangerous high: embalming fluid abuse

Many h shoe p 12, and

By Kathleen F.
USA TODAY

By JOANN LOVIGLIO
The Associated Press
PHILADELPHIA —Embalming fluid is becoming an increasingly popular drug for users looking for a new and different high—one that often comes with violent and psychotic side effects.

Users — mainly teenagers and people in their 20s — are buying tobacco or marijuana cigarettes that have been soaked in the fluid, then dried. They cost about $20 apiece and are called by nearly a dozen names nationwide, including "wet," "fry" and "illy."

"The idea of embalming fluid appeals

to people's morbid curiosity about death," said Dr. Julie Holland of New York University School of Medicine.
Formaldehyde can be bought in drug stores and beauty supply stores. It is also available in many school science labs. In addition, there have been reports of embalming fluid thefts from funeral homes in Louisiana and New York.

Although there are no national statistics on usage, many drug experts say it appears to have spread from the inner cities to well-to-do neighborhoods and college campuses.

"Whether they live in a million-dollar

house or a $5,000 house, kids who are smoking pot or crack and are looking for a different type of high are turning to wet," said Julie Kirlin, a juvenile probation officer in Reading, about 50 miles from Philadelphia.
Embalming fluid is a compound of formaldehyde, methanol, ethanol and other solvents.

The high depends on what the user is really getting: Often the drug PCP is mixed in.

Twenty Houston-area users interviewed for a 1996 study by the Texas Commission on Drug Abuse said the effects

include visual and auditory hallucinations, euphoria, a feeling of invincibility, increased pain tolerance, anger, forgetfulness and paranoia.

Stranger symptoms reported include an overwhelming desire to disrobe and a strong distaste for meat.

Other symptoms may include coma, seizures, kidney failure and stroke. The high lasts from six hours to three days.

"Fry users are described like those who do a lot of inhalants — they're just spaced-out, dissociative," said Jane Maxwell of the National Institute on Drug Abuse's Community Epidemiology

Work Group. When they've taken PCP, "they come into the emergency room and are just wild. They have to be strapped down in their beds or they destroy the place."

In the Philadelphia suburb of Morrisville, a 14-year-old boy fatally stabbed a 33-year-old neighbor more than 70 times last year after smoking wet.

The boy, who said he took wet to quiet the voices in his head, is serving a seven-year sentence.

"This is a violent drug, and it will turn into a big fire if it's not watched very closely," Kirlin said.

TABLE 7–1 INHALANTS

Product	Chemicals
Volatile Solvents & Aerosols	
Gasoline and gasoline additives	Gasoline and high-octane fuel additives (e.g., STP®)
Airplane glue	Toluene, ethyl acetate
Rubber cement	Toluene, hexane, methyl chloride, acetone, methyl ethyl ketone, methyl butyl ketone
PVC cement	Trichloroethylene
Paint sprays (especially gold and silver metallic paints)	Toluene, butane, propane, fluorocarbons, hydrocarbons
Hairsprays and deodorants	Butane, propane, fluorocarbons
Lighter fluid	Butane, isopropane
Fuel gas	Butane
Dry cleaning fluid, spot removers, typewriter correction fluid, degreasers	Tetrachloroethylene, trichloroethane, trichloroethylene
Nail polish remover	Acetone
Paint remover/thinners	Toluene, methylene chloride, methanol
Local anesthetic	Ethyl chloride
Analgesic/asthma sprays	Fluorocarbons
Volatile Nitrites	
Room odorizers (Locker Room®, Rush®, Liquid Gold®, Ram®, Rock Hard®, Stag®, Stud®, Thrust®, TNT®)	(Iso)amyl nitrite, (iso)butyl nitrite, isopropyl nitrite, cyclohexyl nitrite
Anesthetics	
Nitrous oxide whipped cream propellant ("whippits," laughing gas, "blue nun," nitrous)	Nitrous oxide
Chloroform	Chloroform
Ether	Ether

(Sharp & Rosenberg, 1997)

glue, spray paint, aerosol spray, lacquer thinner, and typewriter correction fluid.

Inhalants have some distinct differences from other psychoactive drugs.

◊ They are **quick acting and have intense effects**. They are absorbed through the lungs and into the bloodstream, which carries them rapidly to the brain. Their intoxicating effects occur within 7–10 seconds and last no more than 30 minutes to 1 hour after exposure has ceased.

◊ They are **cheap, readily available, and widespread**. More than 1,500 chemical products can be inhaled for their psychoactive effects.

◊ Because psychoactive gasses and liquids are present in a wide variety of substances in the home, garage, and workplace, they are **readily accessible to children and adolescents**. They have more direct effects on body tissues than most other psychoactive drugs.

◊ They get inadequate attention from parents, educators, the media, and law enforcement personnel because of the **low status of inhalant abuse as a drug problem**. Derogatory and dismissive attitudes towards solvent abusers compound the difficulty of getting warnings and treatment to potential and existing users.

◊ People who abuse inhalants can display strange, erratic, and unpredictable behavior along with poor judgment.

"At 15 maybe 16 I started doing like nitrous and I only did it at raves, like people would be walking around with a whole bunch of sagging balloons, laughing, and like they were a dollar each and you would just go up to people and say, 'Can I buy balloon?' and you just inhale them."
18-year-old inhalant abuser

HISTORY (*see Chapter 1*)

The practice of inhaling gaseous substances to get high goes back to an-

sols, which can be sprayed to produce a foggy mist, are inhaled for their gaseous propellants rather than for their primary contents. Besides volatile hydrocarbons, some other volatile organic compounds that can be abused are esters, ketones (e.g., acetone), alcohols, and glycols.

◊ **Volatile nitrites:** These drugs, including amyl and butyl nitrite, are used clinically as blood vessel dilators (vasodilators) for heart problems and in the past as over-the-counter room fresheners (butyl and isopropyl). They are also used re-

creationally, often at a party or in sexual situations.

◊ **Anesthetics:** These were developed to block pain or induce unconsciousness during surgical or other medical procedures; however their recreational use was discovered at the same time. Nitrous oxide (N_2O), also known as "laughing gas," is still used as an anesthetic as well as a party drug to make people giddy and high.

The most widely abused products in order of popularity are nitrous oxide, nitrites, gasoline (and its additives),

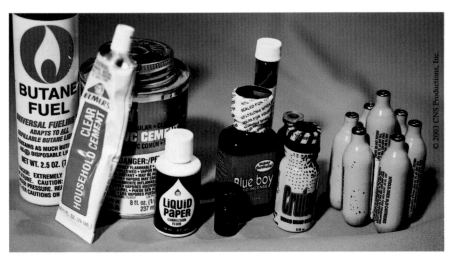

© 2003 CNS Productions, Inc.

The three groups of inhalants are volatile solvents (and aerosols), volatile nitrites, and anesthetics.

● ●

cient times. The Greek Oracle at Delphi was said to breathe in vapors from the earth (naturally occurring carbon dioxide) before uttering her prophecies. The carbon dioxide-induced oxygen starvation produced psychoactive effects (Giannini, 1991). In the Judaic world, spices, gums, herbs, and incense were burned and inhaled during religious ceremonies, a practice shared by other Mediterranean, African, and Native American peoples (Swan, 1995).

Our modern version of inhalant abuse began in the late 1700s with the discovery of nitrous oxide (laughing gas), chloroform, and ether. The use of inhalants for anesthesia and recreation occurred simultaneously (Weil & Rosen, 1998). Nitrous oxide became popular and was reportedly used at parties and in bordellos in the United States, France, and the United Kingdom (Smith, 1974). There were public exhibitions in the 1800s where a middle upper-class audience could inhale nitrous oxide and get high.

Later, at the beginning of the twentieth century when petroleum began to be refined and manufactured into new products—solvents, thinners, and glues to name a few, many more substances began to be inhaled for their intoxicating or euphoric effects. In the 1930s sniffing carbon dioxide (used to make

seltzer bubbles) had a brief fling with popularity as did gasoline sniffing (Giannini, 1991). **After World War II the abuse of glue and metallic paints rose dramatically**, particularly in the midwestern United States and in Japan. The practice persists as a drug abuse problem into the twenty-first century; **inhalants are responsible for about 700 to 1,200 deaths each year in the United States** (Drug Abuse Warning Network, 2003). The actual number of deaths is thought to be underreported

since medical examiners sometimes mistake death from inhalant abuse for suicide, suffocation, or an accident.

EPIDEMIOLOGY

Inhalant abuse often has an episodic pattern with brief outbreaks in particular schools or regions. **Abuse is most prevalent among adolescents.** However, adults also abuse inhalants, including painters, chemical company workers, health care professionals (especially in dentistry and anesthesiology), and others who have access to inhalants at work.

Inhalant abuse continues to be a worldwide problem according to a World Health Organization (WHO) report. **Internationally it afflicts primarily the young, the poor, street children, recent migrants to cities, and children exposed to chemicals daily,** such as children of cleaners or shoemakers. **The inhalant of choice in many countries is gasoline** because of its wide availability (World Health Organization [WHO], 1998).

Use by Sex & Age

Generally more young people than adults abuse inhalants (Table 7-2) and among 12–17-year-olds, more young men than young women although over-

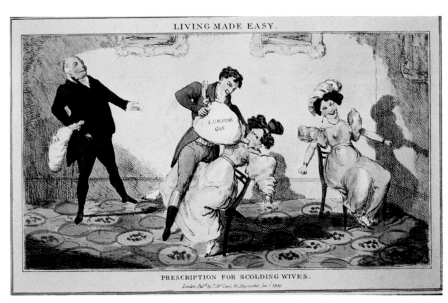

This 1830 print from England with its caption, "Living Made Easy," depicts a "gas frolic."
Courtesy of the National Library of Medicine, Bethesda, MD

● ●

TABLE 7–2 PERCENTAGE OF AMERICANS WHO HAVE USED INHALANTS—2001

Age	Ever Used	Last Year	Last Month
12–17	8.6%	3.5%	1.0%
18–25	13.4%	2.5%	0.6%
26 & up	7.1%	0.2%	0.1%
Total users 12 & up	18,219,000	1,922,000	539,000

Source: National Household Survey on Drug Abuse (SAMHSA, 2002)

all, females use slightly more than males. In adult populations the number of abusers declines by two-thirds or more after the age of 25 (Substance Abuse and Mental Health Services Administration [SAMHSA], 2002). Inhalant use in 8th, 10th, and 12th graders has generally gone down since 1995 (University of Michigan, 2003).

Ethnically, earliest use is highest among Hispanics and Native Americans and lowest among Whites although more Whites and Hispanics have used than Blacks (SAMHSA, 2002). In terms of treatment 67% of adolescents admitted for inhalant abuse were White, 20% were Hispanic, 7% were Native Americans/Alaska Natives, and 3% were Black (Drug and Alcohol Services Information System, 2002).

METHODS OF INHALATION

Although there have been reports of people spraying aerosols onto bread and eating the bread or inserting small bottles of inhalants, such as typewriter correction fluid, into the nostrils, there are about 7 common forms of inhalation.

1. **"Sniffing"** is breathing in the inhalant through the nose directly from the container. "Sniffing" puts the vapor into the lungs in contrast with "snorting" that puts solids, like cocaine, in contact with the mucosal lining of the nasal passages.

2. **"Huffing"** is putting a solvent-soaked rag, sock, or other material over or in one's mouth or nose and inhaling ("huffer" is also a term for any inhalant abuser no matter which route is used).

3. **"Bagging"** means placing the inhalant or inhalant-soaked material in a plastic bag and inhaling by nose, mouth, or both. Rebreathing the exhaled air intensifies the effect.

4. **"Spraying"** means spraying the inhalant directly into the nose or mouth.

5. **"Balloons and crackers"** is the use of a pin or other "cracking" device to puncture a can of nitrous oxide or other inhalant while a balloon is placed over the end of the can. The gas in the balloon is then inhaled.

6. Spraying an aerosol into a bag, putting the bag over one's head, and inhaling is another form of use.

7. Pouring or spraying inhalants onto cuffs, sleeves, or collars and then sniffing over a period of time is occasionally used.

Some users heat the solvent to make it more volatile, a particularly dangerous practice that has resulted in explosions, burns, and deaths (Marnell, 1997). Directly breathing and spraying pressurized inhalants into the mouth or nose are particularly toxic methods. These techniques expose an abuser's fragile membranes to the caustic effects of these substances. They also **put a dangerous amount of pressure into the lungs and can freeze tissue** as the substances quickly vaporize taking heat from everything around them. The choices of inhalant and method of inhalation allow great control over the intensity and duration of the effects.

"A Woodland boy died after he tried to get high by sniffing a common water repellent, Scotchguard®, and a 14-year-old friend who also was inhaling the aerosol was arrested on suspicion of involuntary manslaughter. The boys used a plastic bag to inhale the chemicals. They passed the bag back and forth. Suddenly the boy couldn't breathe."

Scripps-McClatchy News Service, September 17, 1998

VOLATILE SOLVENTS

These are mostly **carbon- and hydrocarbon-based compounds that are volatile (turn to gas) at room temperature**. They include such common materials as gasoline and gasoline additives, kerosene, paints (especially metallic paints), paint thinners, lacquers, nail polish remover, spot removers, glues and plastic cements, lighter fluid, and a variety of aerosols.

These volatile solvents are quick acting because they are **absorbed into the blood almost immediately after inhalation and then they move to the heart, brain, liver, and other tissues**. Solvents are exhaled by the lungs (in which case a telltale odor remains on the breath) or excreted by the kidneys (National Institute on Drug Abuse [NIDA], 2000b).

Short-Term Effects

Inhaling these substances produces a **temporary stimulation, mood elevation, and reduced inhibitions**. A solvent like toluene affects the reward/reinforcement center just as cocaine and other psychoactive drugs do (Gerasimov, Ferrieri, Schiffer, et al., 2002). Impulsiveness, excitement, and irritability also occur. Soon the depressive effects begin including **dizziness, slurred speech, unsteady gait, and drowsiness**. These symptoms along with impaired judgment and falling or fainting increase the danger of an accident or injury.

High dosage or individual susceptibility has a greater effect on the central nervous system (CNS)—**illusions, hallucinations, and delusions may develop**. The abuser may experience a dreamy stupor culminating in a short period of sleep. The effects resemble alcohol or sedative intoxication (inhalant abuse has been called a "quick drunk"). The intoxicated state may last from minutes to an hour or more, depending on the kind, quantity, and length of exposure to the solvent inhaled. Headaches and nausea may follow as part of an inhalant hangover.

"I came to the conclusion that the headaches my son had been complaining about were due to 'huffing.' We found empty spray cans out in the woods near the house. Of course when I confronted him he said, 'No way. Headaches must be from not having enough caffeine today.' He was doing bug spray, air freshener, Arid® deodorant, and whipped cream [the propellant]. When he was coming down, he would be real angry and violent. When loaded, he did stupid things."

Mother of a 14-year-old "huffer"

After prolonged inhalation, delirium with confusion, psychomotor clumsiness, emotional instability, impaired thinking, and coma have been reported. Neurological effects from both low-level and high-level (acute) exposure to volatile solvents are usually reversible.

Long-Term Effects

Chronic abuse is characterized by lack of coordination, inability to concentrate, weakness, disorientation, and loss of weight. Because solvents have been shown to affect the hippocampus, a memory center, long-term use will impair memory (NIDA, 2000b). Chronic abuse can involve extremely high concentrations of fumes, sometimes thousands of times higher than industrial exposure, so some mental and neurological effects can be irreversible though not progressive after abuse ceases. Magnetic resonance imaging (MRI) scans of the brains of

toluene and other volatile solvent abusers showed abnormalities in several areas of the brain that translated to low levels of general intellectual functioning particularly those involving working memory and executive cognitive functions, which include the inability to focus attention, plan, solve problems, and control one's behavior (Rosenberg et al., 2002). Chronic abuse of toluene can result in dementia, spastic movements, and other CNS dysfunction whereas occupational exposure to toluene has not produced these effects.

Complications may result from the effect of the solvent or other toxic ingredients, such as lead in gasoline. **Injuries to the brain, liver, kidney, bone marrow, and particularly the lungs** may result either from heavy exposure or because of individual hypersensitivity. Blood irregularities and chromosome damage can result as well as cardiac arrhythmia, respiratory arrest, or asphyxia due to occlusion of the airway. Chronic abuse of some of these solvents can produce ulcers around the nose and mouth as well as cancerous growths (Dinwiddie, 1998; Sharp & Rosenberg, 1997).

"I have a friend that does the spray cans and his brother overdosed on it. His mom found his older brother in his room with a plastic bag over his mouth from inhaling and he had all the gold paint all over his mouth and his nose and that's what he looks like now; he just looks totally just like a bum, you know, kinda stupid, and his eyes are half way shut all the time. He's just out of it. He's still my friend but I hate to see a person like that, you know."

19-year-old recovering drug user

Toluene (methyl benzene)

The most abused solvent is toluene because it is found in so many substances: glues, drying agents, solvents, thinners, paints, inks, and cleaning agents. Several studies have suggested that toluene has an extremely

high abuse potential (Sharp, Beauvais, & Spence, 1992). Chronic abuse can affect balance, hearing, eyesight, and, most often, problems with neurological functions and cognitive abilities. In one study **65% of chronic abusers of toluene in spray paint had neurological damage** (Hormes, Filley, & Rosenberg, 1986). Heavy abuse can result in deafness, trembling, and dementia. Other severe abnormalities include midrange hearing loss and changes to the white matter of the CNS. "Texas shoeshine," spray paint containing toluene, is widely abused often among painters. Kidney disorders are sometimes the result of toluene abuse (O'Brien, 2001).

Trichloroethylene (TCE)

This most common solvent is used in typewriter correction fluids, paints, metal degreasers, and spot removers. Like two other volatile solvents, toluene and acetone, trichlorethylene (TCE) **causes overall depression effects and moderate hallucinations**. The toxic effects of TCE have been known for 50 years and are similar to those of toluene. It was once even used as an anesthetic despite dangerous side effects. The effects of low-to-moderate doses of TCE are generally reversible but at higher doses various neuropathies (any disorder affecting the nervous system) occur (Sharp & Rosenberg, 1997). Some of these neuropathies can be permanent.

N-Hexane & Methyl Butyl Ketone (MBK)

Used as a solvent for glues and adhesives, as a diluent for plastics and rubber, and in the production of laminated products, n-hexane has caused neurological damage. Similarly methyl butyl ketone (MBK), used as a paint thinner and solvent for dyes, causes some of the same damage. There are **numerous reports of brain damage from occupational exposure as well as from deliberate recreational use**. Recovery in severe cases can take as long as 3 years (Sharp & Rosenberg, 1997).

Alkanes

The smaller molecules of **this class of hydrocarbons are gases at room temperature**. The most common alkanes include methane, ethane, butane, and propane. They are inhaled for their effects but unfortunately can also cause cardiac arrhythmias and sudden death (Siegal & Wason, 1990). The larger molecules of this class include hexane and pentane and are very neurotoxic (NIDA, 2000b).

Gasoline

Gasoline sniffing, especially common among solvent abusers on Native American reservations, introduces various components of gasoline into the system including solvents, metals, and chemicals. **Effects include insomnia, tremors, anorexia, and sometimes paralysis** (Beauvais, Oetting, & Edwards, 1985). When leaded gas is inhaled, symptoms can also include hallucinations, convulsions, and the chronic **irreversible effects of lead poisoning** (brain, liver, kidney, bone marrow, and lung damage). Internationally gasoline is the substance of choice because even in remote areas gasoline is not under

scrutiny and it is cheap (especially if siphoned from a car or truck) (WHO, 1998).

Alcohols

Ethanol, methanol, and isopropanol are the most commonly abused alcohol solvents. Remember the feeling when inhaling deeply from a brandy snifter? When inhaled too deeply and for too long a period of time rather than drunk, alcohols can cause a mild high along with nausea, vertigo, weakness, vomiting, headaches, and abdominal cramping. Isopropanol, found in paints, rubbing alcohol, formaldehyde, and perfumes, can induce severe CNS depression (Giannini, 1991).

Warning Signs of Solvent Abuse

Though solvent abuse is difficult to spot, there are still various warning signs. They are

◇ **headaches;**

◇ **chemical odor** on the body and clothes or in the room;

◇ **red, glassy, or watery eyes and dilated pupils;**

◇ **inflamed nose, nosebleeds, and rashes** around the nose and mouth;

◇ **slow, thick, or slurred speech;**

　　◇ **staggering gait, disorientation, and lack of coordination;**

　　◇ pains in the chest and stomach;

　　◇ fatigue;

　　◇ nausea;

　　◇ shortness of breath;

　　◇ loss of appetite;

　　◇ intoxication;

　　◇ irritability and aggression;

　　◇ seizure;

　　◇ coma.

"I felt like really stupid. I couldn't like focus on anything, you know, When I'd be in school I mean I got an F in

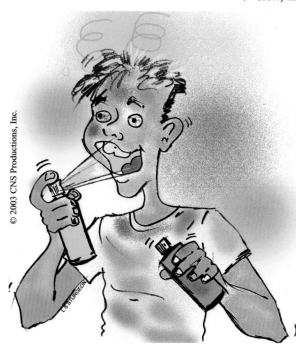

Peter was sure his secret was safe.

Spanish class and I'm Mexican, you know. I know Spanish very well but that stuff just really got me very stupid. But now it's like I feel much better, you know, I can, I can focus on everything."
17-year-old inhalant abuser

VOLATILE NITRITES

The first of the nitrites, amyl nitrite, was discovered in 1857. It was used to relieve angina (heart pains). The substances known as "aliphatic nitrites" or "alkyl nitrites" could be made with any convenient organic chemical, so the family of nitrites expanded to include **isoamyl, butyl, isobutyl, isopropyl, and most recently cyclohexyl nitrites.** Restrictions exist on all but cyclohexyl nitrite.

These inhalants dilate blood vessels, so the heart and brain (as well as other tissues) receive more blood. Effects start in 7–10 seconds and last for about 30 seconds to 1 minute. Blood pressure reaches its lowest point in 30 seconds and returns to normal at around 90 seconds. Nitrites are sometimes called "poppers" because amyl nitrite used to come in glass capsules wrapped in cotton that were broken open (with an audible pop) and sniffed (Weil & Rosen, 1998). Besides angina, amyl nitrite can be used to treat cyanide poisoning.

"Amyl nitrite, you crack 'em, inhale 'em, and you are off to the races; your head, your whole body is just enveloped. I don't know how to describe it better. My whole body, my vision, everything would be blurred around the edges. Sounds are muffled. I would use them with partners, with girlfriends in intimate moments, and it would heighten the experience in some aspects."
42-year-old recovering "huffer" and psychedelic abuser

On inhalation there is a **feeling of fullness in the head, a rush, mild euphoria, a dizziness, and giddiness.**

(First-time abusers have reported feeling panic attacks.) As the effects wear off, the user might experience headaches, nausea, vomiting, and a chill (because of dilation of blood vessels near the skin) (Wood, 1994). Excessive abuse can cause oxygen deprivation, fainting or passing out, and temporary asphyxiation. An extreme increase in heart rate and palpitations can make nitrite inhalation extremely unpleasant. First aid for the headaches includes abstinence. Overdose treatment requires removing the abuser from exposure and insuring that respiration and blood flow are maintained. Occasionally CPR is used. Chronic abuse causes methemoglobinemia, a condition that reduces the ability of the blood to carry oxygen.

Nitrites, **thought to enhance sexual activity**, are sought after especially by some male homosexuals for their euphoric and physiological effects that include relaxation of smooth muscles such as the sphincter muscle. Repeated abuse may alter blood cells and impair the immune system thus increasing susceptibility to HIV infection. There is some evidence that nitrites inhibit the functioning of the white blood cells. Nitrites are also converted to nitrosamines in the body—nitrosamines are potent cancer-causing chemicals.

Warnings have been issued about using poppers, Viagra®, and methamphetamine in combination (particularly at rave clubs and gay bathhouses) since the first two substances lower blood pressure and the combination of all three drugs can cause fainting or even death ("Viagra, Poppers," 1999). Tolerance develops rapidly to the effects of nitrites.

"Heart would race— just boom, boom, boom, boom in your chest. It feels like all the blood was rushing to your head. I've seen myself in the mirror after doing it—bright red. I don't imagine that that is a good sign."
42-year-old nitrite abuser

Nitrites, amyl nitrite in particular, have a sweet odor when fresh but a wet dog or spoiled banana odor when stale. Amyl nitrite is only available by prescription and although butyl and propyl nitrites were banned in the United States, variants of these formulations are still sold as room odorizers, tape head cleaners, and even sneaker cleaners (see Table 7-1). Street supplies of the drug also come from diverted legal sources or are smuggled in from other countries (DrugScope, 2003). Nitrites have been popular in England for quite a while among teenagers. One study found that 20% of 16-year-olds in northwest England had used nitrites.

ANESTHETICS

At the end of the eighteenth century newly discovered volatile substances were found to have anesthetic as well as euphoric effects. Experimentation began in both directions with substances such as chloroform, ether, oxygen, and nitrous oxide. Abuse of nitrous oxide was reported among Harvard medical students starting in the nineteenth century.

Abuse continues today by young experimenters as well as among middle class and affluent groups. A few dentists, doctors, anesthesiologists, hospital workers, and health care professionals abuse nitrous oxide, halothane, and other anesthetics, e.g., ether, ethylene, ethyl chloride, and cyclopropane.

Nitrous Oxide (N₂O)

The rave and party scene has brought back an interest in the abuse of nitrous oxide (N_2O) principally because of its dramatic **rapid onset and equally rapid dissolution of effects**. Ecstasy, the most well-known club drug (psycho-stimulant) is said to enhance the effects of nitrous oxide.

Nitrous oxide, discovered by Dr. Joseph Priestly in 1776, was popularized by the physician Sir Humphrey Davy for its anesthetic/analgesic effects and for its euphoric effects. Davy talked about a pleasurable thrilling in the chest and extremities along with auditory and visual distortions. He also wrote about his recreational use of the gas. In 1869 the gas was first used to effervesce or aerate drinks (Lynn, Walter, Harris, Dendy, & James, 1972). Medically, nitrous is used most often by dentists and since the pain-numbing effects are short acting, the gas is delivered continuously during oral surgery or other dental procedures.

The most commonly abused form of nitrous oxide is **sold in small pressurized metal or plastic canisters** intended for home use to charge whipping cream bottles. These Whip-It!® or EZ Whip® cartridges are sold in boxes of 10, 12, or 24 for about 50 cents a canister. **Large commercial tanks are also diverted from medical or dental suppliers** for abuse (they are painted blue thus called "blue nuns"). Both contain nitrous oxide under great pressure and should not be directly inhaled from their containers. Also the rapid vaporization of the gas will cause freezing to oral, nasal, or lung tissues if inhaled directly from the source container. Most often a source container is used to **inflate a balloon and users then inhale the nitrous from the inflated balloon**. Large tanks come with valves and fittings that can be adapted to fill balloons but the smaller Whip-It!® containers must be opened with a metal device called a "cracker" that is sold for about $10.

Nitrous oxide is abused for its mood-altering effects. Within 8–10 seconds of inhaling from a balloon, the gas produces desired effects including

◇ **dizziness, giddiness, and disorientation**, often accompanied by **silly laughter**;

◇ a throbbing or pulsating **buzzing in the ears**;

◇ occasional **visual hallucinations**.

"I did nitrous, the silver caps; you put it in balloons and then you put it up to your mouth and you breathe in three times. And as soon as you let go man, you feel like your head is gonna pop and again the 'whawha' sound and it felt like my head was in a bell that just rang. I was shaking laughing and my face was pale again and my lips were blue and I did that so much that night I ended throwing up."
16-year-old "huffer"

Nitrous can also cause

◇ **confusion and headache;**

◇ **a sense that one is about to collapse or pass out;**

◇ **impaired motor skills and fainting** that can result in traumatic injuries such as a broken nose or arm.

"People who fall normally have injuries on their knees and their hands because it's a natural reaction to break your fall. These people [nitrous users] would literally hit the ground face first and for a person who's 6 ft. tall, that's a long fall. We have a number of broken noses and broken teeth and we would always say to them, 'Have you been doing nitrous oxide?' 'Oh no, no, no, no, no.'"

Glen Razwyck, Director, Haight Ashbury Rock Medicine

These feelings quickly cease when the gas leaves the body. **The maximum effect lasts only 2 or 3 minutes** though experienced users seem to feel physical effects somewhat longer than novice users, possibly a form of reverse tolerance where less and less gas is needed to produce the same effects. Cognitive functioning is diminished during the peak of the high but returns to normal within 5 minutes. If used more extensively, the impaired thinking can last.

"I'd go to school and my head just wouldn't be there and it wouldn't be there for weeks on end. It would be gone, it would be in a daze the whole time. You wouldn't be able to concentrate. You had to shake it off or something; it just didn't go away."

22-year-old "huffer"

Long-term exposure can cause central and peripheral nerve cell and brain cell damage due to lack of sufficient oxygen since nitrous oxide replaces oxygen in the blood. Symptoms of long-term exposure include loss of balance and dexterity, weakness, and numbness in the arms and legs. Further,

nitrous oxide abuse can lead to physical dependence in some users and has been a major addiction problem for dentists over the past few decades.

"Me and my friend went on a nitrous binge that went on for like about 3 weeks. We had spent easy 80 bucks each on just nitrous, doin' like 100 canisters a day and did that for about 3 weeks and ever since then I've had, I have balance problems still from that."

18-year-old nitrous abuser

Most of the nerve damage is seen in users who employ dental gas masks or some other inhalation devices that expose them to the gas continuously over long periods of time depriving their nerve cells of sufficient oxygen. There is also a significant potential of seizures, cardiac arrhythmias, and asphyxia leading to central or peripheral nerve damage and even death. Although N_2O is not classified as a controlled substance, **possession with intent to use the gas for purposes other than medical, dental, or commercial purposes is a misdemeanor in most states.**

Halothane

Halothane is a prescription surgical anesthetic gas sold under the trade name Fluothane®. Its effects are extremely rapid and powerful enough to induce a coma for surgery. Because of its limited availability, it has been most often abused by anesthesiologists and hospital personnel.

DEPENDENCE

The *Diagnostic and Statistical Manual of Mental Disorders (DSM-IV-TR)* classifies inhalant disorders as inhalant dependence and abuse, intoxication, induced delirium, dementia, psychotic disorder, mood disorder, and anxiety disorder. These are based on abuse of volatile solvents (hydrocarbon or other volatile compounds). *DSM-IV-TR* classifies abuse of nitrites and anesthetics as psychoactive substance dependence not otherwise specified (American Psychiatric Association, 2000).

Though tolerance to volatile solvents will develop, the **liability for physical and psychological dependence and addiction to these inhalants is less than for other depressants**; although younger children get into long-term abuse of inhalants more often than adults perhaps because of the availability and low cost.

Breaking the habit or treating the compulsion can be difficult because most users are young and immature and because **continued use can cause cognitive impairments that hinder comprehension and recovery**. There have been isolated reports of withdrawal symptoms after cessation of long-term use (hallucinations, chills, cramps, and occasionally delirium tremens). A cross-tolerance to other depressants, including alcohol, will develop with long-term use. Interestingly, among drug addicts **inhalant abuse is looked down upon as low class and inferior to other highs**.

PREVENTION

The dangers of inhalant abuse have not been publicized as widely as the dangers of alcohol, tobacco, and other drugs. Parents and young people may not be aware of the risk of sudden death or brain damage from inhaling volatile substances. **Law enforcement officers, health care workers, teachers, and parents need to be trained to recognize signs and symptoms of inhalant abuse** and which youths are particularly at risk. Further it is necessary to be aware of or monitor the potentially abusable substances that are used in common household or business products.

SPORTS & DRUGS

INTRODUCTION

"It's no secret what's going on in baseball. At least half the guys are using steroids. They talk about it. They joke about it with each other."

Ken Caminiti, former Major League baseball player and 1996 MVP

Bechler's death tied to ephedra

Drugs taint Games

Top Romanian gymnast loses gold; husband's

Cyclist admits to drug use

Associated Press

A French cycling star told a

Wells: drug use rampant in Majors

'Half' Players agree to testing for steroids

Marijuana added to IOC banned list

OLYMPICS

Snowboard snafu brings issue to fore

By Mike Dodd
USA TODAY

SYDNEY, Australia — If snowboarders talk about passing the pipe at the next Olympics, they'd better be referring to the half-pipe race course...

NFL suspends two over failed drug tests

Two NFL players, including Atlanta's Ray Buchanan, one of the league's top cornerbacks, were suspended Wednesday for four games for violating the league's substance-abuse policy.

The Associated Press

NEW YORK — Baseball players ended decades of opposition Wednesday by agreeing to be checked for illegal steroids starting next year.

With that statement and other comments in the June 3, 2002, issue of *Sports Illustrated*, retired baseball player Ken Caminiti started a firestorm of controversy about drug use in baseball. He said he used, particularly during his MVP season in 1996, and saw nothing wrong with it (Sports Illustrated [SI], 2002). Later on he modified what he said and stated that it was much less than half the players who used but the debate had already begun. The question of steroid testing became part of the contract between the Players Association and the club owners although most other sports organizations already had testing programs. To further the controversy, pitcher David Wells, in his 2003 autobiography *Perfect I'm Not! Boomer on Beer, Brawls, Backaches and Baseball,* estimated that 25–40% of all Major Leaguers use steroids and/or amphetamines (Bodley, 2003). That same year Tony Gwynne, the great hitter for the San Diego Padres, estimated that half of Major Leaguers used amphetamines (mostly in green tablets called "greenies").

Drugs have often been a part of professional and amateur athletics, some legally and some illegally. There are three main categories of drugs used in sports:

◊ **therapeutic drugs** (e.g., analgesics, muscle relaxants, antiinflammatories, asthma medications) used for specific medical problems and administered with proper medical supervision;

◊ **performance-enhancing drugs (ergogenic drugs)** such as steroids, growth hormones, blood-doping drugs, and stimulants, some legal and some illegal. Most are banned from competition;

◊ **recreational and mood-altering drugs**, both legal and illegal (e.g., cocaine, marijuana, alcohol, tobacco), used to induce euphoria, reduce pain or anxiety, lower inhibitions, escape boredom, or simply to enhance the senses.

It is the performance-enhancing drugs that are unique to athletics and that cause the most problems although many athletes will try a wide variety of legal drugs to enhance their times, strength, and distance. A study by the International Olympic Committee (IOC) of more than 2,000 athletes at the 2000 Olympic Summer Games in Sydney, Australia discovered that each competitor had taken between 6 and 7 legal medications in the previous 3 days. The medications included vitamins, cold tablets, anti-inflammatories, and food supplements. One athlete used as many as 29 different medications and supplements.

Some athletes perceive drugs, often illicit ones, as the quick way to put on pounds and muscle, to increase stamina, to get up for a game, to relieve pain, or to keep up with other athletes suspected of using drugs. Since many drugs used in sports create feelings of confidence and excitement, drugs themselves can motivate athletes to abuse them.

HISTORY

The use of drugs in sports is not new. Greek Olympic athletes in the third century B.C. ate large amounts of mushrooms or meat to improve their performance. About the same time, athletes in Macedonia prepared for their events by drinking ground donkey hooves boiled in oil and garnished with rose petals. Roman gladiators took

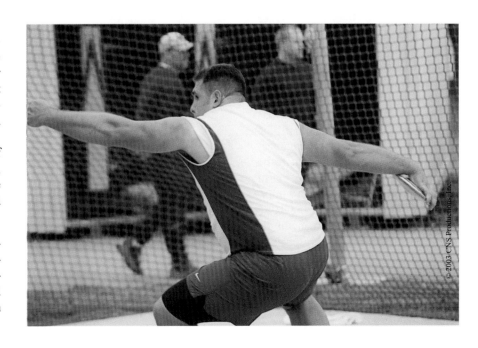

stimulants (betel nuts or ephedra) to give them endurance (Hanley, 1983). Aztec Indians found a stimulant in a native cactus that lasted up to 3 days that they used for running. By the 1800s, cyclists, swimmers, and other **athletes used opium, morphine, cocaine, caffeine, nitroglycerin, sugar cubes soaked in ether** (Dutch canal swimmers), **and even low doses of strychnine** (marathoners). **Boxers drank water laced with cocaine** between rounds. Long-distance runners were followed on bicycles by doctors who gave them a mixture of brandy and strychnine (Wooley, 1992).

Amphetamines, which were developed in the 1930s, increased alertness and energy for competition. In World War II, amphetamines were used by various countries to delay fatigue and increase endurance of their troops. When veterans returned home to the playing fields, some continued to rely on the drugs to give themselves a competitive edge or increase their athletic endurance.

International Politics

The male hormone testosterone had been isolated in the 1930s and was used in its pure form or in compounds to help injury victims heal and survivors of World War II concentration camps gain weight. During the Cold War era, **the Soviet weightlifting team used steroids in the 1952 Olympics to garner medals.** When this information was revealed in 1954 to the U.S. weightlifting coach, the argument was soon made that the United States team should also have access to steroids if they wanted to have a chance of staying ahead of the Soviets and the rest of the Communist bloc (Todd, 1987). **The use of performance-enhancing drugs was thought to be the only way that Americans could maintain their competitive edge in international athletics.** At the 1956 Olympics, the Soviets and many of the Communist-bloc countries, especially East Germany, were rumored to be using anabolic steroids not only in weightlifting and strength sports but in swimming as well. Use of ergogenic drugs continued in succeeding Olympics.

"The [East German] athletes themselves came out and told that these coaches and scientists forced these drugs on them. And then they found the records of that. I've seen their health problems afterwards. They would have medical problems that they, of course, wouldn't openly say but many of them suffered from that a lot."

Suha Tukman, coach and former 1972 Olympic swimmer for Turkey

By 1958 steroids were available and abuse by athletes had become widespread even in the face of growing evidence of negative side effects. At first they were abused by bodybuilders and weightlifters who wanted to increase weight and strength and later by many athletes to accelerate their training and development. Typical dosages have been greatly increased from 30–40 milligrams (mg) per day in the 1970s to 20–300 mg per day in the 1990s. In the 1994 World Championships, winning swimmers from The Peoples Republic of China were accused of using performance-enhancing drugs and subsequently a number of them tested positive.

Over the last 50 years bicycle riders have used a wide variety of substances and techniques to increase their endurance and strength: nitroglycerin, caffeine, amphetamines, strychnine, cocaine, heroin, and most recently EPO (erythropoietin) and blood doping. A cyclist died at the 1960 Rome Olympics and another in 1967 at the Tour de France, both due to amphetamines (Thomason, 1982). At the 1998 Tour de France, two teams were ejected for using EPO and steroids.

Commercialization of Sports

Beginning in the 1950s, the excellence of an athlete's performance began to matter less and less. With televised sports events, the explosive growth of professional sports, larger and larger salaries, and big money for commercial endorsements of products, the public's attitude changed from respect for athletic excellence to envy of athletes' salaries and an expectation that for that kind of money they had better be a winner. **Many coaches echoed this attitude of winning at any cost.**

"Winning is not the most important thing, it's the only thing."

Vince Lombardi, Green Bay Packers coach, 1956–1964

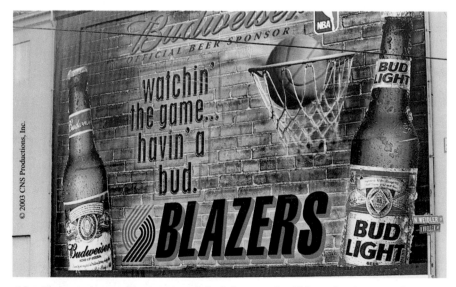

Advertisements that combine sports and alcohol are as plentiful as advertisements that combine sex and alcohol.

TABLE 7–3   NATIONAL COLLEGIATE ATHLETIC ASSOCIATION (NCAA) SURVEY OF DRUG USE BY STUDENT-ATHLETES

ERGOGENIC DRUG USE

	Amphetamines			Anabolic Steroids			Ephedrine	
Men's Sports	**1985**	**1993**	**2001**	**1985**	**1993**	**2001**	**1997**	**2001**
Baseball	8.1%	1.7%	2.7%	3.5%	0.7%	2.3%	3.3%	3.3%
Basketball	4.4%	0.7%	1.4%	3.6%	2.6%	1.4%	1.4%	3.0%
Football	10.1%	2.9%	4.2%	8.4%	5.0%	3.0%	5.3%	3.4%
Tennis	10.7%	0.0%	2.2%	3.6%	0.0%	0.6%	2.9%	3.8%
Track/Field	3.5%	1.1%	1.4%	4.7%	0.0%	1.2%	2.4%	2.8%
Women's Sports								
Basketball	10.8%	1.0%	2.0%	0.8%	0.4%	0.7%	1.8%	5.6%
Softball	10.9%	4.7%	3.9%	0.8%	0.4%	0.8%	1.1%	2.5%
Swimming	7.8%	4.7%	3.3%	1.0%	0.8%	1.3%	0.5%	3.4%
Tennis	11.3%	2.5%	2.7%	0.0%	0.3%	0.0%	1.9%	2.6%
Track/Field	4.9%	2.1%	1.6%	1.2%	0.6%	0.6%	0.9%	1.8%

SOCIAL DRUG USE BY NCAA DIVISION

	Division I					Division II				
Drug	**1985**	**1989**	**1993**	**1997**	**2001**	**1985**	**1989**	**1993**	**1997**	**2001**
Alcohol	85.3%	87.1%	86.3%	79.2%	78.3%	90.9%	90.9%	89.1%	79.7%	77.7%
Cocaine/crack	14.2%	4.6%	0.6%	1.2%	1.8%	1.5%	7.0%	1.9%	2.0%	1.5%
Marijuana/hashish	32.2%	24.7%	17.6%	26.4%	25.3%	37.9%	31.2%	22.5%	29.2%	24.1%
Smokeless tobacco	18.6%	27.2%	24.3%	21.7%	16.1%	23.2%	28.8%	30.6%	23.8%	18.7%
Cigarettes	na	na	na	na	21.3%	na	na	na	na	23.8%
Psychedelics	—	—	—	4.6%	4.3%	—	—	—	6.1%	5.5%

Over the past 30 years **the financial and social pressures to win have encouraged athletes to try drugs as a way to gain an advantage**. "Do what you have to but just win, baby, win" became our society's best advice to athletes. Many athletes earn more from endorsements than from salary, making winning even more crucial in their minds.

Extent of Abuse

At the beginning of the twenty-first century, some athletes continue to use and abuse substances that cover a very large diverse group of drugs, chemicals, and other substances, many of which are not psychoactive but are being misused in the context that they are taken. The actual extent of the problem is hard to judge as people are reluctant to admit use because use will get them suspended or kicked out of athletics or make them not desirable as a spokesperson for a product.

In the past when many perform-ance-enhancing drugs were legal, use was extremely high. In the '70s over half of the National Football League (NFL) players admitted to using amphetamines on a regular basis. A 15-year study published in 1985 reported that 20% of college athletes said they used anabolic steroids compared with 1% of nonathlete students though anecdotal evidence in football and other strength sports suggests the numbers were much higher. The number of people using performance-enhancing substances has dropped because of increased drug testing (National Collegiate Athletic Association [NCAA], 2003b).

"There is a misconception that athletes use drugs [other than steroids] more than the rest of the college student body and that's not true. The studies show that student-athlete use of drugs is actually at a level less than the rest of the student body."
Frank Uryasz, former Director, NCAA Sports Sciences

In 2001 it was estimated that at least 400,000 junior high and high school students had tried steroids (University of Michigan, 2003). Another report indicates that as collegiate testing for steroids becomes more stringent, **young athletes are encouraged to bulk up on them during high school and then go clean when they get to college**. This is particularly disturbing because anabolic steroids stunt bone development and disrupt hormonal function in adolescents and teenagers.

To understand the physical, mental, legal, and moral consequences of drug use in sports, it is necessary to examine the drugs themselves. Although there are literally hundreds of drugs and techniques that are used in connection with sports, we have focused on the most used and abused. The three categories of drugs used in sports (therapeutic, performance-enhancing, and recreational or mood-altering) are based on athletes' motives and the context in which use occurs more than the pharmacological properties of the substances.

THERAPEUTIC DRUGS

These are **drugs used for specific medical problems**, usually in accordance with standards of good medical practice, and fall into four main groups:

◇ analgesics (painkillers) and anesthetics,

◇ muscle relaxants,

◇ anti-inflammatories,

◇ asthma medications.

Analgesics (painkillers) & Anesthetics

These drugs are normally used to deaden pain. They include both **topical anesthetics** that desensitize nerve endings on the skin (alcohol and menthol or local anesthetics, such as procaine and lidocaine) and **systemic analgesics**, such as aspirin, ibuprofen, and acetaminophen (Tylenol®) for mild-to-moderate pain or narcotic (opioid) analgesics for moderate-to-severe pain. The most common opioids used in sports are **hydrocodone (Vicodin®, the most prescribed)**, meperidine (Demerol®), morphine, codeine, and propoxyphene (Darvon®). These drugs are either ingested or injected. Besides the pain-killing effects, opioids can cause sedation, drowsiness, dulling of the senses, mood changes, nausea, and euphoria.

"Pain is something you can play with. Everybody experiences pain at one time in their life or another and your body's just telling you something. Injury is a totally different situation. You don't participate when you're injured."

Bob Visgar, strength coach, Sacramento State University

For athletes, **the biggest danger from these drugs results from their ability to block pain without repairing the damage**. Normally pain is the body's warning signal that some muscle, organ, or tissue is damaged and that it should be protected. If those signals are constantly short-circuited, the user

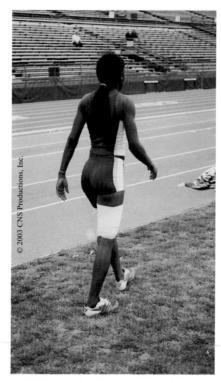

When injured, athletes who continue to compete by masking the pain with drugs can aggravate the injury.

becomes confused about what the body is saying. In addition, since tolerance develops so rapidly with opioids, increasing amounts become necessary to achieve pain relief. The problem is that **tissue dependence can develop**, along with the analgesic effects, making it easier for the user to slip into compulsive use.

Muscle Relaxants

Muscle relaxants are drugs that depress neural activity within skeletal muscles. They are used to treat muscle strains, ligament sprains, and the resultant severe spasms and to control tremors or shaking. Some athletes also use them to control performance anxiety. This class of drugs includes skeletal muscle relaxants, such as carisoprodol (Soma®) and methocarbamol (Robaxin®), and benzodiazepines, such as diazepam (Valium®) or clonazepam (Klonopin®) (Brukner & Khan, 2002; Arnheim & Prentice, 1993).

As with analgesics, the performance enhancement of these drugs is minimal because the drugs are depressants and can also cause sedation, blurred vision, decreased concentration, impaired memory, respiratory depression, and mild euphoria especially if overused. Skeletal muscle relaxants are **occasionally abused for their mental effects** although in recent years there has been an increase in the abuse of carisoprodol. Benzodiazepines and barbiturates have a higher dependence liability since accelerating use causes tolerance and tissue dependence. The benzodiazepines also stay in the body for a long period of time causing prolonged and even undesired effects.

Anti-Inflammatory Drugs

These drugs control inflammation and lessen pain. Anti-inflammatory drugs come in two classes: **NSAIDs (nonsteroidal anti-inflammatory drugs)**, typically aspirin, ibuprofin (Motrin® or Advil®), indomethacin (Indocin®), phenylbutazone (Butazoliden®), or sulindac (Clinoril®), and **corticosteroids, such as cortisone and Prednisone®** (corticosteroids are different than androgenic-anabolic steroids described below) (Physicians' Desk Reference [PDR], 2003).

With the corticosteroids, side effects are a significant consideration. Prolonged use can cause water retention, bone thinning, muscle and tendon weakness, skin problems such as delayed wound healing, vertigo, headaches, and glaucoma. Psychoactive effects are minimal at low doses but severe psychosis results from excessive high-dose use.

As with analgesics and skeletal muscle relaxants, when athletes are using anti-inflammatory drugs, a careful examination must be done to insure that the injury is not serious and that practice or play can continue without risk of aggravating the injury. They should not be used solely to enable the athlete to resume activity but **should be part of the overall healing process**. Ice, elevation, rest, physical therapy, and other treatment measures must accompany pharmacological relief of pain and inflammation.

Asthma Medications (beta$_2$ agonists)

Asthma affects 10% of the general population and is aggravated by heavy exercise in sports that require continuous exertion, e.g., cycling, rowing, middle- to long-distance running. It is also aggravated by the excess stress that comes from preperformance anxiety. A lesser condition, exercise-induced asthma (EIA), has been found. **The incidence of EIA is 11–23% in athletes** (Fuentes & DiMeo, 1996; Rupp et al., 1993). Because asthma is so widespread in athletics, permission to use certain asthma medications is given. Medications used to control asthma include beta$_2$ agonists like clenbuterol (banned) and albuterol (limited use). Beta$_2$ stimulation also increases muscle energy and growth but to a lesser extent than steroids. Asthma medications like ephedrine are stimulants and are therefore banned in sports. These drugs can

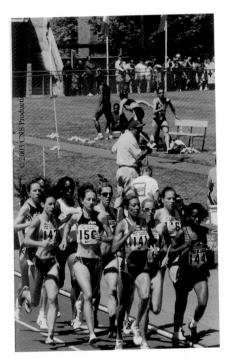

Often the difference between winning and coming in fifth is a fraction of a second. Athletes look for any edge, occasionally an illegal one.

slightly increase oxygen intake by bronchodilation that is helpful to the asthmatic. Other asthma medications such as theophyline and cromolyn are freely allowed by both the IOC and National Collegiate Athletic Association (NCAA) (Rosenberg, Fuentes, Wooley, Reese, & Podraza, 1996).

ANABOLIC STEROIDS & OTHER PERFORMANCE-ENHANCING (ergogenic) DRUGS

To this very broad general category of drugs we will add other substances and even techniques used to enhance performance. **Most of these drugs, substances, and techniques are banned by various sports-governing bodies such as the IOC and the NCAA.**

The goals that motivate users make these drugs different from alcohol and other psychoactive drugs. These ergogenic and energy-producing drugs, substances, and techniques are thought to possess various capabilities for boosting an athlete's performance (e.g., muscle building, fatigue delay). They are also abused to enhance self-image by adding muscle mass (bulking up) and shaping one's physique. Young adolescents might want them to hasten maturity or to develop a "buff" look. Unfortunately one of the side effects is to limit growth. The final reason performance-enhancing drugs are used is to increase confidence and aggression.

Anabolic-Androgenic Steroids (AAS or "roids")

"It's a performance-enhancing drug. I mean, that's what it did. It enhanced my performance. There were a few side effects but for the most part I had pretty good results from them as far as gaining strength and power."
24-year-old weightlifter

The most abused performance-enhancing drugs today, **anabolic-androgenic steroids (AAS) are derived from the male hormone testos-**

terone or are synthesized. Anabolic means "muscle building," androgenic means "producing masculine characteristics," and steroid is the chemical classification of the natural and synthetic compounds resembling hormones like testosterone and cortisone. AAS are used clinically to treat testosterone insufficiency, osteoporosis, certain types of anemia, some breast cancers, endometriosis, and a few other conditions (Lukas, 1998).

For the athlete, these drugs have marked benefits that include **increases in body weight, lean muscle mass, and muscular strength. The drugs can also increase aggressiveness and confidence**, traits that are of value in many sports.

Many students use AAS strictly to enhance personal appearance. As with any drug that's misused, less desirable side effects occur such as bone weakness, tendon injury, cancer, sexual

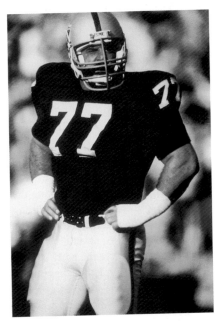

Lyle Alzado played football for the Raiders in the 1980s. He was one of the few players to speak out publicly about his use of performance-enhancing drugs. He blamed his use of human growth hormone and steroids for the brain cancer that eventually killed him. He said, "If I had known I would be this sick now, I would have tried to make it in football on my own, naturally." He died in 1992 at the age of 42.
Courtesy of Peter Alzado

problems, and even feminization in males or masculinization in women. So far no pharmacological process has been able to separate the desirable muscle-building properties of AAS from their undesirable or dangerous hormonal side effects.

"The men I knew who used steroids the most were 5'8" and under and they talked about how they were the runts of the class and the 98-pound weakling at the beach. Steroid use is one way they felt they could overcome that."
Ex-weightlifter

Patterns of Use. Steroid users may take from 20–200 times the clinically prescribed daily dosage. Instead of 75–100 mg per week, weightlifters, bodybuilders, and other illicit users have taken 1,000–2,100 mg per week (Mottram, 2002; Yesalis, Herrick, Buckley, et al., 1988). Some athletes practice **steroid stacking** by using three or more kinds of oral or injectable steroids and by alternating between cycles of use and nonuse.

"Basically I go on about 10 weeks, then I'll go off for a little while. So I would kind of cycle it to where it would peak me out at a certain time in the season."
24-year-old weightlifter

Cycling steroids means taking the drugs for a 4- to 18-week period during intensive training and then stopping the drugs for a period of several weeks to several months to give the body a pharmacological rest and then beginning another cycle. Some athletes cycle to escape detection. Studies have reported that **82% of those using "roids" during a training cycle combined 3 or more different anabolic steroids** in that time and 30% used 7 or more. Of special concern is the fact that up to 99% of "roid" users have injected the drug and most increase their dosage during the course of their training (Galloway, 1997).

Physical Side Effects. In men the initial masculinization effect in-

cludes an increase in muscle mass and muscle tone. Most users also report an initial bloated appearance. However, long-term use results in **suppression of the body's own natural production of testosterone**. As a consequence **long-term male steroid users develop more feminine characteristics** (e.g., swelling breasts, nipple changes), decreased size of sexual organs, and an impairment of sexual functioning (Pope & Katz, 1994). In the *Sports Illustrated* interview, Ken Caminiti said he used steroids so heavily that his testicles shrank and retracted and his body stopped producing its own testosterone. It took 4 months after stopping for his testicles to drop on their own (SI, 2002).

In females similar gains in muscular development may be considered beautiful to some but **long-term use by women results in masculinizing effects**, increased facial hair, decreased breast size, lowered voice, and clitoral enlargement.

"Outwardly you have people experience the bad acne. With women, I've seen a change in the facial jaw line—their voices, too. There are definitely things that, as a woman, are not in your

favor. And the lasting results, too, are something that I often wonder why a person chooses to go that route."
Female bodybuilder

If injections of steroids are taken to supplement oral doses and the needles are shared, users are liable to contract or transmit the HIV virus that can lead to AIDS. They are also at risk for other blood-borne pathogens like hepatitis B and C.

Mental & Emotional Effects. Anabolic-androgenic steroids can make users feel more confident and aggressive while using. Some researchers think that the confidence "roids" induce is as sought after as the physical effects. As use continues, **emotional balance starts to swing from confidence to aggressiveness, to emotional instability, to rage, and back to depression or to psychosis**. This "roid rage" can lead to irrational behavior (Pope & Katz, 1994).

"After a dinner date, this one guy attacked me in my apartment. He was in the middle of a 'roid' cycle. I put up a great fight and he gave up but if he

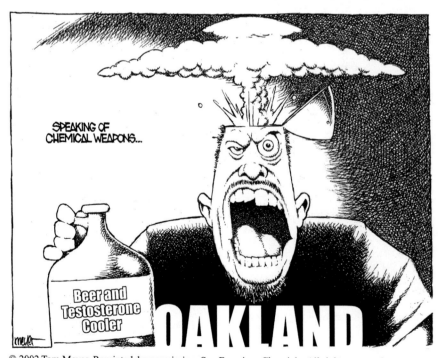

was determined, there was no way I could have overpowered him. I don't know if it was the drugs or he was just crazy."
Female college student

The **"roid rage" is more likely to occur in people who already have a tendency to anger** or who take excessive amounts of steroids. One study of 12 bodybuilders compared to a control group found much higher tendencies towards paranoid, schizoid, antisocial, borderline, histrionic, and passive-aggressive personality profiles due to use. Before use the two groups were about equal in regards to abnormal personality traits (Cooper, Noakes, Dunne, Lambert, & Rochford, 1996).

Compulsive Use & Addiction. About one-third of the users experience a sense of euphoria or well-being (at least initially) that contributes to their continued and compulsive abuse of "roids." In a survey of hard-core AAS users in their senior year in high school, 38% said they wouldn't stop using even if it were proven beyond a doubt that AAS cause permanent sterility, liver cancer, or heart attacks (Kusserow, 1990).

Various surveys of weightlifters found that **distinct withdrawal symptoms are strong signs of dependence and abuse.** Withdrawal symptoms include craving, fatigue, dissatisfaction with body image, depressed mood, restlessness, insomnia, no desire to eat, headaches, and lack of sexual desire (NIDA, 2000b). Even between cycles, users will continue with low doses to avoid withdrawal. As with other drug use, compulsive use of steroids makes the user more likely to use other psychoactive drugs to enhance performance, as a reward, or in social situations.

"It was addicting, mentally addicting. I just didn't feel strong unless I was taking something. When I retired, I kept taking the stuff. I couldn't stand the thought of being weak."
Lyle Alzado, former NFL star (deceased)

Do Steroids Work? In 1984 the American College of Sports Medicine stated that **steroids can increase mass and muscle strength when combined with diet and exercise**. A 1996 study by Dr. Shalender Bhasin of Charles R. Drew University in Los Angeles showed large measurable increases in strength and weight due to steroids in a double blind study involving 43 male volunteers. When steroid use was combined with exercise, the gains in muscle size and strength were significantly greater (Bhasin, Storer, Berman, et al., 1996). What the study didn't cover was the use of multiple steroids and the use of excessive amounts of steroids over long periods of time.

"I took steroids from 1976 to 1983. In the middle of 1979, my body began turning a yellowish color. I was very aggressive and combative, had high blood pressure and testicular atrophy. I was hospitalized twice with near kidney failure, liver tumors, and severe personality disorders. During my second hospital stay, the doctors found I had become sterile. Two years after I quit using and started training without drugs, I set six new world records in power lifting, something I thought was impossible without the steroids."
Richard L. Sandlin, former assistant coach, University of Alabama (U.S. Congress, 1990)

Supply & Cost. Athletes obtain steroids in different ways: from the black market (through gyms, mail order companies, or friends) or illicitly from doctors, veterinarians, or pharmacists. **Serious users spend $200 to $400 per week** on anabolic steroids and other strength drugs, so a single cycle can cost thousands of dollars. Some professional athletes spend $20,000 to $30,000 a year. At a conservative estimate, the black market for steroids grosses up to $300 to $500 million a year (NIDA, 2000a). Most of the product comes from underground laboratories in the United States and foreign countries.

"We all knew who was using. We exchanged information on any new drugs that were on the market. We got our steroids through the gym owner. In fact he would inject them for us in the rear."
28-year-old weightlifter

STIMULANTS

Central nervous system stimulants often start out as performance boosters but the basic pharmacology of most stimulants often makes use self-defeating. The IOC and all other sports organizations have banned the use of any kind of amphetamine and most other strong stimulants in competition. Stimulants used in sports include methamphetamines, diet pills, methylphenidate, ephedrine, caffeine, nicotine, occasionally cocaine, and some herbal or dietary supplements.

Amphetamines

"As a pitcher, I won't ever object to a sleepy-eyed middle infielder 'beaning up' [using amphetamines] to help me win. That may not be the politically correct spin on the practice but I really couldn't care less."
David Wells, Major League pitcher

Amphetamines are referred to as "sympathomimetics" because they mimic and stimulate the effects of the sympathetic nervous system, that part of the nervous system that controls involuntary body functions including blood circulation, respiration, and digestion. Some use amphetamines (meth, Adderall®, "crank") as a way of getting up for competition. Initially many users feel energetic and alert. Athletes also take amphetamines to make themselves more aggressive and confident. Some take them after an event to sustain the competitive high. Studies have shown that amphetamines will increase strength by about 3–4% and endurance by 1.5% in low doses (Rosenberg et al., 1996). Other studies have shown that **much of the increase in**

TABLE 7–4 ANABOLIC-ANDROGENIC STEROIDS (AAS)

Chemical Name (DEA schedule)	Trade Name
U.S. Approved	
Adanazol (no schedule)	Danocrin® (tablet or capsule)
Boldenone undecylenate (Schedule III)	Equipoise® (injection)
Fluoxymesterone (Schedule III)	Halotestin® (tablet or capsule)
Methyltestosterone (Schedule III)	Android®, Metandren®, Testred®, Virilon® (tablet or capsule)
Nandrolone phenpropionate (Schedule III)	Durabolin® (injection)
Nandrolone decanoate (Schedule III)	Deca-Durabolin® (injection)
Oxandrolone (Schedule III)	Oxandrin® (tablet or capsule)
Oxymetholon (Schedule III)	Anadrol-50® (tablet or capsule)
Stanozolol (Schedule III)	Winstrol® (tablet or capsule)
Testolactone (Schedule III)	Teslac®
Testosterone cypionate (Schedule III)	Depo-Testosterone®, Virilon IM® (tablet or capsule)
Testosterone enanthate (Schedule III)	Delatestryl® (injection)
Testosterone propionate (Schedule III)	Testex®, Oreton Propionate®
Veterinary	
Boldenone	Equipoise®
Mibolerone	Cheque Drops®
Stanozolol	Winstrol-V®
Zeranol	Ralgro®
Not U.S. Approved	
Bolasterone	Finiject 30®
Ethylestrenol	Maxibolan®
Mesterolone	
Methandrostenolone	Dianabol® (tablet or capsule)
Methenolone	Primobolan®
Methenolone enanthate	Primobolan Depot®
Norethandrolone	Nilexor®
Oxandrolone	Anavar®
Oxymesterone	Oranabol®

(Other anabolic steroids or agents on the IOC and NCAA lists of banned substances include clostebol, metandienone, metenolone, -19-norandrostenediol, -19-norandrostenedione, clenbuterol, dromostanolone, dehydrochlormethyl-testosterone, dehydroepiandrosterone [DHEA]).

performance comes from the focusing effects of amphetamines and the increase in aggressiveness rather than specific muscular changes as seen with anabolic steroids. Improvement seems to be in complex tasks that require concentration.

Tolerance to amphetamines develops quite rapidly and as it develops, the beneficial effects diminish. Negative effects include anxiety, restlessness, and impaired judgment. In some cases amphetamine users (e.g., football players) can overreact to plays and literally overrun the action. The increase in aggressiveness caused by amphetamines can get out of hand causing injury to the users and their opponents. Physically, heavy use can bring on heart and blood pressure problems, exhaustion, and malnutrition. There have been reports of fatal heat stroke among athletes since these strong stimulants redistribute blood away from the skin thereby impairing the body's cooling system (Mottram, 2002). Mentally, high-dose use can bring on paranoia and even amphetamine psychosis.

Caffeine

This mild stimulant is found in coffee, tea, cola-flavored beverages, and cocoa. It also comes in tablet form and can be very toxic in high doses. It increases wakefulness and mental alertness at blood levels of 10 milligrams per milliliter (mg/ml) by stimulating the cerebral cortex and medullar centers. It also increases endurance slightly during extended exercise and increases muscle contraction (Spriet, 1995). The increased endurance supposedly comes from its ability to increase the body's fat- and sugar-burning efficiency and reduce the sense of fatigue. Various studies have demonstrated this increased endurance. Unfortunately side effects such as increased digestive secretions (that can cause stomach discomfort) or increased urination (and possibly dehydration) can also occur (Weinberg & Bealer, 2001).

The IOC puts a limit on caffeine of 12 mg/ml, about three strong cups of coffee, just before competition (International Olympic Committee [IOC], 2003). Some athletes have been using a combination of caffeine, ephedrine or ephedra, and aspirin to try and increase endurance even though the cardiovascular effects can be risky.

Ephedra (ma huang) & Ephedrine

Ephedra (ma huang), a mild stimulant, is a traditional Chinese herb that comes from the ephedra bush. The active ingredients are ephedrine (a bronchodilator) and, to a lesser extent, pseudoephedrine (a nasal decongestant), substances that can also be synthesized in laboratories. Ephedra contains about 6% ephedrine. Ephedra and ephedrine are found in hundreds of legal over-the-counter cold and asthma medications as well as in some herbal teas, energy drinks, energy bars, energy pills, and especially diet medications. The over-the-counter products use suggestive names, e.g., Xenadrine RFA-1®, Metabolife®, Ripped Fuel®, Diet Fuel®, Stacker 3®, Natural TRIM®, and Truckers Luv It®. Ephedra and ephedrine are used by themselves or in combination with other mild stimulants (e.g., kola nut, guarana, both of which contain caffeine) to supposedly increase strength and endurance and/or promote weight loss. Being able to treat asthma and upper respiratory infections comes from ephedra's and ephedrine's ability to ease bronchial spasms and relieve swelling in mucous membranes. For dieters, they suppress appetite and stimulate the thyroid gland. When taken in excess or by susceptible individuals, they can cause jitteriness, anxiety, headaches, high blood pressure, cardiac arrhythmia, poor digestion, and overheating.

The death of Baltimore Orioles pitching prospect Steve Bechler on February 17, 2003, rekindled the debate about the use of the stimulant ephedra (and ephedrine) in sports. Bechler, who lived with high blood pressure and a slight liver abnormality, was exercising after having supposedly taken three tablets of an over-the-counter diet aid that contained ephedra and caffeine. He died from a combination of heat stroke and multiple organ failure reportedly aggravated by the ephedra. Recently there had been a sharp increase in the use of the drug in sports but the publicity over the recent deaths forced the Food and Drug Administration (FDA) to warn 24 manufacturers of ephedra products to stop their various marketing campaigns aimed at athletes. The FDA also proposed labels warning that ephedra can cause heart attacks and strokes or even kill. In an analysis of reports to the American Association of Poison Control Centers, ephedra accounted for 64% of herb-related adverse reactions in 2001, a figure that is startling since only 1% of herbal products sold contain ephedra (Bent, Tiedt, Odden, & Shlipak, 2003).

Ephedrine is banned by the NFL, the IOC, and the NCAA but so far not by the NBA, NHL, or Major League baseball. However as a result of Bechler's death, ephedra and ephedrine were banned in the minor leagues and players will be tested for the drug. In addition the players union sent a warning notice to its members about use of

the drug. The NFL Players Association says that football players need dietary supplements and unfortunately many that have been used contained ephedrine (Wood, 2002). In urine testing for ephedrine and methylephedrine, the limit is 10 micrograms per milliliter and for pseudoephedrine and phenyl-propanolamine, the limits are 25 micrograms per milliliter (IOC, 2003).

A study of 36 female weightlifters who used ephedrine showed that many had used the drug for years, mostly in high doses, and about 20% exhibited signs of dependence. Eating disorders appeared to be especially prevalent among them (Gruber & Pope, 1998).

Tobacco

The nicotine in cigarettes is a **mild stimulant but does little for performance except perhaps for increasing alertness**. Like other stimulants, it also constricts blood vessels thus raising blood pressure. After the mild stimulation it often acts as a relaxant. Unfortunately smoking reduces lung capacity thus hindering performance and endurance.

Smokeless tobacco (spit tobacco) has many of the same effects as cigarettes except for the reduction in lung capacity. **Chewing tobacco was a mainstay of baseball** dugouts and the image of the baseball player with a large wad of chewing tobacco in his cheek, spitting in the dugout, was common. Fortunately it is becoming less popular partly due to an increasing number of players who speak out about their health problems over the years due to their habit, e.g., Brett Butler, the ex-Dodger leadoff man, underwent surgery for throat cancer that he feels was caused by chewing tobacco.

"You know the first time you try chewing tobacco, it is absolutely disgusting. You get dizzy because of all the nicotine rushing into your bloodstream. I saw some baseball player from the '50s—he had to have a big old chew in his mouth, so now, like half of his face is gone."
28-year-old weightlifter

In 1994 the NCAA banned the use of all tobacco products during NCAA-sanctioned events.

HUMAN GROWTH HORMONE (HGH)

Human growth hormone (HGH) is a polypeptide hormone produced by the pituitary gland that stimulates growth in children. It is used by athletes to increase muscle strength and growth because it was thought that the side effects were less damaging than those of steroids. Studies have found that HGH reduces fat by altering lipolytic effects; it also **increases muscle mass, skin thickness, and connective tissues in muscles** (Schnirring, 2000). Some studies have found that it has little effect on muscle development in those with normal HGH production. Gigantism and acromegaly (abnormal bone growth) along with **metabolic and endocrine disorders have been widely reported. Abuse is also associated with cardiovascular disease, goiter, menstrual disorders, decreased sexual desire, and impotence** while it decreases lifespan by up to 20 years (Jacobson, 1990). HGH used to be harvested from human cadavers but techniques for synthesis were developed in 1986. Cadaver HGH usually contains contaminants, unlike synthetic HGH that is pure. HGH is banned by both the United States Olympic Committee (USOC) and the NCAA although it is difficult to detect because it is found naturally in the body.

OTHER PERFORMANCE-ENHANCING DRUGS & TECHNIQUES

Androstenedione & Dehydroepiandrosterone (DHEA)

In an interview with Mark McGwire in 1998, a reporter asked about a bottle of medication on his locker shelf. The first baseman for the St. Louis Cardinals, on his way to smashing the 37-year-old home run record, identified it as androstenedione, **a natural hormone that is a direct precursor in the biosynthesis of testosterone**, the basic male hormone. At the time the so-called dietary supplement was legal in Major League baseball but banned by the IOC, the NFL, the NCAA, and professional tennis. McGwire said the supplement merely helped him train longer by energizing muscles but that the real work was the thousands of hours he spent training (Patrick, 1998). In response to his position as a role model, in 1999 McGwire announced he had stopped using the supplement. He still hit 65 home runs in 1999.

Androstenedione is produced in all mammals by the gonads and adrenal glands and metabolized in the liver into testosterone. An 8-week study of healthy men with normal testosterone levels was done. Half of the 20 subjects used androstenedione and half used a placebo but they all did resistance training for the 8 weeks. They found no change in testosterone levels between the 2 groups but there was a higher level of estradiol, a female hormone, in the group that used the drug. There was also no difference in strength between the 2 groups. Unfortunately there was an increase in high-density cholesterol in the group that got the hormone (King, Sharp, Vukovich, et al., 1999). In women, according to an older study, there was a 4- to 7-fold increase in their testosterone level (Mahesh & Greenblatt, 1962). The logical conclusion of both studies would be that **in people with low testosterone, the substance would increase levels of the male hormone and increase endurance and muscle size but in those with normal levels, it probably would not.**

A somewhat similar hormone, dehydroepiandrosterone (DHEA) has been tried in an attempt to increase gonadal and peripheral testosterone as well as estrogen production since it is a precursor for those hormones. Over-the-counter sales were banned in 1985. Studies have found little effect from the substance but it has shown some unwanted side effects such as reduced natural testosterone production and liver damage (Earnest, 2001).

Beta Blockers (propranolol [Inderol®] & atenolol [Tenormin®])

Beta blockers are normally prescribed by physicians to lower blood pressure, decrease heart rate, prevent arrhythmias, and reduce eye pressure. They work by blocking nerve cell activity at the brain, heart, kidney, and blood vessels. They keep adrenaline from binding onto beta receptors on the heart. **Their ability to block nerve cell activity in the brain calms and steadies the body** (Gordon et al., 1991). Beta blockers are also used to control the symptoms of a panic attack or performance fright. Because of their ability to calm the brain and tremors, they are sought by some athletes involved in riflery, archery, diving, ski jumping, biathlon, and pentathlon (Fuentes, Rosenberg, & Davis, 1996). Beta blockers are also banned by the IOC and most athletic organizations for specific events.

Beta blockers can cause fatigue, lethargy, gastritis, occasional nausea, vomiting, and temporary impotence. A great danger in the use of these drugs is their potential to intensify some forms of asthma and heart problems that can be fatal to the user.

Erythropoietin (EPO)

In 2002 when American cyclist Lance Armstrong won the Tour de France for the fourth time, there were baseless accusations by a few disgruntled participants and some of the press that he had used **EPO, a blood oxygen booster, to increase endurance**. Accusations of drug use in endurance sports have been around for dozens of years and bicycling has been particularly susceptible. In the 1998 Tour de France several competitors were expelled from competition when drugs, including EPO, were found in their rooms and team trucks ("Another Two Teams," 1998). EPO works because it is a synthetic version of the human peptide hormone that stimulates bone marrow to produce more red blood cells that carry oxygen to muscles. It is used as a substitute for blood doping and there is evidence that it increases performance in endurance sports. It takes 2–3 weeks after beginning injections for full manifestation of the effects.

The dangers from unsupervised EPO administration result from the thickening of the blood that can lead to clots that might cause stroke or heart attack. Sweating, edema, and the ac-

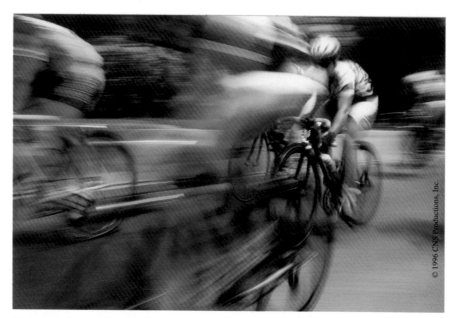

Because endurance is critical in bicycle racing, some racers try to increase the oxygen-carrying capacity of their blood either by blood doping (transfusing stored blood) or the use of erythropoietin (EPO), a drug that increases the oxygen-carrying red blood cells.

© 1996 CNS Productions, Inc.

companying increase in blood viscosity magnify this **potential danger of blood clots**. A number of deaths among European cyclists from blood manipulation have been reported over the last 15 years. EPO is banned by the NCAA, the USOC, and most every other sport.

Blood Doping

While not involving a drug, blood doping **does increase endurance by transfusing extra blood in order to boost the number of red blood cells available to carry oxygen**. Normally about 2 units of the athlete's own blood or someone else's with the same blood type are withdrawn, frozen to minimize deterioration, and then reinfused 5 or 6 weeks later (about 1–7 days before competition) after the athlete's blood volume has returned to normal. **Blood doping is used in endurance sports**, usually cycling, long-distance running, and cross-country skiing. Tests have shown that blood doping lowers performance times for a 5-mile race by an average of 45 seconds and a 3-mile run by about 24 seconds (Williams, Wesseldine, Somma, & Schuster, 1981; Goforth, Campbell, Hodgdon, & Sucec, 1982).

Because doping involves blood transfusion, dangers include poor storage, viral or bacterial infections, and even fatal reactions due to mislabeling. No test yet exists to accurately detect blood doping, so athletes have a clear-cut decision to make: to cheat or not to cheat.

Creatine

Creatine, an amino acid, is a nutritional supplement created naturally in the body and also found in fish and meat. It is used by athletes to delay muscle fatigue, store energy that can be used in short bursts, extend workout time, and help muscles recover faster. Three pounds of meat contain 5 grams of creatine. Sales have exploded in recent years. The use of creatine in muscle energy metabolism has been researched for the past 100 years (Rosenberg et al., 1996). A recent study in which athletes were given 20 grams of creatine suggests the supplement helps the

body store energy and helps muscles to recover faster. The creatine was coupled with 6 weeks of resistance training while the control group did only resistance training. Cyclists increased their endurance from 30 minutes to 37 minutes (Becque, Lochmann, & Melrose, 2000).

"It gives you energy so your muscles don't get tired and just takes away some of the soreness that enables you to work out longer and harder."
College football player

Creatine supplementation also seems to benefit sprint disciplines of running, swimming, cycling, and other power exercises. Its overuse by athletes has been shown to produce severe dehydration, stomach cramps with nausea and diarrhea, along with muscle pulls, strains, and damage. Also there is an increasing concern that creatine causes undue stress on the kidneys.

"The greatest danger that I see with nutritional supplements is that there's the tendency of athletes to try to overuse them to compensate for other things. For example, if a certain supplement supposedly works at one dosage, a lot of times an athlete will take two or three times that because they think that will give them more of an effect."
Lawrence Magee, M.D., Director of Sports Medicine, University of Kansas

Since it is classified as a nutritional supplement, **creatine is sold over the counter and is not yet banned by any sports agency**.

Diuretics

Diuretics (e.g., furosemide, ethracrynic acid, and toresemide) are drugs that increase the rate of urine formation thus speeding the elimination of water from the body. Athletes use these drugs

◊ **to lose weight rapidly**, which is important in sports where people compete in certain weight classes;

◊ **to avoid detection of illegal drugs** during testing by increasing urination (Arnheim & Prentice, 1993).

The main danger from diuretics is dehydration that when coupled with exercise can lead to heat stroke and organ damage.

"I was given a diuretic a week before I was to compete with instructions not to drink more than ½ cup of water per day. I probably lost 12 lbs. of water that week. I left the dorm the morning of my competition and my neighbor across the hall didn't recognize me because my face was so drawn. I wouldn't have placed second if the gym owner hadn't given me the diuretic."
Competitive wrestler

GHB (gamma-hydroxybutyrate)

This supplement was sold in the 1980s and the early 1990s as a **fat burner, anabolic agent, sleep aid, muscle definer, and psychedelic**. It is touted as an amino acid that acts like a diuretic to reduce anabolic steroid water weight gain and raise levels of HGH. Abuse at raves and other parties has become more widespread accounting for a number of visits to emergency rooms because of excess use that can cause respiratory depression, occasionally coma, and a dramatic slowing of the heart rate. GHB has also been used by sexual predators as a date rape drug. It is now illegal in the United States (*see Chapter 4*).

Soda Doping

Some athletes believe that ingesting alkaline salts (sodium bicarbonate) about 30 minutes prior to exercise **delays fatigue by decreasing the development of acidosis**. It seems somewhat effective for shorter events, 30 seconds to 10 minutes, rather than endurance activities (Rosenberg et al., 1996).

Weight Loss

Getting to a specific weight is necessary or strongly desired in a number of sports, especially wrestling, gymnastics, and horse racing (jockeys usually weigh under 125 lbs.). Athletes trying to make their weight will **use diuretics, laxatives, exercise, fasting, self-induced vomiting, and excess sweating** in a sauna. This is done in spite of the evidence that dehydration significantly diminishes performance. Some athletes will lose 3–5% of their total body weight in a couple of days.

"We can definitely see that gymnasts are worried about their weight. I mean we walk around in leotards and we still say we're fat and there's probably not an ounce of fat on any of our bodies."

19-year-old college female gymnast

Besides dieting and exercise, **stimulants are used to control weight**. Diet pills (prescription and over-the-counter), illegal amphetamines, tobacco, and caffeine are used. After a few months of continuous use, most diet pills and amphetamines don't work as well and the rising tolerance and development of tissue dependence can trigger abuse and addiction. Many amphetamine addicts started using the drug to lose weight. **Bulimia (eating and purging) and anorexia (starvation eating) can also be the result of the desire to stay thin or make a weight.** The NCAA recently changed training rules for wrestlers as a result of an increasing number of injuries and deaths due to dehydration and excess weight loss. Wrestlers are not allowed to use any mechanism for shedding weight during training. The NCAA also allowed greater flexibility in weight, permitting up to a 7 lb. variance in the listed weight categories.

The flip side of anorexia is a newly defined disorder called "muscle dysmorphia" that is a preoccupation with body development—no matter how sculptured their body is, they look in a mirror and still see the 98 lb. weakling, so they continue to lift weights and often take supplements and steroids.

Miscellaneous Performance-Enhancing Drugs

◇ **Adrenaline and amyl or isobutyl nitrite:** This combination is taken by weightlifters just prior to their performance to increase strength. The downside includes dizziness (a dangerous side effect with a 400 lb. barbell over one's head), rapid heart beat, and hypertension.

◇ **Bee pollen:** This supplement is sold in pellets that consist of plant pollens, nectar, and bee saliva that contain 30% protein, 55% carbohydrates, some fat, and minerals. The anecdotal reports claim that it increases energy levels and performance, boosts immunity, relieves stress, and improves digestion. Most scientific studies do not show any performance or energy benefits and for someone allergic to bee stings, an inadvertent stinger or other contaminant could be dangerous. However it is not banned by the IOC or the NCAA (IOC, 2003).

◇ **Calcium pangamate:** This nonvitamin (its deficiency is not linked to any disease), also called "vitamin B_{15}" or "pengamic acid," supposedly keeps muscle tissue better oxygenated but this desired effect is supported by testimonials rather than scientific research. It is reportedly a carcinogen.

◇ **Cyproheptadine (Periactin®):** Used for colds and allergic reactions, this antihistamine (serotonin and histamine antagonist) is believed to cause weight gain and increase strength. Some users believe that this prescription drug acts like steroids but in fact the increase in muscle size comes from excess caloric intake caused by serotonin's effect on appetite. Side effects include decreased performance, sweating, and sedation.

◇ **HCG (human chorionic gonadotropin):** HCG, clomiphene, or tamoxifen are occasionally used after anabolic steroid treatment to try to restart the body's own testosterone production. Toxic effects on the liver and reproductive system have been reported.

◇ **Ornithine and arginine:** These amino acids are taken to try to increase muscle mass because they supposedly cause the release of growth hormone. High doses can lead to kidney damage.

◇ **Primagen:** This drug increases steroid production in the body and is mainly used by European athletes.

◇ **Vitamin B-12:** This vitamin is injected supposedly to ward off illness and provide extra energy. It's also used to mitigate the effects of heavy drinking.

In a study of 11 poison control centers in the United States, their hot lines received more than 2,300 calls about dietary supplements. Around 500 of the callers had mild-to-severe symptoms that were believed to be caused by the supplements. There were probably many more problems that were never called in to the poison control center. The symptoms reported ranged from seizure, arrhythmias, and liver dysfunction. Four deaths were thought to be supplement related (Palmer, Haller, McKinney, et al., 2003).

THE RECREATIONAL/MOOD-ALTERING USE OF DRUGS BY ATHLETES

Many of the more common psychoactive drugs, legal and illegal, are used to enhance performance as well as **to adjust moods, help the user fit into social situations, comply with peer pressure, imitate the behavior of older role models, or conform to one's image of an athlete.** Athletes may also turn to drugs to help **cope with the demands of a heavy schedule** (practice, travel time, course work), to reduce stress, to compensate for loneliness, or to fill up time on long road trips.

"I don't think you could find too many college programs—basketball programs, football, track, any sport—

that their athletes don't drink. And I'm sure that there are a lot of people who smoke weed, too."

21-year-old college basketball player

Stimulants

Many stimulants, such as amphetamines, caffeine, and tobacco, are not only used to enhance performance but are also used recreationally. The **advantages and problems with these drugs are the same as with use by nonathletes** as discussed in Chapter 3.

Cocaine, one of the strongest stimulants, isn't often used as a performance enhancer for two reasons. First, it is short acting, 30 minutes to 1 hour, so one would have to reuse during the game for a consistent effect; second, the spike of energy and euphoria is too intense for the sustained effort needed in a game.

"When you have played before 70,000 people and come off the field, you're back down to normal so to speak. You want to get back up there with cocaine. It replaces that high with an artificial stimulation. But the comedown from cocaine is very, very draining, emotionally, physically, and nutritionally. It's totally different than coming down from the natural high."

Delvin Williams, former NFL rushing back, recovering cocaine user

Outfielder Darryl Strawberry has had multiple brushes with the law for cocaine possession, domestic violence, alcohol abuse, and parole violation. The cocaine and alcohol problems limited the successes of his 16-year career with the Mets, Dodgers, Giants, and Yankees.

Sedative-Hypnotics

Some athletes will use drugs such as alprazolam (Xanax®), barbiturates, and even opioids as self-rewards for enduring the stress they experience while performing before so many people. They also use these drugs as a tranquil-izer **to unwind after the excitement of competition** or to counteract the effects of stimulants used to enhance their performance. Regarding performance-enhancing effects, depressants are counterproductive although their painkilling effects can benefit recovery.

Alcohol

"We were 16 and 17 years old and our club coach told us, 'If you can go get hammered the night before the game and still come out and play awesome and play to your maximum performance, go ahead. But if you can't, and you know your body, and you know you won't be able to play well enough if you get drunk the night before, don't do it.'"

20-year-old college soccer player

In general, **alcohol can negatively affect reaction time, coordination, and balance** although studies suggest that low-dose alcohol consumption does not produce impaired performance in all people. The NFL drug policy states that alcohol is "without question the most abused drug in our sport." The problem is how to alert athletes to the health and performance consequences of a drug that has general social, legal, and moral acceptance in society.

"When you have a problem with alcohol or marijuana, things of that nature, you'll see a decline in their academics. You'll see a decline in athletics. You just see a decline in everything. And we see it as coaches and the players see it, so we try to address it right away."

Patti Phillips, college women's soccer coach

The NCAA specifically bans alcohol for riflery competition. It is however not banned by the USOC since it does not generally enhance performance. The problems with alcohol in sports are its **excess use as a reward for performance, its use as a way to unwind, or its use as a consolation prize**. Excess use causes the same problems that are found in the general population. A survey by the NCAA found similar levels of drinking among student-athletes as among the general population but one study found a 5 times greater incidence of acquaintance rape involving athletes and alcohol was involved in most of the cases (Bausell, Bausell, & Siegel, 1994).

"Women are more vulnerable sexually when they've had too much to drink. They're more likely to be raped, date raped, or otherwise. Study after study has shown that. Male athletes, when they've had too much to drink, tend to become extraordinarily aggressive."

Judith Davidson, Ph.D., Athletic Director, Sacramento State University

Alcohol is generally not tested for unless the athlete exhibits abuse and addiction problems, such as occurred with Bob Welch, the ex-Dodger pitcher who was in and out of alcohol rehabilitation half-a-dozen times before he left baseball permanently.

Unfortunately student-athletes are less likely than other college students to turn to treatment professionals in their university or community for help with substance abuse problems, especially alcohol.

Marijuana

Marijuana can either stimulate or depresses the user depending on the strength of the drug and the mood of the smoker. The most consistent effect of marijuana use is an increase in pulse rate of about 20% during exercise (Arnheim & Prentice, 1993). **In general, marijuana hinders not helps performance.** Marijuana

◇ lowers blood pressure, which has caused fainting spells in football linemen who have to go quickly from a down position to a standing one many times during a game;

◇ inhibits sweating, which has caused heat prostration and strokes in athletes;

◊ impairs the ability of users to follow a moving object like a ball in play (decreased tracking ability);

◊ hinders the ability to do complex tasks, such as hitting a golf ball;

◊ diminishes hand-eye coordination;

◊ decreases oxygen intake since it is smoked;

◊ is a banned substance that will result in a 1-year loss of eligibility from any NCAA sport;

◊ is illegal and can destroy an athlete's career.

Since marijuana is extremely fat-soluble and lasts so long in the body, **impairment can persist for a day or two after casual use and longer after cessation of chronic use**.

In a study at a major university, athletes who admitted using marijuana thought they were doing well and performing well but when an objective study was made of their performance, those that smoked marijuana did much worse—they dropped more passes, committed more errors, and suffered more injuries during their college career.

Currently the NCAA bans all marijuana use more for ethical and moral reasons than for performance reasons. The IOC also bans marijuana use. Their testing cutoff level is 15 nanograms per milliliter as compared to a higher cutoff level for nonsports situations.

TESTING

In an effort to reduce the use of illicit drugs in sports, various **drug-testing programs have been instituted by sports organizations and even individual colleges**. The NCAA has two drug-testing programs. The first, started in 1986, tests at all NCAA championships and at post-season football bowl games. The second program is a year-round anabolic steroid testing program that started in 1990. Banned drugs can be therapeutic, performance enhancing, and recreational, including anabolic steroids, diuretics, beta blockers, alcohol, methamphetamines, most street drugs, and even high levels of caffeine. The first positive test causes

the student to lose eligibility for 1 year and a second positive test to lose college eligibility permanently. In a survey of NCAA schools, only 56% of all respondents had a drug/alcohol education program for student-athletes. Three-fourths of the respondents said they refer student-athletes with problems to community agencies (NCAA, 2003a, b).

Testing for the Olympics over the years has generated much controversy. In 1999 the IOC reached agreement on the creation of a world antidrug agency to coordinate drug-testing programs, intensify research, create educational programs, and publish an annual list of banned substances.

ETHICAL ISSUES

Using illegal drugs and using drugs illegally to improve athletic performance is against the rules in all sports and is illegal in most states. **Drugs undermine the assumption of fair competition on which all sports rest** and they violate the very nature of sport, which since the time of the Greeks was a measure of personal excellence, the result of a sound mind in a healthy body. The public wants the outcome of athletic contests to be determined by discipline, training, and effort.

There is a real threat today that the public will walk away from sports if they perceive that winning is based on access to the latest pharmacology and schemes to evade drug testing. Drugs can also rob the athlete of feelings of self-accomplishment and tarnish the pride of winning. Because our society treats sports figures as heroes and role models, drug-abusing athletes diminish all of us.

"If I could take a drug and set the world record out of reach for everybody and the tradeoff would be I would be dead in 5 years, I definitely wouldn't do it. I mean because to me, why is it so important? I want to have a chance to grow old and play with my grandkids and my great-grandkids."

Allen Johnson, 1996 Olympic Gold Medallist, 110-meter hurdle

MISCELLANEOUS DRUGS

UNUSUAL SUBSTANCES

It's amazing what substances and methods some people will use to get high. They include smoking aspirin, chewing dandelion root, drinking gasoline, rubbing alcohol, or hydrogen peroxide, putting Ambusol® (topical anesthetic) in the eye, and smoking toad secretions.

Other psychoactive substances are provided by street chemists who either synthesize drugs that were once legally available, such as Quaaludes® and PCP, or produce illegal drugs, including MDMA, MDE, and methcathinone (synthetic khat). The danger is that street drugs have not been tested and are not made under any kind of control. Irregular doses, incomplete chemical reactions, or contaminants in the manufacturing process can have disastrous effects on an unsuspecting user. For example, in the 1980s a group of heroin users who had been sold a supposedly synthetic Demerol® derivative, MPPP, were later found to have an 80% incidence of Parkinson's disease symptoms (rigid muscles, loss of voluntary body control) caused by contamination of the chemical MPTP that is used in the chemical process. Street drugs can also be dozens of times stronger than the expected dose.

Gasoline

In spite of the toxicity of leaded or unleaded gasoline, a few people have been known to mix it with orange juice and drink it. They call it "Montana Gin," a particularly lethal beverage. Most often gasoline fumes are inhaled for their effects.

Embalming Fluid (formaldehyde)

Mortuaries have been broken into and robbed of their embalming fluid. It can either be directly abused (**inhaled for its depressant and psychedelic effects**) or it can be used in the manufacture of other illicit drugs. Some abusers soak marijuana joints or cigarettes in the fluid and smoke them. Called "clickers," "clickems," "fry," "wet," or "illy," the mixture gives a PCP-like effect. PCP is sometimes mixed in with the fluid in the joint. Effects include visual and auditory hallucinations, a feeling of invincibility, pain tolerance, anger, paranoia, and memory problems. The effects last from 6 hours to 3 days (Loviglio, 2001).

Formaldehyde, the main ingredient of embalming fluid, is a known carcinogen. The fluid also contains methanol, ethanol, and other solvents. Recently formaldehyde has also been used in the illicit manufacture of methamphetamine.

Raid®, Hairspray, & Lysol®

Abusers puncture the aerosol cans, draining out the liquid that they swallow mainly for its alcohol content. These items are rarely abused in the general population but find more use in rural isolated areas where access to alcohol is limited. Recently inner-city youths have been spraying Raid® onto marijuana and rolling it into a joint for smoking. It is said to increase the effects of marijuana; this combination is called "canaid."

Kava

Kava is made from the roots of the *Piper methysticin* plant, which is found in the islands of the South Pacific (Oceana) and in South America. The roots are chewed or crushed into a soapy liquid and drunk. This milky exudate of the root contains at least six chemicals, such as alpha-pyrones, that **produce a drunken state, similar to that of alcohol, when used in larger quantities**. Users claim that the effects of smaller quantities are more pleasurable and relaxing than the effects of alcohol, without the hangover. Kava is used as an antianxiety drug much as a drink of alcohol is used in rest homes to relax the elderly clients. In fact one of the sites of action in the brain is the same one affected by benzodiazepines. Antianxiety effects are found at the 70 mg level while 125–250 mg induces

sleep and 500 mg or more can induce drunkenness and stupor.

Kava is also sold as an herbal supplement to relieve anxiety, stress, and insomnia. In 2000, kava in pill form became popular bringing in about $30 million in sales. There have been reports that in just a few people liver damage can occur especially in those with preexisting liver problems. One theory is that the use of the root in commercial preparations, not in traditional preparations, added a more toxic substance to the mix.

In the Fiji Islands kava is served in half coconut shells as a welcome libation for visitors. The cup is passed around and no business is discussed until the relaxing qualities of the drink make everyone amenable to reason. Visitors unfamiliar with the drink find the taste somewhat unpleasant and numbing to the lips and tongue. In addition, since human saliva is an important ingredient in the preparation of this drug, its use has not found popularity in other cultures.

Camel Dung

Some Arab countries produce hashish by force-feeding ripe marijuana plants to camels. Their four-chambered stomachs convert the marijuana into hashish camel dung.

Toad Secretions (bufotenine)

The *Bufo* genus of toads (Colorado River, Sonoran Desert, Cane, and others) secretes a psychedelic substance from pores located on the back of their necks. This substance, bufotenine, is milked and harvested onto cigarettes that are then smoked to induce a psychedelic experience.

HERBAL PREPARATIONS & SMART DRUGS/DRINKS

Herbal Preparations

Recently the FDA sent letters to three companies warning that certain ingredients in their food products might not be generally recognized as safe. The ingredients were the herbs echinacea, ginkgo biloba, and Siberian ginseng. Preliminary warnings are becoming more common as more and more substances call themselves "food additives" rather than "herbal medications." The FDA also seized 20 different products from an importing com-

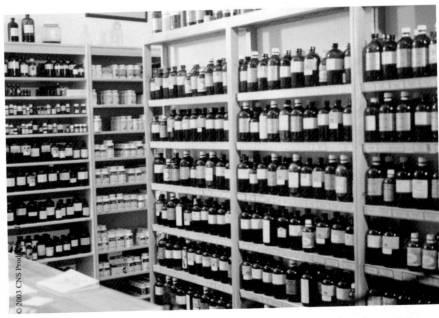

Many herbal medications contain the same active ingredients as a number of prescription and over-the counter medications. This herbal medicine shop carries more than 500 different herbs and preparations.

pany that made false health claims about their dietary supplements (Food and Drug Administration, 2003).

The line between the safety of an over-the-counter medication or dietary supplement vs. a prescription drug is often very thin. Herbal preparations are not examined as closely as what are called "medications" because they have been used for thousands of years and are considered safe or advertised as dietary supplements. What has happened is that some of these herbal preparations have been found to contain actual drugs such as Valium® or indomethacin (Indosin®). There has been much debate over what is a medicine or an herb or a supplement or even a vitamin. Is there a real difference or simply a legal difference? **The biggest distinction is that there are specific manufacturing, distribution, and testing procedural techniques between herbal preparations and prescription or over-the-counter medications.** There needs to be more consistency in labeling and testing of herbal preparations particularly if they are imported from countries where there is little oversight.

Smart Drugs/Drinks

Smart drugs ("SDs") are the drugs, nutrients, drinks, vitamins, extracts, and herbal potions that manufacturers, distributors, and proponents think will boost intelligence, improve memory, sharpen attention, increase concentration, detoxify the body (especially after alcohol or other drug abuse), and energize the user. **They are also promoted as natural, healthy, and legal substi-**

tutes for club drugs or other illegal substances. Popular smart drugs have included Cloud 9®, Brain Tonix®, Brain Booster®, Nirvana®, SAMe® (S-adeno-sylmethione), and many others. Proponents range from AIDS activists to health faddists, New Agers, antiaging seekers, and members of the technoculture who feel they are on the edge of a new field of mental development.

For some consumers, smart drinks are nonalcoholic, usually a mixture of vitamins or powdered nutrients and amino acids in a fruit drink, purchased in a smart bar for $4 to $6. More recently smart drinks and drugs have contained combinations of medications usually prescribed for Parkinsonism, Alzheimer's disease, or dementia. It is felt that these drugs more effectively rebalance the brain after abusing drugs. **It is also claimed that they will slow or reverse the aging process.** The consumers are typically young (17–25) urban students or professionals looking for an intellectual edge or more stamina to work or party harder.

Vitamin supplements and nutrient products, once purchased through ads in New Age magazines, are now also sold through health food stores. Critics of these supplements and products attribute their success to either a placebo effect (only the expectation not the product produces the effect) or to the caffeine, ephedra (ma huang), and the sugar that are part of the ingredients. Smart drugs containing stimulants could lead to problems for someone with high blood pressure, heart problems, or in those prone to stroke especially when taken in high doses.

Nootropics

Investigation of New Age smart drugs like hydergine, vasopressin, ginkgo biloba, 5-HT, piracetam, ginseng, and acetyl-L-carnitine has led to the proposal for a **new classification of these drugs as nootropics (acting on the mind).** Substances in this new psychotropic drug class would be those that improve learning, memory consolidation, and memory retrieval without other central nervous system effects and with low toxicity, even at extremely high doses (Dean & Morgenthaler, 1991).

Americans import nootropic drugs from Europe where many can be purchased that are not yet approved by the FDA for sale in the United States. Critics of these and other prescription drugs, including researchers, doctors, and the FDA, point out that, at the very least, claims for the efficacy of the drugs have not been substantiated. Advocates argue that these and other smart drugs improve mental ability for people suffering from debilitating mental disorders (e.g., Alzheimer's) and that they can enhance mental capacity in normal people too. Nootropic drugs include those prescribed for some mental or medical disorders (but not FDA approved for the nootropic uses that are advocated). These substances include ergoloid mesylates, selegiline hydrochloride, phenytoin (Dilantin®), and vasopressin. Other nootropics are prescription drugs not approved in the United States for any use, such as piracetam, aniracetam, hydergine, fipexide, metformin, tacrine, vinpocetine, and oxiracetam (The Vaults of Erowid, 2003).

OTHER ADDICTIONS

COMPULSIVE BEHAVIORS

"If you're a drug addict, or a food addict, or an alcoholic, or a sex addict, it's not about the addiction, it's about all the other things in your life that you're doing."

36-year-old recovering compulsive overeater

Compulsive gambling, overeating, shopping, sexual behavior, Internet use, and TV watching, along with pathological lying, shoplifting, hair pulling, and fire setting, all offer opportunities for **repetitive compulsive behaviors.** Some of these disorders are classified as impulse control disorders (e.g., compulsive gambling, hair pulling) while

some have their own classification (eating disorders). Some people confuse impulse control disorders with obsessive-compulsive disorders.

The hallmark of **impulse control disorders** as listed in the *DSM-IV-TR* is a **failure to resist an impulse that is harmful to the individual or others but often starts out as pleasurable.**

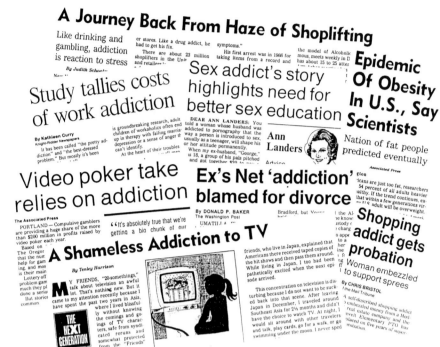

A Journey Back From Haze of Shoplifting

Like drinking and gambling, addiction is reaction to stress

By Judith School...

Study tallies costs of work addiction

By Kathleen Curry
Knight-Ridder Newspapers

Sex addict's story highlights need for better sex education

DEAR ANN LANDERS: You told a woman whose husband was addicted to pornography that the way a person is introduced to sex, usually as a teenager, will shape his or her attitude permanently.
When my ex-husband, "George," us 18, a group of his pals pitched and got together $20 to p...

Ann Landers
Advice

Epidemic Of Obesity In U.S., Say Scientists

Nation of fat people predicted eventually

Associated Press

Video poker take relies on addiction

The Associated Press
PORTLAND — Compulsive gamblers are providing a huge share of the more than $200 million in profits raised by video poker each year.

Ex's Net 'addiction' blamed for divorce

By DONALD P. BAKER
The Washington Post
UMATILLA

A Shameless Addiction to TV

By Tenley Harrison

Shopping addict gets probation

Woman embezzled to support sprees

By CHRIS BRISTOL
The Mail Tribune

THE NEXT GENERATION

The other major hallmark is an increasing sense of tension or arousal before actually committing the act, often followed by gratification, pleasure, relief, and then remorse and guilt over the consequences of that act (McElroy, Soutullo, & Goldsmith, 1998).

The hallmark of **obsessive-compulsive disorders**, including hand washing, checking things, ordering, counting, and praying, is **repetitive activities whose goal is to reduce anxiety or distress not to provide pleasure or gratification** (APA, 2000).

Substance abuse disorders were classified as impulse control disorders until recently when they received their own categories. A number of studies of compulsive shoppers showed that about 37% had substance use disorders at some time in their lives (Christenson, Faber, De Zween, et al., 1994; McElroy, Keck, Pope, et al., 1994).

Addictive behaviors alter brain chemistry in much the same was as psychoactive drugs do.

"Every thought we have, every single thought we have, every action we do has an impact on the brain. I mean the brain in some ways causes it but then the thought or the behavior actually loops back and impacts the brain, so you can actually get a high from a sexual act, you can get a high from the excitement that comes from stealing things, you can get a high from being in a gambling environment, which is likely related to dopamine and people then start to chase the high."

Dr. Daniel Amen, Director, Amen Clinic for Behavioral Medicine

The reasons that people engage in compulsive behavior are the same reasons that they engage in compulsive drug use: to get an instant rush, to forget problems, to control anxiety, to oblige friends, to alter consciousness, to self-medicate, and so forth. Above all, they desire to change their mood—alter their state of consciousness (Nakken, 1996).

At the Department of Radiology at Massachusetts General Hospital, functional MRI scans of the brain showed that the same areas of the brain were activated by abusing drugs, anticipating a desired food, or gambling. The same regions of the brain (e.g., nucleus accumbens, extended amygdala, or-

bitofrontal cortex) responded to the prospects of winning and losing money while gambling as responded to the use of cocaine in cocaine addicts (Breiter, Aharon, Kahneman, Anders, & Shizgal, 2001).

It is instructive to **compare the major hallmarks of drug addiction to those of compulsive behavioral addiction.**

Drug users

◇ use and think about using most of the time (**compulsion**);

◇ need greater amounts of the drug with continued use (**tolerance**);

◇ experience symptoms when abstinence begins (**withdrawal**);

◇ continue use despite adverse medical, social, family, and legal consequences (**abuse**);

◇ do not accept that they have a problem (**denial**);

◇ have a strong tendency to use again after quitting (**relapse**).

If one takes these elements of drug addiction and replaces the word "using" with the words "eating," "gambling," "surfing the Internet," "shopping," "watching TV," or "having sex," then it is easier to see that compulsion isn't limited to psychoactive substances.

Compulsive gamblers

◇ are always playing a poker machine, buying lottery tickets, trying to raise money, or thinking about where they are going to gamble (**compulsion**);

◇ gradually increase the amount bet whether it's at a machine or a high-stakes poker table (**tolerance**);

◇ feel intensely restless and discontent when not gambling (**withdrawal**) (Rosenthal & Lesieur, 1992);

◇ continue gambling though they lose most of their pay check each month through slot/poker machines, lotteries, or table games (**abuse**);

◇ think they can control their gambling and their only problem is a cash flow problem (**denial**);

◇ will gamble again particularly if they have money in their pocket (**relapse**).

"Food does for me what alcohol and drugs and other things do for other people. If I'm feeling angry and I eat, it takes the anger away. If I'm feeling lonely or sad and I eat, it takes care of the feelings. If I feel inadequate or empty, I fill myself with food, or I used to. I don't do it any more. It's just a drug to me."

36-year-old recovering compulsive overeater

Another example of the relationship between compulsive drug use and compulsive behaviors is that in 12-step groups that help people with compulsive behaviors, the members use literature taken directly from Alcoholics Anonymous. Even the structure of the meetings is similar, as is the philosophy that tries to get people to understand that **addiction involves lack of control over the behavior and tries to make them see the necessity of changing their lifestyle and beliefs** (Nakken, 1996).

"I have to work on my behavior. How do I act with my husband? How do I act with my children? How do I act in relationships? My addiction carries over to all that—carries over to my whole life. So I had to change the way I treat people, the way I treat myself."

36-year-old recovering compulsive overeater

HEREDITY, ENVIRONMENT, & COMPULSIVE BEHAVIORS

Apparently, like substance abuse, **compulsive behaviors can be triggered by genetic predisposition, by environmental stresses, and by the comfort, reassurance, or escape provided by the repetitive behavior itself.** Increased dopamine levels in those involved in the behaviors suggest a common biochemical thread.

HEREDITY

Twin studies have already identified a genetic connection to alcoholism

and other drug addictions. **Other twin studies have shown a connection between heredity and compulsive behaviors that doesn't involve psychoactive drugs.**

Compulsive overeating was the first addiction shown to be partly hereditary. A study by the National Institutes of Health of 400 twins over a period of 43 years found that **"cumulative genetic effects explain most of the tracking in obesity over time."** This means that a much higher-than-normal percentage of twins born to obese parents but subsequently raised in totally different households ended up obese. The researchers also found that **"shared environmental effects were not significant" in affecting the twins' weight gain** (Bouchard, 1994). Five studies of adopted children bolstered this finding by discovering that the family environment, such as size and frequency of meals, the amount of food in the house, and the level of exercise of the family, plays very little or no role in determining the obesity of children. They found that **only dramatic environmental differences could mitigate the influence of a genetic profile that made one susceptible to obesity**. Twin studies of risk takers have also found a genetic component that resulted in a higher percentage of children of risk takers being risk takers themselves.

By the mid-1990s genetic connections between alcohol abuse, compulsive drug use, and other compulsive behaviors were starting to be confirmed by research efforts. Kenneth Blum, John Cull, Eric Braverman, David Comings (researchers at various universities) and others have postulated a genetic basis not only for alcoholism but for people with other addictive, compulsive, and impulsive disorders, such as compulsive overeating, pathological gambling, attention-deficit disorder, and Tourette's syndrome (compulsive verbal outbursts or strong muscular tics). They call this genetic predisposition the "reward deficiency syndrome" (Blum, Cull, Braverman, & Comings, 1996; Blum et al., 2000).

Specifically their studies indicate that **a marker gene associated with**

the most severe forms of alcoholism also has a strong association with several addictive compulsive behaviors. This is only one of several yet-to-be discovered marker genes that indicate an imbalance of certain neurotransmitters in the reward/pleasure center. They found that, whereas this marker gene (DRD_2 A_1 allele gene) appears in only 19–21% of nonalcoholic, nonaddicted, and noncompulsive subjects, it exists in

◇ 69% of alcoholic subjects with severe alcoholism;

◇ 45% of compulsive overeaters;

◇ 48% of smokers;

◇ 52% of cocaine addicts;

◇ 51% of pathological gamblers;

◇ 76% of pathological gamblers with drug problems;

◇ and 45% of the people with Tourette's syndrome.

In addition a study of children with attention-deficit disorder found that 49% had the marker gene compared to only 27% of the control group (Blum et al., 2000).

These findings suggest that a biochemical deficiency or anomaly draws some people to compulsive behaviors. The researchers postulate that carriers of this A_1 allele gene have a deficiency of dopamine receptors in the reward/reinforcement center. What the dopamine receptor site deficiency means is that activities that will normally give people a surge of satisfaction, pleasure, and satiation by releasing dopamine do not give that same level of satisfaction to people with a lack of dopamine receptor sites. Such people are more likely to seek out substances and activities that release additional dopamine (e.g., alcohol, drugs, repetitive compulsive behaviors). **The release of extra amounts of dopamine caused by repetitive compulsive behaviors stimulates the reward/reinforcement center to a greater degree than normal.** People with this lack of receptors all of a sudden feel pleasure that they normally don't experience.

It is important to note that there isn't just one marker gene for compul sive drug use and compulsive behaviors. This is because there are several neurotransmitters involved that can alter the reward reinforcement sites in the brain (*see Chapter 2*). For example, in the urine and spinal fluid of pathological gamblers, researchers have discovered higher-than-normal levels of norepinephrine, the neurotransmitter that produces stimulation, alertness, and confidence. Scientists funded by the National Institute of Mental Health discovered abnormal functioning in serotonin and norepinephrine in acutely ill bulimic and anorexic patients further suggesting a link between these disorders at the level of neurotransmitters and their brain receptors (Health, 2003).

ENVIRONMENT

It is fairly easy to understand how environment could intensify the following compulsive behaviors:

◊ compulsive gambling: **an abundance of state lotteries, slot and poker machines, Internet betting, legal off-track betting, and the growth of gambling casinos** in and outside of New Jersey and Nevada;

◊ compulsive overeating: **plentiful fast-food restaurants, a lack of daily physical activity**, an abundance of fats and sugars in food that can induce a certain euphoria, parents who overfeed their children, chaotic childhoods that make people search for an instant escape;

◊ compulsive sexual activity: **an abundance of sexual situations in the media**, an abundance of latch key kids without supervision or without close emotional family connections, an overabundance of easily accessible erotic material and pornography on the Internet;

◊ Internet addiction: **a rapidly expanding network of games, gambling, and chat rooms**;

◊ compulsive shopping: **the ease of obtaining credit, the endless barrage of advertisements** and catalogues, shopping networks urging people to buy, accessibility to Internet shopping and auction sites, and a materialistic view of life.

A history of physical, emotional, and sexual abuse in the lives of many that practice these compulsive behaviors also suggests the importance of environmental conditioning and reinforcement.

"Almost all addicts, and I've talked to thousands of them in groups and individually, have said that they have a background in which they felt inferior, inadequate, guilty, ashamed, rejected, unwanted, all of that captured in this point phrase, 'No matter what I did, it was never enough.'"

Dewey Jacobs, Ph.D., psychologist, addictions specialist, and lecturer

COMPULSIVE BEHAVIORS

It is also easy to understand how **engaging in the activity itself could lead to compulsive acting out**.

◊ Having a big win while gambling imprints the brain in much the same way a potent dose of cocaine would (Shaffer, 1998).

◊ The compulsive eater strains the digestive system with excessive food, particularly fats and sugars, and changes the body's chemistry, so **the person eats to change mood rather than sustain life** (Carr & Papadouka, 1994).

◊ The compulsive shopper walking through the mall or phoning The Home Shopping Network® imprints the brain, so it can anticipate buying a coveted item thereby **kindling a surge of pleasure with no regard for financial responsibility** or even the need for such an item.

◊ The sexual compulsive's repeated use of pornography and participation in other **compulsive sexual behaviors can make him/her avoid normal relationships**.

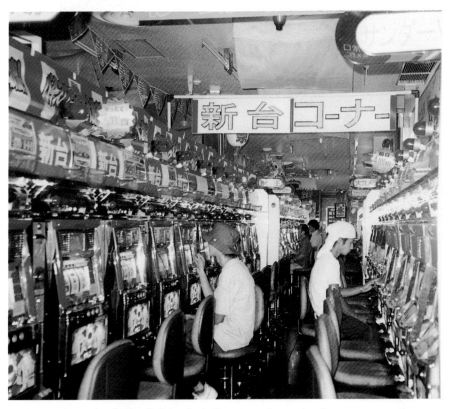

In Japan a form of pinball called "pachinko" is extremely popular. Japanese men and women spend endless hours on these machines to win a variety of prizes. Pachinko parlors are as popular as casinos and slot machines are in the United States.
© 2002 Darryl Inaba

COMPULSIVE GAMBLING

"If I won all the money in the world, I'd have to move to a different world. If I won all the money in the world, there'd be no action, there'd be no game because, uh, there'd be no other players."
38-year-old recovering compulsive gambler

Gamblers Anonymous (GA), a 12-step recovery group, has a rigorous definition of gambling. Their literature states "**any betting or wagering, for self or others, whether for money or not, no matter how slight or insignificant, where the outcome is uncertain or depends upon chance or skill constitutes gambling**" (Gamblers Anonymous [GA], 1998). This includes

◇ poker, blackjack, craps, roulette wheels, and pai gow;

◇ standard slot machines and video poker slot machines;

◇ horse and dog races;

◇ jai alai;

◇ bingo and raffles;

◇ state-run lotteries and keno games;

◇ sports betting, both legal and illegal;

◇ office pools and bets on the golf course;

◇ school ground games, e.g., lag pennies, flip coins;

◇ bar games, e.g., liar's dice;

◇ stock speculation such as day trading, commodities, and options;

◇ and most recently, online gambling.

In the present day there are more opportunities for gambling than ever before and the sheer availability of all these outlets, mostly legal now, are triggering problem and pathological gambling in greater and greater numbers of people. **The problems that result from pathological and problem gambling are as severe as any drug-based addiction.**

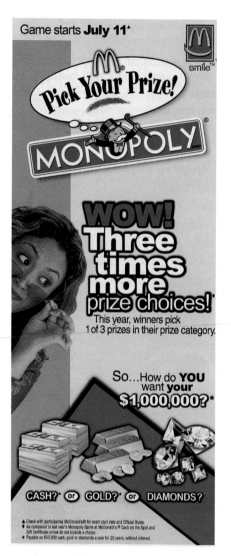

Lotteries, giveaways, sports contest, raffles, and a dozen other gambling opportunities are available everywhere. The ironic thing about the McDonald's Monopoly giveaway is that a criminal ring rigged the contest and allegedly siphoned off more than $20 million to confederates. This emphasized that even the most upright organizations and gambling opportunities can be duped or rigged.

• •

"You go over it and over it and over it in your mind and say, 'How could you be this stupid? How could you not have any inkling of what was happening to you? How could you be so bright in academia and so stupid in your everyday life?'"
53-year-old recovering poker player

HISTORY

Gambling in Ancient Civilizations

The record of gambling by Homo sapiens predates recorded history. Archeologists have unearthed prehistoric gambling bones from 40,000 B.C. called "astragali," small four-sided rolling bones from the ankles of small animals. They were used to make decisions on matters believed to be in the gods' hands, e.g., rain or drought. Six-sided dice made from pottery, wood, and ivory were used as early as 1400 B.C. in Iraq and India. Other gaming artifacts, like throwing sticks, have been found in ancient Britain, Greece, Rome, and in Mayan ruins in pre-Columbian America. The casting of lots is recorded in the *Bible* as a means of ending disputes or distributing property. It also records that **Roman soldiers cast lots for the robes that Jesus wore at the Crucifixion**. Crusading knights in medieval Europe gambled at dice (Herman, 1984).

Along with the desire to gamble came prohibitions against gambling; many of the upper classes kept gambling from the lower classes, e.g., Roman emperors kept "dicing" to themselves. Churchmen sermonized against gambling in the Middle Ages and Louis IX of France made dice illegal in 1255. Henry VIII made public gaming houses unlawful in England because he thought they distracted young men from the arts of war. This prohibition lasted until the 1960s when private gambling clubs proliferated in Great Britain (Fleming, 1992).

Gambling in America

Three waves of gambling have swept the United States. The first wave was in revolutionary times. Lotteries, popular for centuries in both Asia and Europe, were imported to the American colonies in the 1700s where, among other things, their proceeds were used to support roads, build schools (e.g., Harvard University), hospitals, and other public works. Betting on horse races, cockfights, and dog fights was popular among gentry and farmers alike. Gambling financed some of the Revolutionary War though certain antigambling laws were later passed by a number of the original 13 colonies as corruption and scandal brought lotteries to an end (Clotfelter, Cook, Edell, & Moore, 1999).

The second wave began at the end of the Civil War in 1865 with the expansion of the western frontier. Riverboat gambling on the Mississippi, saloon card games, roulette wheels, and dice games became part of the lore of the Wild West. But again, scandals and Victorian morality caused their demise around 1910.

The third wave began in the 1930s with the legalization of gambling in Nevada and the opening of racetracks in 21 states. New Hampshire rediscovered the state lottery in 1964 but it wasn't until the late 1970s that gambling really took off with the opening of casinos in Atlantic City, the expansion of lotteries to 38 states, off-track betting, riverboat casinos, and finally the legalization of gambling casinos on Native American lands.

For much of the nineteenth and twentieth centuries, gambling continued to be popular though it was considered immoral and preyed on human weakness. Gamblers have also been considered decadent, irresponsible, or insane. But in the last 40 years **gambling has become a respectable pastime and has become legal.** By the mid-1990s all states except Hawaii and Utah had established some kind of gambling. In addition the Indian Gaming Regulatory Act that had been approved in 1988 had caused a construction explosion of Indian-run casinos. By 2001, **198 of the 554 Native American tribes in the United States had 320 gambling facilities in 28 states.** Gaming revenues from 1988 to 2001 went from $220 million to $12.7 billion, the total being more than that of Las Vegas and Atlantic City combined (Barlett & Steele, 2002; National Indian Gaming Commission, 2003).

State-supported lotteries were established through the 1980s and 1990s to supplement tax dollars and generate jobs. From 1974 to 2002 the public increased its wagers on legal gambling from $17 billion to over $500 billion per year, generating profits in 2002 of $50–$60 billion. Some argue that legalized gambling imposes a very regressive tax on low-income gamblers. The poor devote $2^{1}/_{2}$ times more of their income on gambling than the middle class (National Opinion Research Center, 1999).

"I could be behind on bills for my electric, my rent, whatever . . . telephone, and I'll be like, 'Well I don't have the money,' but if I get the urge to go gamble, I'll find a way that day to come up with a couple of hundred dollars. Amazing what you can do."
23-year-old compulsive sports gambler

With the increasing accessibility of the Internet in the 1990s and 2000s, **online gambling is exploding.** Revenues from a variety of games, including poker, roulette, dice, and even online poker machines, went from $445 million in 1997, to $919 million in 1998, $3 billion by 2001, and an estimated $6 billion in 2003 and $10.2 billion in 2005 (Sinclair, 1999; Christiansen Capital Advisors, 2003). In Congress the **House Justice Subcommittee is trying to put limits on Internet gambling**—Congress has yet to decide. Just recently PayPal®, an online payment firm that handles payments between businesses and subscribers, was fined $200,000 for handling hundreds of millions of dollars in gambling web site payments. This one company has 525 separate gambling web site accounts. Fortunately a number of credit card companies are refusing to act as a conduit for offshore gambling companies because of lawsuits and the fact that pathological gamblers run up a lot of unpayable bills whether online or in regular gambling venues.

"Well I certainly started to realize when I went into such debt on credit cards that I was running to the mailbox so that my husband wouldn't see 22 credit cards with $10,000 and $20,000 limits maxed out."
53-year-old recovering poker player

Unfortunately most states have not adequately studied compulsive gambling nor have they established prevention or treatment programs. Critics contend that except for a few states with funded programs (e.g., Oregon, Louisiana), **governments encourage gambling and legitimize it but do not address the problem of gambling addiction.** The gambling industry often sees excess concern over compulsive gambling as an impediment to its growth since **the majority of states' and casinos' gambling income derives from problem gamblers.** In a study in Connecticut 47% of casino patrons were compulsive or problem gamblers (WEFA Group, 1997). In Minnesota 2% of the gamblers generated 63% of the state's revenue (Tice, 1993). A study of 7 states found that over half of their revenue came from problem or pathological gamblers even though they represented only 1–5% of the public at large (Lesieur, 1997).

"I worked in a dozen casinos over the years and was a compulsive gambler. And I tell you, in every place I worked, a healthy percentage of the employees were compulsive gamblers. At one place, at the end of the day, the casino would pay us half our salary in cash and of course those of us who got paid usually gambled—and lost. We were cheap employees and the casino knew it."
45-year-old compulsive gambler

The media directly or indirectly supports gambling by publishing odds, sports scores, players' injury reports, winning lottery numbers, stories of big winners, and ads for gambling excursions. CNN Headline News offers a sports ticker listing running scores across the bottom of the screen. There is also simultaneous picture-in-picture coverage of multiple games.

EPIDEMIOLOGY

There is controversy over estimates of the number of gamblers and the number of gamblers with problems. A meta-analysis study at the Harvard Medical School estimated that **125 million adult Americans gamble and of those, 2.2 million are pathological gamblers and 5.3 million are problem gamblers** (Shaffer, Hall, & Bilt, 1999). In addition there are about 1.1 million pathological adolescent gamblers (National Research Council, 1999). Another study by the University of Chicago estimated the total number of adult gamblers at 148 million, pathological gamblers at 2.5 million, problem gamblers at 3 million, and **at risk for problem gambling at 15 million** (NORC, 1999). In a different study the number of pathological gamblers was estimated at 3.6 million by 2002 due to the proliferation of gambling outlets (Califano, 2001). **Male compulsive gamblers outnumber female compulsive gamblers 2 or 3 to 1** (Cunningham-Williams & Cottler, 2001). Women more than men seem to use gambling as a means of escape from depression, traumas, or relationship problems.

A recent trend has been the increase in older gamblers. One survey of residential and assisted-care facilities found that 16% of the seniors go to casinos at least once a month on facility-sponsored trips while the casinos themselves offer day trips to two-thirds of the facilities.

"The greatest thing that compelled me toward gambling was the fact that I had lost all structure in my life. I just felt like life has come to an end. I am no longer important. I am no longer needed. I have retired. The world is running on just fine without me."
67-year-old recovering female compulsive gambler

College students have a higher rate of pathological gambling than the general population—$5\frac{1}{2}$%, with 15% reporting at least some problems associated with gambling. College male pathological gamblers outnumbered their female counterparts approxi-

mately 4 to 1, suggesting that problem gambling surfaces at an older age for women. Among college students, pathological gamblers were absent more often and got lower grades than other students (Lesieur, Cross, Frank, et al., 1991). Even high school students can get caught up in gambling. A Canadian study of grades 7–13 found 5.8% met the criteria for past-year problem gambling and an additional $7\frac{1}{2}$% met the criteria for at-risk gambling (Adlaf & Ialomiteanu, 2001).

CHARACTERISTICS

There are 4 specific types of gamblers.

1. There are the **recreational/social gamblers** who are able to separate gambling from the rest of their lives. Those are the majority of gamblers.

2. There are **professional gamblers** and they are able to take losses as part of the game. It's a business for them and they are able to make a living at it. They are few and far between.

3. There are **antisocial gamblers** who will steal to gamble and have no conscience.

4. Finally there are **pathological gamblers** (compulsive gamblers) who are obsessed with gambling, getting the money to gamble, and figuring out ways to stay in action.

There are two subtypes of pathological gamblers, the action-seeking gamblers and the escape-seeking gamblers. The **action-seeking compulsive gambler** is the stereotype of the gambler—always in action, frenetic, excited although they also want to escape.

"More than anything, I just wanted to be a big shot. I didn't care if I was winning or losing or if you saw me go back to the same place day after day after day. Somebody was going to think, 'God, this kid is a high roller or something because he's here every single day.'"
23-year-old recovering action-seeking compulsive gambler

The other type that is growing in numbers, the **escape-seeking compulsive gambler**, is often drawn to slot machines especially poker machines.

"There were no feelings. That's why I played it. There were no feelings. Blocked all the feelings. Blocked all the stress. Blocked all the anxiety. There were no feelings."
42-year-old recovering escape-seeking compulsive slot machine player

Like other addictions, pathological gambling seems to be a progressive disorder requiring more gambling episodes and larger bets to engender excitement and relieve anxiety. The similarity to substance addictions is emphasized by the fact that there is a high rate of other addictions among pathological gamblers; other behavioral and substance addictions occur in 25–63% of pathological gamblers (NORC, 1999).

"I didn't see that one was just making the other worse. The more drugs and alcohol I did, it seemed that I wanted to gamble more. The more I gambled, if I lost, especially, then I wanted to do more drugs."
24-year-old recovering compulsive gambler

Symptoms of persistent recurrent pathological gambling (positive diagnosis with five or more of the following) are

◇ preoccupation with gambling (reliving past experiences, planning future ones);

◇ gambling with increased amounts of money;

◇ repeated unsuccessful efforts to control, cut back, or stop gambling;

◇ restlessness and irritability when attempting to control, cut back, or stop;

◇ gambling as an escape;

◇ attempts to recoup previous losses (chasing);

◇ lying to others to conceal gambling;

◇ illegal acts to finance gambling;

◊ jeopardization or loss of job, relationship, or educational or career opportunity;

◊ reliance on others to get bailed out of pressing debts (APA, 2000).

A pathological male gambler often begins gambling as an early adolescent. Female pathological gamblers typically begin later in life. They both are more likely than the general population to have a parent who was a problem gambler. One study found the risk of heavy or compulsive gambling was 65% if the father gambled, 30% if the mother gambled, and 40% if a sibling gambled (Lesieur, Blume, & Zoppa, 1986).

Dr. Robert Custer, a clinician at the Brecksville, Ohio VA Hospital treatment unit, the first unit for compulsive gamblers, described three phases of gambling—winning phase, losing phase, and desperation phase. To these three, researchers Henry Lesieur and Robert Rosenthal added a giving-up phase (Lesieur & Rosenthal, 1991).

Winning Phase

Initially gambling is recreational and pleasurable for the action-seeking gambler. Bets are small and consequences negligible. The feelings that come from playing and winning or breaking even seem to satisfy the gambler.

"For me it was a rush, you know— nothing like alcohol, nothing like anything I've ever experienced. It was nervousness yet excitement and if you won, you know, the excitement turned into happiness. If you lost, you didn't feel too good unless there was another race to bet on and you had more money."
23-year-old recovering sports gambler

Skills improve and the gambler becomes more confident and even overconfident in his/her abilities. The winning phase can last 1 year or 10 years. A winning phase doesn't really exist for escape gamblers, such as poker machine, slot machine, keno, bingo, and lottery players, if they play on a regular basis. They will have days where they win but overall they will lose. For them a good day is breaking even while staying in action for hours at a time. **The key to escape for all gamblers is to stay in action as long as possible— winning is secondary.**

Early on for 70–80% of both action and escape gamblers, **there was a big win that fueled the craving to gamble.** The amount could have been anywhere from a few hundred to tens of thousands of dollars; it's all relative. The big win to the gambler is like the first intense rush to the cocaine user— never forgotten and forever chased.

"I had a winning phase that lasted me for probably 12 to 15 years and I actually lived on my gambling. I thought I was a semiprofessional but I still did it in the closet."
42-year-old recovering male compulsive gambler

A gambler with a susceptibility to compulsion **begins to devote more time and wager more money.** Stakes increase from a nickel and dime poker, to $5–$10, to table-stake games while blackjack goes from $2 a hand to $20 on two different hands; sports bets escalate from $5 on the Super Bowl to $100 on 10 different football games on the weekend. A $2 bet on the favorite at the racetrack ends up with $20 on the trifecta and $100 on every other race. Day traders start by depositing $500 to cover their trades and soon up it to tens of thousands of dollars if they have a run of luck, good or bad. The player comes to rely more and more on the high to deal with undesired moods and relationships or other problems.

"The longer you could stay in action, the more you could, for me anyways, the more I could escape from the reality of what my life really had become."
43-year-old recovering action-seeking gambler

They begin to believe in luck and magic to solve their problems. **They remember their wins and minimize their losses.** Their self-esteem is boosted by their gambling ability and the camaraderie of other gamblers. Gambling increases heart rate significantly and remains elevated during gambling; cortisol, the stress hormone, also increases (Hauffa, Schedlowski, Pawlak, Stadler, & Exton, 2000).

Losing Phase

"I would talk less and less to the people around me. I would play for hours and hours and hours till I was practically in a stupor. We don't stop to eat, we don't stop to drink anything, we don't stop to go to the bathroom, we don't leave the machine for an instant."
63 year old recovering female compulsive gambler

A losing phase for both action and escape gamblers often starts with **a losing streak that is inevitable due simply to the laws of chance** but if the gambler's tolerance has increased and they are betting large sums, the suddenness of heavy indebtedness can be startling. **They try to recoup their losses and they begin chasing their money.** A sports gambler may listen to three or four games simultaneously while a compulsive stock or commodities speculator may call for quotes frequently or be glued to a quote screen. A poker machine player will stick at a machine and spend hundreds of dollars because they just know that machine is ready to pay off. Again, the point is to stay in action. Social, job, and family tensions multiply. Gamblers may deny there is a problem or lie to conceal the amount of money involved or the frequency of the gambling. Now emotional satisfaction, ego, self-esteem, and money are involved. The magic is gone and for the action gambler, the emotional anguish of appearing to be a loser can be overwhelming. Chasing brings other changes in the gambler: depression, lying, isolation, and irritability. **But even when losing, gamblers still rely on gambling for their emotional satisfaction.**

"My mind told me, 'Yes, you're going to lose,' but your mind also tells you, 'But

if you do this, you don't have to feel either.' As long as you don't have to feel the price you're paying, whether it be weight gain or whether it be for the money, is almost worth it at that point."

44-year-old recovering compulsive gambler

As losses multiply, the gambler tries to recover financially by gambling more, tries unsuccessfully to cut back, swears he or she will never gamble again (but always does), and often seeks a bailout to get out of trouble.

Desperation Phase

In the end stages, which may take decades to develop or might just take a year especially with machine players, **compulsive gamblers often lose jobs, max out credit cards, borrow from friends and family, and even turn to illegal activities like theft, embezzle-**

ment, and drug dealing. Their desperation causes them to play badly because they lose patience and common sense. They play too many hands in poker, they get mad at the poker or slot machines and swear they won't let a machine beat them, and their sense of being lucky turns into a lament that they are the unluckiest people in the world.

"After 15 years, it got really bad in dollars, hundreds of thousands of dollars lost, loss of my marriage, my self-esteem of course, my vehicles, my homes. At one other point in time, I lost my mother's home. I don't even know how I got them [my parents] to sign on the dotted line."

43-year-old recovering gambler

Gamblers often bankrupt their families and suffer divorce or separation because of deteriorating family re-

lations, long absences from home, arguments over money, and indifference to the welfare of family members and others.

Giving-Up Phase

At this stage, pathological gamblers **stop thinking they will win it all back and just want to stay in action so they don't have to think**. Gamblers can experience elated moods when they win and **mania, depression, panic attacks, insomnia attacks, health problems, and suicidal thoughts or actual attempts when they lose**. One study of Gamblers Anonymous members found severe depression in 72% of those who say they have hit bottom; **suicide attempts occurred in 17–24% of them** (Linden, 1985). In Gulfport, Mississippi suicide attempts went from 24 in 1992 before casinos came in, to 85 in 1995 after casinos opened, and 137 in 1996.

"Every time I get out from the casino I want to kill myself. Then it's going to be over. Then it's going to end. I tried to kill myself twice. I took my car to the mountains. I just wanted to—I decided I didn't want the pain anymore."

38-year-old recovering compulsive gambler

Often the problems become so overwhelming that they can precipitate the final crisis that hopefully leads the compulsive gambler into treatment rather than to suicide.

VIDEO POKER MACHINES

There are some things that make some games more potent and more powerful than others according to Robert Hunter, an expert in the field of pathological gambling. For the average gambler it means the game is more exciting or more interesting. For the 5% who are pathological gamblers what makes a game exciting for the average person makes it deadly for them:

◇ **immediacy**, finding out right now if you're winning or losing;

◇ an **ability to increase both the time and money** to play longer as well as increase the amounts of bets;

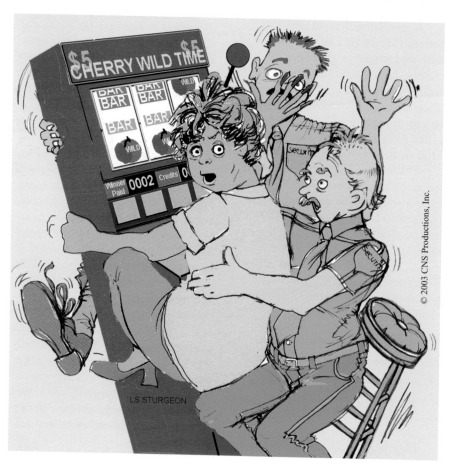

© 2003 CNS Productions, Inc.

LS STURGEON

Hilda thought that for $38,000 she should own the machine. Casino management disagreed.

◊ the **ability to lose yourself in the game**, to block out external stimuli, to get lost and focus solely on what's in front of you;

◊ the **perception of a skill component**. It's only perception of the skill component because how do you outwit a microchip?

If you think of those four qualities, then **there's not a form of gambling in the world that maxes out all four of those except video poker**, the crack cocaine of gambling. What probably ties for second place in this addictive hierarchy are cards and dice and traditional casino table gambling. **In states with video poker machines 70–80% of people entering treatment listed video poker as their game of choice.**

GAMBLERS ANONYMOUS

Gamblers Anonymous (GA) was formed in 1957 on the model of Alcoholics Anonymous. **Their basic concept is to let problem/compulsive/ pathological gamblers help themselves by developing spirituality and ultimately changing the way they live in order to stop gambling.** At present it is almost the only stopgap and hope between compulsive gamblers and their addiction.

GA lists several characteristics of the compulsive gambler including inability and unwillingness to accept reality, emotional insecurity, and immaturity. These traits lead the compulsive gambler into a dream world that can lead to destruction.

"A lot of time is spent creating images of the great and wonderful things they are going to do as soon as they make the big win . . . . When compulsive gamblers succeed, they gamble to dream still greater dreams. When failing, they gamble in reckless desperation and the depths of their misery are fathomless as their dream world comes crashing down. Sadly they will struggle back, dream more dreams,

and of course suffer more misery. No one can convince them that their great schemes will not someday come true. They believe they will for without this dream world, life for them would not be tolerable."
Gamblers Anonymous Combo Book (GA, 1998)

The above statement is read as part of each meeting. Members also read and answer the 20 questions in the little yellow meeting booklet that reminds gamblers of the havoc their addiction has had on themselves and their families. It is also a good self-test for those who are not sure if they are problem or pathological gamblers.

TREATMENT

(*See Chapter 9 for information about treatment of compulsive gambling.*)

TABLE 7–5   THE 20 QUESTIONS OF GAMBLERS ANONYMOUS

1. Did you ever lose time from work or school due to gambling?
2. Has gambling ever made your home life unhappy?
3. Did gambling affect your reputation?
4. Have you ever felt remorse after gambling?
5. Did you ever gamble to get money with which to pay debts or otherwise solve financial difficulties?
6. Did gambling cause a decrease in your ambition or efficiency?
7. After losing did you feel you must return as soon as possible and win back your losses?
8. After a win did you have a strong urge to return and win more?
9. Did you often gamble until your last dollar was gone?
10. Did you ever borrow to finance your gambling?
11. Have you ever sold anything to finance gambling?
12. Were you reluctant to use "gambling money" for normal expenditures?
13. Did gambling make you careless of the welfare of yourself and your family?
14. Did you ever gamble longer than you had planned?
15. Have you ever gambled to escape worry or trouble?
16. Have you ever committed, or considered committing, an illegal act to finance gambling?
17. Did gambling cause you to have difficulty in sleeping?
18. Do arguments, disappointments, or frustrations create within you an urge to gamble?
19. Did you ever have an urge to celebrate any good fortune by a few hours of gambling?
20. Have you ever considered self-destruction or suicide as a result of your gambling?

Most compulsive gamblers will answer yes to at least 7 of these questions (GA, 1998).

COMPULSIVE SHOPPING

The inability to handle money in a responsible manner is the hallmark of almost any addict. To the addict, money is a means to buy drugs, keep gambling, sit at a bar longer, buy as much binge food as needed, or purchase things that stimulate, sedate, or alter one's mood. The craving can overwhelm common sense. The addict does what feels good at the time—immediate gratification or immediate relief from anxiety and pain. For this reason, budgets, layaway shopping, avoiding debt or loans are generally not in the addict's vocabulary.

Compulsive shopping (oniomania) is often a manifestation of the personality factors that are present in most addicts. The *DSM-IV-TR* puts compulsive

Anorexia and bulimia are overwhelmingly female disorders especially when compared to compulsive overeating. An estimated 90–95% of anorexics and bulimics are women (Kaplan & Garfinkel, 1995). **Women have been socialized to regard their self-worth as closely tied up with their physical appearance**, especially size and weight. Girls in high school in particular have a distorted perception of how they look; 36% of 12th graders think they are overweight while in reality only 6.3% are. The same distortion of thinking is found in the 9th, 10th, and 11th grades as well (Centers for Disease Control, 2002). Secondly both bulimia and anorexia involve collateral elements of low self-esteem, depression, and secrecy. The illness is often triggered by a stressful event like the break-up of a relationship, social rejection, or going off to college.

Today anorexia and bulimia seem **more common in developed nations with an abundance of food** and media promotion of thin-body beauty ideals for women. But recent studies of schoolgirls in Cairo, Egypt found rates for anorexia and bulimia about the same as those in England. At the Hospital for Anorexia and Bulimia in Buenos Aires, Argentina hundreds of emaciated teenage girls are patients. More than 70 new ones arrive each week. Almost 1 in every 10 Argentinean teenage girls suffers from clinical anorexia or bulimia ("Argentina Struggles," 1997). The globalization of pop culture seems to have spread these disorders.

Certainly in the United States anorexia and bulimia are quickly increasing. From the mid-1950s to the mid-1970s, cases of anorexia grew by 300% (NOAH, 1996; Fairburn & Beglin, 1990). Currently, according to one survey of the health care professionals at 490 colleges and universities, it is estimated that **anywhere from 10–20% of college women have an eating disorder** ("Wasting Away," 1999).

Anorexia nervosa is most frequent in young women from 14–18 years old. It afflicts an estimated 0.5–1% of women in their late teens and early adulthood. Women over 40 seldom develop anorexia (APA, 2000). The illnesses can however strike all age groups from children to the elderly. A high incidence of anorexia in males is found in high school and college wrestlers who must maintain a certain weight to stay in a category. There is also a high incidence among rowers.

"It was our coach who taught us how to throw up to maintain our weight in high school on the wrestling team. We'd go to smorgasbords, eat a bunch, throw up in the bathroom, eat again, throw up again. Most of the team did it. Of course we weren't supposed to tell anybody but about a year and a half later, word got out and he was fired."
College wrestler

Females involved in sports who are at risk include gymnasts, runners, swimmers, dancers, cheerleaders, and figure skaters, many of whom are prodded or compelled by teachers, coaches, and trainers to maintain a certain weight no matter what.

A complex of disorders afflicting women athletes has been called the "female athlete triad." It consists of

◇ an eating disorder such as anorexia or bulimia but also includes elimination of certain food groups and abuse of weight control methods such as dieting, fasting, and use of diet aids and laxatives;

◇ irregular menstruation, i.e., missing more than one period;

◇ osteoporosis or irreversible loss of bone density, which can result in pain or fractures (Beals & Manore, 2002).

It is not clear whether eating disorders precede or follow women's participation in sports. Any extreme method of weight loss has physiologic and psychologic consequences. Even moderate dieting increases the risk of eating disorders in adolescent girls (Daee et al., 2003).

ANOREXIA NERVOSA

Historically anorexia existed in the Middle Ages as the "holy anorexia" during which monks and nuns piously starved themselves to achieve a control over the desires of the flesh and an ideal of holiness. Over the last 3 centuries there have been numerous descriptions of anorexia that are quite similar to the modern day definition (Bell, 1985; Morton, 1694).

Definition

Although anorexia means "without appetite," the condition has less to do with loss of appetite than with what one expert calls "**weight phobia.**" Some anorexics, the so-called anorexia restrictors, will **maintain weight by limiting their food intake through dieting, fasting, the use of amphetamines and other diet pills, and excessive exercise**. Binge-eating/purging types limit weight by purging through the use of diuretics, laxatives, or enemas (APA, 2000). Some people even control weight through liposuction (surgical removal of fat). Sometimes the line between anorexia and bulimia becomes blurred. **Bulimic symptoms appear in 30–80% of all anorexics.**

People afflicted with anorexia nervosa are afraid of weight gain and eventually may lose from 15–60% of their weight. They will not maintain a normal body weight and **they have a distorted perception of their body's shape and size** often feeling, even when emaciated, that their body or parts of it are overweight. Their emotional state is tied to their weight. They let the scale dictate how they feel about themselves. Often there is ignorance or denial of the seriousness of low body weight. Peer approval may aggravate the condition by praising the anorexic and encouraging "the look," which confers high status among adolescents (Aronson, 1993).

Causes

Some psychologists see anorexia as a compensatory behavior for people who are too concerned with following directions and pleasing others. Young females may be considered good girls and be model students, academically talented, good athletes, and **may have a** tendency to perfectionism but they lack self-esteem and a sense of self. A refusal to eat gives them a measure of control in their lives and continuous loss of weight can be an index of their discipline, achievement, self-esteem, and status among their peers.

"I didn't have a sense of myself or my body growing up but I tried to be so perfect. But whenever I do anything, I feel I'm going to be criticized for it, especially by my mother. I mean, even when she's not around, I still hear her. And she's not a bad person. So the only thing I could control was my eating. And the more they tried to get me to eat, the more I could say no. I thought that if I could control my eating, I could control the rest of my life."

19 year old recovering from anorexia

Additional **characteristics of anorexia include delusions and compulsions**: delusions are persistent unshakable ideas that one is unattractive or overweight; compulsions are rigid self-imposed rituals, such as weighing food, dividing it into small pieces, or eating in a prescribed order.

Family studies, including twin studies, indicate a higher prevalence of anorexia if one has an immediate relative who is anorexic (Treasure & Cambell, 1994). Just recently research at the University of Pennsylvania identified a susceptibility to anorexia on chromosome one (Grice & Kaye, 2002). One theory suggests that **what initially may begin as a strict diet, in about 3 months begins to change brain chemistry**, so that more of the body's natural opiates (endorphins) are produced and the person becomes addicted to those brain chemicals (Marazzi & Luby, 1989). The act of eating something precipitates a kind of opiate withdrawal encouraging further abstinence.

Effects

Semistarvation strains all the body systems especially the heart, liver, and brain. Dehydration from vomiting depletes electrolytes, a dangerous condition that can lead to arrhythmias and even cardiac arrest. In addition mild anemia, swollen joints, constipation, and light-headedness can also occur. Females can decrease their estrogen levels and males, their testosterone levels. Amenorrhea (absence or abnormal cessation of menstruation) often occurs in women practicing anorexia. It can take several months into treatment before a normal menstrual cycle is reestablished. Other disturbances include stomach cramps, dry skin, and lanugo (a downy body hair that develops on the trunk). There is also a growing belief that the early use of amphetamines and other strong stimulants to control weight will disrupt normal weight control mechanisms.

With anorexia nervosa additional dangers are osteoporosis, sterility, miscarriage, and birth defects. **Death rates among anorexic patients have been estimated at 4–20%** over the life of the disease, with risks increasing as weight loss approaches 60% of normal. The most frequent causes of death are heart disease, especially congestive heart failure, and suicide (APA, 2000). More recent studies suggest that gray matter volume deficits remain even after the patient has received sufficient nutrition for a period of time (Tamburrino & McGinnis, 2002).

Treatment

Most severely ill anorexic patients have to be admitted to a hospital because of the extreme weight loss, disturbed heart rhythms, extreme depression, and often suicidal ideation. It usually **takes 10–12 weeks for full nutritional recovery**. For the hospitals and clinics that treat this eating disorder, the rate for full recovery is about 40%. **In one study the recovery rate among 84 anorexic women after 12 years was 54%** based on the restarting of menstruation (41% based on the criterion of general well-being); the mortality rate was 11% (Helm et al., 1995). A first priority in treatment is to prevent death by starvation. Severely ill patients are monitored for body weight, serum electrolytes, and diet as the patient is returned to normal nutrition. Fluoxetine (Prozac®), other antidepressants, and MAO inhibitors have been tried to help patients **improve eating behavior by treating the underlying depression**. Generally though, antidepressant drugs have had marginal effects in aiding recovery (Jacobi, Dahme, & Rustenbach, 1997).

For an adolescent a weight gain of 4 oz. (0.1 kg) per day is the goal. The patient is generally monitored by staff for 2–3 hours after eating to prevent self-induced vomiting.

One of the first problems in treatment is convincing the patient that anorexia is a potentially fatal problem. Often it is a parent who brings a young woman to treatment. The client will think that her anorexic body weight is normal or even that she is overweight. Programs involve stabilizing the patient and psychological counseling to alert the anorexic to the problem and its causes; to devalue an overemphasis on thinness, weight, dieting, and food; to build self-esteem; and to promote healthy behaviors. They also involve family therapy to provide the family with understanding, support, and the ability to cope.

BULIMIA NERVOSA

Definition

Although bulimia means "ox hunger" ("I'm so hungry I could eat an ox"), the term generally is used to designate the eating disorder **characterized by eating large amounts of food in one sitting [bingeing] followed by inappropriate methods of ridding oneself of the food.** These methods may include self-induced vomiting (used by 80–90% of those with this disorder), use of diuretics or laxatives, fasting, and excessive exercise. These methods of eliminating food are used primarily to keep from gaining weight (APA, 2000).

"It was like depression, you know. I'd just keep eating all day and so I got to the point where I was gaining weight

too fast. I spoke with a friend about it and she said, 'Do like I do, throw it up.' I went into this mad trip of eating everything I could shove down my throat and then if I felt bad about it or if I felt any guilt at all, I could throw it back up and all the guilt would go away."

28-year-old recovering bulimic

People with bulimia often are ashamed of their behavior, do it secretly, and consume food rapidly. Although a slightly overweight condition may precede bulimia, those suffering from the disorder often are within a few pounds of normal weight. People with bulimia may feel loss of control during binges and guilt after them. Bulimia was first described in 1979 (Russell, 1979).

Generally a binge means "an abnormally large amount of food on the order of a holiday meal, eaten in 2 hours or less but definitely more than other people would eat in the same timespan." Continuous snacking during the day does not constitute a binge. Diagnosis of bulimia requires that bingeing and purging occur at least twice a week for 3 months. Although many binge eaters prefer sweet high-caloric foods like ice cream, soft drinks, and cookies, bulimia has more to do with the amount of food than the types of food. During binge episodes there may be **a feeling of frenzy, of not being in control, and a sense of being disconnected from one's surroundings.** Between binges low-calorie foods and drinks are often consumed to control weight.

Causes

As with anorexia, there are multiple causes of bulimia. Because the disease spans different races and classes, it is clear that environmental pressures to be slim are extremely influential. For example, when television was widely introduced in 1995 in the Pacific Island nation of Fiji, only 3% of girls reported they vomited to control their weight. Three years later the number had grown to 15%. In addition the study

found that 74% of the Fijian girls reported feeling "too big or fat" while almost two-thirds reported dieting in the past month. In the past, before the slender bodies of TV stars such as those on *Melrose Place* or *Ally McBeal* were on television, extreme thinness was a sign of illness. About 84% of women were what insurance charts consider overweight but there was an acceptance of that look (Becker et al., 1999).

Some claim that the socialization of women to an ideal of excessive thinness begins with the Barbie® dolls young girls receive; dolls that if extrapolated into an adult female's measurements would produce a woman with a 36 in. bust, an emaciated 18 in. waist, and 33 in. hips. The average model's measurements are 36-23-33. The contemporary "starved" look popularized by the 92 lb., 5'6" Twiggy has given way to the "heroin chic" ultrathin look of current actresses such as Lara Flynn Boyle. One study found that **between 1979 and 1988, the weights of models and beauty pageant contestants averaged 13–19% below the average weights of women in relevant age groups** (Wiseman et al., 1992).

The biochemical changes involved with bulimia can make the disorder self-perpetuating. There is evidence that metabolism adapts to the bulimic cycle and slows down, so more weight is gained with the same intake of food. This increased weight gain is then seen as even more reason to continue to binge and purge. There is also evidence that purging through vomiting or laxatives produces higher levels of natural opioids (endorphins), so people suffering from bulimia become addicted to the body's own natural drugs (Gold et al., 1997).

Effects

Effects and health consequences are less severe with bulimia if it does not progress into anorexia. Problems include **dental complications and a greater liability for alcohol and drug abuse** than other people, even those suffering from anorexia. Dependency on laxatives for normal bowel move-

ments can result along with a **high rate of depression and a greater risk of suicide**.

Because of the frequency of vomiting, bulimia puts people at risk for **stomach acid burns to the esophagus and throat** resulting in chronic sore throat and greater risk of cancer. When vomiting is practiced with either bulimia or anorexia, the tooth enamel can be permanently eaten away by acid. There is also a high incidence of cavities and front teeth can appear ragged, chipped, and mottled. Dental professionals are often the first to spot bulimic activities. The back of the fingers and hands can become scarred from abrading the skin on the teeth while pushing the hand down the throat to induce vomiting.

"Bingeing and purging is the choice of my best friend and it's easy to see the signs: the skin on a finger eaten away and yellow from the acids in the vomit. You feel guilt for eating even a salad with no dressing. If you eat only once a day, your mind screams at you to not eat, to say no. The guilt of eating anything almost consumes you. I used to do it, too."

19-year-old female college student

As with anorexia, **heart problems, such as arrhythmias, can develop as can electrolyte imbalances** and irregular menstrual periods or no periods at all. Additional problems are caused by the abuse of syrup of ipecac. This medication, usually taken to induce vomiting in cases of accidental poisonings, is often used on a regular basis by bulimics and can cause heart problems, tears in the esophagus or stomach lining, vomiting blood, seizures, or even death.

Psychological effects include loneliness and self-imposed isolation, difficulty in dealing with any activities involved with food, irritability, mood changes, and depression.

Treatment

Bulimia presents special problems. As with other eating disorders, bulimia is **best treated in its early stages**. Unfortunately people with bulimia often are in a normal weight range, so their problem may escape detection for years. After diagnosis a decision is made to treat an individual in a hospital or on an outpatient basis.

Because of the multiple problems involved, a **multidisciplinary integrated treatment is generally used**.

◇ An **internist** advises on medical problems.

◇ A **nutritionist** provides help with diet and eating patterns.

◇ A **psychotherapist** provides emotional support and counseling and may begin therapy that involves changing attitudes and behaviors.

◇ A **psychopharmacologist** may counsel on which psychoactive medications might be effective (NOAH, 1996). In recent years antidepressants have been used, especially selective serotonin reuptake inhibitors, along with monoamine oxidase inhibitors (Goldbloom, 1997).

The Karolinska Institute in Sweden found that conditioning methods that focused on physical symptoms, not on psychological problems, were the most effective treatment for those with bulimia as well as anorexia. When patients were trained to eat, recognize satiation, not exercise after eating, and some other behavioral conditioning, remission rates were 75% (Bergh, Brodin, Lindberg, & Södersten, 2002).

Family and group therapies are extremely useful to provide understanding and emotional support to the patient. Group therapy may provide great relief for a person who doesn't need to keep the disorder secret any longer. Family, friends, and colleagues can help an ill person start and complete treatment and then provide the encouragement to make sure the disorder does not reoccur. There are also self-help and peer-support groups organized specifically for bulimia but these are currently less effective than groups for compulsive overeating.

BINGE-EATING DISORDER (including compulsive overeating)

"During your life, my child, see what suits your constitution,
do not give it what you find disagrees with it;
for not everything is good for everybody,
nor does everybody like everything.
Do not be insatiable for any delicacy,
do not be greedy for food;
for overeating leads to illness,
and excess leads to liver attacks.
Many people have died from overeating;
control yourself, and so prolong your life."
Sirach 37, 27, The Bible

The prevalence of obesity in the United States is increasing. One major study found that **obesity (more than 30 lbs. overweight) increased from 15% of the population in 1980 to 31% in 2000**. That figure is expected to rise to 38% by 2008 (Helmich, 2003). The greatest increase was found in 18–29-year-olds, in those with some college education, those of Hispanic ethnicity, and those from the south Atlantic states. In addition the prevalence of diabetes, one of the main consequences of obesity, was 7.3% (Mokdad et al., 2001). A study by the Centers for Disease Control also found that about **65% of the U.S. population was overweight (10–30 lbs.) or obese in 2003 compared to 45% in 1991**.

Internationally, for the first time in history, there are as many people overweight as underweight, about 1.1 billion of each in a worldwide population of 6 billion. In Europe overweight people outnumber those who are underweight by a ratio of 9 to 1, in North America, 12 to 1, and in Latin America, 5 to 1, while in Africa they are about equal and in Southeast Asia there are 5 times as many underfed as overfed people (Gardner & Halweil, 1999).

Definition

There is much debate on how to define obesity. For example:

◇ Is obesity a specific syndrome or is it a symptom of a number of conditions such as metabolic disorders, psychological disorders, or simply situational factors (there are too many fast-food restaurants and people don't get enough exercise)?

◇ Is obesity an outcome of the metabolic changes wrought by excessive

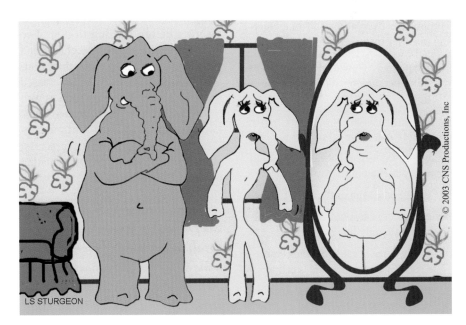

Georgia, haven't you hit your goal weight yet?

© 2003 CNS Productions, Inc

LS STURGEON

eating and overuse of refined carbohydrates?

◇ Is obesity the result of childhood traumas and damaged self-image that occurred in infancy?

◇ Is obesity genetically determined as was suggested when scientists created fat mice simply by genetic manipulation?

The current *DSM-IV-TR* says that binge-eating disorder affects 4.6% of the community at large and 28.7% of those in a weight-loss program (Spitzer, Yanovski, Wadden, et al., 1993). **Binge-eating disorder is marked by recurrent episodes of binge eating without use of vomiting, laxatives, or other compensatory activities.** A pattern of frequent eating and snacking over a period of several hours is a symptom of this condition.

Certain foods and excessive intake activate the mesolimbic dopaminergic reward system during ingestion of food and not only give pleasure but block out unwanted emotions (Blum et al., 2000). This chapter will use the phrase "compulsive overeater" and acknowledge that there are several causes of obesity but the main ones are remarkably similar. With compulsive overeating or binge-eating disorder, **people eat in response to emotional states rather than to hunger signals.** Symptoms of compulsive overeating and binge-eating disorder include the following:

◇ frequent episodes of eating what other people consider large quantities;

◇ feeling a lack of control while overeating or bingeing;

◇ eating rapidly and swallowing food without chewing;

◇ eating when uncomfortably full;

◇ eating large amounts when not feeling physically hungry;

◇ eating alone because of being embarrassed by how much one is eating;

◇ feeling disgusted and distressed when one is overeating;

◇ having a preference for refined carbohydrates including high-sugar

junk food as well as high-fat foods (APA, 2000).

"Eating at 3 o'clock in the morning; sneaking food when my husband was asleep and my kids were in bed; hiding food so my kids wouldn't know I had it because I didn't want to share it with them; and it would be junk, it would be cakes and cookies and sweet stuff, sugars. That was probably the height of it and feeling so lousy about myself because of the weight."
Recovering binge eater

People with a binge-eating disorder feel that **they cannot control the amount eaten, the pace of eating, or the kind of food eaten. They will only stop when it becomes painfully uncomfortable.** Most who suffer from this disorder are obese but those with normal weight can suffer this disorder as well.

Causes

Food is used to modify emotions, especially anxiety, solitude, stress, and depression. Eating controls anxiety since **food has a calming and sedating effect.** Dieting may trigger binge-eating disorder in some cases but in one study nearly 50% of all cases had the disorder before starting to diet. Two different studies of adolescents found that depressed mood more than doubled the risk of obesity and increased the risk of bulimia and anorexia as well (Goodman & Whitaker, 2002; Johnson, Cohen, Kotler, Kasen, & Brook, 2002). Unfortunately weight gain may increase stress, guilt, and depression thus perpetuating the overeating cycle.

"I was molested, sexually abused at 12, and I remember feeling really uncomfortable about my body after that and using food to just feel comfortable and maybe as a layer of protection to keep people away; not wanting to look good because then I might have to interact with the opposite sex and maybe have

some kind of altercation. I was just afraid of men after that."
36-year-old recovering compulsive overeater

Effects

People who compulsively overeat are generally overweight and may suffer from those conditions associated with obesity, including

◇ **high cholesterol, diabetes, high blood pressure, gall bladder disease, and heart disease;**

◇ greater risk for stroke, gout, arthritis, and according to a recent study, a 15–60% greater risk of cancer (Calle, Rodriguez, Walker-Thurmond, & Thun, 2003);

◇ **higher rates of depression** than the population at large.

Psychological problems often develop. People who binge eat

◇ **become distressed, develop a negative body image**, and avoid going out in public or gathering socially;

◇ allow their **self-esteem to suffer badly** because of the way they look or think they look.

Scientists at the University of Pennsylvania identified a fat-cell hormone they call "resistin" that blocks the effectiveness of insulin accelerating the onset of diabetes. If the same hormone is a factor in human weight gain once a person has put on too much weight in the form of fat, this could explain the **high incidence of adult-onset diabetes in 15 million Americans** (Steppan, Bailey, et al., 2001).

Treatment

Many people with this disorder have unsuccessfully attempted to control it; over 90% of dieters return to their original weight or greater within 2 years. Professional treatment personnel generally recognize that both **physiological and psychological causes underlie the disorder** and address those issues while initiating a weight-loss program. Common treatment methods include:

IRS approves deductions for losing weight

By Curt Anderson
ASSOCIATED PRESS

The IRS has previously permitted deductions for weight-loss programs recommended by a

The IRS also recently included smoking-cessation programs as a deductible medical expense, as

cent, also said they would vote for a congressional candidate who supports a balanced budget over

Gene may hold secret of obesity

The Associated Press
NEW ORLEANS — A thrifty gene that helped cavemen survive

to store up fat for later.
They said the gene could be an important explanation of an inher

"This gene was advantageous in times of food scarcity," said Dr.

cially complex in the way people gain weight. Experts believe that perhaps 30 or 40 genes can increase the tendency to obesity.

But these genes operate in concert with each other as well as with people's exercise and dietary habits.

Fat-cell hormone keeps body from using insulin

By ALEX DOMINGUEZ
The Associated Press

mice and found genetic evidence that the same hormone exists in though they have yet to

gold," said Lazar, director of university's Diabetes Center.

A body of work

New diet pill — new health risks

2 hunger hormones identified

By Steve Sternberg

50 to 100 drugs to counter obesity are in early stages

By Nanci Hellmich
USA TODAY

Only diet, exercise will keep weight off

■ Researchers find that successful dieters learn they have

"We are better at getting people to lose weight than to maintain" the

Exercise, diet have huge impact on diabetes

By Anita Manning
USA TODAY

Study: Insulin-sensitizing drug also helps

tracking in tandem ... and now we have the first concrete evidence (that) if you increase activity and decrease

Theory of eat less, live longer evolves

By Tim Friend
USA TODAY

Living longer by eating less — a proven step toward longevity in smaller creatures — also may work for monkeys and people, suggests National Institute on Aging research.

Experiments since the 1930s show that cutting calories by one third transforms short-

lived insects and rodents into lower-kingdom Methuselahs. But, until now, no research has shown whether it might do the same in primates and humans.

Since a study in humans would take almost a century to complete, study leader George Roth and NIA colleagues Donald Ingram and Mark Lane are using monkeys to look for changes in metabolism like

those seen in calorie-restricted rodents.

In today's Proceedings of the National Academy of Sciences, the researchers report that restricting calories by 30%, while still providing a nutritionally balanced diet, slows metabolism and reduces body temperature in monkeys.

"This is the first study to show that you get the same ef-

fect in monkeys as you do in rodents, so it bodes very well that the same metabolic processes might be affected in humans," Roth says.

In simple terms, the effect is like running a car's engine at a lower rpm — there is less tendency to overheat, fuel is used more efficiently and there is less wear on the engine.

If future studies prove calo-

ric restriction works in humans — say from 3,000 a day to 2,100 — the maximum lifespan theoretically could be extended to well over 150 years and the average lifespan could be pushed above 100.

But what about the quality of those extra years? Roth says rodent Methuselahs are just as quick at learning new mazes as when they were young.

◊ counseling that focuses on **changing attitudes and ideals**;

◊ psychiatric treatment that **examines underlying traumas**;

◊ **behavioral therapy** to help monitor and control responses to stress and to change eating habits;

◊ **pharmacological treatment** with antidepressants (e.g., Zoloft®, Paxil®), the opioid blocker naltrexone, and a dozen other drugs;

◊ **self-help groups, such as OA**, to reassure people who overeat that they are not alone and to provide examples and support for positive changes.

Abstinence from all food is impossible, unlike alcohol and other drug dependencies where total abstinence is

possible. The treatment goal is to learn to manage one's intake and to avoid foods that trigger binges, such as refined sugars, chocolate, or carbohydrates. Binge foods are substances that provide a person much greater emotional relief than other foods and they vary from person to person.

Prevention efforts aimed at the environment are being pursued.

◊ A number of school systems such as in Los Angeles are banning sugared/caffeinated soft drinks from school grounds. The FDA wants to require all food sold in schools to meet good nutrition standards.

◊ More detailed labeling is now required by law that lets the consumer know the amount of calories, sugar, fats, sodium, and other crucial nu-

tritional ingredients in anything they eat.

◊ A lawsuit was filed against fast-food restaurants because of the high fat, high sugar content of most of their foods and the unavailability of healthy foods. This is reminiscent of the many lawsuits filed against tobacco companies for selling a dangerous product. The fast-food lawsuit was dismissed.

Pharmaceutical Treatments for Obesity

In the 1950s and 1960s legal amphetamines were the diet drugs of choice while since then, illegal amphetamines remained available. In the '80s and '90s it was a variety of amphetamine congeners, weaker versions of amphetamines, including a combination of diet pills called "fen-phen," that are still the target of massive lawsuits due to alleged heart damage from the drugs. **Many of the diet stimulants proved to have an addictive component creating more problems than they solved.** In the 2000s it is antidepressants: Meridia® (sibutramine, an antidepressant), Xenical® (fat blocker), phentermine HCL (appetite suppressant), and a dozen other substances with varying pharmacological actions. A promising line of research opened in 1999 when the Japanese discovered ghrelin, a hormone that is secreted by the stomach and small intestine to signal hunger. When people diet, the level of this hormone increases, signaling the body that it is starving; hunger is increased, metabolism is made more efficient, and the up-down cycle of dieting is intensified (Cummins et al., 2002). A number of drug companies are planning to look for a drug that will affect this hormone directly.

Some of the other drugs in the developmental pipeline include Axokine®, an injectable drug that makes the user feel full; Rimonabant® to suppress a CNS receptor that regulates food intake; a drug that increases metabolic rate; one from a cactus that suppresses appetite; an enzyme inhibitor that alters brain chemistry suppressing a desire to

TABLE 7–6   COMPULSIVE OVEREATING SELF-DIAGNOSTIC TEST

(The following questions are used by Overeaters Anonymous [OA] to help someone determine whether he or she is involved in compulsive overeating.)

1. Do you eat when you're not hungry?
2. Do you go on eating binges for no apparent reason?
3. Do you have feelings of guilt and remorse after overeating?
4. Do you give too much time and thought to food?
5. Do you look forward with pleasure and anticipation to the time when you can eat alone?
6. Do you plan these secret binges ahead of time?
7. Do you eat sensibly before others and make up for it alone?
8. Is your weight affecting the way you live your life?
9. Have you tried to diet for a week (or longer) only to fall short of your goal?
10. Do you resent others telling you to "use a little willpower" to stop overeating?
11. Despite evidence to the contrary, have you continued to assert that you can diet on your own whenever you wish?
12. Do you crave to eat at a definite time, day or night, other than mealtimes?
13. Do you eat to escape from worries or troubles?
14. Have you ever been treated for obesity or a food-related condition?
15. Does your eating behavior make you or others unhappy?

eat; and another that causes fat to burn more quickly.

In addition other psychoactive medications such as cocaine, coffee, ephedrine-based medications, and especially cigarettes have been tried, often with initial successes that are trumpeted in newspapers and medical TV shows but later do not seem as efficient or effective. The problem is that **many substances will work initially but prolonged use seems to make them lose their effectiveness** due to the body's physiological adaptation like the development of tolerance and a raising of the body's metabolic setpoint. Unfortunately the side effects of certain stimulants can be significant. In general, **diet pills (especially amphetamines and amphetamine congeners) are only recommended for short-term use**, so careful monitoring by physicians and review boards is very important.

SEXUAL ADDICTION

DEFINITION

"Early on we came to feel disconnected from parents, from peers, from our-selves. We tuned out with fantasy and masturbation. We plugged in by drinking in the pictures, the images, and pursuing the objects of our fantasies. We lusted and wanted to be lusted after. We became true addicts: sex with self, promiscuity, adultery, dependency relationships, and more fantasy. We got it through the eyes, we bought it, we sold it, we traded it, we gave it away. We were addicted to the intrigue, the tease, the forbidden. The only way we knew to be free of it was to do it."

(Sexaholics Anonymous, 1989)

Sexual addiction is marked by sexual behavior over which the addict has little control and little choice. Compulsive sexual behavior is practiced by males and females, young and old, gay and straight. **Sexual addiction can include masturbation and pornography (the most frequent behaviors) along with serial affairs, phone sex, or visits to topless bars and strip shows.** Some sexual activity that can be compulsive has legal penalties: prosti-

tution, sexual harassment, sexual abuse, exhibitionism or flashing, child molestation, rape, and incest (Goodman, 1997). The incidence of sexual addiction in some studies is 3–6% (Carnes, 1997; Coleman, 1992). The *DSM-IV-TR* diagnostic manual lists some separate sexual disorders under the heading of paraphilias including exhibitionism, fetishism, frotteurism (clandestine rubbing against another person), pedophilia, sexual masochism, sexual sadism, transvestic fetishism, and voyeurism. These are different from sexual compulsivity.

"Once I got married, the first time, I wanted it all the time. And I masturbated quite a bit, you know. I mean, we had sex all the time but that wasn't enough. And it got to the point where I masturbated four, five, six times a day and wanted to go home and have sex with my wife."

34-year-old recovering sex addict

Collateral addictions include love addictions (romance addiction, the compulsion to fall in love and be in love) **and relationship addiction** (either a compulsive relationship with one person or with multiple relationships).

EFFECTS & SIDE EFFECTS

Compulsive sexual behavior is practiced as **a way to cope with anxiety, stress, solitude, or low self-worth**. The body becomes conditioned to the release of pleasure-giving neurotransmitters, especially dopamine, enkephalins, and endorphins, with the repetitive practice of sexual activity (Goodman, 1997). Unfortunately, compulsive sex is not an effective way of solving problems. Often progressively more time must be spent in the sexual activity to reduce the stress. Damage is done to careers, relationships, self-image, and peace of mind but the activity continues despite all negative consequences.

With sexual addiction, sex becomes the person's most important all-consuming activity and the pursuit of the addiction has been described as trance-like. Part of the elevated mood generated by the activity may involve risk. In addition a special routine or pattern may be followed that increases the excitement. **Usually there is a culminating sexual event (orgasm, exposure, rape, molestation) over which the addict has virtually no control.** It is often followed by remorse, guilt, fear of being discovered, and resolutions to stop the behavior. Throughout, the sexual behavior is pursued with a sense of desperation and the person is demoralized and may suffer from low self-image, self-hatred, and despair over the time and money wasted or the danger of injury/disease involved. Sexaholics Anonymous (SA), Sex and Love Addicts Anonymous (SLAA), and other affiliated groups see compulsive sex as a progressive disease that can be treated.

"I think it was compulsive sexuality because I used to love just a man being with me. I liked the money, for one. I liked the money that men would give me for sex. So I think that anytime I would see someone that I knew personally, not as a prostitute, I would always have that temptation that I wanted to have sex with this person and I would always do it. I would always have sex with men who would be friends of mine or so-called friends."
38-year-old female recovering polydrug abuser and sex addict

Many drugs that influence sexual functioning can

◇ release dopamine (stimulate the reward/reinforcement center);

◇ release norepinephrine and epinephrine (stimulate body functions and increase excitement, e.g., Viagra®);

◇ block acetylcholine (interfere with erection and orgasm);

◇ release or block serotonin (which can stimulate or inhibit sexual activity). Researchers feel that **drugs that act to inhibit or stimulate serotonergic activity can possibly be used to treat sexual addiction or other sexual dysfunctions** (Meston & Gorzalka, 1992).

TABLE 7–7 SEXAHOLICS ANONYMOUS SELF-TEST

(The following is a self-test for those who may not be sure they have a problem with compulsive sexuality or love addiction.)

Test yourself.

1. Have you ever thought you needed help for your sexual thinking or behavior?
2. Have you ever though that you'd be better off if you didn't keep "giving in"?
3. Have you ever felt that sex or stimuli are controlling you?
4. Have you ever tried to stop or limit doing what you felt was wrong in your sexual behavior?
5. Do you resort to sex to escape, relieve anxiety, or because you can't cope?
6. Do you feel guilt, remorse or depression afterward?
7. Has your pursuit of sex become more compulsive?
8. Does it interfere with relations with your spouse?
9. Do you have to resort to images or memories during sex?
10. Does an irresistible impulse arise when the other party makes the overtures or sex is offered?
11. Do you keep going from one "relationship" or lover to another?
12. Do you feel the "right relationship" would help you stop lusting, masturbating, or being so promiscuous?
13. Do you have a destructive need — a desperate sexual or emotional need for someone?
14. Does pursuit of sex make you careless for yourself or the welfare of your family or others?
15. Has your effectiveness or concentration decreased as sex has become more compulsive?
16. Do you lose time from work for it?
17. Do you turn to a lower environment when pursuing sex?
18. Do you want to get away from the sex partner as soon as possible after the act?
19. Although your spouse is sexually compatible, do you still masturbate or have sex with others?
20. Have you ever been arrested for a sex-related offense?

© 1997-2003 Sexaholics Anonymous, Inc.

INTERNET ADDICTION

"I would wait until my wife was asleep, about one or two in the morning, and I would go into the dining room where the computer was, and I would go to the thumbnail porno pictures or play Texas hold-em online. I'd play for a couple of hours, lose a few hundred dollars, try to go back to bed, and wake up tired for the office. It wasn't until I blew $1,700 at online poker and I got a lousy job evaluation that I tried to get help. Unfortunately only Gamblers Anonymous was available but that did help."
28-year-old compulsive gambler/Internet addict

DESCRIPTION

The predecessor to the Internet was the Advanced Research Projects Agency Network (ARPA), a military network started in 1969 that was eventually opened to defense researchers at universities and other companies. In the late 1980s most universities and many companies had come online. In 1989 a

British-born computer scientist, Tim Berners-Lee, proposed the World Wide Web project. When commercial providers were allowed to sell online connections to individuals in 1991, the explosion of the Internet began. Ten thousand new subscribers come online everyday in the United States alone (Greenfield, 1999).

The electronic media, like any business, offered services that users wanted. Of course what many wanted were games, erotic material, and gambling, all pleasurable activities to many but which also had the potential for compulsive/impulsive use, abuse, and addiction. In addition the ease and anonymity of the Internet enabled people to start relationships and do things that they might have avoided in the past. **A survey by ABC News of 18,000 Internet users worldwide found that almost 6% of participants met the criteria for a serious compulsive problem with another 4% having mild-to-moderate problems** (Greenfield, 1999). As the Internet has grown in size and sophistication in the 2000s, some studies show the number of compulsive users is also growing. A study by Dr. Richard J. DioGuardi at St. John's University in Queens found 11% of the students thought they were addicted. An objective study put the number at 15%.

Also called "Internet compulsion disorder" or "Internet addiction disorder," cyberaddiction is marked by compulsive involvement in chat groups, game playing, stocks or commodities market watching, sexual relationships, and other aspects of the Internet. America Online (AOL) established a chat group (room) for those suffering from cyberaddiction, AOL-Anon.

Symptoms of Internet addiction include

◇ logging on every chance there is at home, work, or school;

◇ thinking about the Internet constantly;

◇ needing progressively more time online to get the same satisfaction;

◇ losing track of time while logged on, so that hours go by like minutes;

◇ neglecting responsibilities;

◇ allowing relationships with spouse, family, co-workers, and friends to deteriorate;

◇ posting more and more messages, downloading more and more data;

◇ eating in front of the monitor;

◇ checking e-mail upon arising and before going to bed at night; and getting up in the middle of the night to check it just in case.

Some people experience a stimulant-like rush when online while others speak of being tranquilized by their quiet isolated online time. The two different styles of Internet addiction are similar to the difference between action and escape gamblers; some use it to zone out while some prefer the frequent interaction with others.

Repetitive compulsive use of the Internet induces tolerance and changes in physical and mental states. Symptoms include blurred vision, lack of sleep, twitching mouse fingers, and relationship problems.

According to the Center for Online Addiction, there are a number of areas involving the Internet where problems occur. These include cybersexual addiction, computer relationship addiction, Net compulsions, information addiction, and computer games addiction.

CYBERSEXUAL ADDICTION

The use of the Internet to view an incredible amount of free pornography, along with development of anonymous sexual relationships that can start out with the person masturbating while chatting online or viewing pornography and escalate into phone sex and even meetings in person, is often tied to sexual addiction. **Over 10 million Internet users logged onto the 10 most popular sex sites in 1 month** (Netaddiction, 2003). The difference is that the sheer availability of the medium, along with the anonymity inherent in the Net, feeds into traits found in many people bothered by sexual compulsivity and addiction. The availability also encourages the idea that it's okay and accepted by society.

Many of those with cybersexual addiction **use chat rooms and message boards to find sexual partners**. Unfortunately sexual predators are sometimes involved, preying mostly on children and women. The problem has caused many police departments to create Internet crime units.

As the compulsion increases, compulsive cybersexual "surfers" will become more secretive, hiding their activities from their partner. They can now avoid expensive 900 sex phone lines, visits to X-rated bookstores, and visits to prostitutes. They often will exclude other forms of normal sexual activity.

COMPUTER RELATIONSHIP ADDICTION

If the connections made on the Internet don't particularly aim towards sexual activity but become compulsive, then they could be called "cyberrelationships." The problems begin when the **online relationships draw the Net surfer from his or her real-life relationships**. The online friendships can lead to cyberaffairs often to the devastation of the forgotten partner. As with so many behavioral addictions, when use increases, it squeezes out other parts of the user's life.

INTERNET COMPULSIONS

The biggest problem with Internet compulsions is that of accessibility. **There are hundreds of online casinos, trading companies, and auction houses.** People can lose fortunes or at least their mortgage payments from the comfort of their own home, day or night. While there isn't quite the excitement of going to a casino, the element of control is important: "I can do it when and where I want." Online traders don't have to rely on brokers to buy stocks. They don't need these so-called experts (Netaddiction, 2003). The promise of large winnings and profits is a spur to activity. For some these elements of accessibility and control can lead to compulsive gambling as described earlier in the chapter. The online gambler or trader goes through the same stages as compulsive gamblers: winning, losing, desperation, and giving-up (*see Compulsive Gambling*).

Information Addiction

The ability to access thousands of web sites that cover virtually every subject is attractive to a wide variety of Internet surfers and the number of web sites seems to be growing geometrically. The problem with surfing the web is that it requires little direct human contact. So if **web surfers start young and often find the cyber activity less threatening than dealing with people**, they will be less likely to learn how to deal with people, which will then cause them to rely more and more on the electronic communication. Like other addictions, only a small percentage of users will have a problem.

Computer Games Addiction

Nintendo®, Sony PlayStation®, and other computer game systems are receiving stiff competition from all the games available online or as part of operating programs. The early game of choice was solitaire, played for hours at a time by new computer users. It is still popular but dozens of other games, such as Free Cell and Minefield, have been added along with hundreds of online games that can be played for fun or money. **Game playing is more common among men, teenagers, and children.**

CONCLUSIONS

As useful as seeing the similarities between substance abuse and other all-consuming behaviors can be, **the danger in generalizing the concept of addiction obscures the distinctive characteristics of a specific addiction that need to be addressed in treatment.** For example, in eating disorders and sex addiction, returning to normal levels of behavior is the preferred option, unlike gambling, alcohol, and other drug abuse that stress abstinence. Fortunately psychotherapy, behavioral therapies self-help groups, and psychiatric medications tailored to specific compulsive disorders offer hope for effective treatment and recovery.

CHAPTER SUMMARY

Introduction

1. It is rare that a person will have only one addiction and this includes compulsive behaviors as well as drug addictions.

OTHER DRUGS

Inhalants

2. The three main types of inhalants used for stupefying, intoxicating, and slight psychedelic effects are volatile solvents and aerosols, volatile nitrites, and anesthetics.

3. Inhalants are popular because they are quick acting, cheap, readily available at work and in the home especially to children and adolescents, and problems due to their use are mostly ignored. Abuse is most prevalent among adolescents and the poor.

4. Inhalants can be "sniffed," "huffed," "bagged," or "sprayed." The pressure from gas tanks and the freezing temperatures can damage lungs and other tissues.

5. Volatile solvents (and aerosols) consist of hydrocarbon gases and liquids refined from oil, including gasoline (especially in poor countries) and gasoline additives, kerosene, airplane glue, nail polish remover, lighter fluid, carbon tetrachloride, and even embalming fluid.

6. The effects of volatile solvents that begin in 7–10 seconds through absorption into the capillaries in the bronchi of the lungs and include an initial stimulation, mood elevation, impulsiveness, excitement, irritability, and reduced inhibitions.

7. The initial reactions turn to mostly depressant effects, including dizziness, slurred speech, unsteady gait, drowsiness, and in a number of cases, hallucinations.

8. Prolonged use of volatile solvents, especially leaded gasoline, can cause brain, liver, kidney, bone marrow, and especially lung damage. Death can occur from respiratory arrest, asphyxiation, or cardiac irregularities.

9. The most common solvents include toluene (glues, cleaning agents), trichlorethylene (paints, spot removers), hexane (glues), ketone (paint thinner), alkanes (butane, methane gases), and gasoline. Alcohol-based volatile solvents (some paints and some perfumes) are also abused.

10. Warning signs of solvent abuse include headaches, chemical odor on the body, bloodshot eyes, inflamed nose, slurred speech, and staggering gait.

11. Volatile nitrites include (iso)amyl, (iso)butyl, isopropyl, and cyclohexyl. The major effects, which last 30 seconds to 1 minute, are muscle relaxation, blood vessel dilation, and increased heart rate causing a blood rush to the head. Dizziness and giddiness also occur. Too much can lead to vomiting, shock, unconsciousness, and blood problems.

12. Volatile nitrites (poppers) dilate blood vessels and send a rush of blood to the brain. They also dilate smooth muscles and cause a rush and mild euphoria. They are thought to enhance sexual activity. Since most nitrites are illegal as recreational drugs, some are camouflaged and sold as tape head

cleaner, sneaker cleaner fluid, or as room fresheners.

13. Nitrous oxide, a dental anesthetic, produces a temporary giddiness, buzzing in the ears, disorientation, and occasional hallucinations that last for just a few minutes. Confusion, headache, and passing out are common. Direct inhalation can cause frozen and exploded lung tissue. It is also sold in small canisters used to charge whipping cream bottles. Nitrous oxide is usually transferred to balloons and breathed.

14. Physical and psychological dependence can occur with inhalants. Prevention often involves education and learning how to recognize signs and symptoms.

Sports & Drugs

15. Three classes of drugs available to athletes are therapeutic drugs, performance-enhancing drugs, and recreational drugs.

16. Athletes use drugs, particularly steroids, to build muscle mass, increase stamina, lessen pain, and improve performance.

17. Drug use among athletes dates from early Greece to the present, spurred by the Olympics and Cold War competition. It continues because of increased availability and synthesis of new drugs, a win-at-any-cost attitude, increased financial incentives, and unbridled ambition.

18. Although use of performance-enhancing drugs among collegiate and professional athletes is decreasing (possibly because of increased testing), use continues especially among high school athletes beefing up for college.

19. A danger of various therapeutic pain-killing drugs (e.g., hydrocodone) is that athletes will unknowingly aggravate injuries. Other side effects of analgesics include mood changes, nausea, and tissue dependence. Muscle relaxants are also occasionally abused.

20. The two kinds of anti-inflammatory drugs are NSAIDs and corticosteroids. Side effects of the latter are more serious than those of the former. Though many athletes suffer from exercise-induced asthma, many asthma medications are also banned because of their stimulant effects.

21. Most performance-enhancing substances are banned by athletic organizations.

22. Anabolic-androgenic steroids, synthetic or natural, mimic the male hormone testosterone. Athletes use them to increase weight, strength, muscle mass, and definition. Some use them to boost aggressiveness, confidence, or appearance.

23. The side effects of anabolic steroid abuse (20–100 times normal dosages) are acne, lowered sex drive, shrinking of testicles in men, breast reduction in women, bloated appearance, anger, aggressiveness, and even "roid rage." With excess use (at an average cost of $200–$400 a week), withdrawal symptoms, abuse, and dependence are common.

24. Amphetamines and methamphetamines initially boost the athlete's confidence, energy, alertness, aggression, and reaction time. The negative effects include irritability, restlessness, anxiety, anger, and heart or blood pressure problems.

25. Other stimulants are also used: caffeine, tobacco, and ephedrine are the most common.

26. Abuse of human growth hormone (HGH) (which increases muscle mass) is somewhat common. Even less common is blood doping involving injecting extra blood to increase endurance by increasing the oxygen content of the blood.

27. Androstenedione and DHEA are used to increase endurance and muscle size, beta blockers to steady the body, EPO to increase oxygen, creatine to delay muscle fatigue, and diuretics to lose weight.

28. Weight loss in order to participate in certain events is common in athletics.

29. Recreational drugs are used to adjust moods, reward or console the athlete, and cope with a heavy schedule.

30. Cocaine is occasionally used by athletes for performance and as a recreational drug; alcohol is the most common recreational drug though like marijuana it can hinder performance. Impairment from marijuana lasts days after cessation of use.

31. Drug testing programs have been instituted by all sporting organizations. Drug use imperils the notion of fair competition.

Miscellaneous Drugs

32. Other substances used to get high have included embalming fluid, gasoline, kava, nutmeg, Raid®, and even camel dung.

33. Herbal preparations and dietary supplements have many of the same benefits and dangers as prescription medications.

34. Smart drugs/drinks and over-the-counter medications are often a mixture of herbal drugs, vitamins, powdered nutrients, and amino acids. Some drugs prescribed to treat diseases of aging are also promoted as smart drugs.

OTHER ADDICTIONS

Compulsive Behaviors

35. Repetitive compulsive behaviors are practiced for the same reasons that compulsive drug use occurs.

36. Many of the symptoms of compulsive behaviors are the same as the symptoms of compulsive drug use, such as compulsion, tolerance, withdrawal, abuse, denial, and relapse.

Heredity, Environment, & Compulsive Behaviors

37. Twin studies and other research has shown that heredity plays a

role in compulsive behaviors involving many of the same areas of the brain that are involved in drug abuse.

38. Besides emotional needs created by a chaotic childhood, some environmental influences that can make users more susceptible to compulsive behaviors include a glut of fast-food restaurants, state-sponsored lotteries, and easy-to-get credit cards.

39. Engaging in a compulsive behavior changes brain and body chemistry to make the person more susceptible to repeat the behavior.

Compulsive Gambling

40. Gambling not only includes slot machines, poker, dice, blackjack, lotteries, sports betting, and keno but stock and commodities trading (especially day trading), online gambling, bingo, raffles, and office pools.

41. Although often considered a vice, historically gambling has been used by governments to raise funds, e.g., financing the American Revolution. This was the first of three waves of gambling in the United States. The current wave has 48 states with legalized gambling, especially state lotteries and Indian gaming casinos, mostly to supplement tax revenues.

42. Though estimates vary, about 2.2–2.5 million Americans are pathological gamblers, 3–5.3 million are problem gamblers, and 15 million are at risk for problem gambling.

43. Male compulsive gamblers outnumber female compulsive gamblers 2 to 1 but only a fraction of women, compared to men, seek help. Older compulsive gamblers are growing in numbers as are college student gamblers.

44. The four kinds of gamblers are recreational/social, professional, antisocial, and pathological. The two main types of pathological gamblers are action-seeking gamblers and escape-seeking gamblers.

45. Some characteristics include preoccupation with gambling, betting progressively larger amounts of money, risky or illegal attempts to recoup losses, restlessness and irritability when trying to stop, and jeopardization of family, relationships, and job. Usually an early big win triggers the compulsion.

46. The four phases of gambling are the winning, losing (including chasing losses), desperation, and giving-up phases.

47. The most compulsive form of gambling involves video poker machines.

48. Compulsive gambling is treatable through Gamblers Anonymous (a spiritual program), individual therapy, and abstinence from all gambling.

Compulsive Shopping

49. The inability to handle money is a hallmark of almost any addict.

50. Compulsive shopping (buying) is an impulse control disorder. This means that the behavior relieves depression and tension and gives pleasure. The crash after shopping is like a cocaine crash.

51. The control a compulsive shopper feels along with the respect they feel they are getting counteracts low self-esteem.

Eating Disorders

52. Society's promotion of underweight models and other role models has set up a false ideal of how we should look.

53. The three main eating disorders are anorexia nervosa, bulimia nervosa, and binge-eating disorder.

54. Up to 95% of anorexics and bulimics are female. The rate of eating disorders in high schools and colleges is much higher than for adults.

55. There is a high incidence of comorbid disorders, especially depression, anxiety, substance abuse, and personality disorders.

56. Anorexia is similar to a weight phobia. Dieting, fasting, excessive exercising, and diet pills are used to stay thin. It occurs mostly in girls and young women with a distorted perception of their body. They have a tendency to perfectionism and low self-esteem.

57. Anorexic individuals lose up to 60% of their normal body weight. The health risks are enormous, especially to the heart, liver, and brain, with a mortality rate of 4–20%.

58. Treatment is difficult because anorexics think their low weight is normal. The underlying depression must also be treated. The recovery rate is only about 54% after 12 years from beginning treatment.

59. Bulimics usually look normal but they stay that way by bingeing and then purging (throwing up) the large amounts of food they eat. The also use excessive exercise, laxatives, and fasting to control their weight.

60. Low self-esteem, pursuit of thinness, society's image of the ideal woman, and biochemical changes induced by constant dieting trigger and perpetuate bulimia.

61. Depression, acid burns to the esophagus and throat, heart problems, and electrolyte imbalances are common.

62. Bulimia is best treated in its early stages through psychotherapy, emotional support by family and friends, and self-help groups.

63. Thirty-one percent of the U.S. population is considered obese and 65% are considered overweight. Bingeing without purging is a characteristic of binge-eating disorder.

64. With compulsive overeating, the desire to eat is triggered more by emotional states (to calm, to satisfy, to control pain, and to combat depression) than by true hunger.

65. Health problems due to eating disorders include heart disease, stroke, gout, cancer, arthritis, and especially diabetes. Over 15 million Americans have adult-onset diabetes (type II diabetes).

66. Treatment includes psychotherapy, self-help groups such as Overeaters Anonymous, and behavioral therapy to change eating habits and lifestyle.

67. Prolonged use of any pharmacological treatment, e.g., amphetamines, amphetamine congener diet pills, and antidepressants, results in a loss of its effectiveness to treat eating disorders.

Sexual Addiction

68. Compulsive sexual behaviors, such as love addiction, pornography, masturbation, phone sex, voyeurism, and flashing, are practiced as a way to control anxiety, stress, solitude, and low self-esteem.

69. After a culminating event such as orgasm, the person often feels guilt, remorse, and fear of being caught and resolves to stop the behavior.

70. Sex and Love Addicts Anonymous (SLAA) and Sexaholics Anonymous (SA) are just two of the self-help groups available to aid those with sexual addiction. Psychotherapy, behavior modification, and even psychiatric medications can also be used.

Internet Addiction

71. About 6% of Internet users have a compulsive use problem including cybersexual addiction, cyberrelationship addiction, Internet compulsions, information overload, and computer games addiction.

72. Cyberaddiction often means using the Internet or the computer to the exclusion of a socially interactive lifestyle.

73. Easy access to online casinos, anonymous chat rooms, game playing, and an endless supply of online pornography leads to more isolation and excess stimulation that perpetuate Internet addiction.

Conclusions

74. Although the roots of drug and behavioral addiction are similar, the differences should be understood, e.g., abstinence is the goal for drug addictions but controlled use is necessary for many other behavioral addictions such as eating disorders and sexual relationships.

REFERENCES

Adlaf, E. M., & Ialomiteanu, A. (2001). Prevalence of problem gambling in adolescents: Findings from the 1999 Ontario Student Drug Use Survey. *Canadian Journal of Psychiatry, 45*(8), 752–755.

American Psychiatric Association. (2000). *Diagnostic and Statistical Manual of Mental Disorders* (4th ed., text revision [DSM-IV-TR]). Washington, DC. Author.

Another two teams quit. (1998, July 31). *San Francisco Chronicle*.

Argentina struggles with record anorexia. (1997, July 6). *Washington Post*.

Arnheim, D. D., & Prentice, W. E. (1993). *Principles of Athletic Training* (8th ed.). St. Louis, MO: Mosby-Year Book, Inc.

Aronson, J. K. (1993). *Insights in the Dynamic Psychotherapy of Anorexia and Bulimia: An Introduction to the Literature*. Northvale, NJ: Jason Aronson, Inc.

Barlett, D. L., & Steele, J. B. (2002, December 16). Wheel of misfortune. *Time Magazine*.

Barlow, S. E., Dietz, W. H., Klish, W. J., & Trowbridge, F. L. (2002). Medical evaluation of overweight children and adolescents. *Pediatrics, 110*, 222–228.

Bausell, R. B., Bausell, C. R., & Siegel, D. G. (1994). *The links among alcohol, drugs and crime on American college campuses: A national follow-up study* (Unpublished report). Towson, MD: Towson State University Campus Violence Prevention Center.

Beals, K. A., & Manore, M. M. (2002). Disorders of the female athlete triad among collegiate athletes. *International Journal of Sport Nutrition and Exercise Metabolism, 12*, 281–293.

Beauvais, F., Oetting, E. R., & Edwards, R. W. (1985). Trends in the use of inhalants among American Indian adolescents. *White Cloud Journal, 3*, 3–11.

Becker, A., Grinspoon, S. K., Klibanski, A., & Herzog, D. (1999). Eating disorders. *New England Journal of Medicine, 340*, 1092–1098.

Becque, M. D., Lochmann, J. D., & Melrose, D. R. (2000). Effects of oral creatine supplementation on muscular strength and body composition. *Medicine and Science in Sports and Exercise, 32*(3), 654–658.

Bell, E. (1999, October 29). Presentation at a symposium sponsored by the National Alliance for Research on Schizophrenia and Depression. *Newsday*.

Bell, R. M. (1985). *Holy Anorexia*. Chicago: University of Chicago Press.

Bent, S., Tiedt, M., Odden, C., & Shlipak, M. G. (2003). Ephedra tied to more adverse effects than other herbal products. *Annals of Internal Medicine, 138*(6).

Bergh, C., Brodin, U., Lindberg, G., & Södersten, P. (2002). Randomized controlled trial of a treatment for anorexia and bulimia nervosa. *Proceedings of the National Academy of Sciences, 99*, 9486–9491.

Bhasin, S., Storer, T. W., Berman, N., et al. (1996). The effects of supraphysiologic doses of testosterone on muscle size and strength in normal men. *New England Journal of Medicine, 335*, 1–7.

Blum, K., Braverman, E. R., Cull, J. G., Holder, J. M., Luck, R., Lubar, J., Miller, D., & Comings, D. E. (2000). "Reward deficiency syndrome" (RDS): A biogenetic model for the diagnosis and treatment of impulsive, addictive, and compulsive behaviors. *Journal of Psychoactive Drugs, 32*(1).

Blum, K., Cull, J. G., Braverman, E. R., & Comings, D. E. (1996). Reward deficiency syndrome. *American Scientist, 84*, 132–135.

Bodley, H. (2003, February 28). While perfect, Wells was 'half-drunk.' *USA Today*, p. D1.

Bouchard, C. (Ed.). (1994). *Genetics of Obesity*. Boca Raton, FL: CRC Press.

Breiter, H. C., Aharon, I., Kahneman, D., Anders, D., & Shizgal, P. (2001). Functional imaging of neural responses to expectancy and experience of monetary gains and losses. *Neuron, 30*, 619–639.

Brukner, P., & Khan, K. (2002). *Clinical Sports Medicine*. Boston: McGraw Hill.

Byrn-Austin, S., et al. (2001). Many high school students have eating disorders. The Society for Adolescent Medicine meeting, San Diego, March, 2001 [Online]. Available: *http://www.adolescenthealth.org*

Califano, J. A. (2001). High stakes: Substance abuse and gambling. National Center on Addiction and Substance Abuse [Online]. Available *http://www.casacolumbia.org/newsletter1457/newsletter_show.htm?doc_id=71136*

Calle, E. E., Rodriguez, C., Walker-Thurmond, K., & Thun, M. J. (2003). Overweight, obesity, and mortality from cancer in a prospectively studied cohort of U.S. adults. *The New England Journal of Medicine, 348*(17), 1625–1638.

Carnes, P. (1992). *Out of the Shadows: Understanding Sexual Addiction* (2nd ed.) Minneapolis: CompCare Publishers.

Carr, K. D., & Papadouka, V. (1994). The role of multiple opioid receptors in the potentiation of reward by food restriction. *Brain Research, 639*(2), 253–260.

Centers for Disease Control. (2002). Youth risk behavior surveillance —- United States, 2001 [Online]. Available: *http://www.cdc.gov/mmwr/preview/mmwrhtml/ss5104a1.htm*

Christiansen Capital Advisors. (2003). E-gambling: The economic impact of a burgeoning industry [Online]. Available: *http://www.cca-i.com/Testimony%20NGC%207-01.ppt*

Christenson, G. A., Faber, R. J., De Zween, M., et al. (1994). Compulsive buying: Descriptive characteristics and psychiatric comorbidity. *Journal of Clinical Psychiatry, 55*, 5–11.

Clotfelter, C. T., Cook, P. J., Edell, J. A., & Moore, M. (1999). *State Lotteries at the Turn of the Century: Report to the National Gambling Impact Study Commission*. Chapel Hill, NC: Duke University.

Coleman, E. (1992). Is your patient suffering from compulsive sexual behavior? *Psychiatric Annual, 22*, 320–325.

Cooper, C. J., Noakes, T. D., Dunne, T., Lambert, M. I., & Rochford, K. (1996). A high prevalence of abnormal personality traits in chronic users of anabolic-androgenic steroids. *British Journal of Sports Medicine, 30*(3), 246–250.

Cummins, D., Weigle, D. S., Frayo, R. S., Breen, P. A., Ma, M. K., Dellinger, E. P., & Purnell, J. Q. (2002). Plasma ghrelin levels after diet-induced weight loss or gastric bypass surgery. *New England Journal of Medicine, 346*(21), 1623–1630.

Cunningham-Williams, R. M., & Cottler, J. B. (2001). The epidemiology of pathological gambling. *Seminar in Clinical Neuropsychiatry, 6*, 155–166.

Daee, A., Robinson, P., Lawson, M., Turpin, J. A., Gregory, B., & Tobias, J. D. (2003). Psychologic and physiologic effects of dieting in adolescents. *Southern Medical Journal, 95*(9), 1032–1041.

Dean, W., & Morgenthaler, J. (1991). *Smart Drugs & Nutrients*. Santa Cruz, CA: B&J Publications.

Dinwiddie, S. H. (1998). The pharmacology of inhalants. In A. W. Graham & T. K. Schultz (Eds.), *Principles of Addiction Medicine* (2nd ed., pp. 187–194). Chevy Chase, MD: American Society of Addiction Medicine, Inc.

Dittmar, H. (1997). Compulsive shopping [Online]. Available: *http://www.sussex.ac.uk*

Drug and Alcohol Services Information System. (2002). The DASIS Report: Adolescent admissions involving inhalants [Online]. Available: *http://www.samhsa.gov/oas/2k2/inhalTX/inhalTX.pdf*

DrugScope. (2003). Nitrites [Online]. Available: *http://www.drugscope.org.uk/druginfo/drugsearch/ds_results.asp?file=\wip\11\1\1\nitrites.html*

Earnest, C. P. (2001). Dietary androgen supplements: Separating substance from hype. *The Physician and Sports Medicine, 29*(5). Also [Online]. Available: *http://www.physsportsmed.com/issues/2001/05_01/earnest.htm*

Fairburn, C. G., & Beglin, S. J. (1990). Studies of the epidemiology of bulimia nervosa. *American Journal of Psychiatry, 147*, 495–502.

Fleming, A. M. (1992). *Something for Nothing: A History of Gambling*. New York: Delacorte Press.

Fuentes, R. J., & DiMeo, M. (1996). Exercise-induced asthma and the athlete. In R. J. Fuentes, J. M. Rosenberg, & A. Davis (Eds.), *Athletic Drug Reference '96* (pp. 217–234). Durham, NC: Clean Data, Inc.

Fuentes, R. J., Rosenberg, J. M., & Davis, A. (1996). *Athletic Drug Reference, '96*. Durham, NC: Clean Data, Inc.

Galloway, P. G. (1997). Anabolic-andro-

genic steroids. In J. H. Lowinson, P. Ruiz, R. B. Millman, & J. G. Langrod (Eds.), *Substance Abuse: A Comprehensive Textbook* (3rd ed., pp. 308–318). Baltimore: Williams & Wilkins.

Gamblers Anonymous. (1998). *Gamblers Anonymous Combo Book*. Los Angeles: Gamblers Anonymous.

Gardner, G., & Halweil, B. (1999). Underfed and overfed: The global epidemic of malnutrition. Worldwatch Paper 150 [Online]. Available: *http://www.worldwatch.org/pubs/paper/150.html*

Gerasimov, M. R., Ferrieri, R. A., Schiffer, W. K., et al. (2002). Study of brain uptake and biodistribution of toluene in non-human primates and mice. *Life Sciences, 70*(23).

Giannini, A. J. (1991). The volatile agents. In N. S. Miller (Ed.), *Comprehensive Handbook of Drug and Alcohol Addiction*. New York: Marcel Dekker, Inc.

Goforth, H. W. Jr., Campbell, N. L., Hodgdon, J. A., & Sucec, A. A. (1982). Hematological parameters of trained distance runners following induced erythrocythemia. *Medicine and Science in Sports and Exercise, 14,* 174.

Gold, M. S., Johnson, C. R., & Stennie, K. (1997). Eating disorders. In J. H. Lowinson, P. Ruiz, R. B. Millman, & J. G. Langrod (Eds.), *Substance Abuse: A Comprehensive Textbook* (3rd ed., pp. 319–329). Baltimore: Williams & Wilkins.

Goldbloom, D. S. (1997). Pharmacotherapy of bulimia nervosa. *Medscape Women's Health, 2*(1).

Goodman, A. (1997). Sexual addiction. In J. H. Lowinson, P. Ruiz, R. B. Millman, & J. G. Langrod (Eds.), *Substance Abuse: A Comprehensive Textbook* (3rd ed., pp. 340–354). Baltimore: Williams & Wilkins.

Goodman, E., & Whitaker, R. C. (2002). A prospective study of the role of depression in the development and persistence of adolescent obesity. *Pediatrics, 110*, 497–504.

Gordon, N. F., et al. (1991). Effect of beta-blockers on exercise physiology: Implication for exercise training. *Medical Science Sports Exercise, 23*(6), 668.

Greenfield, D. N. (1999). *Virtual Addiction*. Oakland, CA: New Harbinger Publications.

Grice, D. E., & Kaye, W. H. (2002). *American Journal of Human Genetics, 70*, 787–792.

Gruber, A. J., & Pope, H. G. (1998). Ephedrine abuse among 36 female weightlifters. *American Journal on Addictions, 7*(4), 256–261.

Hanley, D. F. (1983). Drug and sex testing: Regulations for international competition. *Clinical Sports Medicine, 2,* 13–17.

Hauffa, M. G., Schedlowski, M., Pawlak, C., Stadler, M. A., & Exton, M. S. (2000). Casino gambling increases heart rate and salivary cortisol in regular gamblers. *Biological Psychiatry, 48*(9), 948–953.

Health. (2003). Anorexia and bulimia [Online]. Available: *http://www.health.com/health/wynks/Anorexia_BulimiaWYNK2000-MAL/whatishappening.html*

Helm, K., et al. (1995). Breaking the dieting habit. *Psychology Today, 28*(2).

Helmich, N. (2003, February 7). Obesity rate could reach nearly 40% in five years. *USA Today*, p. 4A.

Herman, R. D. 1984. Gambling. *Encyclopaedia Britannica* (Vol. 7, pp. 866–867). Chicago: Encyclopaedia Britannica.

Herzog, D. B., Dorer, D. J., Keel, P. K., et al. (1999). Recovery and relapse in anorexia and bulimia nervosa. A 7.5 year follow-up study. *Journal of the American Academy of Child and Adolescent Psychiatry, 38,* 829–837.

Herzog, D. B., Nussbaum, K. M., & Marmor, A. K. (1996). Comorbidity and outcome in eating disorders. *Psychiatric Clinics of North America, 19,* 843–859.

Hormes, J. T., Filley, C. M., & Rosenberg, N. L. (1986). Neurologic sequelae of chronic solvent vapor abuse. *Neurology, 36,* 698–702.

International Olympic Committee. (2003). Prohibited classes of substances and prohibited methods, 2003 [Online]. Available: *http://multimedia.olympic.org/pdf/en_report_542.pdf*

Jacobi, C., Dahme, B., & Rustenbach, S. (1997). Comparison of controlled psycho- and pharmacotherapy studies in bulimia and anorexia nervosa. *Psychotherapiek Psychosomatik, Medizinische Psychologie, 47,* 346–364.

Jacobson, B. H. (1990). Effect of amino acids on growth hormone release. *Physical Sports Medicine, 18*(1), 63.

Johnson, J. G., Cohen, P., Kotter, L., Kasen, S., & Brook, J. S. (2002). Psychiatric disorders associated with risk for the development of eating disorders during adolescence and early adulthood. *Journal of Consulting Clinical Psychology, 70,* 1119–1128.

Kaplan, A. S., & Garfinkel, P. R. (1995). General principles of outpatient treatment—eating disorders. In G. O. Gab-

bard (Ed.), *Treatments of Psychiatric Disorders* (Vol. 2). Washington, DC: American Psychiatric Press.

Kaye, W. H., Pickar, D. M., Naber, D., & Eben, M. H. (1982). Cerebrospinal fluid opioid activity in anorexia nervosa. *American Journal of Psychiatry, 139,* 643–645.

King, D. S., Sharp, R. L., Vukovich, M. D., et al. (1999). Effect of oral androstenedione on serum testosterone and adaptations to resistance training in young men. *Journal of the American Medical Association, 281*(21).

Kusserow, R. P. (1990). *Adolescents and Steroids: A User's Perspective*. Washington, DC: Office of Inspector General, Office of Evaluations and Inspections, Department of Health and Human Services.

Lesieur, H. R. (1997). *Measuring the Costs of Pathological Gambling*. Revision of the presentation to the Tenth International Conference on Gambling and Risk Taking, Montreal, Quebec.

Lesieur, H. R., Blume, S. B., & Zoppa, R. M. (1986). Alcoholism, drug abuse and gambling. *Alcohol Clinical Experimental Research, 10*(1), 33–38.

Lesieur, H. R., Cross, J., Frank, M., et al. (1991). Gambling and pathological gambling among university students. *Addictive Behaviors, 16,* 515–527.

Lesieur, H. R., & Rosenthal, R. J. (1991). Pathological gambling: A review of the literature. Prepared for the American Psychiatric Association Task Force on DSM-IV. *Journal of Gambling Studies, 7*(1), 5–39.

Linden, R. D. (1985). Pathological gambling and major affective disorder: Preliminary findings. *Journal of Clinical Psychiatry, 47,* 201–203.

Loviglio, J. (2001). Newest dangerous high: Embalming fluid abuse. *Medford Mail Tribune*, p. 3B.

Lukas, S. E. (1998). The pharmacology of steroids. In A. W. Graham & T. K. Schultz (Eds.), *Principles of Addiction Medicine* (2nd ed., pp. 173–186). Chevy Chase, MD: American Society of Addiction Medicine, Inc.

Lynn, E. J., Walter, R. G., Harris, L. A., Dendy, R., & James, M. (1972). Nitrous oxide: It's a gas. *Journal of Psychedelic Drugs, 5*(1), 1–7.

Mahesh, V. B., & Greenblatt, R. B. (1962). The in vivo conversion of dehydroepiandosterone and androstenedione to testosterone in the human. *Acta Endocrinology, 41,* 400–406.

Marazzi, M. A., & Luby, E. D. (1989). Anorexia nervosa as an auto-addiction. *Annual of the New York Academy of Science, 575,* 545–547.

Marnell, T. (Ed.). (1997). *Drug Identification Bible*. Denver: Author.

McElroy, S. L., Keck, P. E. Jr., Pope, J. F. Jr., et al. (1994). Compulsive buying: A report of 20 cases. *Journal of Clinical Psychiatry, 55,* 242–248.

McElroy, S. L., Satlin, A., Pope, H. G. Jr., Hudson, J. I., & Keck, P. E. Jr. (1991). Treatment of compulsive shopping and antidepressants: A report of three cases. *Annals of Clinical Psychiatry, 3,* 199–204.

McElroy, S. L., Soutullo, C. A., & Goldsmith, R. J. (1998). Other impulse control disorders. In A. W. Graham & T. K. Schultz (Eds.), *Principles of Addiction Medicine* (2nd ed., pp. 1047–1062). Chevy Chase, MD: American Society of Addiction Medicine, Inc.

Mellan, O. (1995). *Overcoming Overspending*. New York: Walker and Company.

Meston, C. M., & Gorzalka, B. B. (1992). Psychoactive drugs and human sexual behavior: The role of serotonergic activity. *Journal of Psychoactive Drugs, 24*(1), 1–40.

Mjoseth, J. (1999). Overzealous shopping: A higher prevalence of compulsive shopping among women may be attributable to their response to low levels of serotonin. *APA Monitor, 30.*

Mokdad, A. H., Bowman, B. A., Ford, E. S., Vinicor, F., Marks, J. S., & Koplan, J. P. (2001). The continuing epidemic of obesity in the United States, 1991–2000. *Journal of the American Medical Association, 286*(10), 1195–1200.

Morton, R. (1694). *Phthisological: Or a Treatise of Consumptions*. London: Smith and Walford.

Mottram, D. R. (Ed.). (2002). *Drugs in Sport* (3rd ed.). London: Routledge Press.

Nakken, C. (1996). *The Addictive Personality*. Center City, MN: Hazelden.

National Center on Addiction and Substance Abuse. (2002). CASA Conference. Food for thought: Substance abuse and eating disorders [Online]. Available: *http://www.casacolumbia.org/newsletter1457/newsletter_show.htm?doc_id=47194*

National Center on Addiction and Substance Abuse. (2003). Big differences in why girls vs. boys use cigarettes, alcohol and drugs [Online]. Available: *http://www.casacolumbia.*

org/newsletter1457/newsletter_show.ht m?doc_id=147504

National Collegiate Athletic Association. (2003a). NCAA drug-testing program [Online]. Available: *http://www.ncaa. org/library/sports_sciences/drug_testing_program/2002-03/drugTesting Program.pdf*

National Collegiate Athletic Association. (2003b). NCAA study of substance use habits of college student-athletes [Online]. Available *http://www.ncaa. org/library/research/substance_use_habits/2001/substance_use_habits.pdf*

National Drug Intelligence Center. (2003). Intelligence brief: Huffing [Online]. Available: *http://www.usdoj.gov/ndic/pubs/708/#What*

National Indian Gaming Commission. (2003). Tribal data overview [Online]. Available: *http://www.nigc.gov/nigc/nigcControl?option=TRIBAL_DATA*

National Institute of Mental Health. (2001). Eating disorders: Facts about eating disorders and the search for solutions [Online]. Available: *http://www.nimh. nih.gov/publicat/eatingdisorder.cfm#ed5*

National Institute on Drug Abuse. (2000a). Anabolic steroid abuse [Online]. Available: *http://www.drugabuse.gov/ResearchReports/Steroids/Anabolic Steroids.html*

National Institute on Drug Abuse. (2000b). Inhalant abuse. NIDA Research Report [Online]. Available: *http://www.nida. nih.gov/ResearchReports/Inhalants/Inh alants.html*

National Research Council. (1999). Pathological gambling: A critical review. *Committee on the Social and Economic Impact of Pathological Gambling.* Washington, DC: National Academy Press.

Netaddiction. (2003). Center for Online Addiction [Online]. Available: *http:// Netaddiction.com*

Neumark-Sztainer, D., et al. (2000). Disordered eating in adolescents linked to sexual and physical abuse. *International Journal of Eating Disorders, 28,* 249–258.

NOAH. (1996). Eating disorders: Anorexia and bulimia nervosa [Online]. Available: *http://www.noah-health.org/english/illness/mentalhealth/eatingdisorders.html*

NORC (1999). Gambling impact and behavior study. Report to the National Gambling Impact Study Commission [Online]. Available: *http://govinfo.library.unt.edu/ngisc/index.htm*

O'Brien, C. P. (2001). Drug addiction and drug abuse. In J. G. Hardman & L. E. Limbird (Eds.), *Goodman's & Gilman's Pharmacological Basis of Therapeutics* (10th ed.). New York: McGraw Hill.

Palmer, M. E., Haller, C., & McKinney, P. E., et al. (2003). Adverse events associated with dietary supplements: An observational study. *Lancet, 361,* 101–106.

Patrick, D. (1998, August 24). McGwire taking hits over use of power pill. *USA Today.*

Physicians' Desk Reference. (2003). *Physicians' Desk Reference (PDR).* Montvale, NJ: Medical Economics Company.

Pope, H. J., & Katz, D. L. (1994). Psychiatric and medical effects of anabolic-androgenic steroid use. A controlled study of 160 athletes. *Archives of General Psychiatry, 51*(5), 375–382.

Rosenberg, N. G., et al. (2002). Neuropsychologic impairment and MRI abnormalities associated with chronic solvent abuse. *Journal of Toxicology Clinical Toxicology, 40*(1), 21–34.

Rosenberg, N. G., Fuentes, R. J., Wooley, B. H., Reese, T., & Podraza, J. (1996). Questions and answers–What athletes commonly ask. In R. J. Fuentes, J. M. Rosenberg, & A. Davis (Eds.), *Athletic Drug Reference '96.* Durham, NC: Clean Data, Inc.

Rosenthal, R. J., & Lesieur, H. R. (1992). Self-reported withdrawal symptoms and pathological gambling. *American Journal of Addictions, 1,* 150–154.

Rupp, N. T., et al. (1993). The value of screening for risk of exercise-induced asthma in high school athletes. *Annual Allergy, 70,* 33–39.

Russell, G. (1979). Bulimia nervosa: An ominous variant of anorexia nervosa. *Psychological Medicine,* 429–448.

Schnirring, L. (2000). Growth hormone doping: The search for a test. *The Physician and Sports Medicine, 28*(4) [Online]. Available: *http://www.physsports med.com/issues/2000/04_00/news.htm*

Sexaholics Anonymous. (1989). *Sexaholics Anonymous.* New York: SA Literature.

Shaffer, H. (1998, February 28). Lecture to casino executives, Las Vegas gaming convention. *Medford Mail Tribune.*

Shaffer, H. J., Hall, M. N., & Bilt, J. V. (1999). Estimating the prevalence of disordered gambling behavior in the United States and Canada: A meta-analysis. *Journal of Public Health, 89,* 1369–1376.

Sharp, C. W., Beauvais, F., & Spence, R. (1992). Inhalant abuse: A volatile research agenda. *NIDA Research Mono-graph Series No. 129, NIH Publication No. 93-3480.* Rockville, MD: National Institutes of Health.

Sharp, C. W., & Rosenberg, N. L. (1997). Inhalants. In J. H. Lowinson, P. Ruiz, R. B. Millman, & J. G. Langrod (Eds.), *Substance Abuse: A Comprehensive Textbook* (3rd ed., pp. 246–263). Baltimore: Williams & Wilkins.

Siegal, E., & Wason, S. (1990). Sudden death caused by inhalation of butane and propane. *New England Journal of Medicine, 323*(23), 1638.

Sinclair, S. (1999). Gambling in the United States [Online]. Available: *http://www. casino-gambling-reports.com/Gambling Study/Gambling/page14.htm*

Smith, G. (1974). *When the Cheering Stopped.* Toronto: MacLeod.

Spitzer, R. L., Yanovski, S., Wadden, T., et al. (1993). Binge-eating disorder: Its further validation in a multi site study. *International Journal of Eating Disorders, 13,* 137–153.

Sports Illustrated (2002, June 3). Steroids in baseball. *Sports Illustrated,* pp. 35–49.

Spriet, L. L. (1995). Caffeine and sports. *International Journal of Sports Nutrition, 5,* S84–S99.

Steppan, C. M., Bailey, S. T., et al. (2001). The hormone resistin links obesity to diabetes. *Nature, 409,* 307–312.

Substance Abuse and Mental Health Services Administration. (2002). *Summary of findings from the 2001 National Household Survey on Drug Abuse.* Rockville, MD: Substance Abuse and Mental Health Services, Office of Applied Studies.

Swan, N. (1995). Inhalants. In J. H. Jaffe (Ed.), *Encyclopedia of Drugs and Alcohol* (Vol. 2, pp. 590–600). New York: Simon & Schuster MacMillan.

Tamburrino, M. B., & McGinnis, R. A. (2002). Anorexia nervosa. A review. *Panminerva Medicine, 44,* 301–311.

The Vaults of Erowid. (2003). Nootropics: "Smart drugs" [Online]. Available: *http://www.erowid.org/smarts/smarts.sh tml*

Thomason, H. (1982). Science and sporting performance: Management or manipulation. In B. Davies & G. Thomas (Eds.), *Drugs and the Athlete.* Oxford: Clarendon Press.

Tice, D. J. (1993, February). Big spenders. *Saint Paul Pioneer Press* (Special Reprint Section).

Todd, T. (1987). Anabolic steroids: The gremlins of sport. *Journal of Sports History, 14,* 87–107.

Treasure, J., & Campbell, I. (1994). Editorial: A biological hypothesis for anorexia nervosa. *Psychiatric Medicine, 24*, 3–8.

U.S. Congress. (1990). Hearing before the Subcommittee on Crime of the Committee on the Judiciary, House of Representatives, March 22, 1990. *Abuse of Steroids in Amateur and Professional Athletics.*

U.S. Food and Drug Administration. (2003). Dietary supplements [Online]. Available: *http://www.cfsan.fda.gov/%7 Edms/ds-warn.html*

University of Michigan. (2003). Monitoring the Future Study. 2002 data from in-school surveys of 8th, 10th, and 12th grade students [Online]. Available: *http://monitoringthefuture.org/data/02d ata.html#2002data-drugs*

University of Sussex. (1997). Shopping addicts need help. Bulletin in the University of Sussex newsletter [Online]. Available: *http://www.sussex.ac.uk/press_ office/bulletin/17jan97/item5.html*

Viagra, poppers are a fatal combination. (1999, June 22). *San Francisco Chronicle.*

Volkow, N., et al. (2002). Synapse, June 1, 2002 [Online]. Available: *www.drugabuse.gov/MedAdv/02/NS-05.html*

Wang, G. J., Volkow, N. D., Logan, J., Pappas, N. R., Wong, C. T., Zhu, W., Netusil, N., & Fowler, J. S. (2001). Brain dopamine and obesity. *Lancet, 357,* 354–357.

Wasting away: Eating disorders on campus. (1999, April 12). *People Magazine.*

WEFA Group. (1997). *A Study Concerning the Effects of Legalized Gambling on the Citizens of the State of Connecticut.* Prepared for State of Connecticut, Department of Revenue Services, Division of Special Revenue.

Weil, A., & Rosen, W. (1998). *From Chocolate to Morphine.* Boston: Houghton Mifflin Company.

Weinberg, R. A., & Bealer, B. K. (2001). *The World of Caffeine.* New York: Routledge.

Williams, M. H., Wesseldine, S., Somma, T., & Schuster, R. (1981). The effects of induced erythrocythemia upon 5-mile treadmill run time. *Medicine and Science in Sports and Exercise, 13,* 169–175.

Wiseman, C. V., et al. (1992). Cultural expectations of thinness in women: An update. *International Journal of Eating Disorders, 11*(1).

Wolf, N. (1992). *The Beauty Myth: How Images of Beauty Are Used Against Women.* New York: Anchor Books/ Doubleday.

Wood, R. W. (1994). Inhalants. In J. H. Jaffe (Ed.), *Encyclopedia of Drugs and Alcohol* (Vol. 2, pp. 590–595). New York: Simon & Schuster MacMillan.

Wood, S. (2002, November 21). Upshaw defends dietary extras. *USA Today*, p. 1C.

Wooley, B. H. (1992). Drugs of abuse in sport. In R. Banks, Jr. (Ed.), *Substance Abuse in Sport: The Realities* (2nd ed., pp. 3–12). Dubuque, IA: Kendall/Hunt Publishing Company.

World Health Organization. (1998). *Volatile Solvent Use: A Global Overview,* WHO/ HSC/SAB/99.7. Geneva: Substance Abuse Department, World Health Organization.

Yesalis, C. E., Herrick, R. T., Buckley, W. E., et al. (1988). Self-reported use of anabolic-androgenic steroids by elite powerlifters. *Physiology of Sports Medicine, 16,* 91–100.

Drug Use & Prevention:
From Cradle to Grave

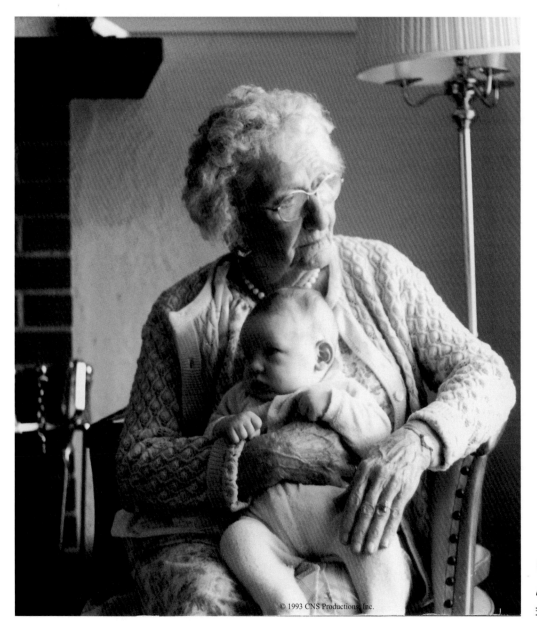

© 1993 CNS Productions, Inc.

D rug abuse prevention is a lifetime project.

- **Introduction:** Since drug use affects people from cradle to grave, many drug educators believe that prevention should be taught from cradle to grave.

PREVENTION

- **Concepts of Prevention:** Historically substance abuse prevention has included a wide range of philosophies from total prohibition, to temperance, to harm reduction. Scare tactics, drug information programs, skill-building programs, and resiliency programs have been some of the methods used over the years.
- **Prevention Methods:** The three main prevention methods are supply reduction (enforce legal penalties and interdict drugs), demand reduction (reduce craving for drugs), and harm reduction (minimize harm without requiring abstinence).
- **Challenges to Prevention:** The impediments to prevention efforts include the abundance of legal drugs, the availability of street drugs, the relatively slow rate of success of prevention programs, the difficulty of properly evaluating these efforts, and the lack of adequate funding.

FROM CRADLE TO GRAVE

- **Patterns of Use:** A pattern of earlier age of first use and high levels of overall use are associated with future development of drug problems. Drug abuse is not restricted to any age, race, gender, or level of intelligence.
- **Pregnancy & Birth:** Drugs cross the placental barrier and affect the fetus more strongly than the mother. The infant can be born addicted and go through dangerous withdrawal. Drug effects continue after birth.
- **Youth & School:** Alcohol is still the number one problem in schools, tobacco is second, marijuana third, and the use of stimulants like methamphetamine and ecstasy has risen rapidly. Increased alcohol abuse is being countered by recognizing risk factors, bolstering resiliency, and using normative assessment. Prevention efforts are effective when taught throughout all grades.
- **Love, Sex, & Drugs:** Psychoactive drugs are used to lower inhibitions in order to enhance sexual activity. Initially some drugs may increase sensation but with continued use they can diminish sexual performance and pleasure. Sexual violence, such as date rape, is strongly associated with drug use. High-risk sex practices, aggravated by lowered inhibitions and contaminated needles, spread sexually transmitted diseases (STDs), e.g., HIV/AIDS, hepatitis, and gonorrhea.
- **Drugs at Work:** Employee assistance programs (EAPs) help control substance abuse in the workplace that costs businesses and society more than $160 billion a year in lost productivity, lost earnings, and increased health care.
- **Drug Testing:** Preemployment testing, testing of people in treatment, military testing, sports testing, and random testing of workers responsible for public safety (e.g., pilots, nuclear technicians) are the most widely used forms of drug testing.
- **Drugs & the Elderly:** The elderly are more susceptible to the pharmacological effects of drugs. Alcohol abuse and prescription drug abuse are the biggest problems.
- **Conclusions:** To be successful, a prevention program must be specific to age, ethnicity, and cultural group and the message must be consistent. It should also be practiced throughout everyone's lifetime.

321

Forced Rehab for Drug Abusers Can Be Effective, Studies Show

Associated Press
Washington

The research comes as the White House's drug policy office seeks to triple the nation's drug

dent of Families Against Mandatory Minimums, a Washington group that works to change mandatory

Canada plans injection site for drug users

Drug testing for welfare recipients OKd

ACLU says it will appeal ision in Michigan

By Dee-Ann Durbin
Associated Press

NG, Mich. — A federal ha ourt Friday cleared the m

Kids' anti-drug program working, study shows

Participants better at saying no,

Bush's new drug policy: crack down on U.S. demand

By EDWIN CHEN
Los Angeles Times
WASHINGTON — President Bush ordered a major shift of emphasis in the war on drugs Thursday, vowing debted" and

During his rema declared his unequ legalization of dru

"So we'll continue to do the best we can to interdict supplies," Bush said while tour community center.

to educate and train parents in effective drug prevention." He is seeking $25 million over five years for such a corps. Bush said he intends to in

Inmates number over 2 million, a record for USA
By Richard Willing
USA TODAY
Population

Strategies sought to fight hepatitis C

Amphetamine use rises in workplace

Tests show 17

By Del Jones
USA TODAY

While overall drug use down, use of amphetam addictive the drug tests on employees Cocaine remains th choice, but its use is slow newer, potent and highl

College blackout drinkers face more risks

Accidents, injuries are more common

By Kathleen Fackelmann
USA TODAY

had experienced a memory blackout during the two weeks prior to the survey; 40% said they had experienced at least one such bl

People experiencing a memory blackout can talk, have sex, drive a car or get into a fight and

blood-alcohol concentration rises quickly

Drugs trigger withdrawal of student financial aid

Convictions make people ineligible; even law's author hopes to change it

By Maureen Groppe
Gannett News Service

The millions of college students heading to campus this fall might not include an estimated 28,230 who were denied federal financial

students and financial-aid officers who say it hurts poor and minority students disproportionately because they are more likely to have a conviction and less likely to have the independent means to forgo financial aid

Education assistance denied to thousands

A federal law that took effect last year prohibits students from receiving federal drug aid for college if they have been convicted of possessing an illegal drug in the past year or of selling drugs in the past 2 years.

Applied for federal aid for 2001-02 school year | 7,583,207
conviction | 28,230

"I definitely feel it's very unfair," he says. "I know walking around on this campus there have been people convicted of crimes far worse than choosing to partake in a little marijuana smoking."

A drug conviction is the only crime that will make a student ineligible for aid.
Setiuck was able to get help from Kris Sperry

"It sort of blew us away," Heller says. "It has been the driving force in creating the largest anti-drug movement since Vietnam."
Today, the group has 156 local chapters and has gotten 66 student governments, the U.S. Student Association and the Association of Big Ten Schools to pass resolution calling for the harsh repeal. The group has held a national drug war created scholarships

Tarnishing the Golden Years With Addiction

Scientists urge worldwide AIDS vaccine effort

Program would override cost, frustration of development

By Sabin Russell
Chronicle Medical Writer

As the search for an effective AIDS vaccine continues to sputter, a group of top international scientists called today for the creation of a new global program

project was launched.

Virus outfoxing science

Scientists typically work independently, often in highly competitive pursuits of common targets. But two decades into the human immunode-

Just one binge puts fetus at risk

By DAIH

— A single drinking binge by n can be enough to permabrain of her unborn child, study of the effects of alcohol

nents in the study were conv rats, experts said the findnation of why children born can suffer learning disabilin disorders.

Smoking in films promotes habit

Youth influenced by actors, study says

By Emma Ross
Associated Press

LONDON — Youngsters who watch movies in which actors smoke a lot are three times more likely to take up the habit than

smoked a cigarette at the time they were recruited.
The adolescents were asked at the beginning of the study which movies they had seen from a list of 50 movies released between 1988 and 1999.

Study shows alcohol kills baby brain cells

"We call this a brain growth spurt period," said Dr. John W. Olney, a Washington University School of Medicine researcher and senior author of the study.
During this brain growth spurt, said Olney, a single prolonged contact with alcohol — lasting for four hours or more — is enough to kill vast

grammed to commit suicide. This is the body's way of eliminating surplus cells.
But, based on the rat studies, alcohol severely disrupts the glutamate-GABA signals and this, in turn, causes nerve cell suicide at about 15 tim the normal rate, he said.
Neuron cells that normally die during br development are about 1.5 percent of the to but in rat pups exposed to alcohol just days a birth, said Olney, the dead neurons ranged 5 to 30 percent of the total.
"Our study showed that it only required round of intoxication of about four hours fo

---

INTRODUCTION

"Preventing addiction should be easy but it's been a difficult process because moral issues become involved with the medical issues. We should have the ability to prevent this condition as well as to treat it. Unfortunately many of the things that people look at from an addictive standpoint seem to concentrate on the illegality, on the police scene, on interdiction, and on stopping drugs at the border. The more we try to stop drugs from coming into the United States, the more drugs it seems are available. From this standpoint, the war on drugs has been an utter and complete failure."

Darryl Inaba, Pharm.D., CEO, Haight Ashbury Clinics

Psychoactive drugs and addictive behaviors affect people's lives from conception to death. For example:

◇ a fetus absorbs heroin through the umbilical cord when an addicted mother injects the drug;

◇ a 14-year-old is offered MDMA at a party so he can get "rolling";

◇ a college coed troubled by bulimia makes herself throw up five times a week;

◇ a young mother with three children hides in her room to smoke crack;

◇ while having sex, a 28-year-old IV methamphetamine user infects his girlfriend with the HIV virus he got through a contaminated needle;

◇ an office worker takes alprazolam (Xanax®) to cope with job stress and anxiety while a co-worker with major depression is prescribed Prozac®, an antidepressant, to help him function;

◇ a mother, whose children have grown, battles boredom by compulsively playing poker machines;

◇ a 50-year-old salesman on the road smokes and drinks to cope with loneliness;

◇ a 74-year-old borrows a prescription painkiller from a neighbor to relieve arthritic pain.

Since drug use and abuse affects all ages, **prevention and treatment programs should also be continued throughout people's lifetimes**. Some strategies include

◇ encouraging pregnant mothers to attend prenatal care programs to teach them how drugs affect their fetuses;

◇ limiting the use of club drugs at parties through greater public scrutiny of such events;

◇ offering counseling on eating disorders in high schools and colleges;

◇ using outreach workers to encourage drug users to practice safe sex and use clean needles in order to prevent HIV or hepatitis C infection;

◇ coercing a heavily drinking salesman into an employee assistance program (EAP);

◇ holding seminars to enlighten senior citizens about drug cross reactions.

If the basic premise of practicing prevention at every age is accepted, then the questions that need to be answered are, "What are the different theories and methods of prevention?" "Which prevention methods work?" and "How should they be implemented throughout people's lives?"

PREVENTION

CONCEPTS OF PREVENTION

PREVENTION GOALS

Each **society has to decide exactly what it is trying to prevent** and since there is such a diversity of cultures, that decision can be difficult. **Is the society trying to prevent any use of any psychoactive drug, just trying to ban illicit drugs, or simply trying to limit the damage caused by use, abuse, and addiction?** In the United States and most countries, a combination of these three concepts is employed. Thus prevention needs to have several goals. They include

◇ keeping the disease of addiction from ever having a chance to develop by teaching skills that will help the individual to resist drug use, make wise decisions, and resolve inner pain and conflict—all aimed at instilling resiliency and creating alternatives to drug use;

◇ stopping inappropriate or potentially destructive use as soon as possible where it has begun;

◇ in more advanced stages of abuse and addiction, reversing the progression, restoring people to health, and helping them find an alternate way of thinking and living.

"I set out on a mission to rebuild myself. I said, 'Okay, now what would you do if you had to rebuild a car? Well you would take everything apart and you'd start all over.' So what I had to do was shed all the negativity and step down naked so to speak and just build myself up all over again. And this time,

not making mistakes and not making the bad choices that I made before."
48-year-old recovering addict

Traditionally there have been 3 methods used to achieve the above goals:

1. **reduce the supply** of illegal drugs available in society. This is usually done through interdiction of drugs supplies, legislation against use, and legal penalties for possession, distribution, and use;

2. **reduce the demand** for all psychoactive drugs, legal and illegal. This is done through treatment of drug dependency, education, emotional development, moral growth, and individual or community activities;

3. **reduce the harm** that drugs do to users, relatives and friends of users, and society as a whole. This more controversial alternative is done through such methods as promoting temperance, instituting needle exchanges with outreach components, using drug substitution programs (e.g., methadone maintenance), providing resources to lessen the consequences of abuse (e.g., designated drivers, needle exchange programs), and decriminalizing drug use.

Historically **supply reduction and harm reduction (temperance) have been the most widely used methods**. In the twentieth century, with the recognition of addiction as a disease process, demand reduction has become a viable method of prevention. Almost one-half of the projected $11.7 billion in federal funds requested for drug control in 2004 is allocated for demand reduction (Office of National Drug Control

Policy [ONDCP], 2003a). Note that the figures do not include the costs of incarceration and parole, which would almost double the budget.

"A common fault in drug policy has been anticipating or promising dramatic results within an unrealistically brief period. Reducing and stopping drug use requires fundamental changes in the attitudes of millions of Americans and that shift in attitude is more gradual than we would wish. The National Drug Control Strategy promotes a steady pressure against drug use and underscores why drug control must be lifted out of partisan conflict."
Barry R. McCaffrey, former Director, Office of National Drug Control Policy

"We know that treatment works. But we also know that there are too many Americans who, for a variety of reasons, cannot access the treatment they need. By giving people a choice and the means to help connect them with effective treatment, we will be able to more directly help drug users who have recognized their problem.
John P. Walters, Director Office of National Drug Control Policy (ONDCP, 2003b)

HISTORY

Temperance vs. Prohibition

Attempts to regulate drugs, particularly alcohol, have wavered between moderation of use and prohibition. In the United States, eighteenth- and early nineteenth-century attempts to regulate alcohol consumption initially focused on the ideal of temperance. **The guid-**

TABLE 8–1   NATIONAL DRUG CONTROL BUDGET 1995–2004

FUNCTIONAL AREAS	1995	1997	1999	2001	2004 (est.)
Demand Reduction					
Drug abuse treatment	$2,175.80	$2,188.70	$2,230.80	$2,549.40	$2,941.90
Drug abuse prevention	1,104.10	1,162.30	1,461.90	1,598.10	1,496.30
Prevention research	178.60	206.50	249.90	326.80	411.80
Treatment research	262.00	309.60	373.50	489.00	611.00
Total Demand Reduction	**$3,720.50**	**$3,867.00**	**$4,316.10**	**$4,963.40**	**$5,461.00**
Supply Reduction					
Domestic law enforcement	$1,993.40	$2,284.30	$2,542.20	$2,925.30	$3,036.10
International	232.50	389.90	746.30	617.30	1,078.90
Interdiction	1,099.30	1,106.70	2,155.60	1,895.30	2,103.30
Total Supply Reduction	**$3,325.20**	**$3,780.90**	**$5,444.10**	**$5,437.90**	**$6,218.30**
TOTAL BUDGET	**$7,045.70**	**$7,647.90**	**$9,760.10**	**$10,401.30**	**$11,679.30**

(Over the years an additional $6–$10 billion has been spent in the federal, state, and local criminal justice systems.)

(ONDCP, 2003a)

ing assumptions of temperance were that heavy drinking and especially drunkenness were destructive, sinful, and immoral but moderate use could improve health and mood. Initial efforts consisted of convincing drinkers to switch from distilled spirits (hard liquor) to beer, wine, and fermented cider (White, 1998).

By the 1850s the ideal of total abstinence had replaced that of temperance. This ideal eventually led to passage of the Eighteenth Amendment to the Constitution forbidding the manufacture, sale, and transportation of alcohol (Jaffe, 1995).

This conflict between moderate use of alcohol/psychoactive drugs and moral/legal abhorrence of any use of any amount persists to the present day. Historically with alcohol, the concept of complete prohibition, or lately zero tolerance, seems to run on a 70-year cycle: 1780, 1850, 1920, 1990. (Over the last 15 years, all states raised their drinking age to 21 while some states decreased the allowable blood alcohol concentration (BAC) from .10 down to .08. In 1995 Louisiana became the first state to lower the drinking age back to 18 years. Currently several states have enacted zero tolerance laws that suspend driver licenses of youths under 21 convicted of driving with a

BAC of just .01, the equivalent of about half a beer.

Did Prohibition Really Fail?

Popular belief over the decades has been that **Prohibition, enacted into law in 1917 by the Eighteenth Amendment** (enforced starting in 1919 **and repealed in 1933**), was ineffective. An examination of medical records concerning diseases caused by excess alcohol consumption as well as criminal justice records shows that **Prohibition did reduce health problems, domestic violence, crime, and consumption.**

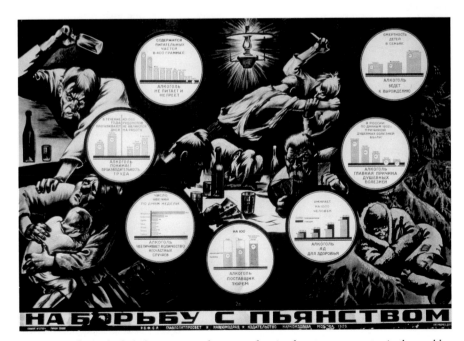

Attempts to limit alcohol abuse were and are prevalent in almost every country in the world. This Russian anti-alcohol poster from 1926 coincided with Prohibition in the United States.
Courtesy of the National Library of Medicine, Bethesda, MD

◊ Admissions to mental hospitals for alcoholic psychosis in Massachusetts fell from a rate of 14.6 per 100,000 in 1910, to 6.4 in 1922, and 7.7 in 1929. In New York the rate fell from 11.5 in 1910, to 3.0 in 1920, and rose back up to 6.5 in 1931 (Aaron & Musto, 1981).

◊ Nationally death rates from cirrhosis of the liver went from 14.8 per 100,000 in 1907, to 7.1 in 1920, and stayed below 7.5 through the rest of the 1920s (Jaffe, 1995).

◊ In addition there were decreased legal costs of jailing drunks, less domestic violence, and less crime in general.

◊ Per capita alcohol consumption dropped in half and did not climb back to pre-Prohibition levels until 20–30 years after Prohibition was repealed.

◊ As bootlegging increased the supply of alcohol in the late 1920s, medical problems increased again but still stayed way below pre-Prohibition levels.

The myth that Prohibition created organized crime wasn't really true. **Criminal organizations existed long before Prohibition; although organizational techniques were refined during this era** and prepared the mobs to step into smuggling and distribution of illicit drugs.

Even though Prohibition did reduce illness and crime, or possibly because it did, concern for and treatment of the alcoholic decreased. Prohibitionists thought that all they needed to do was ban alcohol and the problems would be solved (Lender & Martin, 1987). They also tried to criminalize drinking itself even though Prohibition only banned the "manufacture, sale, and transportation of intoxicating liquors." There was support for Prohibition from President Hoover and most state governors in 1928 and if the Great Depression hadn't occurred in the 1930s, the Eighteenth Amendment might have lasted years longer. **The need for increased tax revenue, the activities of the anti-Prohibition forces called the**

"Wets," and the general public's desire to drink again caused its repeal.

Scare Tactics & Drug Information Programs

Concerted attempts to lessen substance abuse didn't begin in earnest until the 1960s when recreational drugs came out of the ghettos and barrios and began to affect middle-class kids. A number of grassroots prevention movements began in the '60s and '70s as the percentage of Americans who had used any illicit drug went from 2% in 1962 to 31% in 1979 (Rusche, 1995; Substance Abuse and Mental Health Services Administration [SAMHSA], 2002).

These early prevention programs assumed that young people lacked knowledge about the dangerous effects of psychoactive drugs. **Knowledge-based programs were established to teach students about pharmacological effects, causes of addiction, health effects of drug use, and legal penalties.** Providing factual information with a heavy dose of scare tactics was considered enough to reduce drug use. Often the scare tactics overwhelmed the information or made the truth suspect to students. Unfortunately early scare tactics also presented nonfactual or distorted information about drugs, destroying the credibility of the message.

"In the early 1970s the government asked a group of treatment professionals, including myself, to review 297 drug education films that were available. We found that we could barely recommend even 1 or 2 of the films because most of them had bad information, relied only on scare tactics, or were just poorly made."
Darryl Inaba, Pharm.D., CEO, Haight Ashbury Clinics

Although factual information produced documentable increases in knowledge and changes in attitude and is still thought to persuade some young people into rational abstention, **there is little evidence that drug information alone causes changes in behavior.**

"I received only one drug education lesson in my 9th grade health class. They talked a lot about all the different types of drugs and drug use. The class actually made me quite aware that I was missing out on a whole lot of drugs. By the time I ended up in therapeutic boarding school, I knew a lot about drug use and abuse but only because of the extensive drug history I had."
Recovering 21-year-old college student

The role of knowledge in comprehensive prevention programs is still unknown. Some studies indicate that among certain adolescent audiences, factual information actually stimulates experimentation (Moskowitz, 1989). It has been suggested that adolescents' feelings of invulnerability, a limited view of the future, and an indifference to long-term health consequences all frustrate information-only approaches. School-centered knowledge-based programs may also miss students who skip school frequently and are most at risk for health and crime problems associated with drug abuse. However, **good prevention efforts greatly lessen drug problems at a fraction of the cost of supply reduction efforts.** These programs often suffer from underskilled teachers and trainers, or they are not appropriate to the developmental level of targeted students, or they are too brief.

Skill-Building & Resiliency Programs

Prevention efforts then expanded to address the psychological and developmental factors that might predispose individuals to turn to drugs and the social skills that might protect them from experimentation and abuse. The more risk factors that youths have, the more likely they are to abuse drugs (Hird, Khuri, Dusenbury, & Millman, 1997; Bry, McKeon, & Pandina, 1982). Increasing skills that effectively address these risks may result in a solid prevention strategy.

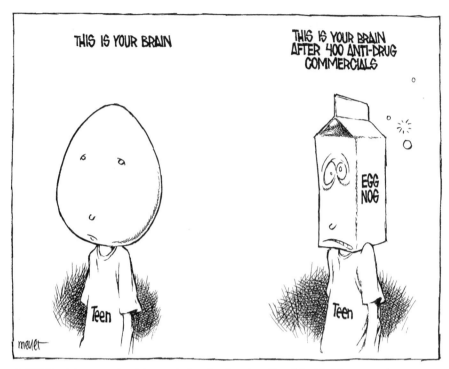

THIS IS YOUR BRAIN

THIS IS YOUR BRAIN AFTER 400 ANTI-DRUG COMMERCIALS

EGG NOG

Teen

Teen

meyer

© 1997 Tom Meyer. Reprinted, by permission, San Francisco Chronicle. All rights reserved.

◊ **General competency building:** The aim is to teach people how to adjust to life through **training in self-esteem, in socially acceptable behavior, and in decision-making, self-assertion, problem-solving, and vocational skills.** Programs employing these prevention strategies continue to report positive results but once training ceases, the gains are soon lost. Periodic booster shots throughout a student's educational career improve the effectiveness of this kind of prevention education.

◊ **Special coping skills:** Coping skills, like parenting classes, stress management, and even breathing classes, are taught to help people face stressful situations. Coping skills are seen as ways of **developing the self-reliance, confidence, and inner resources needed to resist drug use**.

◊ **Reinforcing protective factors and resiliency:** These are ways to **build on natural strengths that people already have available.** The factors that seem to increase re-siliency are optimism, empathy, insight, intellectual competence, self-esteem, direction or purpose in life, and determination (Kumpfer, 1994). These factors, along with supportive friends and family and opportunities to belong to meaningful groups in their own communities, all emphasize that coping resources are usually available to most people.

◊ **Support system development:** The purpose of this method is to **provide easy access to sympathetic resources such as telephone reassurance for the elderly** who are living alone or homework hotlines for students struggling with the stress of school. Stress reduction leads to decreased drug and alcohol abuse.

Changing the Environment

Gradually prevention programs began to look beyond individuals to the social and environmental influences on drug use, such as family and peer group values and practices as well as media influences. Community organization was stressed as a way to ensure cultural sensitivity and to provide local control over prevention efforts, like billboard and advertising distribution controls. Some community programs focused on societal and organizational change, such as altering practices in schools, work situations, organizations, cultures, and society at large. **These community-based systems-oriented programs have been effective in getting entire neighborhoods to take responsibility for preventing substance abuse.**

Typical community coalition activities include

◊ **assessing the needs** of the community and the patterns of drug abuse;

◊ **coordinating existing services** to avoid costly redundancy and fill in the service gaps;

◊ **changing laws and public policy** to reduce availability of alcohol and tobacco;

◊ **increasing funding** for family, school, and community prevention services;

◊ **community-wide training and planning.**

(Kumpfer, Goplerud, & Alvarado, 1998)

Public Health Model

As the complexity of prevention efforts increased, a model was needed to better understand the relationships between all elements in society. The result was the public health approach to prevention.

The public health model holds that addiction is a disease in a **genetically predisposed host** (the actual user) who lives in a **contributory environment** (the actual location and the social network of the host) in which an **agent** (the drug or drugs) **introduces the disease. Therefore prevention is designed to affect the relationship of these three factors to control addiction** (Hoffman, 1998).

For example, programs to regulate cigarette advertising are designed to limit the pervasiveness of the agent in the environment. Programs to raise the drinking age or to have drug-free zones around schools are designed to limit the host's access to the agent. National antismoking, drunk driver, and HIV risk reduction campaigns, which constitute the bulk of the highly visible programs, seek to limit the influence of the environment on the host.

Other prevention activities aimed at the environment-host relationship are designed to reinforce the emotional strengths and protective elements already existing in people's lives or to improve the economic and emotional environment of those most at risk.

Family Approach

Recently a family-focused approach has been embraced by treatment and prevention specialists. The family approach makes sense since susceptibility to addiction often stems from family dynamics. **Family support, skills training, and therapy, along with parenting programs, seem to reduce the risk factors** that lead to drug abuse and addiction (Kumpfer et al., 1998). Certainly any process that reduces abuse, decreases parental use of drugs, and helps the family members improve their relationships with each other must be of benefit to a potential abuser. Unfortunately much of the focus is on the potential addict rather than on the total environment and relationships that have the greatest effect on susceptibility to addiction.

PREVENTION METHODS

Whatever model is used, a good way to understand the effectiveness of the various approaches to prevent drug abuse and addiction is to examine supply, demand, and harm reduction in more detail.

SUPPLY REDUCTION

Supply reduction seeks to decrease drug abuse by reducing the availability of drugs through regulation, restriction, interdiction, and law enforcement. Supply reduction is the responsibility of

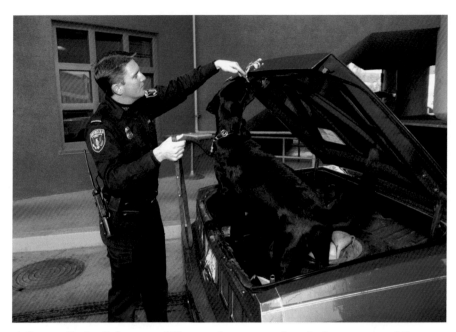

A Customs Canine Enforcement Officer conducts a secondary check on an automobile entering the United States from Mexico. Since the 9/11 attack on the World Trade Center, borders have been tightened to guard against terrorism but the spillover has been felt by drug smugglers.
Courtesy of the U.S. Customs and Border Protection and James R. Tourtellotte

◇ state and local police departments;

◇ the Department of Justice (including the Federal Bureau of Investigation [FBI], the Bureau of Prisons, the Immigration and Naturalization Service [INS], and the Drug Enforcement Administration [DEA]);

◇ the Treasury Department (including the Bureau of Alcohol, Tobacco, and Firearms [ATF], the Internal Revenue Services [IRS], and the Customs Service);

◇ the Department of Transportation (including the U.S. Coast Guard and the Federal Aviation Administration [FAA]);

◇ the Department of Defense.

This complex network of agencies is coordinated by the Office of National Drug Control Policy (ONDCP).

Some of the supply reduction activities include

◇ **interdicting drug smugglers** by air, sea, and highway;

◇ **increasing law enforcement activities at border crossings**;

◇ interdicting and **limiting the supply of precursor chemicals** used in the manufacture of illicit drugs (e.g., ephedrine, a precursor of methamphetamines);

◇ identifying, disrupting, and **dismantling criminal gangs and organized crime**;

◇ supporting and **passing more severe laws** while trying to make sentencing policies fair;

◇ funding the addition of community police officers;

◇ supporting local and state police in high-intensity drug-trafficking areas (HIDTA) as well as coordinating intelligence information and activities;

◇ **disrupting money laundering activities and seizing assets** of drug dealers to limit the profits from illegal drug activities;

◇ breaking up domestic and foreign sources of supply by supporting eradication and the antidrug efforts of countries like Colombia, Pakistan, and Mexico;

◊ enacting treaties and other international agreements to work conjointly towards supply reduction goals.

(ONDCP, 2003b)

Legislation & Legal Penalties

Historically laws to control the use of opium and other drugs did not exist in America prior to the nineteenth century. It wasn't until 1860 that the first antimorphine law was passed and not until 1906 that the Pure Food and Drug Act was approved by Congress. In 1914 the Harrison Narcotics Act was approved, enacting the first major drug controls. Since then laws such as the Comprehensive Drug Abuse and Control Act of 1970, the Sentencing Reform Act of 1984, and the Anti-Drug Abuse Acts of 1986 and 1988 established federal guidelines for mandatory minimum sentences including a minimum 5-year sentence for possession of 5 grams of cocaine base. Note that many believe these latter acts to be discriminatory against African Americans since possession of a greater quantity of powder cocaine results in significantly more lenient sentences. Other legislation has included the Federal Controlled Substance Analogue Act of 1986 (controls designer psychostimulants), Omnibus Drug Act of 1988 (prosecutes money laundering, smuggling drugs and precursor chemicals, etc.), various asset forfeiture laws, chemical precursor laws, and most recently the Illicit Drug Anti-Proliferation Act, enacted in 2003 to protect youth from club drugs such as ecstasy (Drug Enforcement Administration [DEA], 2003c). To curtail drug availability, stiffer penalties that include **long prison terms and asset forfeiture** are given to suppliers (those who manufacture, smuggle, and distribute). On the other hand, in the past 15 years **increased jail time just for use has increased dramatically**. Legal penalties increase for each conviction for possession. In most states, laws also make it illegal just to possess syringes (Carlson, 1998). Such laws, however, increase the possibility that injection drug users will share needles and increase exposure to blood-borne viruses like HIV and hepatitis C.

Women have been prosecuted because they used dangerous substances during their pregnancy ("Hands Off," 1998). Prosecution can be counterproductive in that pregnant drug abusers might be less likely to present themselves for prenatal treatment of drug abuse and even normal prenatal care if they fear that they will be jailed or lose their babies. Lack of prenatal care seems to have greater long-term adverse effects on the baby than use of cocaine (Klein & Goldenberg, 1990). Pilot programs in New York City and in Michigan have tied welfare payments to drug testing as a way of routing clients into treatment ("Plans to Link," 1999).

"I was thinking about going out but then I thought, 'You're gonna have to take the UA [urine drug test], and then your UA's gonna come up dirty, and then there goes your son, there goes your daughter, and the baby that's in your stomach.' You lose your house, hell that was just too much work. I decided not to get loaded."
32-year-old woman in recovery

The so-called three strikes and you're out law requires a life sentence for three convictions (originally to get habitual violent criminals off the street but later expanded to other crimes). As a result of this and other laws, **the prison population (federal, state, and local) has more than tripled between 1980 and 2002 to approximately 2 million. Nearly 55% of the inmates in federal prisons were sentenced for drug offenses in 2003**, down from 60% in 1998 (U.S. Department of Justice [DOJ], 2003). Today between 60% and 80% of those in all prisons are there for drug-related crimes such as use and possession, for crimes committed under the influence of alcohol or other drugs, and for crimes committed to raise money for a drug habit. More than **half of the inmates reported drug use while committing the offense** that put them in prison (Mumola, 1998; ONDCP, 2000; DOJ, 2002).

Sales to minors or sales near schools may earn a perpetrator up to twice the

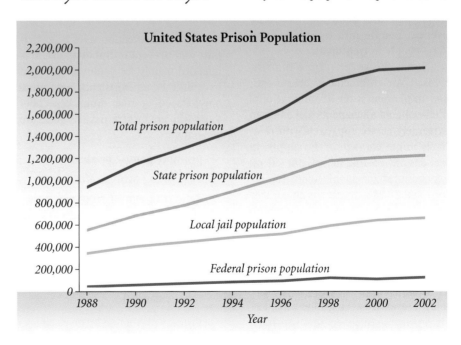

Figure 8-1 •

Nearly one in four inmates in state and local prisons or jails is incarcerated for violating a specific drug law. In federal prisons that figure is close to 60%.
2003 Bureau of Justice Statistics Bulletin (DOJ, 2003)

usual sentence. Supply reduction legislation sometimes extends to laws against products made from hemp and to advertising or sales of drug paraphernalia, the devices used to prepare or consume drugs, such as roach clips and bongs sold in so-called head shops (DEA, 2003a). Governments also promulgate laws that regulate the sale of legal prescription drugs and the availability of alcohol and nicotine. Recent proposals target even more precursor chemicals used to manufacture drugs illegally (e.g., ephedrine, ether, sulfuric acid).

Outcomes of Supply Reduction

The success of supply reduction approaches to the drug problem are debatable. Clearly the estimated 10–15% of drugs that are kept off the market means that a significant amount of illegal drugs never reach the streets (DEA, 2003b; ONDCP, 2000). The number of people imprisoned for drug crimes cuts down on the use and distribution of drugs and an unknown number of people are dissuaded from becoming involved with drugs by the threat of imprisonment. **Advocates of supply reduction say strict policies and strong penalties delay the impulse to use, get people into treatment, and keep people in treatment.**

Some, however, argue that increased law enforcement, court costs, and implementation of international drug-policing agreements make this an **extremely costly approach with relatively minor impact on the supply.** In fact despite a 5-fold increase in federal expenditures for supply reduction efforts since 1986, cocaine is about 25% cheaper today than a decade ago (ONDCP, 2003a).

One of the bright spots in law enforcement is the **increased use of drug courts to avoid clogging the justice system with thousands of minor drug-use arrests.** First-time offenders are diverted to treatment thus **shifting a supply reduction technique to a demand reduction strategy.** Further, treatment outcome studies suggest that mandated treatment of drug abuse by law enforcement results in better outcomes than those achieved through voluntary treatment (Anglin, Prendergast, & Farabee, 1998; Nurco, Hanlon, Bateman, & Kinlock, 1995).

DEMAND REDUCTION

The second major area of current prevention strategy has focused on reducing the demand for drugs. Those pursuing demand reduction believe that the health and crime problems associated with drug abuse could be greatly lessened to a fraction of the cost of supply reduction efforts if any of 3 conditions were met:

1. if individuals never develop an interest in using psychoactive drugs,

2. if those using never progress to abuse or addiction,

3. or if those who abuse drugs or are addicted to them can get treatment and stop their continued use of drugs.

These conditions translate into three levels of demand reduction (prevention) programs that have been developed to decrease drug abuse.

Primary Prevention

Primary prevention **tries to anticipate and prevent initial drug use.** It is intended mainly for young people who have little or no experience with alcohol, tobacco, or other drugs, especially those who are most at risk. Its goals are generally to

◇ **promote nonuse or abstinence**;

◇ **help young people refuse drugs**;

◇ **delay the age of first use**, especially of the legal drugs alcohol and tobacco;

◇ encourage healthy nondrug alternatives to achieving altered states of consciousness (Friday night nonalcoholic dances).

Primary prevention involves education about harmful consequences of psychoactive substance use along with personal skill-building exercises designed to prevent or delay experimentation with abusable drugs. **It attempts to instill resistance by teaching skills in coping, decision making, conflict resolution**, and other abilities that assist young people from ever using psychoactive substances (Hazelden Foundation, 1993). It also undertakes to build self-esteem by examining the roots of susceptibility to addiction and helping children handle the confusion, anger, or pain of growing up. In a broad sense primary prevention also includes nonpersonal strategies such as legislation, policy formulation, and school curriculum design meant to prevent or delay first use.

Though the importance of primary prevention is universally accepted, outcome evaluation of its effectiveness gives mixed reviews of program results. Controversy also exists over the best way to accomplish this important level of prevention (Kumpfer et al., 1998).

Recently the ONDCP designed a set of principles upon which prevention programming can be based.

Primary prevention is the most important level of demand reduction. Many studies over the past several years have demonstrated that the age of first use is the strongest predictor of future drug or alcohol problems. Youths who begin drug experimentation at age 10–12 are 4 to 5 times more likely to have future drug or alcohol problems than those who delay their first use to age 16–18. Others who delay their first use of drugs or alcohol until after the age of 25 rarely develop any drug problems (De Wit, Offord, & Wong, 1997).

Secondary Prevention

Secondary prevention **seeks to halt drug use once it has begun.** It strives to keep experimental, social/recreational, and habitual use, along with limited abuse, from turning into prolonged abuse and addiction by taking action when symptoms are first recognized. It educates people about specific health effects, legal consequences, and effects on a family. It can also provide counseling.

Secondary prevention **adds intervention strategies to education and skill building.** Once drug use is recog-

TABLE 8–2   EVIDENCE-BASED PRINCIPLES FOR SUBSTANCE ABUSE PREVENTION

A. Address appropriate risk and protective factors for substance abuse in a defined population.
  1. Define a population (e.g., by age, gender, race, neighborhood).
  2. Assess levels of risk, protection, and substance abuse for that population.
  3. Focus on all levels of risk with special attention to those exposed to high risk and low protection.
B. Use approaches that have been shown to be effective.
  4. Reduce the availability of illicit drugs and of alcohol and tobacco for the underaged.
  5. Strengthen antidrug use attitudes and norms.
  6. Strengthen life skills and drug refusal techniques.
  7. Reduce risk and enhance protection in families by strengthening family skills.
  8. Strengthen social bonding and caring relationships.
  9. Ensure that interventions are appropriate for the populations being addressed.
C. Intervene early at important stages and transitions.
  10. Intervene at developmental stages and life transitions that predict later substance abuse.
  11. Reinforce interventions over time with repeated exposure to accurate and age-appropriate information.
D. Intervene in appropriate settings and domains.
  12. Intervene in appropriate settings that most affect risk, including homes, schools, and peer groups.
E. Manage programs effectively.
  13. Ensure consistency and coverage of programs and policies.
  14. Train staff and volunteers to communicate messages.
  15. Monitor and evaluate programs to verify that goals and objectives are being achieved.

(ONDCP, 2000)

nized, a number of different intervention techniques are employed to engage the user in educational and counseling processes that encourage abstinence and provide skills to avoid further use or abuse.

Drug diversion programs (e.g., drug courts) used at this level of prevention for first-time drug offenders have proven to be useful and cost-effective. Drug diversion programs route those arrested for possession or use to education and rehabilitation programs instead of jail.

Secondary prevention is somewhat handicapped by two actions typical of drug abusers and even casual users: concealment that makes use more difficult to detect and denial that prevents the user from acknowledging that there is a problem. On average it takes 2 years for parents to recognize drug use and abuse in their children.

Also complicating secondary prevention is the lag phase, the time between first use of a drug and the development of problematic use. The lag phase is particularly long for tobacco since it may take decades for severe health problems to develop after initial smoking begins. Because most drug users describe their initial use of drugs to be enjoyable and problem free, denial and a sense of personal invulnerability to adverse consequences, along with the lag phase, make them less likely to believe that information about harmful effects applies to them.

"I didn't have a clue. Why couldn't I handle this? I never really attributed all the problems that I had to the drinking because I was a periodic drinker, so I could go for periods of abstaining. But once I started, there was always going to be repercussions. So it was hard for me to identify the problems in the beginning."
42-year-old recovering alcoholic

Tertiary Prevention

Tertiary prevention **seeks to stop further damage from habituation, abuse, and addiction to drugs and to restore drug abusers to health.** It joins drug abuse treatment with strategies employed in primary and secondary prevention, such as intervention and drug diversion programs. Tertiary prevention seeks to end compulsive drug use with such strategies as

◇ **group intervention** to engage a person in a treatment program focused on detoxification, abstinence, and recovery;

◇ **cue extinction therapy** that desensitizes clients to people, places, or things that trigger use;

◇ **family therapy** (especially for younger users), group psychotherapy, or residential treatment in therapeutic communities;

◇ **psychopharmacological strategies** like methadone maintenance and drugs that reduce craving;

◇ **promotion of a healthy lifestyle**;

◇ **development of support and aftercare systems**, often 12-step programs.

Advocates of demand reduction, while admitting that interdiction decreases the availability of drugs, point out that young people reported alcohol and other drugs to be more available in 2001 than students did in 1980 (University of Michigan, 2003).

"In our experience over the past 30 years, the best and most cost-effective prevention strategy is treatment on demand."
Darryl Inaba, Pharm.D., CEO, Haight Ashbury Clinics

Treatment of alcoholism and drug addiction has been extensively researched and has consistently been documented to be effective. **Treatment**

(tertiary prevention) results in abstinence or decreased drug use in
40–50% of cases, a great reduction in
crime (74%), and a savings of $4–$20
for every $1 spent by a community
(Gerstein et al., 1994). Despite these results, funding for treatment programs
consistently falls short of meeting the
needs of those seeking treatment. (The
Haight Ashbury Detox Clinic in San
Francisco alone has over 400 people on
their waiting list every month. Only
20–30% of those on its waiting list ever
come into treatment at the Clinic possibly because they initially came for help
at their most vulnerable and treatable
moment.)

Drug courts have further increased
treatment demand without providing
more treatment resources. A drug court
is a collaboration of the court, prosecution, public defenders, probation officers, treatment providers, and sheriff's
department to coordinate treatment and
facilitate processing of convicted drug
offenders. As of 2000, there were 508
drug courts operating with another 281
planned. Drug courts make sense since
incarceration costs between $20,000
and $50,000 a year per prisoner vs.
$2,500 for a well-run drug court pro-
gram (National Criminal Justice Reference
System, 2000).

HARM REDUCTION

Harm reduction is a prevention
strategy that recognizes the difficulty
of getting and keeping people in recovery. It focuses on techniques to minimize the personal and social problems associated with drug use rather
than making abstinence the primary
goal.

One example of a harm reduction
tactic is providing clean syringes to addicts. A panel jointly convened by the
National Research Council (NRC) and
the National Institute of Medicine
(NIM) found that bleach distribution
and needle exchange efforts can reduce the spread of the AIDS virus
without increasing illegal drug use. It
is interesting to note that the study did
not say "does reduce" or "has reduced,"
only that it "can reduce" the spread of

AIDS (National Research Council, 1995). As
of 1999, 47 U.S. states had laws that
make it illegal for injection drug users
to possess syringes (Blumenthal, Kral,
Erringer, & Edlin, 1999). The controversy
continues as to whether needle exchange itself actually works. More than
131 needle exchange programs provide
more than 19 million syringes to IV
drug users in the United States (Centers
for Disease Control [CDC], 2001). In Australia with a population one-tenth that
of the United States, 10 million syringes are exchanged from 4,000 outlets. Less than 5% of Australian drug
users are HIV positive compared to an
estimated 14% in the United States
(Wodak & Lurie, 1997). The estimated
smaller number of HIV infections in
Australia saved about $220 million in
drug-related expenses at a cost of $8
million for the 10 million needles and
syringes (Feacham, 1995).

"The reason why we are so intent on
needle use is because it's the route to
the heterosexual population and to
babies. If you can stop the needle from
infecting heterosexual men, then you
stop most of the cause of the spread of
HIV to heterosexual women and to
babies."

John Newmeyer, Ph.D., drug epidemiologist, Haight
Ashbury Clinic

Another example of harm reduction involves substituting a legal drug
addiction for an illegal one as in
methadone maintenance programs.
These programs have been shown to
decrease crime and health problems in
the user. About 205,000 patients were
enrolled in 950 methadone maintenance programs and 250 methadone
detoxification clinics, about 12–30% of
all heroin addicts in the United States
(depending on the survey) (American Association for the Treatment of Opioid Dependence, 2003). A study by the University of
Pennsylvania found that comprehensive methadone treatment combined
with intensive counseling reduced illicit drug use by 79%. Clients were also
five times less likely to get AIDS (Metz-

ger, Woody, McLellan, et al., 1993). Addition-
ally criminal activity was reduced by
57% while full-time employment increased by 24% (Hubbard, Craddock, Flynn,
Anderson, & Etheridge, 1997).

In the broad sense of reducing the
harm of use without promoting abstinence, some harm reduction tactics for
alcohol and tobacco have already been
used. Examples include designated
driver programs, encouraging eating
when drinking, regulating alcohol and
tobacco advertising, and providing
users with information on less harmful
ways to use drugs.

These legal drug prevention tactics
receive some criticism because they
may be misapplied. For example,
someone gets even drunker when there
is a designated driver, or someone uses
moderation as an excuse to break abstinence, or someone augments methadone with alcohol and other drugs to
try to get a rush. Harm reduction
practices and proposals that are very
controversial include

◇ responsible use education that accepts some level of experimental or
   social use and seeks to inform people of ways of using drugs that minimize dangers;

◇ decriminalization or even legalization of all abused drugs;

◇ treatment of addicts merely to reduce their habits to manageable
   levels;

◇ permitting addicts to totally design
   and manage their intervention and
   treatment processes.

Some harm reduction tactics also
seem to be in conflict with federal drug
policy based on zero tolerance (no use
of illegal drugs). Changes in laws and
policies will probably not be forthcom-
ing soon since many elected officials
are afraid of appearing soft on crime
and drugs. War on drugs advocates fear
that any attempt at decriminalization or
legalization would introduce the kind
of ambiguity about drugs that prevailed
in the 1970s, creating confusion about
whether drug use is undesirable. (See
Chapter 9 for further discussion of
harm reduction.)

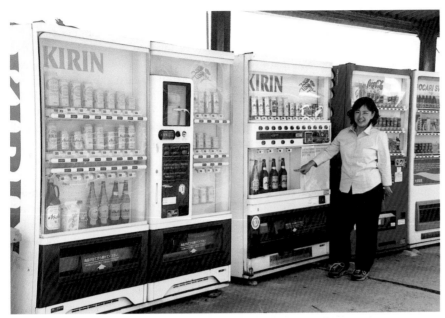

In Japan, beer is available in vending machines. In other countries, especially the United States, this kind of environmental availability of alcohol would be unheard of but in Japan, it is acceptable and not often abused by underage drinkers.

© 2002 Dr. Darryl Inaba

●●●

"I had a parole officer who told me to leave those other drugs alone. Drinking is OK or smoking a little pot now and then but I have come to believe that I can't take any mood-altering chemical into my body today and still remain in recovery. That is still what I stick to and believe in."

Recovering heroin addict

CHALLENGES TO PREVENTION

LEGAL DRUGS IN SOCIETY

For all the effort put into prevention of illicit drug use, we are still primarily an alcohol-drinking, tobacco-smoking, prescription and over-the-counter drug-using society. **The social and health problems from alcohol abuse, along with the health problems from tobacco abuse, are far greater than those of illicit drugs.** Wisely drug abuse prevention efforts over the last decade have increased the emphasis on alcohol and tobacco abuse and most recently on behavioral addictions such as gambling, eating disorders, and sexual addiction that also have devastating effects on society.

Legal drugs such as tobacco and alcohol are widely available and actively marketed by sophisticated advertising campaigns that attempt to show the fun to be found in psychoactive drugs and that try to establish brand recognition and brand loyalty at an early age. Joe Camel® and the Budweiser® frogs were examples of familiar cartoon-like characters that targeted young potential smokers and drinkers. Each year alcohol companies spend over $2 billion and tobacco companies over $11.2 billion on advertising and promoting their products (Federal Trade Commission, 2003). This is not surprising since alcohol sales are about $100 billion per year and tobacco sales over $46 billion per year (U. S. Department of Agriculture, 1999). (There is something to be learned here. If advertising was successful by targeting age-specific and culture-specific populations, prevention groups can do the same by customizing their messages.)

Billions more are spent advertising over-the-counter and prescription drugs thus promoting the concept that there is a chemical solution for any ailment or discomfort. This two-tiered approach, acceptable and unacceptable drugs, breeds cynicism and disbelief of prevention messages in adolescents and young adults. If prevention messages aren't consistent, they are usually ineffective.

One of the realities of prevention is that there is no quick fix. If modern attempts to reduce smoking began with the first health warnings issued in the mid-1950s, then the success of the **antismoking efforts have taken almost a half a century** and are still developing. First knowledge must change, then attitudes, and finally practices. These changes can take a generation or more. When change comes, it can be profound—no smoking in public buildings, restaurants, offices, etc. was unheard of a few decades ago. In 2003 the state of New York passed a ban on smoking in virtually all businesses and indoor locations except in one's home or car, in cigar bars, and at Indian casinos. California and Delaware also have stringent laws.

A second reality of prevention is that the job is never complete. Each year there is a new group entering grammar school, middle school, high school, and college who need to learn or at least be reminded of the potential dangers of smoking and drinking. The high level of adolescent smoking in the last decade is due in part to a diminished antismoking campaign, compared with relatively strenuous efforts conducted in the late '60s through the '70s that included public service ads on TV, limitations on tobacco broadcast advertising, and increased cigarette taxes. (Taxing tobacco does work; an increase of taxes in Oregon reduced per capita cigarette consumption 20% between 1997 and 1999 ["Tobacco Tax," 2000]).

Third, any prevention campaign becomes progressively more difficult. Prevention techniques succeed better with people ready to listen—those already predisposed to heed warnings.

After initial successes it becomes harder to penetrate deeper into any particular generation to change attitudes and behaviors.

Another challenge to prevention is that **no single approach has been shown to work consistently**, probably because there are so many variables that contribute to substance abuse and addiction. There is no doubt that if and when prevention efforts become consistently and documentably successful, they will be cost effective. The difficulty is finding undeniably effective prevention programs.

A recent problem with legal drugs is the **increase in states that allow medical marijuana** or have reduced penalties for possession. As of May 2003 those included Alaska, Arizona, California, Colorado, Hawaii, Maine, Maryland, Nevada, Oregon, and Washington. Five more states are considering legislation to allow medical marijuana (Willing, 2003). There is considerable conflict between the federal government and the individual states over this subject. Overseas, governments are grappling with this issue. Since 2001 in the Netherlands, pharmacies may fill prescriptions for marijuana with the cost being covered by insurance. Before, patients had to buy their own marijuana at one of the country's 800 so-called coffee shops.

FUNDING

Prevention is vastly underfunded especially when compared to the cost of the consequences of alcohol and drug abuse and the moneys committed to tobacco and alcohol advertising. Cocaine-exposed babies alone are estimated to cost the United States $352 million annually (National Institute on Drug Abuse [NIDA], 1998). In 2000 the economic cost of drug and alcohol abuse to the United States was an estimated $160 billion (e.g., lost earnings, health care, crime control). That figure has gone up since then. **In 2000 an estimated $64 billion were diverted from the economy by users to purchase the drugs** while the total national expenditure for primary prevention in the same year was just $8 billion (ONDCP, 2003a).

FROM CRADLE TO GRAVE

PATTERNS OF USE

Since drug use affects us directly or indirectly from cradle to grave, examining the patterns of use of different age groups in our society makes it possible to design prevention programs that have a better chance of success.

USE BY RACE & CLASS

Addicts are often portrayed in the media as inner-city dwellers who are weak, bad, stupid, crazy, immoral, and poor or as the disenfranchised who have nothing else to turn to except drugs. When drug use is studied on a regional basis, the facts show that rural and small urban areas use as much and in some cases more drugs per capita than large urban areas (SAMHSA, 2002). Even in large cities, less than 5% of alcoholics live on skid row in the poor sections of cities. When ethnicity was used as a measure, the differences in overall drug use were minimal, although the use of some specific drugs is higher in certain ethnic, cultural, economic, or social communities (Joseph & Paone, 1997).

The group least likely to have an alcohol problem was African Americans while those of Hispanic origin were least likely to have an illicit drug use problem. Whites and African Americans were about even, percentage wise, in their use of illicit drugs (SAMHSA, 2002). The relatively high rate of African Americans in prisons suggests either that this ethnic group tends to fall prey more readily to the negative aspects of addiction, including dealing, or that they may be the target of greater law enforcement efforts. African Americans with drug problems tend to be incarcerated at a greater rate and receive treatment through the criminal justice system whereas Whites are more likely to get probation and receive treatment from medical and social service programs. In fact African Americans are 57 times more likely to go to prison for drug crimes than Whites.

"They come to Black neighborhoods to cop dope. It's like a pretty regular thing to see White people go slipping around through there at night. Now crack cocaine is not Black or White. Crack cocaine is dope. It doesn't care who it gets. I have sat down with people up here and I have sat down with people from down there and when we do dope, it is all the same."
Recovering cocaine addict

Alcoholics and addicts include not only residents in the inner city but also the most skilled, talented, intelligent, and sensitive individuals in our society. For example, physicians are as likely to be as addicted or possibly slightly more so than members of the general population possibly due to accessibility to drugs and a higher income level (Anthony & Hetzer, 1991; Centrella, 1994). **Intelligence is not a guaranteed protection against addiction.** Members of MENSA, a high-IQ society, also have a relatively high rate of addiction, as do gifted high school students. Members of the American clergy also have a higher-than-average rate of alcoholism. Even nuns have a problem with prescription drug abuse. If people use psychoactive substances, they are liable to addictive disease no matter what race, class, or region of the country they live in. Addiction is an equal opportunity disease.

USE BY AGE

Over the past 35 years **one of the most important changes in drug abuse has been the gradual lowering of the age of drug users**. This is of particular concern since, as we mentioned, one of the most reliable indicators of future addiction problems is early-onset drug use. A 2001 survey by the University of Michigan found that from 1991–2001, the use of marijuana by 8th graders tripled and the use by 10th graders doubled while the use by 12th graders went up 50% although use in the past 3 years has leveled off (University of Michigan, 2003). Another measure of increased use (and possible increased law enforcement) is that the percentage of male juvenile arrestees testing positive for any drug except alcohol went from 22% in 1990 to 48--65% in selected cities in 2001 (Arrestee Drug Abuse Monitoring [ADAM], 2003).

The absolute numbers of Americans who used illicit drugs in the past month (16 million in a population of 223 million, 12 and older) may seem small, however, they have an exaggerated effect on all levels of society especially in regard to economic loss, accidents, assaults, suicides, crime, and domestic or other violence (SAMHSA, 2002; ONDCP, 2003a).

In the rest of this chapter, we will examine the consequences of drug use during pregnancy, in school, on the job (including a section on drug testing), by the elderly, and some of the most dangerous consequences of drug use—sexually transmitted diseases, hepatitis C, and AIDS. We will then examine some of the prevention and early intervention programs designed for those groups.

TABLE 8–3 AVERAGE AGE OF INITIATION OF DIFFERENT SUBSTANCES 1965–2000

(These figures show the mean age of first use among those who have used various drugs.)

Drug	1965	1975	1985	1990	1995	2000
Cigarettes (first use)	15.5 yrs.	15.0 yrs.	15.9 yrs.	15.4 yrs.	15.4 yrs.	15.4 yrs. (est.)
Inhalants	13.4 yrs.	18.2 yrs.	17.6 yrs.	17.6 yrs.	17.9 yrs.	16.2 yrs.
Alcohol	7.6 yrs.	16.8 yrs.	16.6 yrs.	16.9 yrs.	16.4 yrs.	15.9 yrs. (est.)
Hallucinogens	19.0 yrs.	19.6 yrs.	19.1 yrs.	19.2 yrs.	18.0 yrs.	18.6 yrs.
Marijuana/hashish	19.7 yrs.	18.4 yrs.	17.8 yrs.	18.4 yrs.	16.6 yrs.	17.5 yrs.
Heroin	N/A	22.4 yrs.	N/A	24.7 yrs.	20.3 yrs.	22.3 yrs.
Cocaine	N/A	21.4 yrs.	22.1 yrs.	22.9 yrs.	21.1 yrs.	20.0 yrs.

(SAMHSA, 2002)

TABLE 8–4 DRUG USE BY AGE GROUP 2001

Age Group	Used Ever Used	Used Past Year	Used Past Month
12–17 (23 million)			
Any illicit drug	28.4%	20.4%	10.8%
Cigarettes	33.6%	20.0%	13.0%
Alcohol	42.9%	33.9%	17.3%
18–25 (29 million)			
Any illicit drug	55.6%	31.9%	18.8%
Cigarettes	69.0%	46.8%	39.1%
Alcohol	85.0%	75.4%	58.8%
26 & up (171 million)			
Any illicit drug	41.2%	8.2%	4.5%
Cigarettes	71.5%	27.3%	24.2%
Alcohol	86.5%	65.7%	50.8%
Total, 12 & up (223 million)			
Any illicit drug	41.7%	12.6%	7.1%
Cigarettes	67.2%	29.1%	24.9%
Alcohol	81.7%	63.7%	48.3%

(SAMHSA, 2002)

PREGNANCY & BIRTH

OVERVIEW

Drug and alcohol use during pregnancy continues to be a national problem that results in many infants born with physical and mental deficits and even drug-related birth defects. Drug abuse during pregnancy occurs in women of all ethnic and socioeconomic backgrounds. According to the National Institute of Drug Abuse (NIDA), 18.6% of infants were exposed to alcohol at some time during the 9 months of gestation, 4.5% were exposed to cocaine, 17.4% to marijuana, and 17.6% to tobacco (NIDA, 1994; May & Gossage, 2001). **Fetal alcohol syndrome (FAS) is the third most common birth defect and the leading cause of mental retardation in the United States.** Most psychoactive substances may be harmful to the developing fetus. Problems associated with substance abuse during pregnancy are now beginning to be understood.

In the California Perinatal Substance Exposure Study in 1991–1993, the California Department of Alcohol and Drug Programs tried to determine the prevalence of drug-exposed new-

TABLE 8–5   PERCENTAGE OF INFANTS BORN EXPOSED TO DRUGS IN CALIFORNIA 1991-1993

Substance	Asian & Pacific Islander	African American	Hispanic	White	Other	All
Alcohol	5.07%	11.58%	6.87%	6.05%	4.03%	6.72%
Tobacco	1.73%	20.12%	3.29%	14.82%	4.81%	8.82%
Prescription drugs	1.49%	2.38%	1.26%	1.96%	1.31%	1.71%
All illicit drugs	0.39%	11.90%	1.51%	4.92%	1.57%	3.49%
marijuana	0.21%	4.59%	0.61%	3.25%	1.21%	1.88%
cocaine	0.06%	7.79%	0.55%	0.60%	0.20%	1.11%
opioids	0.34%	2.54%	1.06%	1.59%	1.11%	1.47%
amphetamines (illicit & legal)	0.06%	0.19%	0.35%	1.32%	0.24%	0.66%
Total Positives (excluding tobacco)	14.22%	24.02%	9.37%	12.28%	6.76%	11.35%

(Note: Some infants test positive for more than one drug.)

(Source: California Perinatal Substance Exposure Study, 1993 [Noble et al., 1997])

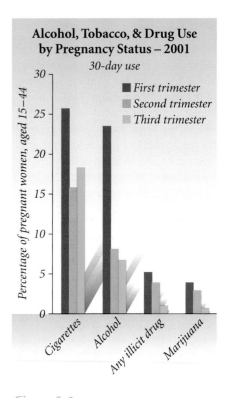

Alcohol, Tobacco, & Drug Use by Pregnancy Status – 2001

Figure 8-2 •

Notice that in the first and second trimesters when the fetus is most vulnerable, drug use, particularly alcohol use, is much higher than just before birth.

National Household Survey on Drug Abuse, 1998 (SAMHSA, 1999a)

borns (Table 8-5). While these rates are high, the actual exposure is probably even higher since most drugs are non-detectable 3 days after exposure. If one looks at drug use at various times during pregnancy, the use of alcohol is higher (Fig. 8-2).

Maternal Risks

"I used after my water broke and I was on my way to the hospital. I got high because I couldn't face bringing another child into domestic violence. And I figured if I got high, at that time, I thought they would take him from me so that he wouldn't have to come home to the violence."

26-year-old recovering addict

Historically the effects of drugs and alcohol on pregnant women and their fetuses have been poorly re-searched or treated. Even when female opium and morphine addicts outnumbered male addicts at the turn of the century, most treatment facilities were aimed at men (Worth, 1991; Young, 1997). In fact, although damage to the fetus due to drinking has been recognized since ancient times, a specific clinical syndrome, FAS, was not identified until

1973 (Jones & Smith, 1973). Starting in the 1980s interest and research on perinatal effects of drugs increased as did funding by the National Institute on Drug Abuse (NIDA), the National Institutes of Health (NIH), and other governmental agencies.

When added to the normal stresses and medical complications of pregnancy, drug and alcohol abuse during this period puts women at even higher risk for medical and obstetrical complications. **Some conditions aggravated by drug use in a pregnant woman include anemia, sexually transmitted diseases, diabetes, high blood pressure, and poor nutrition. In addition, hepatitis C, endocarditis, AIDs and other infections can be contracted from infected needles** (Miller, 1998).

"When I used, my behavior was really dangerous. I'd do things that normal people wouldn't do. I was very promiscuous. I had a lot of unsafe sex. I contracted hepatitis C. I've had numerous STDs. You know, I'd use during all my pregnancies, so my children are affected. The aftereffects still physically affect them you know. It's something I have to live with."

29-year-old recovering mother of four

Eighty percent of children with the HIV virus in the United States were born to mothers who were or are IV drug abusers or sexual partners of IV drug abusers. That figure jumps to 90% worldwide in infants and children. The life expectancy of an infant born with HIV is less than 2 years. Surprisingly in the United States, if AZT (an AIDS drug) therapy is used, only 8% of the newborns will be infected with the virus. If AZT is not used, there is a 25% infection rate (Harris, Thompson, Ball, Hussey, & Sy, 2002). Newer medications lower the rate even more. In underdeveloped countries with less access to AZT and other drugs, that rate jumps to 35–40% (Journal of the American Medical Association [JAMA], 2002; Quinn, 1996; CDC, 1999).

A pregnant addict often has had no prenatal care or medical intervention prior to delivery and often lives a chaotic lifestyle. A further complication of drug use is in pregnant adolescents. Even without the complicating factors of drug use, the infants of adolescent mothers are at higher risk than those born to women over 18. All areas of functioning are affected since the adolescent herself has not yet developed physically, emotionally, or behaviorally (Hechtman, 1989; Kaminer, 1994).

"Across from the hospital where I had my son, when I was supposed to be on my way there, I didn't make it past the park and the hospital was right across the street. I got stuck in the park, and I could literally see the windows of the NICU, know my son's there, but I ended up hangin' out at the park, getting drunk and getting loaded."
27-year-old recovering addict

Fetal &Neonatal Complications

Psychoactive drugs can easily cross the multiple cell layers of the placental barrier, the membrane separating the baby's and the mother's blood (Fig. 8-3), so **a fetus is exposed to the same chemicals that a mother uses. After birth many drugs pass into a nursing mother's breast milk** further exposing a nursing infant to dangerous chemicals.

Because of the fetus's and subsequently infant's metabolic immaturity, each surge of effects caused by the psychoactive drug that the mother injects, ingests, snorts, or smokes may be prolonged in the fetus.

The period of maximum fetal vulnerability is the first 12 weeks. During this first trimester, development and differentiation of cells into fetal limbs and organs occur. This is when drugs pose the greatest risk to organ development. Because the central and peripheral nervous systems develop throughout the entire pregnancy, **the fetus is vulnerable to neurological damage no matter when a woman uses drugs**. The second trimester involves further maturation and continued vulnerability of the organs. Drug exposure at this stage creates a risk of abnormal bleeding or spontaneous abortion. The third trimester includes maturation of the fetus and preparation for birth. Powerful drugs such as heroin or cocaine can cause premature birth. Since drugs can have such a magnified effect on the fetus throughout pregnancy, it is crucial that a pregnant woman abstain from all unnecessary drug exposure.

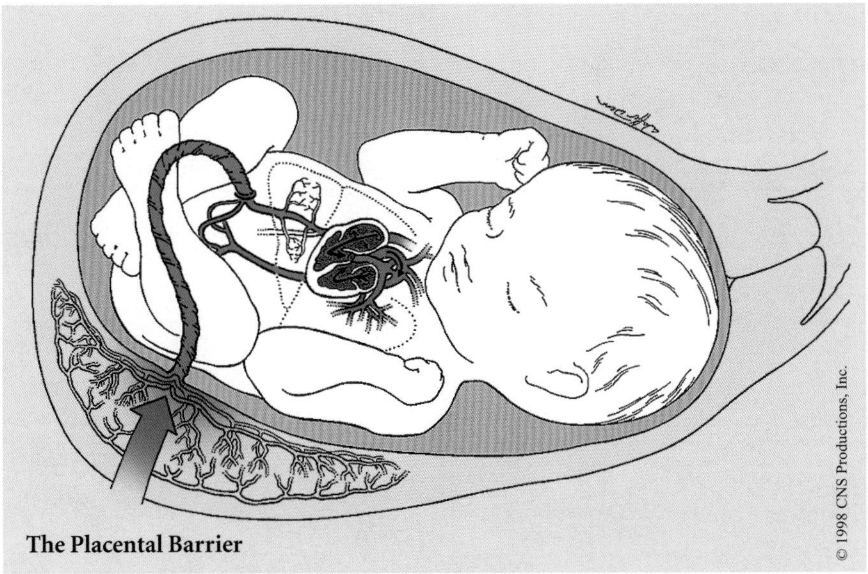

"I was drinking between 3 and 4 liters of wine daily when I was pregnant with her until I was about 8 months. And consequently she was born with fetal alcohol effects. She had a hole in her heart, her digestive system was all messed up, she had projectile vomiting, she didn't gain any weight for about a month. She had to stay in the hospital while I was released. But when she was 3 to 5 she had to have speech therapy."
25-year-old recovering addict

The immaturity of the fetus's metabolic system also causes drugs to remain in the fetus for a longer period and in higher concentrations than in the mother. The problems of fetal drug exposure extend beyond the period of pregnancy. Many babies are born with compromised immune systems due to drug use. **Definite syndromes of neonatal withdrawal, intoxication, and developmental or learning delays have been attributed to a variety of drugs, including alcohol** (Finnegan & Kandall, 1997). In a Florida study the cost of newborn care of those affected by drugs was more than double the normal cost of care for newborns, $11,188 vs. $4,741 (Agency for Health Care Administration, 1999).

Long-Term Effects

"They're older now and some of them have learning disabilities. My oldest son has ADD, my middle son has anger management problems, and because I raised these children in my addiction, you know, they suffer from depression, they have their antisocial skills. I passed the disease of addiction to my oldest son through my behavior and their father's behavior."
29-year-old recovering mother of four

Research is still being done on the long-term effects in drug-exposed children when they enter school. Symptoms range from convulsive disorders

The Placental Barrier

© 1998 CNS Productions, Inc.

Figure 8-3 •

The developing baby is protected by the placental barrier that screens out substances that would affect the fetus. All psychoactive drugs breach this protective barrier and affect the baby usually much more than the mother.

in the most extreme cases, to poor muscular control and cognitive skills, hyperactivity, difficulty concentrating or remembering, violence, apathy, and lack of emotion. The good news is that recent research indicates that **the majority of drug-exposed babies who receive prenatal, perinatal, and postnatal care, along with continued pediatric services, manages to catch up in their development to other nondrug-exposed children after a slow start** (Frank, Augustyn, Knight, Pell, & Zuckerman, 2001). Even without care, some of the effects are reversible. In a study in Ottawa, Canada, children of moderate-drinking mothers showed lower cognitive scores at 36 months but not at 48, 60, or 72 months (Fried, O'Connel, & Watkinson, 1992).

SPECIFIC DRUG EFFECTS

Despite difficulties with scientific research on fetal effects of drug use during pregnancy, scientists have identified prenatal and postnatal symptoms and conditions due to specific psychoactive drugs.

Alcohol (*see Chapter 5 for complete coverage of alcohol's neonatal effects*)

Alcohol is the most widely researched drug in relation to its effect on the developing fetus during pregnancy. **FAS, the best-known condition, is a definite pattern of physical, mental, and behavioral abnormalities in children born to mothers who drank heavily during pregnancy.** Symptoms include retarded growth (reduced height, weight, head circumference, brain growth, brain size), facial deformities (specifically shortened eyelids, thin upper lip, flattened midface, groove in the upper lip), occasional problems with heart and limbs, delayed intellectual development, neurological abnormalities, behavioral problems, visual problems, hearing loss, and balance or gait problems (Sokol & Clarren, 1989; Streissguth, 1997; Mattson, Schoenfeld, & Riley, 2001).

There are a number of other less severe yet much more widespread con-

ditions that mostly involve cognitive abilities, e.g., alcohol-related neurodevelopmental disorder (ARND) and alcohol-related birth defects (ARBD), also known as "fetal alcohol effects" (FAE). Statistics show that **worldwide anywhere from 0.33 to 2.9 cases per 1,000 live births have FAS** although individual countries, such as South Africa, can have a much higher incidence. **The incidence of ARND and ARBD is probably 5–10 times greater than FAS.** In the United States 0.5 to 2.0 cases are the accepted number but the rates of individual groups vary widely: African Americans have an incidence of 6 FAS births per 1,000; Asians, Hispanics, and Whites about 1–2; and Native Americans about

10–30 (May & Gossage, 2001; May, 1996; 1996; Hans, 1998).

Dr. Sterling K. Clarren and his associates at Children's Hospital in Seattle, Washington, located and interviewed 80 mothers of children with FAS. They asked them about 2,000 questions to get a profile of the patients.

"What we learned was really startling—100% of them had been severely physically and sexually abused, about 60% of it occurring before they were adults and the rest as adults. About 80% of them had major mental health diagnoses and not just one but many. The average patient had

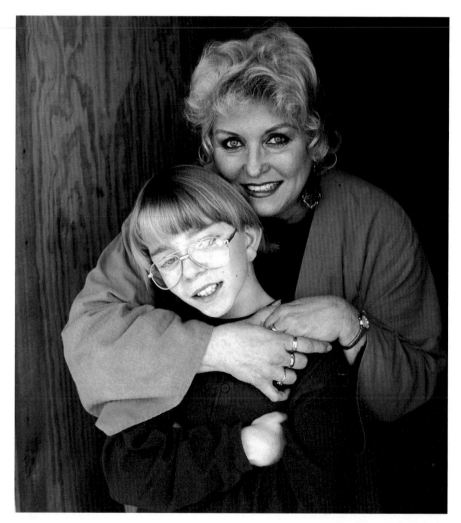

Often the physical effects of alcohol are not as obvious as on this child diagnosed with fetal alcohol syndrome (FAS).

Courtesy of Sterling K. Clarren, M.D., Children's Hospital, Seattle, WA

6 distinct mental health diagnoses made through the DSM-IV system. Some of them had more than 10: schizophrenia, manic depression, phobias, posttraumatic stress disorder, and on and on."

Dr. Sterling K. Clarren (personal communication, 1999)

In addition to FAS and other abnormalities, the rate of sudden infant death syndrome (SIDS) is greatly increased when the mother drinks, either while pregnant or when nursing. A study involving the Indian Health Service found that prevention efforts in the form of a visiting nurse who helped mothers with a drinking problem decreased the incidence of SIDS by 80%.

Cocaine & Amphetamines

Currently in the United States about 200,000 chronic heavy cocaine and crack abusers are women (the number is growing yearly) with their average age in the early 20s, the most fertile childbearing years (SAMHSA, 2002). A percentage of these women use cocaine during pregnancy although the rates vary widely from hospital to hospital and among different ethnic groups. In the 1980s **when cocaine use was at its highest levels, it was estimated that about 4.5% of all U.S. infants were exposed to cocaine in utero** (Gomby & Shiono, 1991). Other studies showed that from 15% to 25% of babies born in some inner-city hospitals are born cocaine affected (Bateman & Heagarty, 1989). The recent increase of amphetamine abuse will certainly result in increased numbers of pregnancies affected by this stimulant.

"I was smoking crack cocaine and drinking alcohol and he used to kick, really really bad. It was like he was having tremors or something inside of my stomach. Needless to say I had him 6 weeks early. And when he came out, he had to go to NICU, he had tubes coming out of everywhere, he could

not breathe. My son was on a heart monitor. And two times out of that 6 months, his heart stopped beating."

24-year-old recovering crack user

The stimulants **cocaine and amphetamines increase heart rate and constrict blood vessels causing dramatic elevations in blood pressure in both mother and fetus**. Constriction of blood vessels reduces the flow of blood, nutrients, and oxygen to the placenta and fetus, sometimes resulting in retarded fetal development, especially when the mother is a habitual user. Increased maternal and placental blood pressure can, in rare cases, cause the placenta to separate prematurely from the wall of the uterus (abruptio placenta) resulting in spontaneous abortion or premature delivery (Derlet & Albertson, 2002).

Acutely elevated blood pressure in the fetus can also cause a stroke in the brain of the fetus. Fetal blood vessels in the brain are very fragile and may be easily damaged by exposure to cocaine and particularly amphetamines. **Third trimester use of cocaine can induce sudden fetal activity, uterine contractions, and premature labor** within minutes after a mother has used (Plessinger & Woods, 1998).

Although there is no specific set of physical abnormalities connected to cocaine or amphetamine use during pregnancy, exposed babies can be growth retarded with smaller heads, genito-urinary tract abnormalities, severe intestinal disease, and abnormal sleep and breathing patterns (Cherukuri, Minkoff, Feldman, Parekh, & Glass, 1989; Behnke, Eyler, Garvan, Wobie, 2001).

Infants exposed to cocaine during pregnancy **often go through a withdrawal syndrome characterized by extreme agitation, increased respiratory rates, hyperactivity, and occasional seizures**. Because these babies are in withdrawal, intoxicated, or both, they are highly irritable, difficult to console, tremulous, and deficient in their ability to interact with their environment. Many of these initial effects disappear within a few weeks after

birth assuming the mother's breast milk is not contaminated with cocaine.

Infants exposed to cocaine, when studied at 3, 12, 18, and 24 months, seemed to require more stimulation to increase arousal and attention but were less able to control higher states of arousal than unexposed children (Mayes, Grillon, Granger, & Schottenfeld, 1998; Lester et al., 2002). A study of 150 cocaine-exposed infants also found that lower levels of alertness and attentiveness were directly related to the amount of cocaine used during pregnancy (Eyler, Behnke, Conlon, Woos, & Wobie, 1998). Many of these infants show some patterns of neurobehavioral disorganization, irritability, and poor language development. These infants may also have a slightly higher incidence of SIDS although it is often hard to separate environmental and nutritional factors from the direct effects of drugs (Finnegan & Kandall, 1997).

There is hope for parents, educators, and others involved with the education and care of these children. **Many abnormal neurobehavioral effects improve over the first 3 years of life.** Recent studies suggest that earlier predictions of severely impaired cocaine babies have been exaggerated (Frank et al., 2001). Cocaine does harm the fetus, especially when the mother is a heavy user but most children prenatally exposed to cocaine will have more normal behavior by the age of 3 than was feared. However, reports of attention-deficit disorder and low frustration levels are related by teachers and parents (Harvard University, 1998). It should also be noted that these studies were on children who had access to good neonatal and pediatric care. It is unclear whether cocaine-affected children will catch up to other nonexposed children without that quality of care.

Opioids

Physical dependence on opioids leads to more continuous use, so the **effects on the fetus seem greater than with binge drugs such as cocaine**. People addicted to heroin, hydrocodone (Vicodin®), oxycodone (OcyContin®), and other opioids have a greater risk for fetal growth retardation, miscarriages, stillbirths, abruptio placenta as well as **severe infections from intravenous use**.

For pregnant heroin users, the periods of daily withdrawal that alternate with the rushes following each drug snort or injection cause dramatic fluctuations in autonomic functions in the fetus believed to harm the fetus and contribute to maternal/fetal complications. Babies born to heroin-addicted mothers are **often premature, smaller, and weaker than normal** (Fulroth, Phillips, & Durand, 1989; Zhu & Stadlin, 2000). Prenatal exposure to heroin has also been associated with abnormal neurobehavioral development. These infants have abnormal sleep patterns and are at greater risk for SIDS. **A 600% increase in SIDS deaths was found in a study of 16,409 drug-exposed infants in New York City** (Kandall, Gaines, Habel, Davidson, & Jessop, 1993).

If a mother becomes truly addicted to opioids, so does the fetus. Depending on the mother's daily dose of shorter-acting opioids, such as heroin, **a majority (60–80%) of opioid-exposed infants exhibit the neonatal abstinence syndrome (withdrawal) 48–72 hours after birth** (Finnegan & Ehrlich, 1990). With longer-acting opioids, such as methadone, it can take 1–2 weeks. Symptoms include hyperactivity, irritability, incessant high-pitched crying, increased muscle tone, hyperactive reflexes, sweating, tremors, irregular sleep patterns, increased respiration, uncoordinated and ineffectual sucking and swallowing, sneezing, vomiting, and diarrhea. In severe cases failure to thrive, seizures, or even death may occur. These withdrawal effects may be mild or severe and may last from days to months (Kandall, 1998).

Since the onset of symptoms varies, close observation of the opioid-exposed neonate is necessary. Most cases of neonatal narcotic withdrawal can be treated with good nursing care, loose swaddling in a side-lying position, quiet and dimly lit surroundings, good nutrition, and normal maternal/infant bonding behaviors. Opioids have

been found in breast milk in sufficient concentration to expose newborns. Only in severe cases is medication required for the infant and then it should be a milder opioid such as paregoric (Kandall, 1993). However **opioid withdrawal in neonates can be fatal** and should therefore be appropriately treated.

Marijuana

Marijuana is used by 5–17% of pregnant women during their pregnancy (depending on the survey). Recent research has found high levels of anandamide in the uterus of mice and suggests that this neurotransmitter, mimicked by marijuana, helps regulate the early stages of pregnancy and perhaps control the pain of childbirth. This study found that high levels of anandamide inhibit the progression of the fertilized egg from blastocyst stage to embryo (Paria, Das, & Dey, 1995; Paria et al., 1999; Schmid et al., 1997). These discoveries might give a better understanding of the process of gestation but they also suggest that the use of marijuana might disrupt the birth process.

Most marijuana exposure in newborns goes undetected or is masked by the use of other drugs that can also cause problems. Some studies have reported reduced fetal weight gain, shorter gestations, and some congenital anomalies; however most studies have found minimal developmental effects in regards to motor skills and mental functioning (Richardson, Day, & Goldschmidt, 1995). However, long-term development studies (Ottawa Prenatal Prospective Study) showed that intrauterine **exposure to marijuana led to poorer short-term memory and verbal reasoning at age 3** (Day, Richardson, Goldschmidt, et al., 1994; Richardson, 1998). Between the ages of 5–6 and 9–12 years, according to the Ottawa study, **marijuana-exposed children scored somewhat lower on verbal and memory performance tests, impulsive/hyperactive behavior, conduct problems, and distractibility**. They also scored lower on tasks associated with executive function—the indi-

vidual's ability to plan ahead, anticipate, and suppress behaviors that are incompatible with a current goal (Fried et al., 1992; Fried & Watkinson, 1997; Fried, Watkinson, & Gray, 1998).

Many of the problems with marijuana have to do with the delivery system—marijuana is smoked and therefore limits oxygen to the body and fetus, irritates alveoli and bronchii, and causes babies to weigh about 3.4 ounces less on average than nonexposed neonates (Zuckerman, Frank, Hingson, et al., 1989; Fried, 1995).

Since there are withdrawal symptoms after ceasing heavy or long-term use of marijuana and since the fetus is also exposed, it is logical to assume that neonates would exhibit withdrawal symptoms. Anecdotal reports relate that these **marijuana-exposed babies have abnormal responses to light and visual stimuli, increased tremulousness, "startles," and a high-pitched cry** associated with drug withdrawal. Unlike infants undergoing narcotic withdrawal, marijuana babies are not excessively irritable.

Prescription & Over-the-Counter Drugs

Over-the-counter and prescribed medications are the most common drugs used by pregnant women. About two-thirds of all pregnant women take at least one drug during pregnancy usually vitamins or simple analgesics such as aspirin. In one study half of a group of newborns had NSAIDs such as ibuprofen, naproxen, and particularly aspirin in their meconium (the baby's first intestinal discharge). In addition the use of NSAIDs was often not reported to the obstetrician and the incidence of pulmonary hypertension was high (Alano, Ngougmna, Ostrea, & Konduri, 2001). Medications to treat maternal discomfort, anxiety, pain, or infection must be prescribed carefully for a variety of prescription drugs are harmful to the human fetus. Sedative-hypnotics are among the most studied of these drugs.

Benzodiazepines accumulate in the fetal blood at more dangerous

levels than in maternal blood at dosages normally safe for the mother alone. Besides high fetal drug concentrations, excretion is also slower. The drugs and their metabolites remain in fetal and newborn systems days or even weeks longer than in the mother, resulting in dangerously high concentrations of the drug, leading to fetal depression, abnormal heart patterns, or rarely, death.

In the Physician's Desk Reference (PDR) under alprazolam, the warnings read:

"Because of experience with other members of the benzodiazepine class, Xanax® is assumed to be capable of causing an **increased risk of congenital abnormalities when administered to a pregnant woman during the first trimester**. Because use of these drugs is rarely a matter of urgency, their use during the first trimester should almost always be avoided."
(Physicians' Desk Reference [PDR], 2003)

Studies have indicated an increased risk of cleft lip and/or cleft palate when diazepam was used in the first 6 months of pregnancy. A newborn addicted to benzodiazepines may exhibit a variety of neonatal complications. Infants may be floppy, have poor muscle tone, be lethargic, and have sucking difficulties. **A withdrawal syndrome, similar to narcotic withdrawal, may also result and may persist for weeks.** Because diazepam and its active metabolites are excreted into breast milk, it has been thought to cause lethargy, mental sedation/depression, and weight loss in nursing infants. Since diazepam and other benzodiazepines can accumulate in breast-fed babies, their use in lactating women is ill advised. Barbiturates are also to be avoided during pregnancy.

Withdrawal symptoms occur in infants born to mothers who receive barbiturates throughout the last trimester of pregnancy. Withdrawal symptoms include hyperactivity, disturbed sleep, tremors, and hyperreflexia. Prolonged withdrawal can be treated through tapering the infant with phenobarbital over a period of 2 weeks.

Anticonvulsants such as phenytoin (Dilantin®) increase a pregnant woman's chances of delivering a child with congenital defects such as cleft lip, cleft palate, and heart malformation. Consequently the physician must carefully weigh the dangers of seizures vs. the chances of congenital defects in the neonate. Pregnancy also alters the absorption of the drug, so there is a chance of more frequent seizures (PDR, 2003).

Even antibiotics such as tetracycline can cause a variety of adverse effects.

"The use of drugs of the tetracycline class during tooth development in the last half of pregnancy, infancy, and childhood to the age of 8 years may cause permanent discoloration of the teeth (yellow-gray-brown)."
(PDR, 2003)

Many over-the-counter medications contain stimulants including caffeine or ephedrine and their use should also be carefully monitored by the pregnant woman and the physician.

Nicotine

In the overall population the percentage of women who smoked in the past month has steadily increased from 5% in the 1920s to 28.2% in 1997 but finally dropped to 23% in 2001. **About 17% of pregnant women smoked cigarettes** compared to 30.5% of nonpregnant women (SAMHSA, 2002). In an earlier study the percentage of pregnant women who were using tobacco at the time they gave birth was 8.82%. The highest rates were among African Americans (20.12%) and Whites (14.2%) (Noble et al., 1997). After birth the rate of smoking rose again back to prepregnancy levels.

Smoking during pregnancy is particularly dangerous because tobacco smoke contains more than 2,000 different compounds including nicotine and carbon monoxide. Both have been shown to cross the placental barrier and **reduce the fetal supply of oxygen**. In addition smoking is a continual activity—one, two, or three packs a day—so the impact on the fetus is constant.

Recent studies now indicate that **women smokers with a heavy habit are about twice as likely to miscarry** and have spontaneous abortions as nonsmokers. Nicotine damages the placenta and has adverse effects on the developing fetus. Stillbirth rates are also higher among smoking mothers (Cook, Petersen, & Moore, 1994).

As with many other psychoactive substances, smoking decreases newborn birth weights. Babies born to mothers who smoke heavily **weigh, on the average, 200 grams (7 oz.) less, are 1.4 centimeters shorter, and have a smaller head circumference** compared to babies from nonsmoking or nondrug-abusing mothers (Martin, 1992). Although the incidence of physical birth defects is very low in babies born to smoking mothers, there is still a significant increase in cleft palate and congenital heart defects. Smoking leads to potential minor brain and nerve defects that may be hard to detect. Because nicotine is toxic and creates lesions in that part of animal brains that controls breathing, it is given as one possible reason for the increase in SIDS (sudden infant death syndrome or crib death) seen in babies born to mothers who smoke heavily (Jaffe & Shopland, 1995).

Babies born to heavy smokers have been shown to have **increased nervous nursing (weaker sucking reflex)** and possibly a depressed immune system at birth, resulting in more pneumonia and bronchitis, sleep problems, and less alertness than other infants. Long-lasting effects of smoking exposure before birth can include **lower IQ and cognitive ability**, along with lower verbal, reading, and mathematical skills (Rush & Callahan, 1989). There is even some small association with smoking during pregnancy and the incidence of attention-deficit/hyperactivity disorder (Milberger, Biederman, Faraone, & Jones, 1998).

Caffeine

An early study of pregnant women found caffeine in 75% of infants at birth. In general, neonates, newborns, and infants have less tolerance for caffeine than adults (Weinberg & Bealer, 2001). In addition pregnant women have decreased ability to metabolize methylxanthines, so the stimulatory effects of caffeine last longer in the fetus. No long-lasting fetal or neonatal effects have been conclusively proven but **physicians recommend avoiding caffeine during pregnancy**. As big a problem as the effect of caffeine during pregnancy is the continued exposure of infants and small children by their parents to caffeine products especially iced tea and colas.

PREVENTION

Since drugs can have such a magnified effect on the fetus throughout pregnancy, **it is crucial that a pregnant woman abstain from all unnecessary drug exposure**. It is estimated that only 55% of women of childbearing age know about fetal alcohol syndrome although as many as 375,000 children every year may be impacted by their mother's drinking and drug use. Reaching pregnant women with appropriate prevention messages through OB/GYN health professionals, prenatal and well-baby clinics, alcohol/drug warning labels, and public service messages is essential to reducing the effects of alcohol and drug use on babies (Hankin, 2002; NIDA, 1994).

Providing treatment to addicted pregnant women is vital. Many professionals know that if a drug-abusing pregnant woman can be gotten off drugs in the third trimester, the baby will not be born addicted and will not have to go through detoxification. Most prevention professionals agree that because the effects of alcohol on a developing fetus are not yet fully known, clear multiple warnings to women not to drink or use drugs if they are pregnant or planning pregnancy should be given. Complete abstinence is the safest choice.

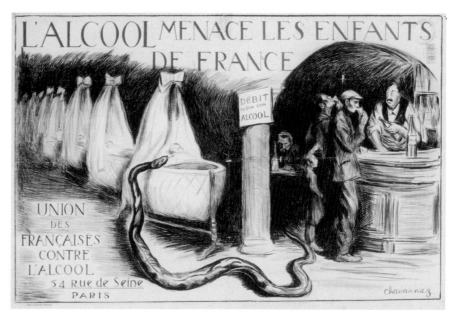

This French prevention poster from the 1920s warns about the impact of parental alcohol use on infants.

Courtesy of the National Library of Medicine, Bethesda, MD

A challenge to prevention exists in some states where mothers have been convicted of drugging babies or have lost custody of their children. Some experts fear that such measures encourage pregnant addicts to avoid prenatal clinics and doctors and to give birth outside hospitals to avoid imprisonment or loss of their children. Other jurisdictions use a treatment alternative to jail. It has been suggested that if women do not have to give up their babies when they enter treatment, the treatment option will be more acceptable and successful.

"These nurses would come in and take my child from me. That was a really painful experience and it's painful now. It gets overwhelming, the feelings of wanting your child, knowing that this little person is very dependent on you, knowing that the meeting of their needs requires you to be clean and sober, requires you to be functional."

29-year-old recovering pregnant addict

YOUTH & SCHOOL

In spite of all the headlines about crack, LSD, and methamphetamine use **among adolescents and college students, the most serious drug problem by far is still alcohol. Tobacco is a close second and marijuana third.**

"In high school we'd have 'keggers.' We found out whose parents wouldn't be home, have a keg delivered, and have the party there. In college the drug scene was a little different. Besides the alcohol, you could get a better selection of drugs: opium, hashish, mescaline, peyote, LSD, but mostly just marijuana. We were too poor in high school for those."

19-year-old college sophomore

A problem with high school, college, and other drug surveys is that many users lie about or minimize their use of drugs even when assured that the survey is confidential. This is part of the denial process. What has been found is that **most figures on current or frequent use of illicit drugs in high** schools and colleges are underreported (Comerci, 1998). In fact underage drinkers account for nearly 20% of the alcohol consumed in the United States.

"We were supposed to put on a skit about drugs and the minute we sat down we said, 'Now what do the parents want to hear about that?' That's the general attitude all my friends have in dealing with these programs, 'What do the parents want to hear from us?' And a lot of the people teaching these drug programs are also telling us what they think our parents want us to hear. It's all very stereotypical."

15-year-old high school student

The other problem with doing surveys is that problematical use means different things for different people and for different drugs. For example, if a college freshman gets drunk only on Friday and Saturday nights, usually leading to a fight or unprotected sex, the student would probably swear that he or she doesn't have a drinking problem. But by the definition of abuse, that kind of drinking is a problem.

With cocaine, if a student goes on a 3-day binge just once a month, spends all available money on the drug, and has nothing left for food or textbooks, that also could be defined as abuse. **The true value of youth surveys is that they show trends in drug use**, so it is possible to see changes from year to year in order to have a sense of where our society is headed. Surveys also give us a rough benchmark for measuring the effectiveness of the prevention efforts we as a society are expending.

ADOLESCENTS & HIGH SCHOOL

How Serious Is the Problem?

In a 2001 report titled "Malignant Neglect: Substance Abuse and America's Schools," the National Center on Addiction and Substance Abuse at Columbia University found that

◇ **substance abuse and addiction will add 10% to the cost of elementary and secondary education** due to violence, special education, teacher turnover, truancy, property damage, injury, and counseling;

◇ the **school environment has the greatest influence on drug and alcohol use**;

◇ **if a student gets to the age of 21 without smoking or using alcohol and other drugs, he or she probably never will**.

The report found that experimentation is not benign. For example, of those students who have ever

◇ tried cigarettes, 85.7% are still smoking in the 12th grade;

◇ been drunk, 83.3% are still getting drunk;

◇ tried marijuana, 76.4% are still smoking pot.

In addition adolescents who use marijuana weekly reported that they were almost six times likelier to cut

class or skip school as those who do not (National Center on Addiction and Substance Abuse [NCASA], 2001).

Fortunately recent surveys show some positive trends: the use of marijuana after rising in the 1990s has begun to decrease as has the use of other illegal drugs. There has also been a large drop in tobacco and alcohol use even though the high prevalence of these legal drugs, with all their attendant health consequences, continues (Fig. 8-4).

Much of the alcohol and other drug use in high schools is experimental, social, or habitual with bouts of abuse. Most students haven't had enough time for addiction to occur. Unfortunately they also **don't have much experience in their drinking and drug-taking habits, so inappropriate use, including intoxication, drunk driving, and unsafe sex is more likely**. Another factor that can lead to inappropriate use occurs when young people drink or take drugs to control emotional turmoil and they don't recognize it as dangerous. Part of the reason is society's be-

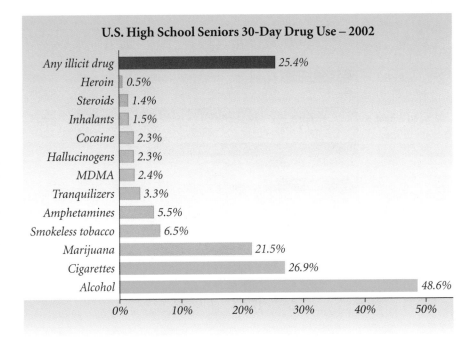

U.S. High School Seniors 30-Day Drug Use – 2002

Drug	Percentage
Any illicit drug	25.4%
Heroin	0.5%
Steroids	1.4%
Inhalants	1.5%
Cocaine	2.3%
Hallucinogens	2.3%
MDMA	2.4%
Tranquilizers	3.3%
Amphetamines	5.5%
Smokeless tobacco	6.5%
Marijuana	21.5%
Cigarettes	26.9%
Alcohol	48.6%

Figure 8-4 •

Since 1992 decreased funding, greater availability of drugs, and a tolerance to drug use led to sharp increases in drug use among high school seniors as well as 8th and 10th graders. Recently the levels of use have begun to drop.

(University of Michigan, 2003)

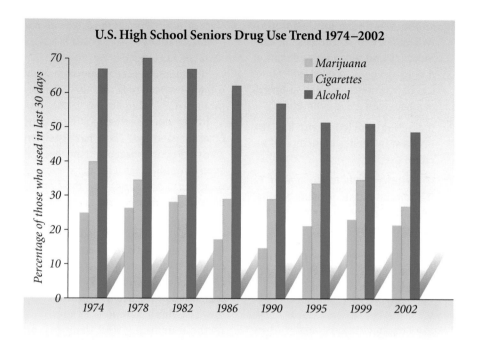

Figure 8-5 •

This graph compares the change in the 30-day use of alcohol, marijuana, and tobacco over the last 28 years by high school seniors.

(University of Michigan, 2003)

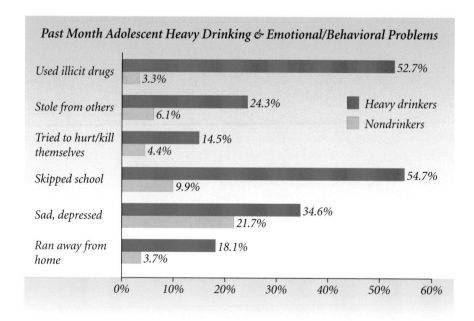

Figure 8-6 •

A survey of 12–17-year-olds showed that heavy drinkers were more likely to have emotional and behavioral problems. Some of the problems led to experimentation and eventually heavy use of alcohol while others were caused by the heavy use itself.

(SAMHSA, 2000)

nign attitude towards legal psychoactive drugs.

Finally, because many **adolescents think of themselves as invulnerable to the consequences of use**, their level of concern is lower than that of older users. Whereas the majority of teenagers who experiment with drugs will

not become addicted, some will and for them the legal, academic, psychological, and physical effects of psychoactive drugs will cause problems:

◇ 70% of teen suicides involve alcohol or drugs;

◇ 50% of date rapes involve alcohol (victim and/or rapist);

◇ 40% of drownings involve alcohol.

Physical immaturity is another problem. Just 3 drinks in the younger user causes significantly more mental impairment than in an adult drinker (NCASA, 2001).

Crime

The biggest effect of alcohol and drug use is on crime. In some cities the youth guidance centers or juvenile halls are clogged because of crimes related to drugs. Nationally, according to the Arrestee Drug Abuse Monitoring Program, in 2001 **more than half of juvenile male arrestees tested positive for one or more illegal drugs**, with marijuana being by far the most frequent (ADAM, 2003). If the authorities had also tested for alcohol, the figures would be much higher. It has been estimated that the cost of youth alcohol abuse is more than $58 billion (e.g., $36 billion in violent crime, $18 billion in traffic accidents).

"I went to jail a lot for being drunk, being on drugs, for committing crimes, lots of assaults and deadly weapons and things like that. I was a whole different person when I was using, you know, I wasn't giving a rat's ass about nobody or nothin'. I was just gang bangin' to the fullest, that was it."
17-year-old high school student

A change in federal law made people ineligible for student financial aid if they have a drug conviction on their record. In 2000 and 2001, of the 7.58 million who applied for federal financial aid for college, 39,647 were denied because of a conviction. Another 42,579 who had a conviction on their record were eligible because they completed a drug treatment program or had another exemption (U.S. Department of Education, 2003).

The Effects of Drugs on Maturation

In the United States, levels of legal and illegal substance abuse among teenagers are estimated to be the highest found in any developed country in the world. If true, this trend is particularly alarming from two perspectives: first, drug use among our youth gives us a preview of future levels of drug abuse in our society and second, **since teenagers are still maturing and developing physically, drugs are generally more toxic and cause disruption of psychological and emotional growth**.

"When you begin to use drugs around 12, 13, or 14, you never have rites of passage. You never get indoctrinated into the adulthood of society. Many people that we talk to who come into treatment actually began using substances at that age, so their rites of passage haven't yet occurred when we see them at 30 or 35. And essentially, we're talking to a 14–15-year-old in a 30- to 35-year-old body and that's where we have to begin."
Counselor, Haight Ashbury Detox Clinic

When drugs or alcohol are commonly used in adolescence to avoid feelings, drown out problems, or as a shortcut to feeling good, then **young people will not fully learn how to deal with their emotions and life's problems without psychoactive substances**. They will not learn patience, they will not learn that emotional pain can be accepted and used to grow on, and they will not learn that being willing to do things you don't want to do is part of the maturation process.

Risk-Focused & Resiliency-Focused Prevention for Adolescents

Recent studies indicate that a number of conditions put adolescents more at risk for substance abuse and other behavioral addictions. These **risks include**

◊ **being subject to physical, sexual, or emotional abuse**;

◊ getting pregnant;

◊ dropping out of school;

◊ living in poverty;

◊ having emotional and mental disturbances;

◊ lacking self-esteem;

◊ getting caught in the juvenile justice system;

◊ being exposed to peer group tolerance or encouragement of drug use;

◊ lacking alternative activities;

◊ being in a school that has no policies, detection procedures, or referral services for users;

◊ being in a family that tolerates use, has no consistent rules, lacks consistent discipline, and has absent and uninvolved parents or especially parents that use drugs (ONDCP, 2000; Juliana & Goodman, 1997).

"I believe both my parents were alcoholics. My brother's an addict and alcoholic. It runs in the family. So I basically followed in my father's footsteps—the drinking, the running around."
Recovering alcoholic

The challenge for prevention specialists is to develop programs that clearly identify the above risks and teach adolescents to deal with them while enhancing the protective elements that promote healthy lifestyles and personal accomplishments. Researchers Steven Glenn, Ph.D. and Richard Jessor, Ph.D. present **4 determinants of future drug use in children** by age 12.

1. **Strong sense of family participation and involvement:** Those children who feel that they are significant participants in and valued by their families seem to be less prone towards substance abuse in the future.

2. **Established personal position about drugs, alcohol, and sex:** Children who have a position on these issues and who can articulate how they arrived at their position, how they would act on it, and what effect their position would have on their lives seem less likely to develop drug or alcohol problems.

3. **Strong spiritual sense and community involvement:** Young people who feel that they matter and contribute to their community and that they are individuals with a role and purpose in society also seem less likely to develop significant drug or alcohol problems.

4. **Attachment to a clean and sober adult role model:** Children who can list one or more nondrug-using adults (other than their parents) for whom they have esteem and to whom they can turn for information or advice seem less prone to develop drug abuse problems. These positive role models, often persons like a coach, a teacher, activities leader, minister, relative, neighbor, or family friend, play a critical role in the formative years of a child's development.

"There is stuff around you in your life, including if you are just bored, that makes you want to experience the effect of a drug. You can change that if you can make yourself happy. When I'm with friends doing something that's fun or even important, then I don't even think about drugs."
16-year-old student

Primary, Secondary, & Tertiary Prevention for Grades K through 12

When prevention programs are planned, they need to keep the risk and resiliency factors in mind and tailor programs not only for the age groups but also for ethnicity, gender, culture, and any other factors that will get the message across.

Primary Prevention. Since the purpose of primary prevention is to **prevent or at least minimize drug experimentation and use**, it needs to start as early as kindergarten. Coordinated efforts among parents, teachers, and other community members are of great value. Parent-teacher sessions and the incorporation of drug prevention lesson plans within the school's overall curriculum are the first steps. School-based prevention programs can teach life skills, resistance education, and/or normative education (Bates & Wigtil, 1994). Unfortunately primary prevention can only focus on a few of the risk factors in an adolescent's or teenager's life, which include personal, genetic, psychological, family, and social problems. For example, zero tolerance policies that punish any use of alcohol or drugs are often used just to identify children for expulsion rather than to place them in appropriate treatment (NCASA, 2001).

A **life-skills program**, Life Skills Training (LST), being taught in grades 7 to 10, focuses on **increasing social skills and reducing peer pressure to drink**. An evaluation of this program showed a decrease in the frequency of drinking and excessive drinking (Botvin, Baker, Dusenbury, Tortu, & Borzin, 1990; Life Skills Training, 2003).

One of the most widely used resistance education programs is **DARE (Drug Abuse Resistance Education)** that consists of **16 or 17 weekly 1-hour sessions conducted by uniformed police officers and presented to 5th or 6th graders**. The program teaches self-esteem, decision-making skills, and peer resistance training. Several studies have shown that the program has modest short-term (1 year) effects on reducing drug use although it improved self-assertiveness and increased knowledge about the dangers of alcohol and other drugs (Ennet, Tobler, Ringwalt, & Flewelling, 1994). A study of students 10 years after they took the course found that the effects of the teaching were not long lasting and actual drug use was not reduced more than control groups (Lyman, Milich, Zimmerman, et al., 1999; NCASA, 2001). In response to criticism and to update their courses, DARE revised its program. It has programs for junior high and senior high students and involves students in more lifelike situations to teach them to handle peer pressure better. There is even a DARE program for parents to involve them in prevention.

Another resistance education program similar to DARE is **AMPS (Alcohol Misuse Prevention Study)** that consists of a four-session curriculum for 5th and 6th graders. It educates as well as **develops peer resistance skills**. Studies of high-risk students who had taken the course found a 50% reduction in use after 26 months and through grade 12 (Dielman, 1995; Littlefield, 2003).

Normative education is a strategy that aims to correct erroneous beliefs about the prevalence and acceptability of alcohol use and drug use among peers. This strategy was found to be a strong adjunct to resistance education causing substantial drops in alcohol use among high school students (Hansen & Graham, 1993).

The most pertinent point about primary prevention is that it needs to be continued not just limited to a 1 yr. attempt at inoculating students against drug and alcohol use. Education and skills-training booster sessions need to continue through high school and into college. The most effective prevention programs seem to be those in which the students are taught self-esteem and confidence and in which they learn not be afraid of their feelings.

Since the roots of most addictions come from the family, family-focused primary prevention is a necessary adjunct to any school-based program. Programs such as parental skills training through the school, reduction in parental use of drugs or alcohol in front of the children, and greater positive participation of parents in their children's lives have a great influence on children's behavior. Results from a study by the Partnership for a Drug-Free America indicate that **parents who have repeated discussions with their children about the risks of illicit drugs and set clear rules do make a difference in adolescent drug use.** About 45% of teenagers who heard nothing at home about drug risks used marijuana in the last year. That figure drops to 33% for those who learned a little at home and 26% for those who learned a lot (Partnership for a Drug-Free America, 1998; Parents' Resource Institute for Drug Education, 2001).

Secondary Prevention. Once experimentation, social use, habituation, and occasional abuse have begun, usually starting in the 7th and 8th grades, **school-based prevention programs need to continue primary prevention but also need to add a number of secondary programs and policies**. Junior high and high schools should include clear formulation and strict policies on substance use. **Teachers and staff should be trained in recognizing drug use** and how to deal with the consequences. Training to enable parents to recognize problems due to drug use in their children, supporting their children, and seeking counseling should also be included. Additional services should include crisis intervention and referral. Other essential (but sometimes neglected) services are follow-up aftercare, support to make sure use does not reoccur, and care that emotional, social, and physical problems leading to substance use are being corrected. Often these services are available through utilization of existing community services rather than hiring new and expensive staff.

At this level some other programs found to be effective in minimizing experimentation with drugs are peer educator programs, prevention curricula, positive role models, Students Against Drunk Driving (SADD), health fairs, and Friday Night Live alternative activities.

"When I was going through my wild stage, I think what changed my mind about drugs was seeing someone who went through their wild days and never stopped. So I think that there is a point when you cross over from experimentation and go on to abusing."
22-year-old former college student

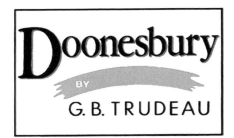
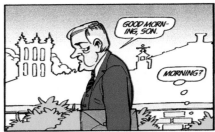
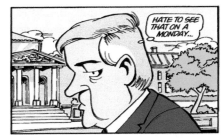
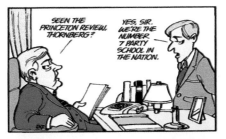
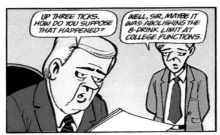
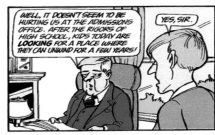
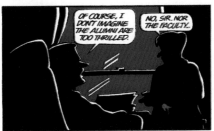
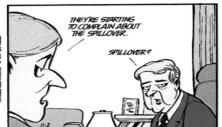
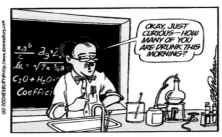

Tertiary Prevention. This program (**for students who have a problem with drugs**) uses student assistance programs, teenage Narcotics/Cocaine/Alcohol/Marijuana/Addictions Anonymous meetings, peer intervention teams, and other activities geared at getting drug abusers into early treatment to limit abuse. **The honesty of peers seems most effective in reaching students who are in trouble.**

Home drug tests provide one way parents monitor drug abuse. They use these drug tests when behavior suggests that family rules have been violated. Teenagers, however, may resent the tests as a breach of trust and an invasion of privacy.

Children of Alcoholics & Drug Abusers. It is estimated that 1 in 4 U.S. children under 18 years old are exposed to alcohol abuse or alcohol dependence in their family (Grant, 2000). So whether it's primary, secondary, or even tertiary prevention, teachers, counselors, and health professionals have to recognize that **children are affected by**

drugs and alcohol even when they don't use. They have to be able to identify and deal with the different roles a child will take in a family since many of these roles will affect future drug use. These roles include

◇ **the hero (model child)**, a hardworking student who tries to bring pride to the family but is still affected by the intense stress of having an addict or alcoholic in the family; also known as the "chief enabler," this type of child often takes over the duties of their dysfunctional parents;

◇ **the problem child** who experiences multiple personal problems, has a tendency to use drugs, and demands attention;

◇ **the lost child** who is extremely shy and deals with problems by avoiding family and social activities;

◇ **the mascot (or family clown)** who tries to ease tension in a dysfunctional family by being funny or cute and has trouble maturing.

(Adger, 1998; Sher, 1997)

COLLEGE STUDENTS

Although illegal drugs appear on college campuses, alcohol is the drug that predominates. In a Carnegie Foundation survey, college presidents ranked alcohol abuse as the quality of campus life issue that was their greatest concern. Drinking is embedded in college traditions and norms. College students are particular targets for advertising by the alcoholic beverage industry since a freshman who prefers a particular brand is expected to generate $20,000–$50,000 in sales over his or her lifetime.

Prevalence

Various reports confirm that **80% of students on most college campuses drink at least some alcohol**. Research by Harvard University Professor Henry Wechsler and his colleagues indicates that

◇ **44.4% of the students surveyed on college campuses binge drink** (5 or more drinks in one sitting for men, 4 or more for women);

◇ about **one-half of binge drinkers are frequent binge drinkers** (5 or more drinks at one sitting 3 or more times in the past 2 weeks);

◇ men bingers outnumber women bingers 48.6% to 40.9% but the number of women binge drinkers has been increasing in recent years;

◇ **the rate of binge drinking is even higher for members of fraternities and sororities**: almost 64.3%. If they live in a fraternity or sorority house, the rate jumps to 75.4%;

◇ fraternity men lag behind nonfraternity men in cognitive development, especially critical thinking skills after the freshman year;

◇ on the positive side, since 1993 the number of abstainers has increased from 16.4% to 19.3% (Wechsler et al., 2002).

In the general population, among 18–20-year-olds, binge drinking has increased by 50% since 1993 (Bellandi, 2003).

Secondhand Drinking

Many problems that occur on campuses are related to **secondhand drinking—the effect binge drinkers and heavy drinkers have on other students**. On campuses where more than 50% of students binge, 86% of nonbinge-drinking students reported being victims of assault or unwanted sexual advances, having sleep and study time interrupted, suffering property damage, having to care for or clean up after a drunken student, or suffering from the general impairment of the quality of life on campus (Wechsler, Kelley, Weitzman, Giovanni, & Seibring, 2000). Recently on many campuses, efforts have been made to protect students from the damage that other people's drinking causes them.

Prevention in Colleges

College drinking games and songs date back to the Middle Ages as do attempts to control the damage students do to themselves and to one another. A sheriff still leads the commencement parade at Harvard graduation ceremon-

ies, a centuries-old tradition to prevent drunken rowdy behavior.

Contemporary college prevention efforts date from the federal Anti-Drug Abuse Act of 1986 that set aside funds for higher education and designated the **Fund for the Improvement of Post-Secondary Education (FIPSE)** as the granting agency that reviewed prevention grant proposals and dispersed funds. Many current drug courses and campus prevention programs derive from that legislation. Newer programs include counter-advertising campaigns of the National Association of State Universities and Land Grant Colleges as well as programs by individual colleges.

Normative Assessment. One prevention approach that has had success is **normative assessment**. This program **aims to change common misperceptions that drug and alcohol use among peers is higher than it really is**. It recognizes that if students think that heavy drinking or drug use is the normal thing to do, they will be more likely to do it themselves. If they recognize that heavy drinking or illicit drug use is not normal, then they are more likely not to use. At Hobart and William Smith Colleges in Geneva, New York, studies found that 68% of the students believed that their peers found frequent intoxication acceptable when in fact only 14% found it acceptable (Perkins, Meilman, Leichliter, Cashin, & Presley, 1999; Perkins & Craig, 2002). In the first 18 months of the program that disseminated the normative assessment information through a variety of media (including screen savers in university computers), there was a 16% reduction in drinking to get drunk, a 21% reduction in frequent heavy drinking, a 31% reduction in missed classes, a 36% reduction in property damage, and a 40% reduction in unprotected sex.

Instead of talking about drug and alcohol use, **normative assessment emphasizes that prevention efforts should talk about not using**. The key is to let students know what constitutes normal use on a particular campus rather than letting their perceptions be formed by sensational stories in the

media or the exaggerations of their friends and classmates.

Other Programs. The following is a list of different **campus strategies directed at controlling alcohol use** and abuse:

◇ **regulate campus drinking** (25% of campuses ban beer, 32% prohibit liquor on campus, and 98% prohibit kegs in dorms) (Wechsler et al., 2000);

◇ **provide alcohol-, tobacco-, and drug-free dorms** (wellness halls) (two-thirds of campuses offer such dorms);

◇ **prohibit alcohol at campus events and fraternity/sorority parties**;

◇ announce and **enforce campus alcohol and other drug policies**;

◇ require that food and nonalcoholic beverages be served when alcohol is available;

◇ provide server training for bartenders at college-sponsored functions;

◇ ban or regulate alcoholic beverage advertising in campus newspapers (50% ban such advertising);

◇ integrate substance abuse education into the curriculum;

◇ have a substance abuse officer and a task force deal with on-campus use and abuse;

◇ establish a higher education prevention consortia in which several campuses pool their knowledge and efforts; about 90 such consortia exist;

◇ create programs to work with the neighborhood and community;

◇ initiate early detection, intervention, enforcement, and referral by residence hall assistants, peer counselors, and the health and counseling centers.

At the college level, primary prevention also includes well-publicized alcohol-free parties, week-long "red ribbon" alcohol- and drug-free celebrations, and active outreach activities especially those promoting safe sex.

In an effective college prevention program, the three levels of drug abuse prevention (primary, secondary, and tertiary) need to be tailored mostly for 17–20-year-olds. Experience has shown that **as most college students mature, their alcohol and drug use becomes more sensible**.

"It's the freshman that are the biggest pain—not all of them. They are free from their parents' supervision for the first time, they are in an exciting but lonely place and they try out their wings. Those are the ones I try to keep an eye on and help but if I'm too strict, they just drink off campus and come back and make noise and throw up. As dorm supervisor I turn a partial blind eye to the older students who have learned how to drink and close their door and have a few beers or wine. I can't burst into their rooms and I don't want to lurk behind doors but I do have to protect the other students. I do know that when the university instituted alcohol-free dorms they were instantly popular."
Resident assistant at university dormitory

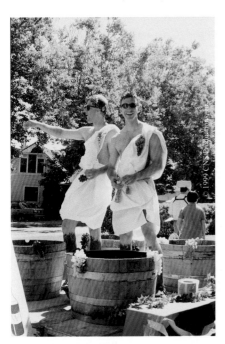

Alcohol is still the number one problem in colleges despite the continued use of marijuana, MDMA, and methamphetamines.

It is crucial to recruit peer counselors or dorm monitors who are themselves clean and sober and will model the kind of attitudes and behavior desirable in a prevention program.

LOVE, SEX, & DRUGS

"The deepest human need is the need to overcome the prison of our aloneness."
Erich Fromm

Over the last few years, the appearance of **Viagra® (sildenafil citrate) to treat erectile dysfunction has been the biggest change in the use of drugs to enhance human sexuality**. It releases nitric oxide that eventually relaxes smooth muscles in the corpus cavernosum erectile tissue allowing greater blood flow. After years of searching, a so-called aphrodisiac that works has been discovered. The rush to find more medications to enhance sexuality continues. However it is important to remember that Viagra® has no effect in the absence of sexual stimulation (PDR, 2003). This limited effect of Viagra® emphasizes the complexity of human sexuality.

Our desire for friendship, affection, love, intimacy, and sex is a primary driving force in men and women. That primary force is affected by drugs in many different and complicated ways. For example, some psychoactive drugs, such as alcohol, marijuana, and ecstasy, lower inhibitions. Others, including cocaine, amphetamines, marijuana, and some inhalants, are used to intensify and otherwise alter the physical sensations of sexuality and to counter low self-esteem or shyness. Often psychoactive drugs **substitute a simple physical sensation, or the illusion of one, for more complex (and yet more rewarding) true emotions**, such as desire for intimacy and comfort, love of children, or release from anxiety. What many psychoactive drugs do is artificially manipulate natural biochemicals, thereby stimulating, counterfeiting, blocking, or confusing physical sensations and true emotions.

Drugs have an impact on all phases of sexual behavior from puberty, through dating, to marital relations. Unfortunately drugs can also trigger sexual aggression, sexual harassment, rape (including date rape), and child molestation. Sexual violence occurs because certain psychoactive drugs can decrease inhibitions, increase aggressiveness, and disrupt judgment, particularly in those already prone to such behavior. **Drugs also encourage high-risk sexual behavior** like multiple partners, anonymous sex, unprotected sex, anal sex, and even prostitution, all of which can spread sexually transmitted diseases, e.g., syphilis, gonorrhea, hepatitis B and C, and HIV disease (El-Bassel, 2000).

"I'm monogamous. I'm with just one boyfriend at a time. I've been with him for 2 months now. The one before, I was with for 4 months."
Teenage high school junior

The 1960s and 1970s signaled an increase in the use and availability of marijuana, amphetamines, and several other psychoactive drugs, all of which affect sexual activity. This easier availability of drugs, along with less severe attitudes towards sexual activity, increased sexual contacts and drug experimentation. In addition the onset of the cocaine and crack epidemic in the 1980s that continued into the 1990s and 2000s encouraged high-risk sexual activity. The mood-altering effects of the drugs, along with the need to make money to buy the drugs, added to the problem.

"These were women that otherwise I would never even have the nerve to approach. Once I've got crack, then I'm someone who's desirable and I can do with these women anything that I want to. And that's what got me involved with crack cocaine."
Crack user

GENERAL EFFECTS

The three main effects of psychoactive drugs on sexual behavior are on desire, excitation, and orgasm. Physically, psychoactive drugs affect hormonal release (testosterone, estrogen, adrenaline, etc.), blood flow, blood pressure, nerve sensitivity, and muscle tension that in turn affect excitation (erectile ability) and orgasm. For example,

◊ heroin desensitizes penal and vaginal nerve endings;

◊ alcohol diminishes spinal reflexes thus decreasing sensitivity and erectile ability;

◊ steroids increase testosterone that stimulates the fight center of the brain making a user more sexually aggressive;

◊ cocaine and amphetamines release dopamine that stimulates our pleasure center in the limbic system, the same system stimulated during excitation and orgasm;

◊ many psychoactive drugs affect the hypothalamus that can trigger hormonal changes.

"It's a very euphoric satisfying kind of effect and it's similar to sex but different. If I have heroin, I don't want or need real sex."
Heroin user

The actual effect of drugs in contrast with their expected effect can vary radically. In a survey conducted at the Haight Ashbury Detox Clinic, **regular drug users said they combined sex and drugs in order to lower their inhibitions, try to make themselves perform better, and increase their fantasies**.

"As a teenager, I was sort of shy and the meth made me feel I was super smart, super pretty, a super person. At that age, I felt very awkward and uncomfortable without the drug."
Recovering meth user

When people combine sex and drugs, the reactions to the various substances are so variable, often escalating into compulsive and addictive behavior, that many of the initial enhanced effects on desire and performance change with time. Diminished sexual performance, even to the point of impotence, is experienced by males who are heavy users of a number of drugs, including heroin and alcohol, as is diminished interest in physical and emotional contact.

Sex and love are such complicated processes and so tied in with our mental state that **people use drugs not only to enhance their sexuality but also to shield themselves from their sexuality and even from any emotional involvement.**

THE DRUGS

Drug-using behavior takes on a life of its own as tolerance, withdrawal, and side effects overwhelm the original intentions of the user. Most of the effects on sexuality are from the drugs' disruption of the neurotransmitters serotonin, dopamine, and norepinephrine. Serotonin affects mood, aggression, and self-esteem; dopamine is believed to help regulate mood, emotional behavior, motor control, and orgasm; while norepinephrine stimulates heart rate and other body functions while increasing motivation and confidence (Peugh & Belenko, 2001).

Cocaine & Amphetamines

Amphetamines and cocaine are popular with heterosexuals but particularly with gay males because for some, use **increases confidence, prolongs an erection, increases endurance, and intensifies an orgasm during initial low-dose use.** Cocaine and amphetamines increase the supply of dopamine and norepinephrine in the nervous system thus inducing a rush of pleasure by affecting centers in the brain involved with sexual activity mostly in the limbic system (Gold & Miller, 1997). The difference between the two drugs has most to do with the duration of action; **methamphetamine lasts hours longer than cocaine and thus prolongs the stimulation**. Men who used methamphetamine were able to sustain sexual functioning (erection, orgasm) longer than men who used cocaine (Werblin, 1998).

One difficulty with judging the effects of cocaine or amphetamines is the variability of the purity of the drug, the amount actually taken, and any drugs taken at the same time, particularly alcohol. However, the myth of stimulant effectiveness on sexual functioning often outweighs the reality when controlled studies (which are limited) are conducted. For example, the view is that crack cocaine enhances sexual pleasure but in fact, particularly in women, it has been shown to induce a loss of sexual pleasure. People mistake desperately selling one's body for drugs with a desire for sex (Henderson, Boyd, & Whitmarsh, 1995). Also, as with all drug use, **preexisting sexual proclivities are directly related to the effect and effectiveness of a drug on sex**. For example, someone who is shy or sexually inhibited will often get a larger boost of confidence from cocaine or methamphetamines. Someone who has unusual sexual practices will be more likely to intensify those practices under the influence of these drugs.

"The kind of feeling you get when you inject it, it's sort of like the feeling when you're making love with your wife. After a while, when you keep doing it, you're impotent and it doesn't have any effect. The opposite sex can do anything they want to you and you won't react."
Recovering cocaine addict

High-dose and prolonged use have quite the opposite effect on sexuality. In men, **heavy or prolonged use often causes delayed ejaculation, a decrease in sexual desire, and difficulty achieving an erection** especially with cocaine. In women, abuse can disrupt the menstrual cycle, cause difficulty in achieving orgasm, and decrease desire (Buffum, 1982; Smith, Wesson, & Apter-Marsh, 1984).

Then too in cocaine or amphetamine abusers, there is a higher inci-

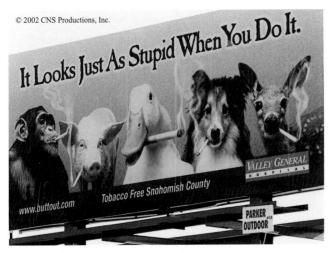
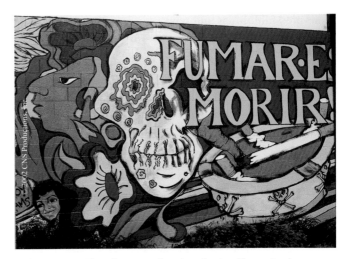

Antitobacco advertising focuses on demystifying the use of tobacco in sexual situations. The ads are produced professionally or simply on community walls.

dence of antisocial and other personality disorders as well as a number preexisting social and emotional problems, so it is often difficult to measure just the effects of the stimulants.

"I was so loaded in the beginning that I would just blank my mind. I didn't want to think he was on top of me or anything because it would bring back [memories of] my stepfather. It would bring back what he was doing. He used his hands all over me."
Recovering 42-year-old crack abuser

Tobacco

From Humphrey Bogart puffing on cigarette after cigarette in *Casablanca* to Brad Pitt smoking in *The Fight Club*, **the use of cigarettes in romantic and sexual situations has been portrayed by the movie industry and encouraged (often with financial incentives) by the tobacco industry**. The image of a cigarette after sexual activity was so common that now it is used satirically to denote sex. Physically nicotine can both stimulate and relax depending on the set (mood and mental state) and setting. In social situations it is a great distracter, something to do while figuring out what to do. However, long-term tobacco use has been associated with lower testosterone and even erectile

dysfunction in men and reduced fertility in women although not nearly to the degree caused by excessive cocaine or alcohol use (U.S. Department of Health and Human Services, 1988; Rosen, 1991: Augood, Duckitt, & Templeton, 1998).

Opioids

Downers are often used to lower inhibitions though **the physiological depressive effects often decrease performance and eventually desire**. Some "nod out" when using, some feel "up." These differences can be explained by selective tolerance of different functions of the body to the effects of opioids. In a study at the Haight Ashbury Clinic in 1982 of men and women who had come in for heroin treatment, the majority of those who had some sexual dysfunction before using reported an initial improvement in sexual activity functioning when they first began to use the drug. Men reported an increased delay in ejaculation while women reported an increase in relaxation and lowered inhibitions. However with continued use, some users became disinterested in sex while others wanted to repeat the experience. **Long-term users reported a decrease in sexual drive and impaired performance.** Reduced testosterone in men led to impotence in some while long-term female users reported men-

strual irregularities, reduced fertility, and frigidity (O'Brien, Cohen, Evans, & Fine, 1992). This is due to inhibition of gonadotropin-releasing hormone that regulates the testes or ovaries (Jaffe, Knapp, & Ciraulo, 1997).

"You start to look more masculine. You feel out of your skin. You can't really feel yourself anymore. The same sort of people you really loved aren't attracted to you anymore."
Female heroin user

In the Haight Ashbury study 60% of heroin addicts reported an overall decrease in desire. While they were high on heroin, that figure jumped to 90%. In another study 70% reported delayed ejaculation when using, which is why some premature ejaculators self-medicate. Further **the overall rate of impotence (inability to become aroused) in one study of male addicts was 39%**, jumping to 53% when they were actually high (Shen & Sata, 1983; Buffum, 1982).

Sedative-Hypnotics

Many sedative-hypnotics, such as the benzodiazepines, barbiturates, and street Quaaludes®, have been called "alcohol in pill form" and touted as sexual enhancers. As with alcohol, it is a case of **lowered inhibitions and relaxation vs. physical depression that makes one unable to perform or respond sexually**.

"Sexually and mentally, everything is so down. If I were a man, I couldn't have an erection. As a woman, I don't have an orgasm. Your mind is just mush but you don't care. The last thing you worry about is sex."
37-year-old benzodiazepine addict

Along with the disinhibition, sedative-hypnotics also impair judgment, making the user more susceptible to sexual advances. As the dose increases, the sedative effects take over making the user physically less able to ward off sexual aggressiveness. The user becomes lethargic and sleepy while experiencing extensive muscle relaxation. **With abuse comes sexual dysfunction and total apathy towards sexual stimulation** (Buffum, 1982).

Flunitrazepam (Rohypnol®). Flunitrazepam, dubbed the "date rape drug," is marketed outside the United States as a sleeping pill. **It causes profound amnesia and lowered inhibitions as well as a decreased ability to resist a sexual assault.** Unfortunately much of the publicity surrounding the drug educated some unscrupulous males in the predatory use of the drug for sex. Flunitrazepam also produces muscle relaxation and has an elimination half-life of 16–35 hours but can accumulate in the system. While not as toxic as barbiturates, it can be dangerous when used with alcohol (NIDA, 1999; Smith, Wesson, & Calhoun, 1995). This benzodiazepine, although legal in approximately 60 countries, is illegal in the United States. Also known as "roofies," "rophies," "ropes," and "roches," it is many times more powerful than Valium® and sells on the street for $5–$10 a pill (Marnell, 1997). (*Also see Chapter 4.*)

GHB (gamma hydroxybutyrate). GHB is a sedative-hypnotic and dopamine enhancer that was originally used as a sleep inducer but is now popular on the rave club scene. It has been touted

as a drug that will **lower inhibitions and make sex more pleasurable**. It was widely available in health food stores in the 1980s and used by body-builders. The problem with GHB is that slight increases in the amount used can mean large differences in the effects. **Doubling the dose that induces a pleasant effect can disrupt coordination, cause sleep, and even induce coma** within 10–20 minutes (Morganthaler & Joy, 1994). It is also often used with other drugs causing synergistic effects that can add dangerous interactions, many of which disrupt sexual activity. Unfortunately the amnestic effects of the drug, which can be therapeutically valuable, lead to its exploitation as a date rape predatory drug like Rohypnol®. GBL, another chemical, is converted to GHB in the body and is marketed as a sexual enhancer. It has been sold as Renewtrient®, Revivarant®, and Vitality® (Peugh & Belenko, 2001).

Alcohol

"One drink of wine and you act like a monkey, two drinks and you strut like a peacock, three drinks and you roar like a lion, and four drinks, you behave like a pig."
Henry Vollam Morton, 1936

More than any other psychoactive drug, alcohol has insinuated itself into the culture of romantic and sexual behavior—champagne to celebrate, the cocktail before sex, or beer swilled before a date. **Alcohol's physical effects on sexual functioning are closely related to blood alcohol levels. Its mental effects however are less strictly dose related and have more to do with the psychological makeup of the user** and the setting in which it is used. Often there are preexisting issues that are dealt with under the influence.

"It was making me feel better about myself. It was like I was a grown woman. I could take any man I wanted. It was like, 'Honey, let's go have a drink,' and there was always

alcohol involved. And we would sit at a bar and then it was easy for them to invite me to a hotel for the night."
42-year-old recovering polydrug abuser

Women & Alcohol. In most societies more taboos and restrictions are placed on a woman's sexuality than on a man's. Many heavy drinkers seem to associate their identity as a woman with their sexual activity. Inevitably, **because alcohol diminishes sexual arousal, women suffer lowered self-esteem and feelings of inadequacy**. Typically the alcoholic denies that what is happening to her sexuality is related to what is happening with her progressive alcohol use.

"I was quite drunk. It was a 'kegger' party and I remember sitting right next to the keg and just drinking constantly all night. I voluntarily went out to a car with a boy. I voluntarily had sex with that boy because I was quite drunk and I guess the thinking was that I wanted someone to hold me, and love me, and make me feel pretty."
24-year-old woman who is a heavy drinker

Even though many women report that alcohol use increases sexual pleasure, quantitative measures of physical sexual arousal and ability to have an orgasm decreased with blood alcohol level increases (Peugh & Belenko, 2001). This seems to emphasize the powerful influence of lowered inhibitions in women on emotions. In men, however, the self-reported feelings and objective measures of physical arousal were more consistent.

In one study of chronic female alcoholics, 36% said they had orgasms less than 5% of the time. They also found that sexual dysfunction was the best predictor of continued problems with alcohol abuse (Wilsnack, Klassen, Schur, et al., 1991). As drinking increases, menstrual disturbances, spontaneous abortions, and miscarriages increase as do the adverse effects on fertility and sexual function (Mello, Mendelson, & Teoh, 1993).

In both men and women, **as the drinking progresses, alcoholic behavior is reinforced and it is difficult for the alcoholic to do anything but drink**. Sex is merely something to do while drinking.

Men & Alcohol. The familiar release of inhibitions both in words and deeds is the key to alcohol's dual effect on a man's sexual activity, i.e., more desire/less performance. In men a blood alcohol level of .05 (about three beers in 1 hour) has a very measurable physical effect on erectile ability and yet legal intoxication in most states is almost twice that amount. On the other hand, mentally even one drink can loosen the tongue. **Physically alcohol diminishes spinal reflexes thus decreasing sensitivity and erectile ability.** Even a few drinks lower testosterone levels; however, the long-term male drinker shows a greater decrease in testosterone, an increase of female sex steroids, such as estradiol, and abnormalities in sex steroid metabolism (Wright, Gavaler, & Thiel, 1991; Zakhari, 1993).

Initially, however, alcohol gives men more confidence because it acts on the area of the brain that regulates fear and anxiety thereby promoting, not decreasing, aggressiveness. As alcoholism progresses many men feel less sexual (possibly due to decreased testosterone and preoccupation with alcohol) and tend to shy away from the bedroom and even become asexual. In one study impotence was reported in 60% of heavy alcohol abusers (Crowe & George, 1989).

"Sure I could have sex without alcohol. I've just never had occasion to do it."
43-year-old problem drinker

Marijuana

Marijuana has been called the "mirror that magnifies" because many of its effects—sensory enhancement, seeming prolongation of time, increased affectionate bonding, disinhibition, diffusion of ego, and sexualized fantasy—suggest a preexisting desire for these sensations.

Most of the reported effects from marijuana are general comments, such as feelings of sexual pleasure, rather than specifics, like prolonged excitation or delayed orgasm. **Marijuana, more than any psychoactive drug, illustrates the difficulty in separating the actual effects from the influence of the mind-set and setting where the drug is used.** If the drug is shared in a social setting, at a party, or on a date, the expectation is that it will make people more relaxed, less inhibited, and more likely to do things they wouldn't normally do.

A problem with excessive marijuana smoking is that **the user often forgets or never learns how to have sexual relations without being high**, so the cycle of excess use is perpetuated. (The loss of sexual interest from hashish use is well-known in other cultures.)

MDMA & MDA (ecstasy, rave)

In the past year 1.4% of the general population and 7.4% of high school seniors used ecstasy (SAMHSA, 2002). Users say MDMA and MDA (at moderate doses), unlike methamphetamines, **calm them, give them warm feelings towards others, and induce a heightened sensual awareness.** The warm feelings supposedly make closer relations with those around them possible.

"I had no inhibitions. I mean it was like whatever sexual compromise or, you know, touching or conversation that I would normally have had boundaries for, I didn't when I took ecstasy."
22-year-old ecstasy user

Although the feelings of closeness and sensuality are enhanced, the ability to have an erection and orgasm are more difficult to achieve (Holland, 2001). The neurological mechanism for some of **the effects of MDMA are caused by its manipulation of serotonin**—reportedly it reverses the reuptake of this neurotransmitter resulting in an excess in the synapse thus it has a more calming effect than methamphetamine.

Supposedly sexual excitement occurs more often when coming down from the drug than while under the influence. However only 25–50% of the users report any of these reactions. A survey of 100 MDMA users found that the drug induced pleasure in touching and physical intimacy rather than sexual experience (Beck & Rosenbaum, 1994). Also most of the reports about the sexual effects of MDMA and MDA are anecdotal and since polydrug use is quite widespread (especially involving amphetamine, marijuana, and alcohol) and an exciting set and setting can enhance the effects, accurate data is lacking. Possible dangers from excess use include high blood pressure, rapid heart rate, overheating, and prolonged **disruption of serotonergic activity in the central nervous system**. For some the emotional revelations brought on by the drug prove to be extremely upsetting.

PCP

PCP is generally not associated with sex but because it is an anesthetic, it has been **used to deaden the pain of some unusual sexual practices** mostly in small segments of the gay community. And even though it is a dissociative anesthetic making communication difficult when under the influence, low doses have been said to enhance sexual desire and performance in some, possibly from the lowering of inhibitions (Buffum, 1988; Peugh & Belenko, 2001).

LSD

The effects of a psychedelic like LSD are so confusing to the senses that it is **not considered to be a sexual enhancer** and as a result few controlled studies have been done. The same is true of psilocybin mushrooms and peyote.

Volatile Nitrites (amyl, butyl, etc.)

Volatile nitrites are vasodilators and muscles relaxants. **If inhaled just prior to orgasm, they seemingly prolong and enhance the sensation.** Abused as orgasm intensifiers by both the gay and straight communities in the

1960s, they too gained the reputation of being yet another "love drug." They are also used because they relax anal sphincter muscles. The side effects, however, of dizziness, weakness, sedation, fainting, and severe headaches often end up diminishing or counteracting the desired effects (Sharp & Rosenberg, 1997; O'Brien et al., 1992).

Nitrous Oxide (laughing gas)

Nitrous oxide has become popular at music clubs and rave parties for the giddiness it produces. However it is **not generally looked upon as a sexually enhancing substance**. One study of 15 dental personnel who abused the substance over a period of time found impotence in 7 cases. The problem eventually was reversed when use of the gas was stopped (Jastak, 1991).

Psychiatric Drugs

Most patients who use psychiatric medications have preexisting emotional problems that can impair sexual functioning. **By treating the mental condition, the drugs can also affect the sexual functioning of the user.** For example, an antidepressant can make a patient more able to engage in intimate relations and sexual appreciation, capabilities that were impaired by the depression.

The neurotransmitter serotonin has been found to be involved with many aspects of sexual behavior. Depending on which serotonin receptor is involved, serotonin can either facilitate or inhibit sexual behavior.

Studies involving tricyclic antidepressants, such as desipramine (Norpramine®) and amitriptyline (Elavil®), **have linked them to decreased desire, problems with erection, and delayed orgasm**. Initially, however, in many cases the relief from depression makes the user more able to be sexually involved. Many of the newer antidepressants, known as "selective serotonin reuptake inhibitors" or "SSRIs," such as **sertraline (Zoloft®), fluoxetine (Prozac®), and paroxetine (Paxil®), also cause delay or inhibition of orgasm and impaired erection ability** (Kline,

1989; Goldberg, 1998). Delayed orgasm often goes away with time. Prozac® has also been associated with a significant incidence of sexual disinterest where sex is possible but interest diminishes (Meston & Gorzalka, 1992; PDR, 2003).

Antipsychotics, such as thioridazine (Mellaril®), **inhibit erectile function and ejaculation**. Chlorpromazine (Thorazine®) and haloperidol (Haldol®) can inhibit desire, erectile function, and ejaculation. Impaired ejaculation appears to be the most common side effect of the major tranquilizers (antipsychotics).

With lithium (used for bipolar disorder), there are some reports of decreased desire and difficulty maintaining an erection as the dosage increases.

Aphrodisiacs

The search for true aphrodisiacs is complicated by the complexity of the sexual response. Are people talking about affection, love, or lust when discussing drugs that enhance sexuality? Are they talking about drugs that change the mental or the physical aspects of sexuality? Is the drug expected to increase desire, prolong excitation, increase lubrication, delay orgasm, or improve its quality? Is a drug that lowers inhibitions an aphrodisiac? Heroin sometimes delays orgasm, cocaine sometimes increases desire or prolongs an erection, and alcohol lowers inhibitions thereby increasing desire.

As mentioned **Viagra® deals mostly with the ability to have an erection by enhancing blood flow** but is not an actual aphrodisiac. Some purported aphrodisiacs, such as Spanish fly or ground rhinoceros horn, work by irritating the urethra and bladder promoting a pseudosexual excitement. But Spanish fly (cantharidin derived from a beetle) is actually toxic. The scent of **pheromones, human hormones discovered in perspiration, has been shown to increase desire and sexual stimulation**. Interestingly pheromones act as aphrodisiacs only if they come from people with differing immune systems. Yohimbine is an alkaloid obtained from several plant sources including the

yohimbe tree in west Africa. This stimulant that produces some hallucinations and a mild euphoria has been used in high doses as a treatment for impotence in men by increasing blood pressure and heart rate thereby increasing penile blood flow. It can produce acute anxiety at low dosages (Morganthaler & Joy, 1994). L-dopa is a precursor to dopamine in the brain and dopamine is the neurotransmitter involved in the mental experience of orgasm. It is used medically to treat Parkinson's disease and was touted as an aphrodisiac during the 1970s; however effective treatment of lost muscle control caused by Parkinsonism may have been more responsible for this aphrodisiac claim.

One problem with purported sexual enhancers is that the body adapts to any drug, so its effectiveness decreases with time. Another problem with illegal substances is that controlled use is difficult and side effects start to overwhelm any benefits. Third, and perhaps most important, the psychological roots of most feelings are quite complex and generally more important to sexual functioning than mere enhancement of sensations. Drugs can distort, magnify, or eliminate feelings involved with erotic activities.

SUBSTANCE ABUSE & SEXUAL ASSAULT

"He definitely had been drinking. However when I replay all the events of that night, I feel like he knew exactly what was going to happen or how he was going to attempt each move that led to me being assaulted [raped]. That included offering me and giving me alcohol. That's the thing I blame myself for. I don't think I was scared until I realized what was happening to me, until I realized that he was raping me. And at that point I started screaming although I did not hear myself screaming at all."
26-year-old woman

One in every three women in this country will be a victim of sexual violence in her lifetime. In one study of **sexual assaults, victims reported using drugs or alcohol in 51% of the cases while substance use by the assailants was found in about 44% of the cases** (Seifert, 1999). Another study found that approximately 60% of sexual offenders were drinking at the time of the offense (Roizen, 1997).

In most cases the male user already has tendencies towards improper or aggressive behavior and the alcohol or other drug is the final trigger. The trigger can also be an emotion such as anger, hate, or in some cases, lust.

"In some men alcohol can disinhibit their aggressive tendencies and they become violent when they drink alcohol but the violence was sitting in them and residing in their psyche way before they picked up that first drink."
Jackson Katz, Executive Director, MVP Strategies Inc. (Male Violence Prevention)

Some generalizations about the effects of psychoactive drugs on sexual behavior and violence can be made.

◇ **Alcohol lowers inhibitions and muddles rational thought**, making the user more likely to act out irrational or inappropriate desires.

◇ **Cocaine and amphetamines increase confidence and aggression**, making the male user more likely to assault his date.

◇ **Sedatives lower inhibitions**, making users more prone to sexual advances or making the woman less able to resist.

◇ **Marijuana makes users more suggestible** to sexual activity and more sensitive to touch.

◇ PCP and heroin make users less sensitive or indifferent to pain and therefore more liable to damage their partners or themselves.

◇ Steroids can increase aggression and irrational behavior.

"I've seen freshman girls drunk, so drunk that they couldn't even stand up, and guys totally grabbing on to them on the dance floor. And it saddens me because we should be able to have that privilege to go out and have fun, drink a few beers or whatever and not have to worry about having someone taking advantage of us that night or waking up in a strange room and not knowing where you are."
22-year-old female who was raped

With date rape the man may just intend to have sex but when he is refused or doesn't get his way, he becomes angry and takes what he feels is his right. In the final analysis **rape is motivated by a need to overpower, humiliate, and dominate a victim not a desire to have sex**.

"Sexual abuse is very much a prevalent thing in domestic violence situations. We estimate through statistics that probably 50% of all women who are battered are raped by their intimate partners."
Karen Darling, Director, Domestic Violence Education Center, Asante Health Services

What also occurs with sexual abuse and domestic violence is that the emotional pain and trauma intensify the need to block one's feelings leading to intensified use of drugs and alcohol.

"I remember being beat up physically and being emotionally abused and drinking a gallon of wine and feeling like I just wanted to be out of it. And for me that was the way to deal with the pain. And I think women tend to do those things—take drugs to be able to continue to have some kind of relationship."
38-year-old counselor at the Haight Ashbury Detox Clinic

SEXUALLY TRANSMITTED DISEASES (STDs)

The World Health Organization (WHO) estimates that worldwide **333 million cases of sexually transmitted diseases occur each year**. About 1% of those will eventually die from their STD. In contrast 42 million people are living with HIV/AIDS. Almost all of them will eventually die from HIV-related diseases (World Health Organization [WHO], 1998).

Epidemiology

The dangers of sexually transmitted diseases, such as **chlamydia, gonorrhea, syphilis, and trichomonas (the four most common)** along with genital herpes, genital warts, and hepatitis B and C, are well-known as are the mortal dangers of HIV disease. However in spite of this knowledge and in spite of a growth in unwanted pregnancies, the practice of unsafe and unprotected sex by high school students, college students, and young adults in the United States continues. **About 85% of all STDs occurs in persons between the ages of 15 and 30.** Very often alcohol and other drugs are involved (CDC, 2003b).

A study by the National Center on Addiction and Substance Abuse at Columbia University that examined the habits of 34,000 teenagers from grades 7–12 found that students who drank and used drugs were 5 times more likely to be sexually active, starting sexual intercourse as early as middle school. They were also 3 times more likely to have had sex with 4 or more partners in the previous 2 years (NCASA, 2000).

The use of crack cocaine, methamphetamine, and marijuana increases high-risk sexual activity due to intensified sensations, lowering of inhibitions, and impaired judgment. In addition the very nature of sexual activity clouds judgment, as do most drugs. Drugs also affect memory, so even if users do something dangerous while under the influence, they might not remember it or if they do, they will see it in a more benign light. They most likely won't appreciate the risks they took thus laying the groundwork for repetition of that behavior.

With this mix it is no wonder that

almost half of all teenagers who are very active sexually have had chlamydia, the fastest-spreading sexually transmitted disease. In fact experts think that as many as 4 million Americans have caught the disease (often without knowing it). Perhaps 20% of all very sexually active men and women have genital herpes. Even syphilis, which had diminished dramatically in the last 50 years, has started to climb again. Surprisingly the number of people infected by the hepatitis C virus (about 4 million) outnumber the HIV-positive population 5 to 1. There were still 41,755 new cases of AIDS in the United States in 2001 (CDC, 2003a).

"This woman was pregnant, she was living on the street, she was prostituting, was HIV positive, and had a $250-a-day habit. I mean she's not a bad looking woman but she was def-

initely into her 'smack' and her cocaine. She told me she had to sleep with at least five guys a day, minimum, to support her habit. I wonder how many people she's given her diseases to."

AIDS patient

The imcreased risk of STDs, including HIV disease, due to trading sex for drugs is all too common among the drug-abusing population who will often do anything to raise money to avoid a cocaine crash or heroin withdrawal.

"I was selling dope and made $3 or $4 thousand a week. I had women coming to me. I never 'tossed' a woman in my life. Those women were coming after me. I mean, you've got to look at both sides of it."

22-year-old recovering crack dealer/user

One thing to remember about sexually transmitted diseases is that there is a delayed incubation period before symptoms show up, so the disease can be unknowingly transmitted to others. There are also some diseases where symptoms aren't evident but the illness is still transmittable.

NEEDLE-TRANSMITTED DISEASES

Many of the same illnesses that are transmitted sexually can also be transmitted through contaminated hypodermic needles when drugs are taken intravenously, subcutaneously, and intramuscularly.

Needle kits are called "outfits," "fits," "rigs," "works," "points," and many other names. Intravenous drug use is also called "mainlining," "geezing," "slamming," or "hitting up." Problems with needle use come from several sources. Besides putting a large

TABLE 8–6   SEXUALLY TRANSMITTED DISEASES

Disease	First Symptoms	Typical Symptoms
Chlamydia or NGU	7–21 days	Discharge from genitals or rectum (nonspecific urethritis)
Pelvic inflammatory disease (PID)	Highly variable	Infection of uterus, fallopian tubes, and ovaries, a potential cause of infertility
Gonorrhea ("clap," "dose")	2–30 days	Discharge from genitals or rectum, pain when urinating, sometimes no symptoms
Herpes simplex I or II (cold sore, fever blister)	2–20 days	Painful blisters/sores on genitals or mouth, fever, malaise, swollen lymph glands
Venereal warts (genital warts)	30–90 days (even years)	Itch, irritation, and bumpy skin growths on genitals, anus, mouth, throat
Syphilis ("syph," "bad blood," "lues")	10–90 days	Primary stage: chancre on genitals, mouth, anus; secondary stage: diffuse rash, hair loss, malaise
Hepatitis B and C (serum hepatitis)	60–90 days	Yellow skin and eyes, dark urine, severe malaise, weight loss, abdominal pain
Trichomonas	7–30 days	Women: vaginal discharge, itching, burning; men: usually no symptoms
Pubic lice ("crabs," "cooties")	21–30 days	Itching, tiny eggs (nits) on pubic hair
Scabies ("7-year itch")	14–45 days	Itching at night, bumps and burrows on skin
Monila (candidiasis, yeast)	Highly variable	White thick vaginal discharge and itching in women, men most often have no symptoms
Bacterial vaginosis (gardnerella, nonspecific vaginitis)	Highly variable	Vaginal discharge, peculiar odor in women, men most often have no symptoms
HIV infection (leads to AIDS)	Many months (up to 5 years)	Weight loss, fever, swollen glands, diarrhea, fatigue, severe malaise, recurrent infections, sore throat, skin blotches

(Venereal Disease Action Council of Portland, Oregon)

amount of the drug in the bloodstream in a short period of time, **needles also inject other substances like powered milk, procaine, or even Ajax® that are often used to cut or dilute drugs. They can also inject dangerous bacteria and viruses.**

Hepatitis A, B & C

Some of the most common diseases transmitted by needles are the various strains of hepatitis, viral infections of the liver. Hepatitis A is often transmitted by fecal matter and is associated more with unsafe sex and poor hygiene than with drug use. The two main types of hepatitis associated with drug use, specifically IV drug use, are hepatitis B and hepatitis C. Hepatitis B is marked by inflammation of the liver and general debilitation but it is treatable with a convalescence of 1–5 months. **More than 75% of IV drug users test positive for hepatitis B.** Of those, about 10% are chronic carriers, guaranteeing the continued spread of the disease (Novick, Haverkos, & Teller, 1997). As discussed in Chapter 4, the blood-borne hepatitis C virus (HCV) is more dangerous and can cause liver disease including cancer. Some people will carry the disease for 10–20 years without symptoms that can develop such as lack of appetite, jaundice, abdominal pain, and a general malaise; however, the only way to be sure is to test for HCV antibodies. Chronic flare-ups can cause inflammation and scarring of the liver.

The hepatitis C virus positive rate in IV drug users is 50–90%. Of those that get infected with HCV, 20–40% will develop liver disease while 4–16% will develop liver cancer (Novick, Reagan, et al., 1997; Cahoon-Young, 1997; CDC, 2003a). The problem with HCV has become so severe that NIDA issued a special alert to increase counseling, treatment, and prevention.

◇ **About 4 million Americans are infected with the HCV virus** with a majority of those young adults aged 20–29 although chronic infections are highest among 30–39-year-olds.

◇ **Between 8,000–10,000 die each year from the disease.**

◇ **Sharing needles is responsible for almost two-thirds of the infections.**

◇ New IV drug users acquire HCV at an alarming rate with 50–80% becoming infected within 6–12 months. (The average incubation period is 6–7 weeks.)

◇ The risk of sexual transmission of HCV is much lower than the risk of IV drug use transmission. About 20% of the cases are supposedly due to sexual activity particularly among those who have multiple partners. In long-term monogamous relationships the rate is very low (0–4%).

◇ The risk of an infected mother passing the infection on to her fetus is about 5–6%.

(NIDA, 2000)

Abscesses, Cotton Fever & Endocarditis

Needle use can also cause abscesses at an infected injection site or it can inject bits of foreign matter in the bloodstream that can lodge in the spine, brain, lungs, or eyes and cause an embolism or other problems. Needle users can also contract cotton fever, a very common disease. The symptoms are similar to those of a very bad case of the flu. Its cause is unknown though some believe that it results from bits of cotton (used to filter the drug) that lodge in various tissues or from infections (viral or bacterial) carried into the body by cotton fibers injected into the blood. Starting in the mid- to late-1990s, more and more cases of necrotizing fasciitis (a flesh-eating bacteria and wound botulism or gangrene) have been reported.

"I started using drugs when I got together with my ex-boyfriend but then I quit using them because I would get these big abscesses on my arms and stuff and my veins—like when I go to the doctor to get blood drawn now, they can't use my veins in my arms."
22-year-old recovering heroin user

Typically veins of the arms, wrists, and hands are used first. As these **veins become hardened due to constant sticking**, the user will inject into the veins of the legs and then the neck. As it becomes difficult to locate usable veins, addicts will also shoot under the skin ("skin popping") or into a muscle in the buttocks, shoulder, or legs ("muscling"). If they become desperate as they run out of places to shoot themselves, they will inject into the foot and males will even inject in the dorsal vein in the penis.

"I'm addicted to needles. Like sticking any needle in my vein will pretty much alleviate my dope sickness even if it's like speed or even water. That would make it go away for a little while—just the part of my brain that would make me think that everything is all right."
17-year-old heroin addict

Another common problem is **endocarditis, a sometimes fatal condition caused by certain bacteria that lodge and grow in the valves of the heart.** IV cocaine users seem to have a higher rate of endocarditis, perhaps because the ups and downs of cocaine require many more injections than heroin or methamphetamines (Wartenberg, 1998).

HIV Disease & AIDS

HIV (human immunodeficiency virus) is the virus that causes AIDS. AIDS stands for "acquired immune deficiency syndrome." AIDS is identified by the incidence of one or more of a group of serious illnesses, such as pneumocystis carinii pneumonia, Kaposi's sarcoma cancer, or tuberculosis, that develop when the HIV virus has taken control of the patient's body and lowered its resistance. However in 1993 a new qualifier to diagnose AIDS was added. AIDS is now also defined as "having a T-cell count below 200." T-cell counts measure the level of effectiveness of one's immune system.

AIDS is fatal because the HIV virus destroys the immune system making it impossible for the body to

fight off serious illnesses. Usually death occurs from a combination of many diseases and infections. Many needle users test positive for the HIV (AIDS) virus because they shared a needle used by someone already infected.

"I know I'm really lucky that I didn't get AIDS 'cause a lot of people that I knew used my needles and then they would put them back in my clean needles and I didn't know that they were using them. And I just thank God that I didn't get any diseases or I'm not dead right now."

22-year-old heroin user

It is impossible to overemphasize the danger of using infected needles because **IV use of a drug bypasses all the body's natural defenses such as body hairs, mucous membranes, body acids, and enzymes**; and the HIV virus itself destroys the body's last line of defense, the immune system. In fact recent research shows that, in and of themselves, opioids and other drugs of abuse can weaken the immune system (Des Jarlais, Hagan, & Friedman, 1997). This, coupled with the malnutrition and unhealthy habits that compulsive drug use promotes, makes the body unable to fight off any illness.

"I told this guy that was sharing some speed with me that I had AIDS and that he should clean the needle but he was so strung out and anxious to shoot up that he pulled a knife on me and made me give him the needle."

Intravenous cocaine user

Worldwide there were 5 million new cases of HIV infection in 2002. Of the 42 million infected with HIV/AIDS, two-thirds are from Sub-Saharan Africa. Most contract the infection by the age of 25 and die before their 35th birthday. By the end of 2002, 27 million people had died from AIDS (WHO, 2003). The three main reasons for the worldwide spread are heterosexual sex, homosexual sex, and drug use (IV

use). Infected drug users also spread the disease to nondrug users through unsafe sexual practices.

By comparison, approximately **800,000–900,000 Americans are infected with the HIV virus or have AIDS while 467,910 have already died from the disease** since it first appeared on the scene in 1981 (CDC, 2003a). Since the beginning of the AIDS epidemic, over one-third of all AIDS cases in the United States have involved intravenous drug use (26% from direct use and 10% from having sex with an IV drug user). Even in Russia and the Ukraine, the use of infected needles has doubled the rate of HIV infection. In 2002 about 700,000 Russians were living with HIV/AIDS (UN-AIDS, 2003).

Intravenous drug use-associated AIDS accounts for a larger proportion of cases among adolescent and adult women than among men. Since the epidemic began, 57% of all AIDS cases among women have been attributed to injection drug use or sex with partners who inject drugs.

Racial and ethnic minority populations in the United States are the most heavily affected by AIDS especially in recent years. Almost 50% of new infections in 2001 were African Americans though they are only 13% of the population. This compares to 19% of the new cases being Hispanic and 30% Caucasian.

Men who have sex with other men are still the greatest cause of AIDS cases in the United States. Among women, 75% of the cases are from heterosexual contact. In 2001 Washington, DC, had the highest new AIDS cases rate while New York was second in rate but first in sheer numbers (Table 8-7).

PREVENTION OF DISEASE

It is important to remember that **communicable diseases start slowly but then rage through the most susceptible groups.** In the case of HIV and AIDS in the United States, the gay community that practiced unsafe sex was the most vulnerable compared to other

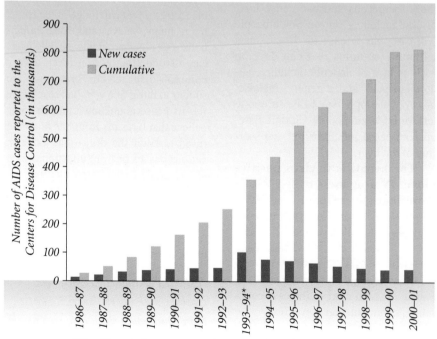

Note: The extra increase over previous years is due to the revised definition of AIDS that includes having a T-cell count under 200.

Figure 8-7 •

The Centers for Disease Control and Prevention keep track of all infectious diseases in the United States.

**TABLE 8–7   NEW U.S. AIDS CASES—NUMBER & RATE
DEC. 31, 2000–DEC. 31, 2001**

Selected States	Cases	Rate per 100,000
New York	7,476	39.3
California	4,315	12.5
Florida	5,138	31.3
Texas	2,892	13.6
New Jersey	1,756	20.7
Pennsylvania	1,840	15.0
Maryland	1,860	34.6
Washington, DC	870	152.1
U.S. total new AIDS cases (12/00–12/01)	**41,755**	**14.7**
Through 1-1-02		
U.S. total HIV/AIDS living	800,000–900,000	
U.S. total AIDS deaths	467,910	
Through 1-1-03		
World: total AIDS/HIV living	42,000,000	
World: total AIDS deaths	27,000,000	

(CDC, 2003a; WHO, 2003)

countries where heterosexual high-risk sexual activity spread the disease.

Once the most vulnerable have been infected, there is usually a lull in the increase of the disease. During such lulls, a false sense of security, along with clouded judgment, builds up a new upwelling of infection. The majority of new cases of HIV in the United States (as in the rest of the world) will be in the heterosexual and drug-using communities. **Continuing public education and public health prevention activities are crucial to stem the spread of AIDS and, for that matter, all sexually transmitted diseases.**

"The only way the attitudes and practices towards AIDS would change is if everybody got these diseases, you hear what I'm saying? It doesn't really sink in unless it strikes close to you. Once the virus is in your own backyard, you become very serious. Kids wanna wear rubbers once they find out their father has it, you know what I mean? People are concerned once they find out their mother has it, or their brother has it, or they have it."

Recovering 43-year-old heroin addict who is HIV positive

Several strategies exist to stop the spread of AIDS, particularly in the drug-using community. Some of them are

◇ improved diagnosis and treatment of STDs;

◇ treatment on demand for drug addiction to encourage users to give up drugs;

◇ needle exchange programs to control transmission of the disease;

◇ creation of outreach activities to get high-risk drug users into contact with the treatment community;

◇ education and counseling programs that teach about the dangers of AIDS and that teach the use of bleach to clean needles;

◇ availability of antiviral drugs such as AZT and other medications for HIV-positive pregnant women and anyone else exposed to the virus (Harris et al., 2002);

◇ vocational training to counteract poverty, a predisposing factor to drug use and HIV infection;

◇ education programs that teach about high-risk sexual activities;

◇ easy access to condoms at a reasonable price;

◇ interdiction and law enforcement activities to limit the flow of drugs into the community (University of California in San Francisco, 1998).

In studies by the Center for Disease Control and other agencies, **drug abuse treatment along with education and needle exchange programs that are tied to outreach components seem to be the most effective HIV disease or AIDS prevention strategies**.

Harm Reduction

In June of 2003 **the health ministry of Canada approved North America's first legal safe injection site for illegal drug users** in Vancouver, British Columbia. Addicts will be able to shoot up under the supervision of a registered nurse. The purpose is to prevent overdoses and provide clean needles to reduce the spread of HIV, hepatitis, and other blood-borne diseases. Health Canada has put the center off limits to police. Similar programs have been tried in Switzerland, the Netherlands, and Australia. Results in those older programs have been mixed. The spread of diseases and overdose deaths has declined somewhat, but addiction rates have not fallen. The director of the White House Office of National Drug Control Policy, John Walters, depicted the program as "state-sponsored personal suicide" (Boston Globe, 2003).

In San Francisco several groups, including the HIV Prevention and Research Center of the Haight Ashbury Free Clinics, have outreach programs meant to contact IV drug users who are not in treatment. **Outreach workers from the Center, armed with AIDS educational materials, free bottles of bleach, and free condoms, go out to the "shooting galleries," crack houses, "dope pads," and other areas** to distribute these materials and provide treatment referrals if requested. Other groups distribute free needles. It's an intervention into drug-related behavior without intervening into drug use. The drug use intervention part of the total policy is handled by the other sections of the Clinic.

The problem with education only in addiction treatment settings about the risks of sharing needles is that it may miss the larger segment of IV drug users who are not ready for treatment (and therefore at highest risk for AIDS). Users alienated by the treatment community or in denial are hard to educate. To keep these people in treatment, some clinics instituted a more tolerant policy towards relapses and towards users who can't clean up during their first few tries. The idea is that at least the user is occasionally in contact with a facility that can intervene, present important information, and eventually get the client into treatment.

Education however does work. In San Francisco, in just a short period of time, drug users' awareness about the dangers of AIDS and the need to clean their needles jumped from a few percent to 85%. The HIV-positive segment of the IV drug-using population in San Francisco is 15–17% compared to 60–80% in New York. Part of this difference in the HIV infection rate between the two coasts seems to be due to the educational effort of the clinics, the San Francisco Health Department, and the gay community. Other differences seem to be the greater presence of "shooting galleries," the limited number of treatment facilities, the difficulty in obtaining clean needles, and language barriers in New York.

Many new drugs besides ziduvodine (AZT), one of the original AIDS drugs, have been developed and are showing promise in slowing or even halting the spread of the HIV virus in the body. Antiretroviral drugs and protease inhibitors seemed more effective but the complicated regimen of dozens of pills that have to be taken daily and the severe side effects have diminished some of the early promise. Recently a group of top international scientists,

supported by the Bill and Melinda Gates Foundation, called for the creation of a new global program to speed the discovery and testing of new AIDS vaccines; a program that would be similar in scope to the $3 billion Human Genome Project (Russel, 2003). Barring the creation of a vaccine, they call for intense prevention and treatment programs.

In addition **studies have shown that people who test positive for HIV who stay clean and sober and maintain a healthy lifestyle with plenty of rest, good food, and exercise will avoid full-blown AIDS for years longer**. And those who have an AIDS diagnosis will live months to years longer. Improved treatment for opportunistic infections that can be so lethal to immune systems weakened by AIDS can also give years of life to infected clients (Haverkos, 1998).

"As I've started going into recovery and learning that I'm worth something and learning that I can have a life even though I'm HIV positive, yeah, it scares me to go back out there 'cause I know that when I use, I have unsafe sex, bottom line. And when I'm high, I'm not going to put on a condom. When I'm high, I will let people do things to me that I normally wouldn't let them do."
Recovering methamphetamine user who is HIV positive

DRUGS AT WORK

"I began to notice that because I was using marijuana on a day-to-day basis, my reactions were slower and my thought processes were certainly slower. In the electronics business, you really have to be thinking sharply."
33-year-old recovering marijuana abuser

The concept of the drug-free workplace that includes preemployment drug testing, employee assistance pro-

grams, and a greater understanding of the effects of drug abuse has led to a reduction in drug use and associated problems in the workplace.

Contrary to the popular picture of the unemployed drug or alcohol user,

◇ **76% of illicit drug users age 18 or older work full or part time;**

◇ **of full-time workers, 5.6 million (7.2%) were heavy alcohol users;**

◇ about 1.6 million of these workers were both heavy alcohol and illicit drug users;

◇ the percentage of all full-time workers who used illicit drugs in the past month fell from 17.5% in 1985 to 6.9% in 2001;

◇ 26.2% of full-time workers had at least 5 alcoholic drinks at one sitting in the last 30 days.

(SAMHSA, 2002)

The highest rates of illicit drug use are in the construction industry and food preparation and among waiters and waitresses, helpers, and laborers. The lowest rates are among police (SAMHSA, 1996).

COSTS

Studies on the impact of alcohol and other drug abuse in the American workplace have resulted in estimates that substance abuse cost our industries about $140 billion in 1995 of which $60 billion was for drug-related costs and $80 billion for alcohol-related costs. The costs have risen since then; estimated at $160 billion (ONDCP, 2000; NIDA, 1998).

Loss of Productivity

Compared to a nondrug-abusing employee, **a substance-abusing employee is**

◇ **late 3–14 times more often**;

◇ **absent 5–7 times more often** and 3–4 times more likely to be absent for longer than 8 consecutive days;

◇ involved in many more job mistakes;

◇ likely to have lower output, make a less-effective salesperson, experience work shrinkage, i.e., less productivity despite more hours put forth;

◊ likely to appear in a greater number of grievance hearings.

(SAMHSA, 1999b; Mangione et al., 1998)

"If you're doing coke, you really don't like authority over you. You want to take your time to do what you have to do and if a person has any kind of input, you have a tendency to rebel. I used to get in trouble a lot."

Recovering cocaine abuser

About 21% of workers report being injured, having to redo work or to cover for a coworker, needing to work harder, or being put in danger due to other's drinking. However 60% of alcohol-related work performance problems can be attributed to occasional binge drinkers rather than alcoholics or alcohol-dependent employees (U.S. Department of Labor [USDL], 1990).

Medical Cost Increases

Substance abusers as compared to nondrug-abusing employees

◊ **experience 3–4 times more on-the-job accidents;**

◊ **use 3 times more sick leave;**

◊ **file 5 times more workman's compensation claims;**

◊ overutilize health insurance for themselves and their family members;

◊ increase premiums for the entire company for medical and psychological insurance;

◊ endanger the health and well-being of coworkers (USDL, 2003).

Legal Cost Increases

As tolerance and addiction develop, a drug-abusing employee often enters into some form of criminal activity. Crime at the workplace brought about by drug abuse results in

◊ **direct and massive losses from embezzlement, pilferage, sales of**
corporate secrets, and property damaged during commission of a crime;

◊ increased cost of improved company security, more personnel, product monitoring, quality assurance, intensified employee testing and screening;

◊ more lawsuits, both internal and external, expanded legal fees, court costs, and attorney expenses;

◊ loss of customer good will and negative publicity from drug use and trafficking at the workplace, employee arrests, the perception that there are more substance abusers than just those arrested, and manipulation of client contracts or goods.

PREVENTION & EMPLOYEE ASSISTANCE PROGRAMS (EAPs)

"Really, what I've found now that I'm clean and sober is that it wasn't those jobs that were intolerable, it was where I was with myself. I needed to look at myself and do some work on myself."

Recovering cocaine user

Workplace Drug Testing

Businesses attempt to control drug abuse in two ways: through drug testing and employee assistance programs (EAPs).

The cost of private sector workplace drug testing has been estimated to range from $300 million to $1 billion per year (White, Nicholson, Duncan, & Minors, 2002). The various drug-testing programs used by industry have shown positive results.

◊ Since 1988 the percentage of **positive drug tests among American workers dropped from 13.6% down to 4.4%** in 2002. However amphetamine positives almost doubled and propoxyphene (Darvon®) positives tripled.

◊ **The most common drug found in those testing positive is marijuana (57.6%)** compared to cocaine (14.6%), amphetamines (7.1%), opiates (5.5%), and benzodiazepines (4.5%). Generally employers do not test for alcohol without cause although it is the most common drug used.

TABLE 8–8   SUMMARY OF RECOMMENDATIONS FOR A DRUG-FREE WORKFORCE

In order to achieve a drug- and alcohol-free workforce, you must take a comprehensive approach. The approach should include:

A Written Policy: Clear and definite guidelines should be written explaining the reasons for a drug policy and actions that will be taken.

An Employee Assistance Program (EAP): Establish an EAP that provides counseling and referral programs to be operated either by your own staff or by a contractor.

Employee Awareness and Education: Education about company policies along with drug education is necessary.

Supervisor Training: Offer supervisors substance abuse training so those closest to the problem can be coached on the signs, symptoms, behavior changes, performance problems and intervention concepts attendant to drug and alcohol abuse.

Drug and Alcohol Testing: Consider a drug and/or alcohol testing program to detect and deter drug and/or alcohol use or abuse. If testing is adopted, it should conform to proper procedures.

Sanctions: Determine the consequences for those who violate the policy.

Appeals Process: Include an appeals process in the program and clearly define it in the policy.

Evaluation: Monitor cost effectiveness and success of the program.

(Adapted from Guidelines for a Drug-Free Workforce [DEA, 2003d])

◇ In safety-sensitive industries such as transportation, the rate of positive drug tests is about half that of the general workforce.

◇ **About 26% of those tested for cause, tested positive for an illicit drug.**

◇ The highest positive rates came from southern rural areas rather than from big cities like New York, Chicago, or Los Angeles.

(Quest Diagnostics, 2003; SmithKline Beecham Clinical Laboratories, 1997)

Employee Assistance Programs (EAPs)

In response to the increased problem of drugs in the workplace and the resultant drain on profits and productivity, many employers have instituted an EAP. **Successful EAPs balance the needs of management to minimize the negative impact that drug abuse has on their business with a sincere concern for the better health of employees.** Once the benefits of EAPs were recognized, many companies initiated programs. In 1980 there were 5,000 EAPs; in 1990 that number had grown to 20,000 and the number of covered employees grew from 12% to over 35%. Today 45% of full-time employees are covered. In large companies with over 500 employees, 70% are covered (Englehart, Robinson, & Kates, 1997).

Designed as an employee benefit, these programs often encourage self-referral by the employee and/or a supervisor's referral as an alternative to more stringent discipline for poor work performance. The successful EAP supports a broad-based strategy to address the full spectrum of substance abuse prevention needs. The most successful EAPs share 2 overall design features.

1. They frame the EAP drug abuse services as part of a **full-spectrum prevention program** that minimizes employee attraction to drugs and helps those with problems get into treatment.

2. They provide a **diverse range of services for a wide spectrum of employee problems** (emotional, relationship, financial, and burnout).

These two design features lessen employees' apprehension about being labeled as a drug abuser. They prevent drug problems before they start and they identify drug problems for employees in denial who don't accept the fact that they have a problem and often first approach the EAP about another problem area. The EAP is comprised of 6 basic components:

1. prevention/education/training;

2. identification and confidential outreach;

3. diagnosis and referral;

4. treatment, counseling, and a good monitoring system (including drug testing);

5. follow-up and focus towards aftercare (relapse prevention);

6. confidential record system and effectiveness evaluation.

(SAMHSA, 1997; Employee Assistance Professionals Association, 1990; Balzer & Pargament, 1988)

In a full-spectrum prevention program, the EAP provides primary, secondary, and tertiary prevention.

Primary Prevention.   In the most effective EAPs, both corporate and individual denial are addressed with a systems-oriented approach to prevention. **Education and training about the impact of substance abuse are provided at all levels** in the corporation: to the administration, unions, and line staff. These segments agree on a single corporate policy on drug and alcohol abuse.

Secondary Prevention.   Both education and training focus on **drug identification, major effects, and early intervention** that are incorporated into the prevention curriculum. The corporation's legal, grievance, and escalating discipline policies are designed in light of EAP goals. Security measures (testing, staff review, monitoring, etc.) are established in a manner that is legal and humane. These meas-

ures operate both as deterrents to use as well as methods of identifying the abusers and getting them help.

Tertiary Prevention.   The EAP formalizes its **intervention approach, allowing for confidential self-referral, peer referral, and supervisor-initiated referral to the EAP**. A diagnostic process is established, along with a number of **appropriate treatment referrals**. Treatment is confidential but the EAP monitors treatment to insure for proper follow-up aftercare and continued recovery efforts. The employment status of workers is evaluated on work performance and not on their participatory effort in the EAP.

Effectiveness of EAPs

Well-conceived successful programs have demonstrated great effectiveness and cost savings to businesses. **For every $1 spent in an EAP, employers save anywhere from $5–$16.** The cost of providing EAP services ranges from $12–$20 per employee per year (USDL, 1990). Several studies in major corporations have documented a 60–85% decrease in absenteeism, a 40–65% decrease in sick time utilization and personal/family health insurance usage, and a 45–75% decrease in on-the-job accidents as well as other cost savings once the EAP system was put into operation.

◇ Northrup Corporation saw a 43% increase in productivity in its first 100 employees who entered an alcohol treatment program.

◇ Employees in the Philadelphia Police Department going through treatment reduced sick days by 38% and injury days by 62%.

◇ In Oldsmobile's Lansing, Michigan, plant, lost man-hours declined by 49%, health care benefits by 29%, sick leaves by 56%, grievances by 78%, disciplinary problems by 63%, and accidents by 82% (Campbell & Graham, 1988).

"I stopped using it [marijuana] and I noticed a major difference in how I felt,

the fact that I was able to get up okay in the morning. You know, I wouldn't drive to work drowsy and my thought processes were a lot clearer. I could even program my VCR."

Phone company worker

There are a number of different types of EAPs, often determined by financial considerations.

◊ **Internal/In-House Programs.** These EAPs are usually found in large companies that can afford the expense. The staff is employed by the organization and counsels employees on-site.

◊ **Fixed-Fee Contracts.** The company contracts with an outside EAP provider for a number of services such as counseling and educational programs.

◊ **Fee-for-Service Contracts.** Outside EAP services are used and paid for only when employees use the service.

◊ **Consortia.** To save money, smaller employers pool their needs and contract with an outside EAP service provider.

◊ **Peer-Based Programs.** Peers and co-workers give education, training, assistance, and referrals to troubled workers. This type of program requires considerable education and training for employees.

(DEA, 2003d)

DRUGS IN THE MILITARY

One example of reducing the use of psychoactive drugs in the workplace is the experience of the military. In a survey of American military, the Research Triangle Institute in North Carolina found that **from 1980–1998, 30-day illicit drug use dropped from 27.6% to just 2.7% of military personnel** (RTI International, 1999). Unfortunately the rate of heavy drinking showed a smaller drop, from 20.8% to 15.4%.

The reasons for the drop are varied. Probably the strongest reason was an **intensified program of urine testing**, starting in the early 1980s, with a posi-

tive result as grounds for referral to rehabilitation or, if that fails, discharge. The military does about 3 million drug tests each year. The message was zero tolerance. **In the past, drug users had been treated and kept in the military but with zero tolerance, they decided that there was no margin for having impaired people.** Discharge has become the preferred option. A second reason for the drop in drug use was that drugs, in general, became less popular in society over that period of time. The drop in smoking from 51% to 30% over the same period was attributed to military smoking bans, an end to free cigarettes for GIs, and stop-smoking programs as well as a general smoking decline in society as a whole. **Heavy drinking still occurs at a higher rate than the general public: 17.1% in the military vs. just 12% in the general public.** The highest rate is in the Marine Corps and the lowest in the Air Force. Part of the difficulty in reaching heavy drinkers who are mostly young enlistees is that there is a high turnover rate in the ranks and historically drinking has been acceptable.

The military has the advantage of being able to discharge almost anyone they define as being dangerous to other military personnel (Rhem, 2001). In addition because it is the military, they can conduct testing whenever and wherever they choose.

During the Vietnam War, drug use, particularly heroin use, was high. It was readily available, stress was intense, and the environment was strange and permissive (Robins, 1993). During the war in the Persian Gulf, drugs and alcohol were difficult to obtain and as a result there were a lot fewer disciplinary problems among the troops (O'Brien et al., 1992).

DRUG TESTING

Increasingly, **drug testing has appeared in all walks of life not just in business**. Drug testing has long been used to determine the blood or breath alcohol level of drivers suspected of

drunk driving. Testing has been expanded to include

◊ pre-employment testing,

◊ reasonable cause testing,

◊ random testing,

◊ post-accident testing,

◊ periodic testing,

◊ rehabilitation testing of ex-convicts or felons on probation or of others suspected of a crime,

◊ testing for compliance in addicts who are in treatment,

◊ testing by medical examiners to determine the cause of death,

◊ testing of welfare recipients to get them into treatment (about 12 states allow this kind of testing).

The federal government issued **mandates in 1988 and 1998 for a drug-free workplace**. Although there is now a consensus that testing is effective, there have been a number of regulations and laws promulgated over the past 10 years that limit random testing.

At present **the most widespread use of drug testing is in the military, in the federal government, in preemployment drug testing, and in drug treatment facilities**. Most medium and large businesses routinely use preemployment testing to keep drug users out because once they are hired, the problems they engender can be very expensive. Because of the many challenges to random testing of those already employed, many businesses are leery of using it. However, **random testing is still used in jobs involving public safety**—jobs such as bus drivers, policemen, and pilots.

THE TESTS

Many different laboratory procedures are used to **test for drugs in the urine, blood, hair, saliva, sweat**, and even different tissues of the body. Each test possesses inherent differences in sensitivity, specificity, and accuracy along with other potential problems. The drugs most often tested for are **amphetamines, cannabinoids, cocaine, opioids, and phencyclidine (PCP)**.

Other drugs commonly tested for are **barbiturates, benzodiazepines, methadone, propoxyphene (Darvon®), methaqualone, MDMA, and ethanol (alcohol)**. Those that can be tested for but usually are not include LSD, fentanyl, psilocybin, MDA, and designer drugs.

Currently some two dozen methods are used to analyze body samples for the presence of drugs. None is totally foolproof. The following are the most common methods (Vereby & Buchan, 1997).

Thin Layer Chromatography (TLC)

TLC **searches for a wide variety of drugs at the same time** and is fairly sensitive to the presence of even minute amounts of chemicals. The major drawback is its inability to accurately differentiate drugs that may have similar chemical properties. For example, ephedrine, a drug used legally in over-the-counter cold medicines, may be misidentified as an illegal amphetamine.

Enzyme-Multiplied Immunoassay Techniques (EMIT), Radio Immunoassay (RIA), Enzyme Immunoassay (EIA)

All immunoassays use antibodies to seek out specific drugs. **EMIT tests are extremely sensitive, very rapidly performed, and fairly easy to operate**. However they cannot usually distinguish the concentration of the drug present. Also, a separate test must usually be run for each specific suspected drug. Immunoassay techniques are used for many home-testing kits. Some can test for several drugs at once (e.g., Ascend Multimmunoassay [AMIA]).

EMIT tests can also mistake non-abused chemicals for abused drugs, e.g., opioid alkaloids in the poppy seeds of baked goods for heroin or another opioid. One of the chemicals in Advil® or Motrin® may be mistaken for marijuana and the form of methamphetamine in Vick's Inhaler® is sometimes identified as "crank." This method is so sensitive that breathing air at most rock concerts will show a positive trace of marijuana even though the testee didn't smoke. This oversensitivity is corrected by raising the sensitivity level of the test so only current users will test positive. This may miss detection of some users.

Gas Chromatography/Mass Spectrometry Combined (GC/MS) & Gas Liquid Chromotography (GLC)

The GC/MS test is currently **the most accurate, sensitive, and reliable method of testing** for drugs in the body. It uses gas chromatography separation and mass spectrometry fragmentation patterns to identify drugs. Being very sensitive, it can detect even trace amounts of drugs in the urine and therefore requires skilled interpreters to differentiate environmental exposure from actual use. However it is very expensive, requires highly trained operators, and is a very lengthy and tedious process in comparison to other methods. The GLC test separates molecules by migration similar to TLC. This process is somewhat less accurate than GC/MS.

Hair Analysis

Hair analysis employs hair samples to detect drugs of abuse. Chemical traces of most psychoactive drugs are stored in human hair cells, so the drugs can be detected as long as the hair stays intact, even decades after the drug has been taken. This gives a picture of the degree of drug use (to differentiate occasional use from chronic use (Karacic, Skender, Brcic, & Bagaric, 2002; Kintz, 1996). RIA techniques are used for screening of hair samples and GC/MS techniques are used for confirmation. More research needs to be done on the accuracy of hair testing although a number of businesses, such as casinos in Nevada, are using it in preemployment drug testing.

Saliva, Sweat, & Breath

Less accurate tests look for traces of drugs in saliva, sweat, or exhaled air. The advantage of these tests is that they are less invasive, however, they are much more prone to contamination by environmental traces of drugs. Saliva and breath tests can be useful in **on-the-spot testing of drivers involved in accidents or suspected of driving under the influence**. Confirmation tests are almost mandatory because of the inaccuracy of the tests and probable court challenges.

DETECTION PERIOD

Many factors influence the length of time that a drug can be detected in someone's blood, urine, saliva, or other body tissues. These include an individual's drug absorption rate, metabolism rate, rate of distribution in the body, excretion rate, and the

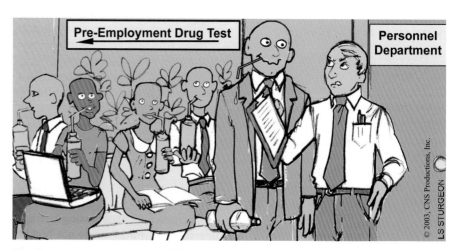

The front page newspaper article on hair and urine testing made the personnel director's job that much harder.

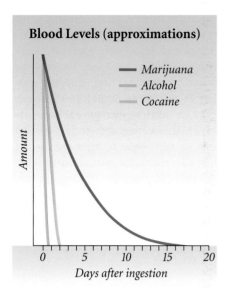

Blood Levels (approximations)

— Marijuana
— Alcohol
— Cocaine

Amount

0   5   10   15   20

Days after ingestion

Figure 8-8 •

This graph compares the length of time cocaine, marijuana, and alcohol remain in the blood. For purposes of testing, there is a cutoff level when testing for certain drugs, so that even when there is still some of the drug in a person's blood or urine, it will not be detected by the standard test.

Detection Period Range

Once sufficient amounts of a drug enter the urine, **the drug can be detected for a certain length of time by urinalysis**. The rough estimates for the more common drugs of abuse are shown in Table 8-9. Again, these are merely rough estimates with wide individual variations. Thus an individual delaying a urine test 5 days because of cocaine abuse will probably, but not definitely, test negative for cocaine.

Redistribution, Recirculation, Sequestration, & Other Variables

Long-acting drugs like PCP and possibly marijuana can be distributed to certain body tissues or fluids, be concentrated and stored there, then be recirculated and concentrated back into the urine. While not common, this can result in a positive test following negative tests and several months of abstinence.

ACCURACY OF DRUG TESTING

Despite many claims of confidence in the reliability of drug testing, independent blind testing of laboratory results continues to document high error rates for some testing programs. For this reason many companies and agencies use **a medical review officer (MRO) to review positive results and rule out any errors in procedure, environmental contamination, or alternative medical explanations**. The MRO usually interviews the testee, checks the chain of custody, or asks for retesting to search for explanations of a positive result since the consequences can greatly affect the person's future. In some cases the MRO will look at indeterminate results where manipulation of the specimens is suspected (e.g., when the urine sample is too dilute suggesting tampering) (Macdonald & DuPont, 1998).

False positive tests could result from the limitations of testing technol-

specific testing method employed. With a wide variation of these and other factors, a predictable drug detection period would be, at best, an educated guess. Despite this, the public interest requires that some specific estimates be adopted. For urine testing, these estimates can be divided into three broad periods: **latency, detection period range, and redistribution**.

Latency

Drugs must be absorbed, circulated by the blood, and finally concentrated in the urine in sufficient quantity before they can be detected. This process, called **"latency," generally takes about 2–3 hours for most drugs except alcohol, which takes about 30 minutes**. Thus someone tested just 30 minutes after using a drug would probably (but not always) test negative for that drug though they might already be under the influence. A chronic user however should have enough chemicals already present to test positive even if tested within 30 minutes of use (Johnson & Quander, 1998).

TABLE 8–9 DETECTION PERIOD RANGE CHART	
Alcohol	$^{1}/_{2}$–1 day
Amphetamines	2–4 days
Methamphetamines	2–4 days
Barbiturates	
amobarbital, pentobarbital	2–4 days
phenobarbital	up to 30 days
Benzodiazepines	
alprazolam (Xanax®),	up to 30 days
clonazepam (Klonopin®)	
Cocaine (coke, crack)	12–72 hours
Marijuana	
single use	1–3 days
casual use to 4 joints per week	5–7 days
daily use	10–15 days
chronic, heavy use	1–2 months
Opioids	
codeine	2 days
hydromorphone (Dilaudid®)	2–4 days
oxycodone (OxyContin®)	2–4 days
propoxyphene (Darvon®)	6–48 hours
heroin (morphine is measured)	2–4 days
methadone	2–3 days
PCP	
casual use	2–7 days
chronic, heavy use	several months

(Stanford, 2003; JAMA, 1987)

ogy. For example, dextromethorphan, found in many cold products, has been misidentified as an opioid. Herbal teas have been implicated in producing a false cocaine-positive result.

Errors also can result from the mishandling of urine and other specimen samples. Tagging the specimen with the wrong label, mixing and preparing the testing solutions incorrectly, errors in calculations, mistakes in coding the samples and solutions, logging and reporting the wrong results, as well as exposure of samples to destructive conditions or to other drugs in the laboratory have all resulted in inaccurate tests.

False negative results, not false positives, constitute the bulk of urine-testing errors. These result from laboratories being overly cautious in reporting positive results and from specimen manipulation by the testee. Many manipulations, some effective and some just folklore, have been used by drug abusers to prevent the detection of drugs in their urine. **Substitution methods include a concealed container, injection into the bladder, catheterization, urine from a clean donor, and even dog urine.**

Attempts to manipulate urine testing have grown to such proportions that "clean pee" (drug-free urine) has become a profitable black market item. Substances such as aspirin, goldenseal tea, niacin, zinc sulfate, bleach, Klear®, water, ammonia, Drano®, hydrogen peroxide, lemon juice, liquid soap, vinegar, and even Visine® have been tried to mask drugs in the urine. Most are ineffective. Further, recent designer drugs create a major problem in drug testing. Many have no standard to test against and some are so potent (the effective dose so small) that they are impossible to identify in the body. Inaccurate tests also result from disease states, pregnancy, medical conditions, interference of prescribed drugs, and individual metabolic conditions.

With the technology available at this time, the best chance for a reliable drug-testing program would include direct observation of the body specimen and rigid chain of custody over the sample. It would also include testing for a wide range of abused drugs and using the most accurate testing methods available (e.g., GC/MS) with a mandatory second confirmatory test via a different method. It would include the use of a MRO along with a detailed medical and social history to interpret lab results.

Consequences of False Positives & Negatives

Concerns about false positive test results are well publicized, debated, and feared. **People could lose their jobs, be denied employment, be disqualified from the Olympics, or even risk prison following an erroneous positive result.** Less publicized or feared, but just as critical, are the false negative results that prevent the discovery of drug abuse and feed the already strong denial process in the user. They permit the addict to become progressively more impaired and dysfunctional until a major life crisis occurs.

Nevertheless **drug testing is still an effective intervention, treatment, and monitoring tool** especially when used to intervene with heavy users and to discourage casual use. Addicts often state that they wished they had been tested and identified before their lives had been destroyed. Drug abusers in treatment often request increased urine testing to help them focus on abstinence and resist peer pressure. They can say, "Hey, I can't use. I have to be tested." **Treatment programs use testing to overcome denial and dishonesty in addicts during early treatment.** Recovering addicts in jobs that expose the public to high risk would not be acceptable without a reliable drug-testing program.

DRUGS & THE ELDERLY

"As I started to get older in life and started to gain more experience in life, I started to realize that I was doing a lot of wrong things and it had affected a lot of other people's lives as well as destroying my own. I tried to hide from that pain."
65-year-old recovering heroin addict

SCOPE OF THE PROBLEM

Overall Drug Use

The number of elderly Americans has doubled since 1950. At present,

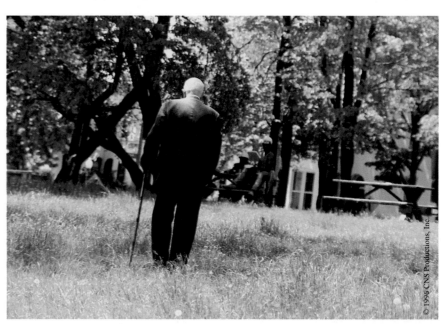

Isolation, ill health, and financial worries are some of the problems that can lead the elderly to drug abuse.

15% of the U.S. population is 65 years or older and that figure will increase to 21% by the year 2030. By 2050, 80 million Americans will be over the age of 65 (U.S. Bureau of the Census, 2002). As the population grows, the problems with drug overuse, abuse, and addiction will grow as well. This is mostly due to the increased use of prescription drugs, over-the-counter drugs, and alcohol. The use of street drugs begins to decrease at ages 21 through 25.

From 363 million filled prescriptions in 1950 to over 3 billion in 2002, the increase in the use of prescribed medications has been fueled by a larger medical care system, greater life span, and the discovery of hundreds of new compounds (IMS Health, 2003; Pharmaceutical Research and Manufacturers of America, 2003). This surfeit of available remedies for the illnesses and problems of the aging process have also increased the chances of adverse reactions from medications along with the chances of abuse of drugs with psychoactive properties. In addition peak use of over-the-counter medications occurs after the age of 65 and these too can have adverse reactions and interactions with other drugs. Since more than four out of five elderly suffer from some chronic disease **by age 65, 83% of them take at least one prescription drug a day, however, an astonishing 30% take eight or more** (Sheahan, Hendricks, & Coons, 1989).

Chemical Dependency

Up to 17% of adults aged 60 and older abuse alcohol and legal drugs (American Society of Addiction Medicine, 1998). Often some elderly abuse psychoactive drugs to deal with physical or psychological problems, their feelings of loneliness, being unwanted, not respected, and rejected by their families and the workplace. Events such as the death of a spouse, retirement, illness, loss of physical appearance, financial worries, and ageism can also increase drug use and abuse. Although most older adults (87%) see physicians regularly, it is estimated that 40% of those who are at risk do not self-identify or

TABLE 8–10		PAST YEAR DRUG USE FOR SELECTED AGES			
Substance	**All Ages**	**21 yrs.**	**55–59 yrs.**	**60–64 yrs.**	**65 yrs. & up**
Any illicit drug	12.6%	35.0%	3.0%	1.9%	0.9%
Tobacco	34.8%	56.4%	30.2%	24.9%	15.0%
Alcohol	63.7%	82.6%	62.2%	58.9%	43.9%

(SAMHSA, 2002)

seek services for substance abuse problems on their own (Raschko, 1990). Unfortunately **physicians have a difficult time identifying alcoholism or drug abuse**. In one study only 37% of alcoholics were identified compared to a 60% identification rate in younger patients (Geller et al, 1989; Fleming, Barry, Manwell, Johnson, & London, 1997). This is partly because most older adults live in the community and fewer than 5% live in nursing or personal care homes where supervision and physician contact is greater (Altpeter, Schmall, Rakowski, Swift, & Campbell, 1994). In addition **many manifestations of drug abuse can be attributed to other chronic illnesses** often present in those over 55 and since so many drugs are being used legally, adverse reactions due to the misuse of psychoactive drugs can be masked. Even family members can misattribute the symptoms of drug abuse to the normal effects of aging or the effects of legal prescription drugs.

To compound these problems, the attitude of society is often one of, "They've lived a full life and made their contribution to society, so why disturb their lives now? If they want to abuse drugs at this age, who will it harm?" This attitude assumes that the unhindered abuse of psychoactive drugs is desirable. But since **addiction is a progressive illness for the elderly as well as the young**, continued use leads to progressive physiological, emotional, social, relationship, family, and spiritual consequences that users find intolerable. Addiction means unhappiness and lack of choice, no matter what the age of the addicted person (Gambert, 1997).

Costs mount up for untreated eld-

erly chemical abusers. **Failure to prevent and then treat chemical abuse among this population leads to huge medical costs** in treating high blood pressure, cardiac and liver disease, gastrointestinal problems, and all the other diseases resulting from the abuse of drugs.

PHYSIOLOGICAL CHANGES

"When I was young, nobody told me what really happens to your body when you grow old and now that I'm here, it's a shock. The physical part I can accept although the constant arthritis makes me an aspirin addict. It's the mental part that's difficult, being closer to the end than the beginning. Wine and beer used to be my favorite psychiatric drug, better than Prozac®, but at my age my liver and body can only handle a couple of drinks and I nod off."
61-year-old male

The human body's **physiological functioning and chemistry are not as efficient in the elderly as they are in young** people and midlife adults. This results in an abnormal response to drugs compared to younger adults. Generally elderly people's enzymes and other bodily functions become less active, conditions that impair their ability to inactivate or excrete drugs (Smith, 1998). **This makes drugs more potent in older people.** For example, Valium® is deactivated by liver enzymes but after the age of 30, the liver slowly loses its ability to make the necessary enzymes. Thus a 10-milligram dose of

Valium® taken by a 70-year-old will result in an effect equal to a dose of about 30 milligrams taken by a 21-year-old.

Older people are also more likely to have concurrent illnesses that may greatly alter the effects of drugs in their bodies or make them **more sensitive to the toxic and adverse side effects**. Conditions like diabetes and liver, heart, and kidney disease all affect or are affected by drug abuse. Further, drugs used to treat these concurrent illnesses, along with a greater use of over-the-counter drugs, give rise to a greater potential for drug interactions.

The drugs most commonly abused by the elderly besides alcohol are prescription sedatives (e.g., Valium®), hydrocodone (Vicodin®), Darvon®, and other opioid analgesics, narcotic cough syrups, and over-the-counter sedatives or sleep aids. One change that has reduced the abuse of psychoactive drugs has been the **increased use of psychiatric medications**, e.g., fluoxetine (Prozac®), sertraline (Zoloft®), and buspirone (BuSpar®). Because older adults are less likely to use psychoactive medications nontherapeutically, many problems with drugs fall into the misuse category. **A major problem is not understanding directions especially when several medications are involved** often from multiple physicians unaware of a colleague's treatments.

Age does not endow a person with immunity to the negative effects of drugs or chemical dependence. **About 6–11% of elderly patients who are admitted to hospitals display symptoms of alcoholism.** This figure goes up to 14% for emergency room admissions, 20% for elderly patients in psychiatric wards, and as high as 49% in some nursing homes, though this high figure may result from the use of nursing homes as short-term alcoholism treatment facilities (JAMA, 1996). Thus prevention education and treatment services targeted for the aged are as important as those for adolescents. Age-related changes significantly affect the way an older person responds to alcohol: a decrease in body water, an increased sensitivity and decreased tolerance to alcohol, a decrease in the metabolism of alcohol in the gastrointestinal tract. For these reasons the same amount of alcohol that previously had little effect can now cause intoxication (Smith, 1995).

PREVENTION ISSUES

Primary Prevention

Because social drinkers and even abstainers can develop late-onset alcoholism, often in response to age-related problems, **older people need to be reeducated about the dangers of excessive use of alcohol and other psychoactive drugs**. Elderly people need to receive information and counseling about ways to manage the problems associated with growing older without using psychoactive drugs at all or at least, in the case of alcohol, in moderation. Community volunteerism, an active social life, continuing education are ways to encourage primary prevention. Information about primary prevention, customized for the elderly, needs to be given to those who provide services to this population, such as nurses, physicians, and social workers.

Secondary Prevention

Secondary prevention for the elderly focuses on **recognition of early stages of alcoholism or drug abuse and appropriate intervention tactics**. Frequently, there is **strong denial by this age group** because many of this generation see alcohol and other drug abuse as a sin or moral failure. Drug abuse tends to be hidden mainly because of the seclusion and solitude many live in, so that a mobile professional staff and vigorous outreach program are necessary. Home visits are particularly effective. It is **important to recognize alcoholism and addiction as primary diseases that must be treated**.

In addition to healthcare workers recognizing signs of addiction, friends and family of older adults along with drivers and volunteers from senior centers who see older adults on a regular basis and are intimately acquainted with their habits and daily routines should also be aware of signs. Other venues and activities where problems can be identified are clubs, health fairs, congregate meal sites, and senior day care programs.

Tertiary Prevention

Treatment frequently involves different procedures from those used with younger clients. This age group is not responsive to abrupt, coercive, confrontational therapies. **The pace of therapy has to be slow, patient, and reassuring.** Bringing in the entire family to create an understanding sympathetic support group helps. Detoxification needs more time as does the period for recovery, often 2 years or more. Thereafter outpatient counseling, peer group work, and a protective environment (safe from alcohol and other drugs) provide continuing care and reinforce recovery (Center for Substance Abuse Prevention, 1998). The least-intensive treatment options are recommended not only to resolve elderly patients' alcohol or other drug problems but also to move them into specialized treatment by helping them overcome their denial or resistance to change.

CONCLUSIONS

The major challenge of prevention efforts is to provide a measurement of long-term effectiveness for the strategies involved. Studies cannot conclusively show the effectiveness of a campaign since so many factors are involved and it can be hard to differentiate inevitable trends in society with specific efforts. However to do nothing is worse. A second, seemingly successful, recent direction is the use of massive advertising campaigns that are more effective, more honest, and more pervasive than earlier efforts. The reasoning is that if multiple ads and marketing campaigns can get people to eat unhealthy food, drink beer, and smoke cigarettes, why can't they do the opposite.

There is profound disagreement about drugs and drug policy in our society. Some see all drugs as inherently evil substances that must be regulated by laws. Some see drug use as a matter of choice (free choice in the case of legal drugs) or eventual decriminalization and even legalization in the case of illicit drugs. Some see drug abuse as a pathological disease requiring treatment.

CURRENT PROMISING DIRECTIONS

As we begin the twenty-first century, prevention is seen as a shared responsibility. The most promising approaches are the ones in which various segments of a community work in unison—youth, merchants, police, professionals, schools, parents, the government, and the media. An entire community arrives at a consensus about what it must do to prevent drug abuse, then agrees on the specific models that would best serve individuals and the whole community.

People are at risk throughout their lives. **If they are going to be exposed from cradle to grave, then prevention efforts also must extend over a lifetime.**

◇ **Early primary prevention can treat a pregnant mother that uses drugs so the child is not born addicted.** Prenatal care programs can provide parenting skills, teaching her to give unconditional love, showing the importance of holding her baby, and making her aware of other resources available to her. Toddlers can be given activities that increase bonding with their parents or caregiver. If the child has been exposed to drugs in the womb, rigorous early care can minimize long-term effects.

◇ **The family is a crucial prevention delivery system in childhood.** Parents may decide not to drink or use especially during their child-rearing years and model life-enhancing behavior.

◇ **Grammar schools can integrate prevention into the curriculum.** Developmental skills can be taught including resistance and decision-making skills. Students can be taught how to process moral dilemmas and how to talk about feelings.

◇ **By middle school** many children stop listening to adults and start listening to other children. **Peer educator programs can identify natural leaders who will serve as models,** leaders, teachers, and guides for in-school peer prevention efforts.

◇ **In high school and college, prevention must assume a higher level of sophistication to counter experimentation, social use, and habituation** since there is greater exposure to drugs. Prevention at this level must make a continual effort involving curriculum infusion, normative education, support services, environmental change, policy formulation and enforcement as well as alternatives to alcohol and other drug use in social occasions.

◇ **For the workforce, prevention needs to be continued through EAPs.** They must be proactive and provide ongoing prevention, referral, and treatment opportunities. Prevention education should be provided in the normal course of job training.

◇ Programs should be developed that address and **publicize many of the health risks of drugs, such as increased potential of sexually transmitted diseases including HIV and hepatitis C** from needle use as well as heart disease from cigarettes.

◇ **For older people preretirement training sessions and grief counseling can help prevent alcohol and other drug use.** Outreach programs need to take the prevention message to the people who are housebound or are not part of the school-workplace-community avenues of access.

◇ **Finally prevention must be adapted to the needs of specific audiences.** A program for a rural midwestern town may not be consistent for a school in inner-city Los Angeles. Secondary prevention designed for experimenters who need to know effects of drugs might actually stimulate experimentation in a primary audience. Since no single prevention program can demonstrate universal reproducible results, modifications of existing programs must be made to fit particular situations.

CHAPTER SUMMARY

Introduction

1. Psychoactive drugs affect people at all ages from the crack-affected baby to the elderly woman who borrows a friend's prescription painkiller. Thus prevention efforts are needed for all age groups.

PREVENTION

Concepts of Prevention

2. The goals of prevention are to prevent abuse before it begins, stop it where it has begun, and treat people where abuse and addiction have taken hold.

3. The three methods of prevention are supply reduction, demand reduction, and harm reduction.

4. Almost one-half of the National Drug Control Budget is aimed at demand reduction.

5. Historically prevention has wavered between temperance and prohibition. In the 1920s and 1930s, Prohibition did reduce problems associated with alcohol although it was repealed 14 years after being put into law.

6. Scare tactics, drug information programs, skill-building and resiliency programs, environmental change programs, normative education, and public health model programs are some of the prevention tactics that have been tried.

7. The public health model uses the concepts of the host (the actual user), the environment (the social climate), and the agent (the psychoactive drug) to explain all the rationale of prevention programs.

8. The most effective prevention programs involve the family.

Prevention Methods

9. Supply reduction by law enforcement and other government agencies, augmented by the passage of antidrug laws, is aimed at reducing the supply of drugs on the streets. The effectiveness of supply reduction is open to debate.

10. Demand reduction tries to reduce people's desire for drugs either through primary, secondary, or tertiary prevention (which includes treatment).

11. Primary prevention for drug-naive people aims at preventing experimentation and social use.

12. Secondary prevention seeks to halt drug use once it has begun through education, intervention, and skill building.

13. Tertiary prevention, usually some form of treatment, seeks to stop further damage from drug abuse and addiction. Through intervention, individual and group therapy, medical intervention, cue extinction, and promotion of a healthy lifestyle, recovery is encouraged.

14. The primary goal of harm reduction is not abstinence but rather reduction of the harm that addicts do to themselves and to society through their use of drugs.

15. Drug substitution programs, designated driver programs, and outreach needle exchange programs are some examples of harm reduction. These programs conflict with zero tolerance government programs.

Challenges to Prevention

16. The legality of alcohol and tobacco, along with heavy advertising, limits the effectiveness and believability of many prevention programs.

17. Prevention that works takes time, must be carried on throughout people's lifetimes, and must be adequately funded.

FROM CRADLE TO GRAVE

Patterns of Use

18. The age of first use of drugs has gotten lower and lower particularly since 1992. Caffeine, cigarettes, inhalants, and alcohol are generally the first drugs used. The earlier people begin drug use, the more likely they are to develop problems.

19. Neither level of intelligence, income, nor social class protects one from abuse and addiction.

Pregnancy & Birth

20. Almost one-third of fetuses are exposed to some psychoactive drug, particularly alcohol, tobacco, and marijuana, during pregnancy.

21. Drugs are particularly dangerous to the fetus because its defense mechanisms, e.g., drug-neutralizing metabolic system, immune system, and body organs, are not yet developed, so each surge of effects from a drug the mother takes gives multiple surges to the defenseless fetus.

22. Eighty percent of children with AIDS are born to addicted mothers who use drugs intravenously.

23. Major problems from drug use during pregnancy include a higher rate of miscarriage, blood vessel damage, severe infant withdrawal symptoms, and a much higher risk of sudden infant death syndrome (SIDS).

24. The problems of drug abuse during pregnancy last well beyond the birth of the baby. Withdrawal, intoxication, and developmental delays are commonplace.

25. Fetal alcohol syndrome (FAS) is the third most common cause of mental retardation in the United States. Other cognitive deficits such as ARND (alcohol-related neurodevelopmental disorder) are even more prevalent than FAS.

26. Cocaine and amphetamines cause increased blood pressure and heart rate, stroke, and premature placental separation.

27. Opioids cause physical addiction to the fetus. Heavy marijuana use, heavy smoking, and over-the-counter drug use also affect the fetus.

28. Prevention includes prenatal education, drug education, and addiction treatment.

Youth & School

29. Alcohol, tobacco, and marijuana are still the major drug problems in high schools and colleges.

30. The levels of substance abuse among youth in the United States are among the highest of any developed country.

31. A sense of invulnerability, the lag time between initial drug use and severe consequences, and especially delayed emotional maturation are major problems with psychoactive drug use in junior high, high school, and college.

32. Identifying risks and teaching resiliency are two important prevention strategies for students.

33. A strong sense of family, established personal positions on drugs, a strong spiritual sense, active community involvement, and attachment to good role models help prevent drug abuse and addiction.

34. Primary, secondary, and tertiary prevention must be continued throughout school and beyond.

35. Heavy drinking and secondhand drinking (e.g., disruptive dorm mates) are the two biggest drug problems in college.

36. Normative assessment (understanding real levels of abuse), having nonalcohol activities, providing alcohol- and drug-free dormitories are good college-level prevention techniques.

Love, Sex, & Drugs

37. Those who use drugs to achieve sexual gratification are usually looking for a quick sensation rather than enduring emotions.

38. Drugs affect desire, excitation, and orgasm often in diverse and contradictory ways.

39. The consequences of combining drugs and sexual activity, usually caused by lowered inhibitions or the need to support a drug habit, are increased sexual activity, high-risk sexual practices, sexual aggression, and an increase in sexually transmitted diseases.

40. Physical effects of drugs on sex include hormonal changes, blood flow and blood pressure changes, nerve stimulation or desensitization, and changes in muscle tension, all of which affect sexual response.

41. Cocaine and amphetamines in low doses can stimulate desire but in high doses they make orgasm more difficult. In females they can either increase or decrease desire and orgasm but in high doses a decrease is much more likely.

42. Opioids generally suppress sexual activity. Sixty percent of users report a general decrease of desire; 90% report decreased desire while they were high.

43. Sedative-hypnotics enhance desire by lowering inhibitions and inducing relaxation. With abuse, sexual dysfunction and apathy have been reported.

44. There has been a cultural link between love, sex, and alcohol. Initially alcohol lowers inhibitions and often increases aggressiveness. Long-term abuse causes a decrease in performance.

45. Because of the distortion of the senses involved with psychedelics, their effect on sexual experience can be very unpredictable.

46. Psychotropic medications, such as antidepressants, may enable patients to engage in sexual activities that their depression or psychosis kept them from doing.

47. The search for a true aphrodisiac may be illusory because sexuality is more a matter of mental attitude than physical sensation.

48. By lowering inhibitions, distorting judgment, and increasing aggressive impulses, alcohol and other drugs contribute to sexual assault.

49. Worldwide 330 million cases of sexually transmitted diseases occurred last year.

50. The use of contaminated needles and the increased incidence of high-risk sexual behavior due to drug abuse have increased the incidence of sexually transmitted diseases, such as chlamydia, pelvic inflammatory disease, gonorrhea, venereal warts, and particularly AIDS.

51. AIDS is a disease that destroys the immune system, so the user is susceptible to any infection. Drugs also lower the body's defenses indirectly.

52. The best AIDS prevention program is substance abuse treatment and education about the dangers resulting from sharing dirty needles or engaging in high-risk sex practices.

53. Other diseases and infections caused by dirty needles include hepatitis B and C, cotton fever, endocarditis, abscesses, malaria, tuberculosis, and syphilis.

Drugs at Work

54. Drug abuse in the workplace costs American business more than $140 billion a year in loss of productivity and increases in medical and legal costs.

55. The most effective answer to drug abuse in the workplace seems to be EAPs (employee assistance programs).

56. Studies show that good EAPs have decreased absenteeism 60–85% and on-the-job accidents 45–75%.

57. Drug education, zero tolerance, and drug testing have drastically reduced drug use in the military.

Drug Testing

58. The major uses of drug testing are preemployment testing, testing to see whether a client in treatment is being abstinent, and testing in jobs that are hazardous to the public.

59. The major types of drug tests are thin layer chromatography (TLC), enzyme multiplied immunoassay technique (EMIT), and gas chromatography/mass spectrometry (GC/MS).

60. The important aspects of testing are the length of time it takes for drugs to leave the body, the accuracy of the various methods, and the consequences of false positives and false negatives.

61. It takes 2 or 3 hours for most drugs to enter the urine and be detectable (latency). Alcohol, the exception, takes 30 minutes.

62. False negative tests can be as damaging as false positives. Failure to recognize a serious addiction can be more serious than damage to one's reputation from a false positive.

Drugs & the Elderly

63. As drug users get older, their bodies become less able to neutralize and metabolize psychoactive drugs.

64. Drug abuse in the elderly is often overlooked. Continuing education, recognition of the signs of abuse,

and appropriate treatment need to be directed at the elderly.

Conclusions

65. Prevention has no simple answer, no one program that will work for everyone.

66. Special programs need to be directed at each age group and then further directed to specific ethnic, cultural, gender, and specific target groups (e.g., geographical area, etc.).

REFERENCES

Aaron, P., & Musto, D. F. (1981). Temperance and prohibition in America: A historical overview. In M. Moore & D. Gerstein (Eds.), *Alcohol and Public Policy: Beyond the Shadow of Prohibition*. Washington, DC: National Academy Press.

Adger, H., Jr. (1998). Children in alcoholic families: Family dynamics and treatment issues. In A. W. Graham & T. K. Schultz (Eds.), *Principles of Addiction Medicine* (2nd ed., pp. 1111–1114). Chevy Chase, MD: American Society of Addiction Medicine, Inc.

Agency for Health Care Administration. (1999). Drug abuse hospitalization costs study, May 1999. State of Florida [Online]. Available: *http://www.floridahealthstat.com/publications/drugabuse.pdf*

Alano, M. A., Ngougmna, E., Ostrea, E. M. Jr., & Konduri, G. G. (2001). Analysis of nonsteroidal antiinflammatory drugs in meconium and its relation to persistent pulmonary hypertension of the newborn. *Pediatrics, 107*(3), 519–523.

Altpeter, M., Schmall, V., Rakowski, W., Swift, R., & Campbell, J. (1994). *Alcohol and Drug Problems in the Elderly: Instructor's Guide*. Providence, RI: Center for Alcohol and Addiction Studies.

American Association for the Treatment of Opioid Dependence. (2002). AMTA. 217 Broadway, New York, NY, 10007. Tel. (212) 566-5555.

American Society of Addiction Medicine. (1998). Substance abuse: Older adults at serious risk, new federal report warns. *News, 13*(3).

Anglin, M. D., Prendergast, M., & Farabee, D. (1998) Effectiveness of coerced treatment for drug abusing offenders, ONDCP Conference of Scholars and Policy Makers [Online]. Available: *http://www.ncjrs.org/ondcppubs/treat/consensus/anglin.pdf*

Anthony, J., & Hetzer, J. (1991). Syndrome of drug abuse and dependence. In L. N. Robins & D. A. Regier (Eds.), *Psychiatry Disorders in America*. New York: The Free Press, Macmillan.

Arrestee Drug Abuse Monitoring. (2003). ADAM annualized site reports, 2001. National Institute of Justice [Online]. Available: *http://www.adam-nij.net/files/2001_AnnualizedSiteReports.pdf*

Augood, C., Duckitt, K., & Templeton, A. A. (1998). Smoking and female infertility: A systematic review and meta-analysis. *Human Reproduction, 13*(6), 1532–1539.

Balzer, W. K., & Pargament, K. I. (1988). The key to designing a successful EAP. *EAP Digest, 1,* 55–59.

Bateman, D. A., & Heagarty, M. C. (1989). Passive freebase cocaine (crack) inhalation by infants and toddlers. *American Journal of Disabled Children, 134,* 25–27.

Bates, C., & Wigtil, J. (1994). *Skill-Building Activities for Alcohol and Drug Education*. Boston: Jones and Bartlett Publishers, Inc.

Beck, J., & Rosenbaum, M. (1994). *Pursuit of Ecstasy: The MDMA Experience*. Albany, NY: State University of New York Press.

Behnke, M., Eyler, F. D., Garvan, C. W., & Wobie, K. (2001). The search for congenital malformations in newborns with fetal cocaine exposure. *Pediatrics, 107*.

Bellandi, D. (2003, January 1). Underage binge drinking climbs by 56 percent. *Medford Mail Tribune*, p. 1A.

Blumenthal, R. N., Kral, A. H., Erringer, E. A., & Edlin, B. R. (1999). Drug paraphernalia laws and injection-related infectious disease risk among drug injectors. *Journal of Drug Issues, 29*(1), 1–16.

Boston Globe. (2003, June 27). Canada plans injection site for drug users. *San Francisco Chronicle*, p. D1.

Botvin, G. J., Baker, E., Dusenbury, L., Tortu, S., & Borvin, E. M. (1990). Preventing adolescent drug abuse through a multimodal cognitive-behavioral approach to substance abuse prevention: Results of a 3-year study. *Journal of Consulting Clinical Psychology, 58*(4), 473–487.

Bry, B. H., McKeon, P., & Pandina, R. J. (1982). Extent of drug use as a function of number of risk factors. *Journal of Abnormal Psychology, 91*(4), 273–279.

Buffum, J. C. (1982). Pharmacosexology: The effects of drugs on sexual function, a review. *Journal of Psychoactive Drugs, 14*(1–2), 5–43.

Buffum, J. C. (1988). Substance abuse and high-risk sexual behavior. *Journal of Psychoactive Drugs, 20*(2), 165–168.

Cahoon-Young, B. (1997). Prevalence of hepatitis C virus in women: Who's getting it, why, and co-infection with HIV. Perspective on the epidemiology. *Treatment and Interventions for the Hepatitis C Virus*. San Francisco: Haight Ashbury Free Clinics.

Campbell, D., & Graham, M. (1988). *Drugs and Alcohol in the Workplace: A Guide for Managers*. New York: Facts on File Publications.

Carlson, B. (1998). Addiction and treatment in the criminal justice system. In A. W. Graham & T. K. Schultz (Eds.), *Principles of Addiction Medicine* (2nd ed., pp. 405–419). Chevy Chase, MD: American Society of Addiction Medicine, Inc.

Centers for Disease Control. (1999). Status of HIV perinatal prevention: U.S. decline continues [Online]. Available: *http://www.cdc.gov/hiv/pubs/facts/perinatl.htm*

Centers for Disease Control. (2001). Update syringe exchange programs [Online]. Available: *http://www.cdc.gov/mmwr/preview/mmwrhtml/mm5019a4.htm#tab2*

Centers for Disease Control. (2003a). HIV/AIDS surveillance report 13(2) [Online]. Available: *http://www.cdc.gov/hiv/stats/hasr1302/table2.htm*

Centers for Disease Control. (2003b).

Sexually transmitted diseases: Treatment guidelines [Online]. Available: *http://www.cdc.gov/STD/treatment/TOC 2002TG.htm*

Center for Substance Abuse Prevention. (1998). *Substance Abuse Among Older Adults* (CSAT Treatment Improvement Protocol No. 26). Rockville, MD: Author.

Centrella, M. (1994). Physician addiction and impairment—current thinking: A review. *Journal of Addictive Disease, 13,* 91–105.

Cherukuri, R., Minkoff, H., Feldman, J., Parekh, A., & Glass, L. (1989). A cohort study of alkaloidal cocaine (crack) in pregnancy. *Obstetrics and Gynecology, 72,* 145–151.

Comerci, G. D. (1998). Office assessment and brief intervention with the adolescent suspected of substance abuse. In A. W. Graham & T. K. Schultz (Eds.), *Principles of Addiction Medicine* (2nd ed., pp. 1145–1146). Chevy Chase, MD: American Society of Addiction Medicine, Inc.

Cook, P. C., Petersen, R. C., & Moore, D. T. (1994). *Alcohol, tobacco, and other drugs may harm the unborn.* Rockville, MD: U.S. Department of Health and Human Services, Public Health Service.

Crowe, L., & George, W. (1989). Alcohol and sexuality. *Psychological Bulletin, 105,* 374–386.

Day, N. L., Richardson, G. A., Goldschmidt, L., et al. (1994). Effect of prenatal marijuana exposure on the cognitive development of offspring at age three. *Neurotoxicology and Teratology, 16,* 169–175.

Derlet, R., & Albertson, T. (2002). Toxicity, methamphetamine [Online]. Available: *http://www.emedicine.com/EMERG/topic859.htm*

Des Jarlais, D. C., Hagan, H., & Friedman, S. R. (1997). Epidemiology and emerging public health perspectives. In J. H. Lowinson, P. Ruiz, R. B. Millman, & J. G. Langrod (Eds.), *Substance Abuse: A Comprehensive Textbook* (3rd ed., pp. 591–596). Baltimore: Williams & Wilkins.

De Wit, D. J., Offord, D. R., & Wong, M. (1997). Patterns of onset and cessation of drug use over the early part of the life course. *Health Education and Behavior, 24*(6), 746–758.

Dielman, T. E. (1995). School-based research on the prevention of adolescent alcohol use and misuse: Methodological issues and advances. In G. M. Boyd, J.

Howard, & R. A. Zucker (Eds.), *Alcohol Problems Among Adolescents: Current Directions in Prevention Research.* Hillsdale, NJ: Lawrence Erlbaum Associates.

Drug Enforcement Administration. (2003a). Drug paraphernalia [Online]. Available: *http://www.usdoj.gov/dea/concern/paraphernaliafact.htm*

Drug Enforcement Administration. (2003b). Drug trafficking in the United States [Online]. Available: *http://www.usdoj.gov/dea/concern/drug_trafficking.html*

Drug Enforcement Administration. (2003c). FAQs about the Illicit Drug Anti-Proliferation Act [Online]. Available: *http://www.usdoj.gov/dea/ongoing/anti-proliferation_act.html*

Drug Enforcement Administration. (2003d). Guidelines for a Drug-Free Workforce [Online]. Available: *http://www.usdoj.gov/dea/demand/dfmanual/index.html*

El-Bassel, N., et al. (2000). Sex trading and psychological distress in a street-based sample of low-income urban men. *Journal of Psychoactive Drugs, 32*(3), 259–267.

Employee Assistance Professionals Association. (1990). Standards for employee assistance programs. *Exchange, 20*(10).

Englehart, P. F., Robinson, H., & Kates, H. (1997). The workplace. In J. H. Lowinson, P. Ruiz, R. B. Millman, & J. G. Langrod (Eds.), *Substance Abuse: A Comprehensive Textbook* (3rd ed., pp. 875–884). Baltimore: Williams & Wilkins.

Ennett, S. T., Tobler, N. S., Ringwalt, C. L., & Flewelling, R. L. (1994). How effective is drug abuse resistance education? A meta-analysis of project DARE outcome evaluations. *American Journal of Public Health, 84,* 1394–1401.

Eyler, F. D., Behnke, M., Conlon, M., Woos, N. S., & Wobie, K. (1998). Birth outcome from a prospective, matched study of prenatal crack/cocaine use. *Pediatrics, 101,* 237–241.

Feacham, R. G. A. (1995). *Valuing the Past . . . Investing in the Future. Evaluation of the National HIV/AIDS Strategy 1993–94 to 1995–96.* Canberra, Australia: Australian Government Publishing Service.

Federal Trade Commission. (2003). Cigarette report for 2001 [Online]. Available: *http://www.ftc.gov/opa/2003/06/2001cigrpt.htm*

Finnegan, L. P., & Ehrlich, S. M. (1990). Maternal drug abuse during pregnancy: Evaluation and pharmacotherapy for neonatal abstinence. *Modern Methods of Pharmacological Testing in the Evaluation of Drugs of Abuse, 6,* 255–263.

Finnegan, L. P., & Kandall, S. R. (1997). Maternal and neonatal effects of alcohol and drugs. In J. H. Lowinson, P. Ruiz, R. B. Millman, & J. G. Langrod (Eds.), *Substance Abuse: A Comprehensive Textbook* (3rd ed., pp. 513–533). Baltimore: Williams & Wilkins.

Fleming, M. F., Barry, K. L., Manwell, L. B., Johnson, K., & London, R. (1997). Brief physician advice for problem alcohol drinkers: A randomized controlled trial in community-based primary care practices. *Journal of the American Medical Association, 277,* 1039–1045.

Frank, D. A., Augustyn, M., Knight, A. M., Pell, T., & Zuckerman, B. (2001). Growth, development, and behavior in early childhood following prenatal cocaine exposure: A systematic review. *Journal of the American Medical Association, 285*(12), 1613–1625.

Fried, P. A. (1995). The Ottawa prenatal prospective study (OPPS): Methodological issues and findings: It's easy to throw the baby out with the bath water. *Life Sciences, 56,* 2159–2168.

Fried, P. A., O'Connel, C. M., & Watkinson, B. (1992). 60- and 72-month follow-up of children prenatally exposed to marijuana, cigarettes, and alcohol: Cognitive and language assessment. *Developmental and Behavioral Pediatrics, 13,* 383–391.

Fried, P. A., & Watkinson, B. (1997). Reading and language in 9- to 12-year-olds prenatally exposed to cigarettes and marijuana. *Neurotoxicology and Teratology, 19,* 171–183.

Fried, P. A., Watkinson, B., & Gray, R. (1998). Differential effects on cognitive functioning in 9- to 12-year-olds prenatally exposed to cigarettes and marijuana. *Neurotoxicology and Teratology, 120,* 293–306.

Fulroth, R., Phillips, B. & Durand, D. J. (1989). Perinatal outcome of infants exposed to cocaine and/or heroin in utero. *American Journal of Disabled Children, 143,* 905–910.

Gambert, S. R. (1997). The elderly. In J. H. Lowinson, P. Ruiz, R. B. Millman, & J. G. Langrod (Eds.), *Substance Abuse: A Comprehensive Textbook* (3rd ed., pp. 692–698). Baltimore: Williams & Wilkins.

Geller, G., Levine, D. M., Mamon, J. A., Moore, R. D., Bone, L. R., & Stokes, E. J. (1989). Knowledge, attitudes, and reported practices of medical students and house staff regarding the diagnosis and treatment of alcoholism. *Journal of the American Medical Association 261,* 3115–3120.

Gerstein, D. R., Johnson, R. A., Harwood, H., Fountain, D., Suter, N., & Malloy, K. (1994). *Evaluating Recovery Services: The California Drug and Alcohol Treatment Assessment (CALDATA).* Sacramento, CA: California Department of Alcohol and Drug Programs.

Gold, M. S., & Miller, N. S. (1997). Cocaine (and crack): Clinical aspects. In J. H. Lowinson, P. Ruiz, R. B. Millman, & J. G. Langrod (Eds.), *Substance Abuse: A Comprehensive Textbook* (3rd ed., p. 188). Baltimore: Williams & Wilkins.

Goldberg, R. J. (1998). Selective serotonin reuptake inhibitors: Infrequent medical adverse effects. *Archives of Family Medicine, 7,* 78–84.

Gomby, D. S., & Shiono, P. H. (1991). *The Future of Children.* Los Altos, CA: Center for the Future of Children.

Grant, B. F. (2000). Estimates of U.S. children exposed to alcohol abuse and dependence in the family. *American Journal of Public Health, 90*(1), 112–115.

Hands off pregnant drug users. (1998, August 1). *USA Today.*

Hankin, J. R. (2002). Fetal alcohol syndrome prevention research. *Alcohol Research & Health, 26*(1).

Hans, S. L. (1998). Developmental outcomes of prenatal exposure to alcohol and other drugs. In A. W. Graham & T. K. Schultz (Eds.), *Principles of Addiction Medicine* (2nd ed., pp. 1223–1236). Chevy Chase, MD: American Society of Addiction Medicine, Inc.

Hansen, W. B., & Graham. J. (1993). Preventing alcohol, marijuana, and cigarette use among adolescents: Peer pressure resistance training versus establishing conservative norms. *Prevention Medicine, 20,* 414–430.

Harris, N. S., Thompson, S. J., Ball, R., Hussey, J., & Sy, F. (2002). Zidovudine and perinatal human immunodeficiency virus type 1 transmission: A population-based approach. *Pediatrics, 109*(4).

Harvard University. (1998). Cocaine before birth. *The Harvard Mental Health Letter, 15*(6), 1–4.

Haverkos, H. (1998). HIV/AIDS, tuberculosis, and other infectious diseases. In A. W. Graham & T. K. Schultz (Eds.), *Principles of Addiction Medicine* (2nd ed., pp. 825–832). Chevy Chase, MD: American Society of Addiction Medicine, Inc.

Hazelden Foundation. (1993). *Refusal Skills.* Center City, MN: Author.

Hechtman, L. (1989). Teenage mothers and their children: Risks and problems. *Canadian Journal of Psychiatry, 34,* 569–575.

Henderson, D. J., Boyd, C. J., & Whitmarsh, J. (1995). Women and illicit drugs: Sexuality and crack cocaine. *Health Care for Women International, 16,* 113–124.

Hird, S., Khuri, E. T., Dusenbury, L., & Millman, R. B. (1997). Adolescents. In J. H. Lowinson, P. Ruiz, R. B. Millman, & J. G. Langrod (Eds.), *Substance Abuse: A Comprehensive Textbook* (3rd ed., pp. 683–691). Baltimore: Williams & Wilkins.

Hoffman, K. (1998). Fitting prevention into the continuum of care. In A. W. Graham & T. K. Schultz (Eds.), *Principles of Addiction Medicine* (2nd ed., pp. 233–245). Chevy Chase, MD: American Society of Addiction Medicine, Inc.

Holland, J. (2001). *Ecstasy: The Complete Guide.* Rochester, VT: Park Street Press.

Hubbard, R. L., Craddock, S. G., Flynn, P. M., Anderson, J., & Etheridge, R. M. (1997). Overview of one-year follow-up outcomes in DATOS. *Psychology of Addictive Behavior, 11.*

IMS Health. (2003). IMS reports 7% growth in retail pharmacy drug sales [Online]. Available: *http://www.imshealth.com/ims/portal/front/articleC/0,2777,6599_18731_41276537,00.html*

Jaffe, J. H. (1995). Prohibition of alcohol. In J. H. Jaffe (Ed.), *Encyclopedia of Drugs and Alcohol* (Vol. 2, pp. 885–888). New York: Simon & Schuster Macmillan.

Jaffe, J. H., Knapp, C. M., & Ciraulo, D. A. (1997). Opiates: Clinical aspects. In J. H. Lowinson, P. Ruiz, R. B. Millman, & J. G. Langrod (Eds.), *Substance Abuse: A Comprehensive Textbook* (3rd ed.). Baltimore, MD: Williams & Wilkins.

Jaffe, J. H., & Shopland, D. R. (1995), Tobacco: Medical complications. In J. H. Jaffe (Ed.), *Encyclopedia of Drugs and Alcohol* (Vol. 2, pp. 1045–1046). New York: Simon & Schuster Macmillan.

Jastak, J. T. (1991). Nitrous oxide and its abuse. *Journal of the American Dental Association, 122,* 48–52.

Johnson, B. L., & Quander, J. D. Esq. (1998). Overview of drug-free workplace programs. In A. W. Graham & T. K. Schultz (Eds.), *Principles of Addiction Medicine* (2nd ed., pp. 1241–1254). Chevy Chase, MD: American Society of Addiction Medicine, Inc.

Jones, K. L., & Smith, D. W. (1973). Recognition of the fetal alcohol syndrome in early infancy. *Lancet, 2,* 999–1001.

Joseph, H., & Paone, D. (1997). The homeless. In J. H. Lowinson, P. Ruiz, R. B. Millman, & J. G. Langrod (Eds.), *Substance Abuse: A Comprehensive Textbook* (3rd ed., pp. 733–743). Baltimore: Williams & Wilkins.

Journal of the American Medical Association. (1987). Scientific issues in drug testing. *Journal of the American Medical Association, 257*(22), 3112.

Journal of the American Medical Association. (1996). Council on Scientific Affairs. Alcoholism in the elderly. *Journal of the American Medical Association, 275*(10), 797–801.

Journal of the American Medical Association. (2002). Preventing mother-to-child HIV transmission. *Journal of the American Medical Association, 288*(2), 245–288.

Juliana, P., & Goodman, C. (1997). Children of substance-abusing parents. In J. H. Lowinson, P. Ruiz, R. B. Millman, & J. G. Langrod (Eds.), *Substance Abuse: A Comprehensive Textbook* (3rd ed., pp. 665–671). Baltimore: Williams & Wilkins.

Kaminer, Y. (1994). Adolescent substance abuse. In M. Galanter & H. D. Kleber (Eds.), *Textbook of Substance Abuse Treatment.* Washington, DC: The American Psychiatric Press.

Kandall, S. R. (1993). *Improving Treatment for Drug-Exposed Infants* (Treatment Improvement Protocol Series). Rockville, MD: Center for Substance Abuse Treatment.

Kandall, S. R. (1998). Treatment options for drug-exposed neonates. In A. W. Graham & T. K. Schultz (Eds.), *Principles of Addiction Medicine* (2nd ed., pp. 1211–1222). Chevy Chase, MD: American Society of Addiction Medicine, Inc.

Kandall, S. R., Gaines, J., Habel, L., Davidson, G., & Jessop, D. (1993). Relationship of maternal substance abuse to sudden infant death syndrome in offspring. *Journal of Pediatrics, 123,* 120–126.

Karacic V., Skender, L., Brcic, I., &

Bagaric, A. (2002). Hair testing for drugs of abuse: A two-year experience. *Arh Hig Rada Toksikol. 53*(3), 213–20.

Kintz, P. (1996). *Drug Testing in Hair.* Boca Raton, FL: CRC Press.

Klein, L., & Goldenberg, R. L. (1990). Prenatal care and its effect on pre-term birth and low birth weight. In I. R. Markets & J. E. Thompson (Eds.), *New Perspectives on Prenatal Care* (pp. 511–513). New York: Elsevier.

Kline, M. D. (1989). Fluoxetine and anorgasmia. *American Journal of Psychiatry, 146*, 804–805.

Kumpfer, K. L. (1994). *Promoting Resiliency to AOD Use in High Risk Youth.* Rockville, MD: Center for Substance Abuse Prevention.

Kumpfer, K. L., Goplerud, E., & Alvarado, R. (1998). Assessing individual risks and resiliencies. In A. W. Graham & T. K. Schultz (Eds.), *Principles of Addiction Medicine* (2nd ed., pp. 207–214). Chevy Chase, MD: American Society of Addiction Medicine, Inc.

Lender, E. M., & Martin, J. K. (1987). *Drinking in America.* New York: Free Press.

Lester, B. M., et al. (2002). The maternal lifestyle study: Effects of substance exposure during pregnancy on neurodevelopmental outcome in 1-month-old infants. *Journal of Pediatrics, 142*(3), 279–285.

Life Skills Training. (2003). [Online]. Available: *http://www.lifeskillstraining. com*

Littlefield, J. (2003). Preventing adolescent alcohol misuse [Online]. Available: *http://ag.arizona.edu/pubs/general/resr pt1999/alcoholuse.pdf*

Lyman, D. R., Milich, R., Zimmerman, R., et al. (1999). Project DARE: No effects at 10-year follow-up. *Journal of Consulting and Clinical Psychology, 67*(4), 590–593.

Macdonald, D. I., & DuPont, R. L. (1998). The role of the medical review officer. In A. W. Graham & T. K. Schultz (Eds.), *Principles of Addiction Medicine* (2nd ed., pp. 1255–1262). Chevy Chase, MD: American Society of Addiction Medicine, Inc.

Mangione, T. W., et al. (1998). *New Perspectives for Worksite Alcohol Strategies: Results from a Corporate Drinking Study.* Boston: JSI Research & Training Institute.

Marnell, T. (Ed.). (1997). *Drug Identification Bible* (3rd ed.). Denver, CO: Drug Identification Bible Publishing.

Martin, J. C. (1992). The effects of maternal use of tobacco products or amphetamines on offspring. In T. B. Sonderegger (Ed.), *Perinatal Substance Abuse: Research Findings and Clinical Implications.* Baltimore: The Johns Hopkins University Press.

Mattson, S. N., Schoenfeld, A. M., & Riley, E. P. (2001). Teratogenic effects of alcohol on brain and behavior. *Alcohol Research & Health, 25*(3), 185–191.

May, P. A. (1996). Research issues in the prevention of fetal alcohol syndrome and alcohol-related birth defects. *Research Monograph 32, Women and Alcohol: Issues for Prevention Research.* Bethesda, MD: National Institute on Alcohol Abuse and Alcoholism.

May, P. A., & Gossage, P. (2001). Estimating the prevalence of fetal alcohol syndrome: A summary. *Alcohol Research & Health, 25*(3), 159–167.

Mayes, L., Grillon, C., Granger, R., & Schottenfeld, R. (1998). Regulation of arousal and attention in preschool children exposed to cocaine prenatally. *Annals of the New York Academy of Sciences, 846,* 144–152.

Mello, N. K., Mendelson, J. H., & Teoh, S. K. (1993). An overview of the effects of alcohol on neuroendocrine function in women. In S. Zakhari (Ed.), *Alcohol and the Endocrine System. NIAAA Research Monograph No. 23,* NIH Pub. 93-3533. Bethesda, MD: National Institute on Alcohol Abuse and Alcoholism.

Meston, C. M., & Gorzalka, B. B. (1992). Psychoactive drugs and human sexual behavior: The role of serotonergic activity. *Journal of Psychoactive Drugs, 24*(1), 1–40.

Metzger, D. S., Woody, G. E., McLellan, A., et al. (1993). Human immunodeficiency virus seroconversion among intravenous drug users in and out of treatment: An 18-month prospective follow-up. *Journal of Acquired Immune Deficiency Syndrome, 6,* 1049–1056.

Milberger, S., Biederman, J., Faraone, S. V., & Jones, J. (1998). Further evidence of an association between maternal smoking during pregnancy and attention-deficit/hyperactivity disorder: Findings from a high-risk sample of siblings. *Journal of Clinical Child Psychology, 27,* 352–358.

Miller, L. J. (1998). Treatment of the addicted woman in pregnancy. In A. W. Graham & T. K. Schultz (Eds.), *Principles of Addiction Medicine* (2nd ed., pp. 1199–1210). Chevy Chase, MD:

American Society of Addiction Medicine, Inc.

Morganthaler, J., & Joy, D. (1994). *Better Sex Through Chemistry: A Guide to the New Prosexual Drugs.* Petaluma, CA: Smart Publications.

Moskowitz, J. (1989). The primary prevention of alcohol problems. A critical review of the research literature. *Journal of Studies on Alcohol, 50*(1), 54–88.

Mumola, C. (1998). *Substance Abuse and Treatment, State and Federal Prisoners, 1997.* Washington, DC: Bureau of Justice Statistics.

National Center on Addiction and Substance Abuse. (2000). *Dangerous Liaisons: Substance Abuse and Sex.* New York: Columbia University.

National Center on Addiction and Substance Abuse. (2001). *Malignant Neglect: Substance Abuse and America's Schools.* New York: Columbia University.

National Criminal Justice Reference System. (2000). Drug court activity update [Online]. Available: *http://www. ncjrs.org/drug_courts/facts.html*

National Institute on Drug Abuse. (1994). *Annualized Estimates from the National Pregnancy Health Survey.* Washington, DC: Author

National Institute on Drug Abuse. (1995). *AZT and Pregnant Women (ACTG 076).* Washington, DC: National Institute of Allergy and Infectious Diseases.

National Institute on Drug Abuse. (1998). Costs to society [Online]. Available: *http://www.nida.nih.gov/Infofax/costs. html*

National Institute on Drug Abuse. (1999). Rohypnol and GHB. NIDA Infofax [Online]. Available: *http://www.nida. nih.gov/Infofax/RohypnolGHB.html.*

National Institute on Drug Abuse. (2000). NIDA Community Drug Alert Bulletin - Hepatitis [Online]. Available: *http:// 165.112.78.61/HepatitisAlert/Hepatitis Alert.html*

National Research Council. (1995). *Preventing HIV Transmission. The Role of Sterile Needles and Bleach.* Washington, DC: National Academy Press.

Noble, A., Vega, W. A., Kolody, B., Porter, P., Hwang, J., Merk, G. A., & Bole, A. (1997). Prenatal substance abuse in California: Findings from the perinatal substance exposure study. *Journal of Psychoactive Drugs, 29*(1), 43–53.

Novick, D. M., Haverkos, H. W., & Teller, D. W. (1997). The medically ill substance abuser. In J. H. Lowinson, P. Ruiz, R. B. Millman, & J. G. Langrod

(Eds.), *Substance Abuse: A Comprehensive Textbook* (3rd ed., pp. 534–550). Baltimore: Williams & Wilkins.

Novick, D. M., Reagan, K. J., Croxson, T. S., Gelb, A. M., Stenger, R. J., & Kreck, M. J. (1997). Hepatitis C virus serology in parenteral drug users with chronic liver disease. *Addiction, 92*(2), 167–171.

Nurco, D. N., Hanlon, T. E., Bateman, R. W., & Kinlock, T. W. (1995). Drug abuse treatment in the context of correctional surveillance. *Journal of Substance Abuse Treatment, 12*(1), 19–27.

O'Brien, R., Cohen, S., Evans, G., & Fine, J. (1992). *The Encyclopedia of Drug Abuse* (2nd ed.). New York: Facts On File.

Office of National Drug Control Policy. (2000). Evidence-based principles for substance abuse prevention [Online]. Available: *http://www.whitehousedrugpolicy.gov*

Office of National Drug Control Policy. (2003a). *National Drug Control Strategy: 2003 Annual Report*. Bethesda, MD: National Drug Clearinghouse.

Office of National Drug Control Policy. (2003b). White House drug czar releases National Drug Control Strategy [Online]. Available: *http://www.whitehousedrugpolicy.gov/news/press03/021003.html*

Paria, B. C., et al. (1999). Fatty-acid amide hydrolase is expressed in the mouse uterus and embryo during the periimplantation period. *Biology of Reproduction, 60,* 1151–1157.

Paria, B. C., Das, S. K., & Dey, S. K. (1995). The preimplantation mouse embryo is a target for cannabinoid ligand-receptor signaling. *Proceedings of the National Academy of Sciences, 92,* 9460–9464.

Parents' Resource Institute for Drug Education. (2001). PRIDE questionnaire report: 2001–2002 national summary grades 6-12 [Online]. Available *http://www.pridesurveys.com/main/supportfiles/natsum01.pdf*

Partnership for a Drug-Free America. (1998). PATS study [Online]. Available: *http://www.drugfreeamerica.org*

Perkins, H. W., & Craig, D. W. (2002). Alcohol education project [Online]. Available: *http://alcohol.hws.edu*

Perkins H. W., Meilman P. W., Leichliter J. S., Cashin, J. R., & Presley, C. A. (1999). Misperceptions of the norms for the frequency of alcohol and other drug use on college campuses. *Journal of American College Health, 47*(6), 253–258.

Peugh, J., & Belenko, S. (2001). Alcohol, drugs and sexual function: A review. *Journal of Psychoactive Drugs, 33*(3), 223–232.

Pharmaceutical Research and Manufacturers of America (PhRMA). (2003). Industry profile, 1998. PhRMA Publications. *http://www.phrma.org/publications/publications/profile02/index.cfm*

Physicians' Desk Reference. (2003). *Physicians' Desk Reference* (54th ed.). Montvale, NJ: Medical Economics Co.

Plans to link welfare benefits to drug testing spark outcry. (1999, October 11). *Alcoholism and Drug Abuse Weekly.*

Plessinger, M. A., & Woods, J. R. Jr. (1998). Cocaine in pregnancy: Recent data on maternal and fetal risks. *Obstetrics and Gynecology Clinics of North America, 25*(1), 99–112.

Quest Diagnostics. (2003). Amphetamine use increases in the general U.S. workforce [Online]. Available: *http://www.questdiagnostics.com/brand/business/DTI_05_2003/dti_index.html*

Quinn, T. (1996). Global burden of the AIDS epidemic. *Lancet, 348,* 99–106.

Raschko, R. (1990). "Gatekeepers" do the case finding in Spokane. *Aging, 361,* 38–40.

Rhem, K. T. (2001). Drug, alcohol treatment available to DoD beneficiaries. American Forces Press Service [Online]. Available: *http://www.defenselink.mil/specials/drugawareness/afpsstory.html*

Richardson, G. A. (1998). Prenatal cocaine exposure: A longitudinal study of development. *Annals of the New York Academy of Sciences, 846,* 144–152.

Richardson, G. A., Day, N. L., & Goldschmidt, L. (1995). Prenatal alcohol, marijuana, and tobacco use: Infant mental and motor development. *Neurotoxicology and Teratology, 17,* 479–487.

Robins, L. N. (1993). The sixth Thomas James Okey Memorial Lecture. Vietnam veterans' rapid recovery from heroin addiction: A fluke or normal expectation? *Addiction, 88*(8), 1041–1054.

Roizen, J. (1997). Epidemiological issues in alcohol-related violence. In M. Galanter (Ed.), *Recent Developments in Alcoholism* (Vol. 13). New York: Plenum Press.

Rosen, R. C. (1991). Alcohol and drug effects on sexual response: Human experimental and clinical studies. *Annual Review of Sex Research, 2,* 119–179.

RTI International. (1999). Worldwide survey reveals reduced usage of alcohol, tobacco, and illegal drugs by U.S. Military

Personnel. Research Triangle Institute [Online]. Available: *http://www.rti.org/page.cfm?nav=391&objectid=AB12BFB4-F306-4667-9CCDF72168A77F27*

Rusche, S. (1995). Prevention movement. In J. H. Jaffe (Ed.), *Encyclopedia of Drugs and Alcohol* (Vol. 2, pp. 856–861). New York: Macmillan Library Reference.

Rush, D., & Callahan, K. R. (1989). Exposure to passive cigarette smoking and child development: A critical review. *Annals of New York Academy of Sciences, 562,* 74–100.

Russel, S. (2003, June 27). Scientists urge worldwide AIDS vaccine effort. *San Francisco Chronicle,* p. A3.

Schmid, P. C., et al. (1997). Changes in anandamide levels in mouse uterus are associated with uterine receptivity for embryo implantation. *Proceedings of the National Academy of Sciences, 94,* 4188–4192.

Seifert, S. A. (1999). Substance use and sexual assault. *Substance Use & Misuse, 34*(6), 935–945.

Sharp, C. W. & Rosenberg, N. L. (1997). Inhalants. In J. H. Lowinson, P. Ruiz, R. B. Millman, & J. G. Langrod (Eds.), *Substance Abuse: A Comprehensive Textbook* (3rd ed., pp. 246–264). Baltimore: Williams & Wilkins.

Sheahan, S. L., Hendricks, J., & Coons, S. J. (1989). Drug misuse among the elderly: A covert problem. *Health Values 13*(3), 22–29.

Shen, W. W., & Sata, L. S. (1983). Neuropharmacology of male sexual dysfunction. *Journal of Clinical Pharmacology Research Communication, 3.*

Sher, K. J. (1997). Psychological characteristics of children of alcoholics. *Alcohol Health & Research World, 21*(3), 247–254.

Smith, D. E., Wesson, D. R., & Apter-Marsh, M. (1984). Cocaine- and alcohol-induced sexual dysfunction in patients with addictive diseases. *Journal of Psychoactive Drugs, 16,* 359–361.

Smith, D. E., Wesson, D. R., & Calhoun, S. R. (1995). Rohypnol: Quaalude of the nineties? *CSAM News. Newsletter of the California Society of Addiction Medicine, 22*(2).

Smith, J. W. (1995). Medical manifestations of alcoholism in the elderly. *International Journal of the Addictions 30,* 1749–1798.

Smith, J. W. (1998). Special problems of the elderly. In A. W. Graham & T. K. Schultz (Eds.), *Principles of Addiction Medicine*

(2nd ed., pp. 833–854). Chevy Chase, MD: American Society of Addiction Medicine, Inc.

SmithKline Beecham Clinical Laboratories. (1997). *SmithKline Beecham Drug Testing Index, 1997.* Collegeville, PA: Author.

Sokol, R. J., & Clarren, S. K. (1989). Guidelines for use of terminology describing the impact of prenatal alcohol on the offspring. *Alcoholism: Clinical & Experimental Research, 13,* 597–598.

Stanford, M. (2003). Ask the Doctor . . . About drug testing [Online]. Available: *http://www.sccgov.org/scc/assets/docs/2275612115.pdf*

Streissguth, A. (1997). *Fetal Alcohol Syndrome.* Baltimore: Brookes Publishing Co.

Substance Abuse and Mental Health Services Administration. (1996). *Drug use Among U.S. Workers: Prevalence and Trends by Occupation and Industry Categories.* Rockville, MD: National Clearinghouse for Alcohol and Drug Information.

Substance Abuse and Mental Health Services Administration. (1997). An analysis of worker drug use and workplace policies and programs [Online]. Available: *http://www.samhsa.gov/oas/wkplace/workpla6.htm#E8E6*

Substance Abuse and Mental Health Services Administration. (1999a). *Substance Abuse and Mental Health Statistics Source Book, 1998.* Rockville, MD: National Clearinghouse for Alcohol and Drug Information.

Substance Abuse and Mental Health Services Administration. (1999b). *Worker Drug Use and Workplace Policies and Programs: Results from the National Household Survey on Drug Abuse.* Rockville, MD: National Clearinghouse for Alcohol and Drug Information.

Substance Abuse and Mental Health Services Administration. (2000). *Patterns of Alcohol Use Among Adolescents and associations with Emotional and Behavioral Problems.* Rockville, MD: National Clearinghouse for Alcohol and Drug Information.

Substance Abuse and Mental Health Services Administration. (2002). Results from the 2001 National Household Survey on Drug Abuse: Volume I. [Online]. Available: *http://www.samhsa.gov/oas/nhsda/2k1nhsda/vol1/chapter2.htm#2.empl*

Tobacco tax has desired effect. (2000, January 14). *Medford Mail Tribune,* p. 6A.

UNAIDS. (2003). Russian Federation: Epidemiological fact sheets on HIV/AIDS [Online]. Available: *http://www.unaids.org/hivaidsinfo/statistics/fact_sheets/pdfs/Russianfederation_en.pdf*

University of California in San Francisco. (1998). Does HIV prevention work? Center for AIDS Prevention Research [Online]. Available: *http://www.caps.ucsf.edu*

University of Michigan. (2003). *Monitoring the Future Study.* Rockville, MD: SAMHSA. Also [Online]. Available: *http://www.MonitoringTheFuture.org.*

U.S. Bureau of the Census. (2002). National population projections [Online]. Available: *http://www.census.gov/population/www/projections/natsum-T3.html*

U.S. Department of Agriculture. (1999). *Tobacco facts.* U.S. Department of Agriculture's Economic and Statistics System. Washington, DC: U.S. Printing Office.

U.S. Department of Education.(2003). Drug convictions may affect your student aid [Online]. Available: *http://www.ifap.ed.gov/dpcletters/attachments/gen00-14a.pdf*

U.S. Department of Health and Human Services. (1988). The Health Consequences of Smoking: 25 Years of Progress. A Report of the Surgeon General. Rockville, MD: Author.

U.S. Department of Justice. (2002). Drugs and crime facts. Bureau of Justice statistics [Online]. Available: *http://www.ojp.gov/bjs/pub/pdf/dcf.*pdf

U.S. Department of Justice. (2003). Prison and jail inmates at midyear, 2002 [Online]. Available: *http://www.ojp.usdoj.gov/bjs/pub/pdf/pjim02.pdf*

U.S. Department of Labor. (1990). *What Works: Workplaces Without Drugs.* Rockville, MD: Author

U.S. Department of Labor. (2003). Working partners [Online]. Available: *http://www.dol.gov/asp/programs/drugs/working-partners/Screen15.htm*

Vereby, K. G., & Buchan, B. J. (1997). Diagnostic laboratory: Screening for drug abuse. In J. H. Lowinson, P. Ruiz, R. B. Millman, & J. G. Langrod (Eds.), *Substance Abuse: A Comprehensive Textbook* (3rd ed., pp. 369–376). Baltimore: Williams & Wilkins.

Wartenberg, A. A. (1998). Management of common medical problems. In A. W. Graham & T. K. Schultz (Eds.), *Principles of Addiction Medicine* (2nd ed., pp. 731–740). Chevy Chase, MD: American Society of Addiction Medicine, Inc.

Wechsler, H., Kelley, K., Weitzman, E. R., Giovanni, J. P. S., & Seibring, M. (2000). What colleges are doing about student binge drinking: A survey of college administrators. *Journal of American College Health, 48,* 219–226.

Wechsler, H., Lee, J. E., Kuo, M., Seibring, M., Toben, F., Nelson, T. F., & Lee, H. (2002). Trends in college binge drinking during a period of increased prevention efforts: 1993-2001. *Journal of American College Health, 50*(5), 203–217.

Weinberg, B. A., & Bealer, B. K. (2001). *The World of Caffeine.* New York: Routledge Press.

Werblin, J. M. (1998). High on sex. *Professional Counselor, 13*(6), 33–37.

White, W. L. (1998). *Slaying the Dragon: The History of Addiction Treatment and Recovery in America.* Bloomington, IL: Chestnut Health Systems/Lighthouse Institute.

White, J., Nicholson, T., Duncan, D., & Minors, P. (2002). A demographic profile of employed users of illicit drugs. In M. A. Rahim, R. T. Golembiewski, & K. D. Mackenzie (Eds.), *Current Topics in Management* (Vol. 6). Amsterdam: Elsevier Science Ltd.

Willing, R. (2003, May 23). Attitudes ease toward medical marijuana. *USA Today,* p. 3A.

Wilsnack, S. C., Klassen, A. D., Schur, B. E., et al. (1991). Predicting onset and chronicity of women's problem drinking. *American Journal of Public Health, 61*(3), 305–318.

Wodak, A., & Lurie, P. (1997). A tale of two countries: Attempts to control HIV among injecting drug users in Australia and the United States. *Journal of Drug Issues, 27*(1), 117–134.

World Health Organization. (1998). Sexually transmitted diseases. WHO Information Fact Sheets [Online]. Available: *http://www.who.int/inf-fs/en/fact110.html*

World Health Organization. (2003). AIDS epidemic update: December 2002 [Online]. Available: *http://www.who.int/hiv/pub/epidemiology/epi2002/en/*

Worth, D. (1991). American women and polydrug abuse. In P. Roth (Ed.), *Alcohol and Drugs are Women's Issues* (Vol. 1). Metuchen, NJ: Women's Action Alliance and the Scarecrow Press.

Wright, H. I., Gavaler, J. S., & Thiel, D. H. (1991). Effects of alcohol on the male reproductive system. *Alcohol Health and Research World, 15*(2), 110–114.

Young, N. K. (1997). Effects of alcohol and other drugs on children. *Journal of Psychoactive Drugs, 29*(1), 23–42.

Zakhari, S. (Ed.). (1993). *Alcohol and the Endocrine System.* NIAAA Research Monograph No. 23. NIH Pub. No. 93-3533. Bethesda, MD: National Institute on Alcohol Abuse and Alcoholism.

Zhu, J. H., & Stadlin, A. (2000). Prenatal heroin exposure. Effects on development, acoustic startle response, and locomotion in weanling rats. *Neurotoxicology and Teratology, 22*(2), 193–203.

Zuckerman, B., Frank, D. A., Hingson, G., et al. (1989). Effects of maternal marijuana and cocaine use on fetal growth. *New England Journal of Medicine, 320,* 762–768.

Treatment

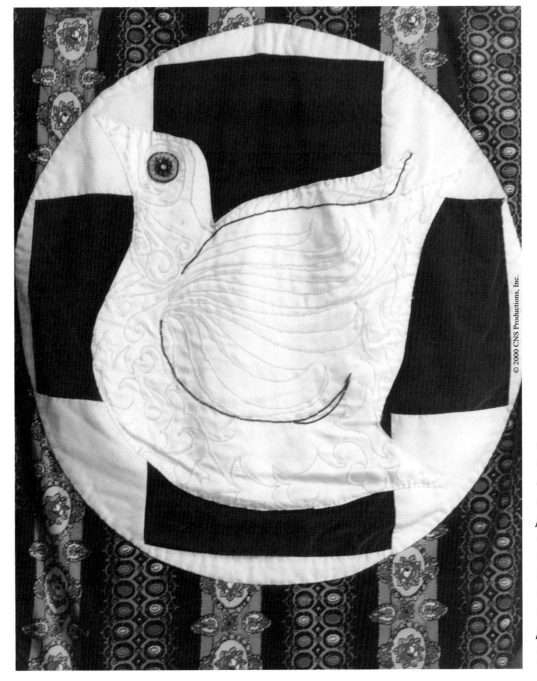

© 2000 CNS Productions, Inc.

T his is the symbol of the Haight Ashbury Free Clinics that opened their doors in 1967 to help take care of the influx of young people during the "Summer of Love." Since that time, they have treated more than 200,000 clients with one of the highest success rates in the country. There are 150 people on the substance abuse treatment staff.

- **Introduction:**
  ◇ **A Disease of the Brain:** The most prevalent mind disorder is substance abuse. It causes more illness, death, and social disruption than any other brain disease. Substance abuse also costs our society more financial loss than any other medical condition.
  ◇ **Current Issues in Treatment:**
    1. There is a rapidly expanding use of medications to treat detoxification, control withdrawal symptoms, lessen craving, and promote short- and long-term abstinence.
    2. Advanced imaging methods and other new diagnostic techniques are being used to visualize the physiological effects of addiction on the human brain.
    3. There is a lack of resources to provide the treatment that has been proven to be effective.
    4. Increasing research supports coerced treatment (e.g., drug courts) as being just as effective in promoting abstinence and recovery from drug addiction when compared to voluntary treatment admissions.
    5. The conflict between abstinence-oriented recovery and harm reduction as philosophies of treatment continues. Historically America has vacillated between temperance, individual abstinence, and societal prohibition.
- **Treatment Effectiveness:** Treatment has a 50% success rate and saves $4 to $20 for every $1 spent on treatment. It also reduces crime by 75%.
- **Principles & Goals of Treatment:** Certain principles for effective treatment include having a wide variety of treatment programs that are readily available, using medications in conjunction with individual and group therapy, and treating any coexisting conditions not just the addiction itself. Goals include motivating clients towards abstinence and reconstructing their lives in ways that exclude drug abuse.
- **Selection of a Program:** Correct diagnosis helps treatment professionals match the client to the best program. Providing a wide range of treatment approaches plus customizing treatment for culture, gender, ethnicity, and other traits dramatically improves outcomes. Programs include medical model detoxification, therapeutic communities, and harm reduction programs. About $1^1/_2$ million people are treated for substance abuse each year.
- **Beginning Treatment:** Breaking through denial is the crucial first step in treatment. Hitting bottom, especially when health, family, work, financial, or legal problems are involved, often gets the user into treatment. Direct intervention with an intervention specialist is also used to get the person into treatment.
- **Treatment Continuum:** Once addiction has occurred, treatment and recovery become a lifetime process.
  ◇ **Detoxification** uses medical care, emotional support, and medications to control withdrawal symptoms, reduce craving, and help the client to begin abstinence.
  ◇ **Initial Abstinence** uses counseling, anticraving medications, drug substitution, and desensitization techniques to rebalance body chemistry, continue abstinence, and prevent relapse due to environmental triggers.
  ◇ **Long-Term Abstinence** involves participation in continued counseling and groups to prevent relapse and begin to change living habits.
  ◇ **Recovery** is a lifelong process that involves rebuilding one's lifestyle to live sober and drug free.
  ◇ **Outcome & Follow-Up** studies are used to judge the effectiveness of treatment programs.
- **Individual vs. Group Therapy:** Individual counseling, peer groups, 12-step groups, facilitated group therapy, and educational groups are all used in treatment.
- **Treatment & the Family:** Treatment should involve the whole family. The problems of codependency, enabling, and being the child of an alcoholic/addict must be addressed.
- **Adjunctive & Complementary Treatment Services:** Abuse and addiction of substances have a negative impact on the user's family and on his or her physical, emotional, social and spiritual well-being. Treatment that effectively addresses all of these components through a comprehensive, integrated, and "wrap-around" service delivery design is being encouraged to increase positive outcomes.
- **Drug-Specific Treatment:** Certain psychoactive drugs call for specialized medical and counseling treatment techniques, e.g., methadone maintenance, stimulant abuse groups, or dual diagnosis groups. A behavioral addiction like gambling is treated with many of the same techniques that are used for substance addiction. Office-based opiate addiction treatment (O-BOAT) using buprenorphine has ushered in a new era of opiate addiction treatment.
- **Target Populations:** Treatment should be culturally specific (i.e., ethnicity, gender, language) since needs vary between men and women, old and young, and among Black, White, Hispanic, Asian, and Native American people.
- **Treatment Obstacles:** Developmental arrest, lack of cognition, conflicting goals, poor follow-through, and lack of facilities are the main problems in treatment.
- **Medical Intervention Developments:** More than 60 medications are being developed, focusing on aspects of treatment such as detoxification, replacement or agonist therapies, antagonist or vaccine effects, anticraving effects, and restoration of homeostasis.

Celebrities rehab their lives — 12 steps at a time

By Ann Oldenburg
USA TODAY

Drug problem requires intervention, compassion

By STEPHANIE SOARES PUMP

Mayor promises drug treatment on demand

NEW YORK, FRIDAY, APRIL 16, 1915

AS FIFTEEN DRUG SLAVES ARE TAKEN IN FOR CURE, 20 MORE ARE SHUT OUT.

Pitiful Begging by Addicts Who Come Late, but the Metropolitan Hospital Can Take No More Just Now of Those Who Find Federal and State Laws Depriving Them of "Dope."

BELLVUE GETS PATIENTS FOR A RIGID TREATMENT.

GUEST OPINION

'3 strikes' law falling heavily on drug users

U.S. CLINIC TO SELL DRUGS TO ADDICTS
August 7, 1919

Drug Fiends Giving 147 of Them in 3 Hos

It is estimated by the police authorities that 500 drug fiends or have surrendered in the last tw

Addicts would get treatment, not jail

By CHARLES E. BEGGS
The Associated Press

SALEM — A bill that's intended to steer more nonviolent drug offenders to treatment instead of jail time won the unanimous endorsement of the Senate on Tuesday.

INTRODUCTION

"One of the reasons you came into recovery was to get away from your old life. Being in the recovery program must be something that you want and desire and once you start desiring it, it sets a fire in your heart and in your mind and you start being more productive and being more aware of how your life was and how beautiful your life can be."

46-year-old recovering addict

"Treatment is effective. Scientifically based drug addiction treatments typically reduce drug abuse by 40% to 60%. These rates are not ideal, of course, but they are comparable to compliance rates seen with treatment for other chronic diseases, such as asthma, hypertension, and diabetes. Moreover treatment markedly reduces undesirable consequences of drug abuse and addiction, such as unemployment, criminal activity, and HIV/AIDS or other infectious diseases, whether or not patients achieve complete abstinence."

Alan I. Leshner, Ph.D., former Director, National Institute on Drug Abuse (National Institutes of Health [NIH], 1999)

A DISEASE OF THE BRAIN

Mental illnesses, nervous system diseases, brain tumors, and physical head traumas come to mind when one thinks of pathological conditions of the human mind but in reality **chemical dependency and addiction are more prevalent than other brain diseases and have a much greater impact on the social fabric of society**. For example, from the ages of 18 to 54, the 1 yr. prevalence rate of

◊ anxiety disorders is 16.4%;

◊ schizophrenia is about 1.3%;

◊ mood disorders (major depression, bipolar disease, affective disorders) is about 7.1%;

◊ any mental disorder is about 21% (U.S. Public Health Service, 1999; Regier, Narrow, & Rae, 1999).

This compares to

◊ **17 million Americans (7% of those aged 12 or older) who abused or were dependent on either alcohol or an illicit drug** during the past year (11 million on alcohol only, 3 million on an illicit drug only, 2 million on both alcohol and an illicit drug);

◊ **nicotine addiction that occurs in about 25% of the population over the age of 12**;

◊ **and gambling addiction that affects 2–6% of adults** (Substance Abuse and Mental Health Services Administration [SAMHSA], 2003a; Kessler, McGonagle, Zhao, et al., 1994; National Institute on Alcohol Abuse and Alcoholism, 2000).

Chemical dependency may also be America's number one continuing public physical health problem.

◊ More than 440,000 Americans die prematurely every year due to nicotine addiction (and another 53,000 from secondhand smoke);

◇ another 130,000 die prematurely from alcohol dependence, abuse, overdose, or from associated diseases;

◇ 6,000–10,000 die of cocaine, heroin, and methamphetamine overdose or dependence;

◇ 35–40% of all hospital admissions are related to nicotine-induced health problems;

◇ 25% of all hospital admissions are related to alcohol-induced health problems (Centers for Disease Control [CDC], 2001, 2002; SAMHSA, 2003b).

These figures are startling when compared to other major health problems like AIDS, prostate or breast cancer, and even stroke, many of which are often the result of drug abuse and addiction.

Psychoactive drug abuse also has profound effects on social systems, family relationships, crime, violence, mental health, and a dozen other areas of daily life. Certainly if we could reduce the impact of addiction, we would have a major impact on the quality of life in the United States and around the world.

CURRENT ISSUES IN TREATMENT

At the start of the twenty-first century 5 aspects of treatment for substance and behavioral addictions dominate research, clinical practice, and discussion.

1. **There is a rapidly expanding use of medications to treat detoxification, control withdrawal symptoms, reduce craving, and promote short- and long-term abstinence.**
   Because addictive use of substances alters brain chemistry, there are increasing efforts to find medications that can correct or lessen the impact of those chemical and structural changes, such as

   ◇ drugs to lessen withdrawal symptoms (e.g., phenobarbital for alco-

hol withdrawal and antipsychotics to control stimulant-induced psychosis);

◇ drugs to lessen craving (bromocryptine for stimulants, naltrexone, buprenorphine, and clonidine for heroin, or naltrexone and acamprosate for alcohol);

◇ substitute medications that are less damaging than the primary substance of abuse including methadone, levomethadyl acetate (LAAM), and more recently, buprenorphine;

◇ nutritional supplements to stimulate neurotransmitter production;

◇ and antidepressants to increase serotonin activity and relieve depression.

2. **Researchers are increasing the use of imaging systems and other new diagnostic techniques to visualize the physiological effects of addiction on the human brain.**
   Until the advent of sophisticated imaging techniques, gene identification technologies, and sensitive neurochemical measurement methodologies, addiction was easy to deny because compulsion was considered a behavioral disorder with few if any physical indicators that could be examined. New imaging techniques have identified multiple brain circuit systems involved in addiction (e.g., reward, motivation, memory/learning, control) and have been able to image those changes (Volkow, Fowler, & Wang, 2003). There are four common imaging techniques used to examine changes in the central nervous system (Meuller, 1999).

   ◇ **CAT (computerized axial tomography)** scans use x-rays to show structural changes in brain tissues due to drugs.

   ◇ **MRI (magnetic resonance imaging)** uses the positioning of magnetic nuclei to give two- and three-dimensional images of brain structures in great detail; it can record subtle alterations of brain tissues due to psychoactive drug use or brain anomalies that indicate a susceptibility to drug abuse. For example, an MRI study at the

University of Southern California showed a smaller prefrontal cortex (11% smaller on average) in those prone to rage and violence, a diagnostic technique that proved as accurate as psychological testing techniques (Raine et al., 2000). There are variations of MRI techniques such as magnetic resonance spectroscopy (31P MRS) that measures abnormal brain activity due to chronic drug use and **fMRI (functional MRI)** that records blood flow changes caused by drugs.

◇ **PET (positron emission tomography)** scans use the metabolism of radioactively labeled chemicals that have been injected into the bloodstream to measure glucose metabolism, blood flow, and oxygenation. This visualizes the effects of naturally occurring neurotransmitters that are affected by drugs.

◇ **SPECT (single photon emission computerized tomography)** scans also use radioactive tracers to measure cerebral blood flow and brain metabolism to show how a brain functions (or doesn't function) when using drugs; they are similar to PET scans but less expensive and easier to use.

(Mathias, 1999)

"There's so much these scans and looking at the brain can offer the field of addiction. We can show children, teenagers, and adults that drugs have an impact on their brain. It's much more powerful than showing them a picture of fried eggs and bacon. It's very helpful in denial to actually sit in front of a computer screen with somebody that has been using drugs and they say, 'Oh, there are really no problems.' And you can say, 'Let's look at yours.' And what I've seen—it's really turned many people around."

Daniel Amen, M.D., Founder, Amen Clinic for Behavioral Medicine

3. **There is a lack of resources to provide the treatment that has been proven to be effective.**

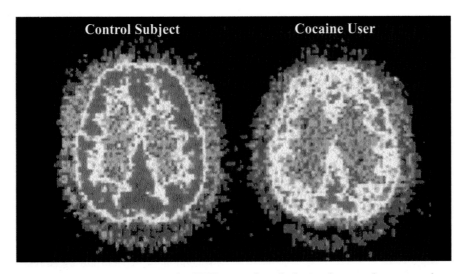

Control Subject | Cocaine User

These positron emission tomography (PET) scans show the brain of a normal person on the left and a cocaine user on the right. PET scans show the brain's use of glucose (red shows high use). The brain of the cocaine user does not use glucose as effectively. Brain imaging helps give visual proof of the effects of drugs and can give clues to effective medications that can be used to promote abstinence.

Courtesy of the National Institute on Drug Abuse

• •

According to one report, **states spend an average of about 13% of their budgets to battle the effects of drug, alcohol, and cigarette abuse** (especially the cost of incarceration, drug courts, and probation for drug offenses). Unfortunately only 4% of that amount is for treatment and prevention in spite of the fact that many states have done outcome studies to assess the cost effectiveness of treatment (National Center on Addiction and Substance Abuse [NCASA], 2001). Studies show that **for every $1 spent on treatment, $4 to $20 are saved, mostly in prison costs, lost time on the job, health problems, and extra social services** (Gerstein et al., 1994; Hubbard, Craddock, Flynn, Anderson, & Etheridge, 1997). Other research has shown the greatly increased effectiveness of matching treatment modalities to each client's needs (McLellan et al., 1997; Nielsen, Nielsen, & Wrae, 1998). Finally, studies have shown that the more services such as health care, psychological care, and social support that are available, the better the outcome (Fiorentine, 1999). The problem is that because of limited community, state, and federal resources, more reliance on managed care, and a general reluctance to spend money on treatment for drug addicts, cities, coun-

ties, and states cannot provide sufficient treatment even for those who desperately want it. In San Francisco and Baltimore, two cities where the concept of treatment on demand was seriously studied, waiting lists for treatment slots still remain excessively high. In 2003 because of budget cuts, the State of Oregon (through the Oregon Health Plan) stopped paying for drug abuse treatment programs such as methadone maintenance. Other states are trying to avoid cutting their methadone and drug treatment programs because they know that would cost more in the long run (Kettler, 2003).

Despite the vast amount of rigorous scientific research validating the effectiveness and benefits of treating addiction, the number of substance abusers treated remained fairly constant from 1992 (1,527,930 treatment admissions) through 2000 (1,599,703 treatment admissions) in spite of a greater need. For example, national data estimates 12–14 million alcoholics alone in 2000 of which only about 724,000 received treatment (SAMHSA, 2003b). That works out to a mere 5% of the total. When considered in the context of an actual decrease in national substance abuse treatment facilities from 15,230 in 1999

to only 13,428 in 2000, the data clearly validates that there is a continued lack of treatment resources (SAMHSA, 2003b). In addition, coverage by health insurers is rare. Employer-provided health benefits for drug addiction treatment fell 50–75% between 1988 and 1998 compared to an 11.5% decline for general health insurance (Galanter, Keller, Dermatis, & Egelko, 2000).

4. **Increasing research supports coerced treatment as being just as effective if not more effective in promoting positive outcomes as voluntary treatment.**

Coerced treatment is that which comes about through mandated participation via the criminal justice system through drug courts, mandatory sentencing, probation/parole stipulations, or through state or federal legislation requiring compulsory treatment. Defendants who complete a drug court program can have their charges dismissed or probation sentences reduced. In 2000 about 508 drug courts were operating in the United States with 281 more in the planning stage. Of the more than 100,000 people who had entered drug courts, 50–65% graduated or remain active participants. These courts keep felony offenders in treatment at about double the retention rate of community drug programs. Two of the reasons are that there is much closer supervision and there is the threat of incarceration (Belenko, 1998; National Criminal Justice Reference System, 2003).

Recent findings of a 5-year Drug Treatment Alternative-to-Prison (DTAP) Program in New York uphold several previous studies in demonstrating the effectiveness of coerced treatment outcomes. The **DTAP study demonstrated a significant reduction in the re-arrest rate (33%), reconviction rate (45%), and return to prison rate (87%)** as compared to prisoners who had not participated in the program. Also 92% of DTAP participants were employed upon completion of the program while only 26% were employed before their arrest (NCASA, 2003; Anglin, Prendergast, & Farabee, 1998). These reports further document

great cost savings from treatment compared to the cost of incarceration for the same length of time. Such findings combined with the success of drug courts and other initiatives led to the passage of Proposition 36 in California and similar legislation in a number of other states like Maryland and New Mexico that mandate treatment for nonviolent drug-addicted criminal offenders.

The growing number of coerced treatment initiatives may actually result in an adverse effect on treatment availability. The downturn in the U.S. economy during the early 2000s resulted in the loss of a number of substance abuse treatment programs. Many treatment slots are currently funded by these new coerced treatment initiatives and reserved for those involved with the criminal justice system (CJS), which further reduces treatment availability for addicts who are not involved with the law even though some of the legislation says the CJS treatment slots will not replace any non-CJS slots.

5. **The conflict between abstinence-oriented recovery and harm reduction as philosophies of treatment continues.**

Most treatment personnel believe that users who have crossed the line into uncontrolled use of drugs or compulsive behaviors can refuse the first drink, injection, or bet but they find it increasingly difficult to refuse the second. For these treatment personnel, abstinence is absolutely necessary for recovery because the very definition of addiction is based on the concept of loss of control. In various studies the **Haight Ashbury Clinic found that when a client slipped, e.g., had a drink, took one hit, or smoked one cigarette, it turned into a full relapse in 95% of the cases** (O'Malley et al., 1992). The full relapse might take an hour, a day, a month, or occasionally longer to reoccur but in 19 out of 20 users who have crossed the line into addiction, it will eventually happen. Even in 1879 a recovering alcoholic and temperance lecturer, Luther Bensen, was aware of his susceptibility to uncontrolled use.

"Moderation? A drink of liquor is to my appetite what a red-hot poker is to a keg of dry powder.... When I take one drink, even if it is but a taste, I must have more, even if I knew hell would burst out of the earth and engulf me the next instant."
Luther Bensen (Bensen, 1879)

Conversely there is a growing group of drug abuse treatment personnel who believe that harm reduction is a viable treatment alternative. The problem with evaluating the effectiveness of harm reduction is that it means different things to different groups. One definition of harm reduction is "a willingness to work for incremental changes rather than to require complete behavior change" (Morris, 1995). Another is "any steps taken by drug users to reduce the harm of their behavior" (Marlatt, 1995; Marlatt & Tapert, 1993).

Harm reduction includes

◇ **drug replacement therapy**, such as methadone maintenance instead of heroin use or methylphenidate maintenance instead of cocaine use;

◇ **needle exchange;**

◇ **the use of less harmful drugs for more harmful ones** (e.g., marijuana instead of heroin);

◇ **testing illegal drugs for users** so they don't use a dangerous substance or additive, e.g., an organization called "DanceSafe" tests samples of ecstasy and occasionally other drugs at concerts and rave parties (DanceSafe, 2003);

◇ **drug decriminalization/legalization** through legislation;

◇ and the most controversial technique, **controlled drinking/drug use through behavior modification.**

Numerous studies have been done on controlled drinking and again the problem is definitions that obscure reported data. What constitutes controlled drinking? Was the patient an alcoholic or problem drinker before starting treatment? Is the patient's self-

reporting of the amount being drunk and the consequences accurate (Peele, 1995)? Long-term follow-up strongly suggests that true controlled drinking does not work (Vaillant, 1995). For some, harm reduction consists of individual techniques that will help advance the addict to full (abstinent) recovery while to others, harm reduction is an all-encompassing philosophy of treatment and drug use.

Finally, it is difficult to measure treatment outcome. Is it measured in days of abstinence, amount of drug used, reduction in hospital visits, improvement in marital and other relationships, or amount of money saved by society? This lack of consensus can further aggravate the argument (Geller, 1997).

More on Abstinence vs. Harm Reduction (temperance, to abstinence, to prohibition)

In his excellent book, *Slaying the Dragon*, on the history of addiction treatment in America, William White shows that this controversy has been around for at least 230 years. The temperance movement started at the end of the eighteenth century as America emerged from its revolution against England and coincidentally changed its drinking habits. From 1792 to 1830, the per capita consumption went from 2.5 gallons of pure alcohol per year to an unbelievable 7.1 gallons or 2 standard drinks for every man, woman, and child every day of the year (Cherrington, 1920). (In 2002, per capita consumption was back down to 2.2 gallons.) **The initial goal of the temperance movement was just to limit the amount drunk but as consumption and public drunkenness increased, that goal shifted from temperance to abstinence,** that is, complete avoidance by the alcoholic of any and all alcoholic beverages (White, 1998). Even then many people thought of alcoholism as a disease.

"The remedy we would suggest, particularly to those whose appetite for drink is strong and increasing, is

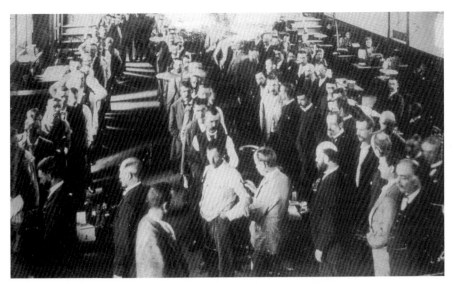

Patients at a Keeley Institute who were addicted to alcohol and other drugs would go for a 4-week cure. Part of the treatment was daily injections of a secret formula to help subdue the pains of withdrawal and keep the patient in treatment. Though the formula was kept secret, various laboratories suggested that the medicine contained a number of ingredients, some of which were psychoactive. These included alcohol, strychnine, willow bark, ginger, ammonia, belladonna, atropine, hyoscine, scopolamine, coca, opium, and morphine.

Courtesy of the Keeley Collection. © 2000, Illinois State Historical Library

a total abstinence from the use of all intoxicating liquors. This may be deemed a harsh remedy, but the nature of the disease absolutely requires it."

From an 1811 temperance pamphlet (Dascus, 1877)

A large segment of the **abstinence movement then expanded the goal to make society as a whole abstinent (prohibition)**, not just those who couldn't limit their consumption. This way alcohol would just not be available, at least legally.

"Our main object is not to reform inebriates, but to induce all temperate people to continue temperance, by practicing total abstinence. The drunkards, if not reformed, will die, and the land be free."

Dr. Justin Edwards, 1824 (Dorchester, 1884).

This shift from simply treating the addict to reforming society confused the perception of the problem of how to treat alcoholism and addiction. The question became "Should a substance that triggers uncontrolled harmful use in 5–10% of the population (25–50%

for tobacco) be banned, allowed, or controlled?" In wanting to allow controlled use of a psychoactive substance by those with a substance problem, some advocates of harm reduction ignore the nature of addiction.

"Most of us have been unwilling to admit we were real alcoholics. No person likes to think he is bodily and mentally different from his fellows. Therefore, it is not surprising that our drinking careers have been characterized by countless vain attempts to prove we could drink like other people. The idea that somehow, someday he will control and enjoy his drinking is the great obsession of every abnormal drinker. The persistence of this illusion is astonishing. Many pursue it into the gates of insanity or death."

Alcoholics Anonymous Big Book (Alcoholics Anonymous, 1934, 1976)

Conversely some advocates of abstinence and/or prohibition overreact to any use of a psychoactive substance, even in that 90% of the population with a lower susceptibility to uncontrolled use. In many of the arguments on the subject, **both sides confuse ideas about the effectiveness of abstinence-based treatment and effective harm reduction techniques with arguments about freedom, politics, and morality**.

The recent advocacy of harm reduction started in the late 1980s and early 1990s in response to the inaccessibility of treatment to many segments of society, e.g., those infected with the HIV virus, hepatitis C, and other diseases who continued to spread the diseases or reinfect themselves through dirty needles, contaminated drugs, and unsafe sex. **Needle exchange programs, free condoms, food incentives, and social service referral information enabled outreach workers to come in contact with homeless street kids, illicit drug users, prostitutes, and others living on the fringes of society** to engage them in prevention efforts that would slow the spread of these diseases. The contact also gave the outreach workers an opportunity to engage them in drug treatment or, at the very least, increase their knowledge of drug abuse and addiction.

The harm reduction people were willing to accept small changes in drug use status in order to protect the addict and society from further infection. What happened was that, as in the past, **the harm reduction concept became an end in itself for certain treatment personnel rather than a transitory step for clients on the way to abstinence and full recovery**. Interest in harm reduction also came from health care insurers and managed care systems that saw it as a more economical way to cover their obligations to provide treatment for chemical dependency problems (Morris, 1995).

One item that has added to the controversy surrounding harm reduction is confusion about the difference between abuse and addiction. The key is that there is a qualitative difference between those two levels of drug use, not just a quantitative difference. **Many of the successes of harm reduction have been in users who had not crossed that line into loss of control that is the hallmark of addiction**, so harm reduction in some of those cases was sustainable. But even there, since addiction is a progressive disease and intensifies with use, continued abuse will often become addiction. **The Haight Ashbury Clinic has an abstinence-based philosophy of treatment that also incorporates many harm reduction techniques.** The rest of this chapter reflects that philosophy.

TREATMENT EFFECTIVENESS

Even though chemical dependency is America's and possibly the world's number one health and social problem, it is also the most treatable. Several studies have confirmed that **treatment outcomes for drug and alcohol abuse result in long-term abstinence along with tremendous health, social, and spiritual benefits to the patient.**

"Everything that I am and everything that I have in me is invested in what I'm doing today in recovery—everything."
56-year-old recovering heroin addict

What is often overlooked when local, state, and federal governments vote on how much money should be allotted for treatment is the undeniable fact that treatment saves money—large sums of money (Fig. 9-1).

TREATMENT STUDIES

The California Drug and Alcohol Treatment Assessment (CALDATA) Study

Studies conducted by the Rand Corporation and the Research Triangle Institute support the findings of the CALDATA Study, the most comprehensive and rigorous study on treatment outcome conducted by the State of California and duplicated by several other states. All of these studies monitored the effect of treatment on several hundred thousand addicts and alcoholics in a variety of programs.

The CALDATA Study monitored 1,850 individuals for a period of 3–5

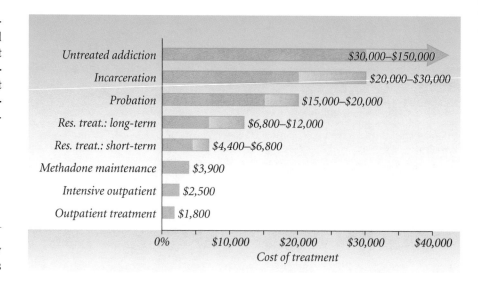

Figure 9-1 •

The cost of treatment for an addict utilizing outpatient treatment is less than one-tenth the cost of incarceration.
(Estimates by authors)

years following treatment. Continual abstinence in these patients approached 50% of all those treated. It further demonstrated that crime was abated in 74% of those treated and that **the state enjoyed actual savings of $7 for every $1 spent on treatment.** For more expensive programs, there was a savings of $4 and for the inexpensive programs, the savings were $12. California spent $209 million on treatment between October 1991 and September 1992 and saved an estimated $1.5 billion, much due to crime reduction and reduced use of health care facilities. The only negative side of the equation was that those in recovery lost income while undergoing treatment and their financial condition did not improve immediately after treatment. The study also looked at a number of variables that, when examined, supported many concepts and practices in the treatment field.

◊ **Treatment was most effective when patients were treated continuously for a period of 6–8 months.**

◊ Shorter periods of time resulted in poorer outcomes and longer treatment duration resulted in continuously better outcomes but not at the same rate. There was a point of diminishing returns.

◊ **Group therapy was shown to be much more effective than individual therapy.**

◊ **Drug of choice also seemed to affect outcomes.** For example, those who listed alcohol as their primary drug of choice had treatment outcomes twice as good as those who listed heroin as their primary drug of choice. Cocaine users' outcomes fell between these two drugs.

◊ **Better treatment outcomes were linked to program modifications directed at being culturally consistent with a specific target population.** For example, programs that targeted women and added child care services to their treatment programs had much better outcomes than generic treatment programs for women. Those programs that added transportation services had better outcomes than those that just had child care. Every additional innovation that was target-group specific improved the outcome of treatment.

(Gerstein et al., 1997; Mecca, 1997)

Drug Abuse Treatment Outcome Study (DATOS)

Another study of the effectiveness of treatment, the Drug Abuse Treatment Outcome Study (DATOS), tracked 10,010 drug abusers in 100 treatment facilities in 11 cities who began treatment from 1991–1993. The study compared pre- and post-treatment drug use, criminal activity, employment, and thoughts of suicide (Hubbard et al., 1997). The four common types of drug abuse treatment studied were outpatient methadone programs, long-term (several months) residential programs, short-term (up to 30 days) inpatient programs, and outpatient drug-free programs. Researchers found that **the use of all drugs after treatment was reduced by 50–70%.** The final level of drug use after treatment was about the same level for all four programs. **Short- and long-term residential programs seemed to have the greatest effect.** As expected, low retention rates were most prevalent in clients with greater problems (Meuller & Wyman, 1997). Unfortunately most patients said they did not receive the services they thought they needed. The study found a decrease in the number of services offered over the past decade (Ethridge, Craddock, Dunteman, & Hubbard, 1995).

The Treatment Episode Data Sets (TEDS)

To supply **descriptive information about the flow of admissions to substance abuse treatment providers**, this survey, part of the Drug and Alcohol Services Information System (DASIS), collects data from all 50 states, the District of Columbia, and Puerto Rico. The information is available through publications or online at *http://www.samhsa.gov/oas/dasis.htm.*

The National Survey of Substance Abuse Treatment Services (N-SSATS)

The National Survey of Substance Abuse Treatment Services (N-SSATS) is an annual **survey of all drug treatment facilities in the United States, public and private.** Unlike the TEDS survey that focuses on the clients who enter treatment, the N-SSATS examines the facilities themselves and their assessment services, continuing care,

transitional services, community outreach, and other services. It is available in publications or online at *http://www.samhsa.gov/oas/dasis.htm#nssats.*

TREATMENT & PRISONS

On December 31, 2001,

◇ **1,962, 220 Americans were in federal, state, and local prisons (10% were women);**

◇ **more than 5 million were on parole or probation** (U.S. Department of Justice [DOJ], 2003b).

In addition,

◇ **about 57% of federal inmates and 21% of state inmates were serving a sentence for a drug offense**; 11.5% were arrested for a drug abuse violation (about 1.6 million arrests, 1.2 million for possession);

◇ **40–65% committed their crime while under the influence of alcohol or drugs;**

◇ of those on probation, 24% were for a drug law violation and 17% for driving while intoxicated;

◇ average time served increased from 22 months to 27 months (Office of National Drug Control Policy [ONDCP], 2003).

The percentage of arrestees testing positive for drugs (not including alcohol) is many times higher than the percentage of drug use in the general population. Despite the high percentage of drug problems among the inmate population, **treatment slots are available for only about 10% of those who have serious drug habits** although 94% of federal prisons, 56% of state prisons, and 33% of jails provide some on-site substance abuse treatment to inmates (DOJ, 2003a; SAMHSA, 2000). Various studies of inmate populations with drug problems found a comparatively low percentage have had contact with the treatment community (Mahon, 1997). About 8% of all admissions for substance abuse treatment are prison inmates (SAMHSA, 2003b).

Earlier studies of prisoners and those involved with the criminal justice system have shown that **drug abuse treatment reduces recidivism dramatically when the treatment is linked to community services** rather than strictly in-jail services (DOJ, 2003a). Since the cost of keeping a felon in jail runs between $25,000 and $40,000 a year, not including any assistance for the felon's family, compensation for human and property damage, and a dozen other liabilities, the savings for

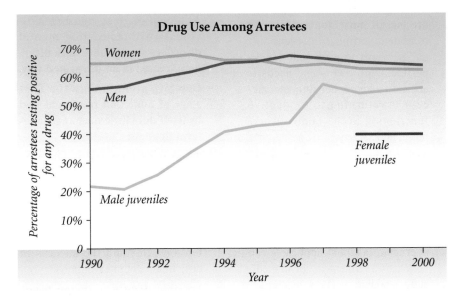

Figure 9-2 •

Testing at jails and prisons is for illicit drugs and excludes alcohol. Besides alcohol the most common drugs found in arrestees are marijuana and cocaine (Arrestee Drug Abuse Monitoring Program [ADAM], 2003).

keeping people out of prisons is quite large. In contrast, outpatient treatment only costs between $1,800 and $4,000 a year depending on the treatment approach (ONDCP, 2001).

"In California during the early '90s, we built nine new prisons but we built no new universities and actually suffered a decrease in drug treatment slots due to reduced funding. Yet 80–85% of our prisoners listed a drug problem as a major reason for their offense. I think we have our priorities backwards."
California education consultant

PRINCIPLES & GOALS OF TREATMENT

PRINCIPLES OF EFFECTIVE TREATMENT

In a 1999 publication by the National Institutes of Health (NIH), *Principles of Drug Addiction Treatment,* 13 principles of effective treatment were listed. These principles are applicable to any treatment facility, program, or therapy.

1. **No single treatment is appropriate for all individuals.** Matching treatment settings, interventions, and services to each individual's particular problems and needs is critical to his or her ultimate success in returning to productive functioning in the family, workplace, and society.

2. **Treatment needs to be readily available.** Because individuals who are addicted to drugs may be uncertain about entering treatment, taking advantage of opportunities when they are ready for treatment is crucial. Potential applicants can be lost if treatment is not immediately available or is not readily accessible.

3. **Effective treatment attends to multiple needs of the individual not just his or her drug use.**

4. **An individual's treatment and services plan must be assessed continually and modified as necessary to ensure that the plan meets the person's changing needs.**

5. **Remaining in treatment for an adequate period of time is critical for treatment effectiveness.** Research indicates that for most patients, the threshold of significant improvement is reached at about 3 months in treatment.

6. **Counseling (individual and/or group) and other behavioral therapies are critical components of effective treatment for addiction.**

7. **Medications are an important element of treatment for many patients, especially when combined with counseling and other behavioral therapies.** Methadone, LAAM (levomethadyl acetate), naltrexone, bupropion, and a number of other medications can help with detoxification as well as short- and long-term abstinence. In 2002 the use of LAAM was associated with cardiac arrhythmias and it is subsequently not being used as much as buprenorphine combined with naloxone (Suboxone®) for the treatment of opiate addiction (Schwetz, 2001).

8. **Addicted or drug-abusing individuals with coexisting mental disorders should have both disorders treated in an integrated way.**

9. **Detoxification is only the first stage of addiction treatment and by itself does little to change long-term drug use.**

10. **Treatment does not need to be voluntary to be effective.** Sanctions or enticements in the family, employment setting, or criminal justice system can significantly increase both treatment entry and retention rates and the success of drug treatment interventions.

11. **Possible drug use during treatment must be monitored continuously.** The objective monitoring of a patient's drug and alcohol use during treatment, such as through urinalysis or other tests, can help the patient withstand urges to use drugs.

12. **Treatment programs should provide assessment for HIV/AIDS, hepatitis B and C, tuberculosis, and other infectious diseases as well as counseling to help patients modify or change behaviors that place themselves or others at risk of infection.**

13. **Recovery from drug addiction can be a long-term process and frequently requires multiple episodes of treatment.** Participation in self-help programs during and following treatment is often helpful in maintaining abstinence. (NIH, 1999)

The problem is that **to fully implement most of the concepts is costly**. Many local, state, and federal governments and health care systems are unable or reluctant to commit the necessary funds to provide a full range of services.

GOALS OF EFFECTIVE TREATMENT

Most treatment experts agree that the two most important goals for treatment outcome are first, to motivate clients towards abstinence from their drugs of abuse and second, to reconstruct their lives once their focus is redirected away from substance abuse. Integrating harm reduction into these goals would mean the willingness to accept incremental behavioral changes that reduce the harm that addiction is causing on one's life while working towards a lifestyle of continuous recovery.

To accomplish these and other goals, several elements need to be addressed through an understanding that **addiction treatment is a lifelong process for the addict**. Treatment merely motivates, initiates, and provides some tools that help them ultimately obtain uninterrupted abstinence from their addiction throughout their lives.

"Well, basically, I'd like to stay off drugs. I'd like to get my family life

together again and have a relationship with my children—a good one—and if nothing else, I'd just like to know that when I do die, I did have a life, you know, aside from being just another dope fiend in the gutter."

24-year-old recovering heroin addict

Primary Goals

Motivation Towards Abstinence. Components of these efforts consist of education, counseling, and involvement with 12-step or self-help groups. This might include harm reduction approaches like methadone maintenance whereby an addict is provided with an alternate medically controlled drug to promote abstinence from the street drug of choice.

Creating a Drug-Free Lifestyle. This covers all aspects of an addict's life, including the ability to address social/environmental issues, like homelessness, relationships, family, and friends, in order to develop drug-free life interactions. They are connected to drug-free activities, like clean and sober dances, and most importantly they learn relapse prevention skills, such as stress reduction, cue resistance, coping, decision making, and conflict resolution.

Supporting Goals

Enriching Job or Career Functioning. Often neglected in treatment, jobs and career comprise a major portion of someone's life. This goal is accomplished through vocational services, management of personal finances, and maintenance of a drug-free workplace.

Optimizing Medical Functioning. Besides treatment of withdrawal and other acute medical problems associated with addiction, many addicts have undiagnosed or existing medical problems that have been neglected through their use of drugs. The comprehensive treatment program includes the ability to assess and treat such conditions.

Optimizing Psychiatric & Emotional Functioning. Many studies suggest that greater than 50% of all substance abusers also have a coexisting psychiatric condition. Identification and appropriate treatment of psychiatric problems are an essential element of the modern treatment program (*see Chapter 10*).

Addressing Relevant Spiritual Issues. Although the inclusion of either spirituality or religious beliefs in addiction treatment is controversial, the most effective long-term treatments of addiction are the spiritually based 12-step Alcoholics Anonymous and other anonymous programs. Further many of the other treatment programs in operation base their interventions on the 12-step traditions. Thus it has become essential for programs to at least help clarify this issue with their clients and provide appropriate referrals (Schuckit, 1994, 2000).

"I don't have hopes of living forever. I never have. I mean, to be my age is a complete shock to me, so it's not about that but the issue is about the quality of life."

40-year-old recovering heroin addict

SELECTION OF A PROGRAM

Most program selections occur on the spur of the moment **based upon cost, familiarity, location, and convenience of access**. The current era of managed health care has made accurate diagnoses and pretreatment assessments essential because they can better match addicts to programs that address their specific needs and thus promote better outcomes.

DIAGNOSIS

Various diagnostic tools can be used to help verify, support, or clarify the potential diagnosis of chemical addiction (Mersy, 1991; Lewis, Dana, & Blevins, 1994). The following are some of the more common ones used.

◇ The **American Psychiatric Association's** *Diagnostic and Statistical Manual of Mental Disorders (DSM-IV-TR)* relies on the pattern and duration of drug use, the negative impact of drugs on the social or occupational functioning of the user, and the pathological effects (e.g., tolerance or withdrawal symptoms) to confirm a diagnosis of dependence (addiction) (American Psychiatric Association, 2000).

◇ The **Selective Severity Assessment (SSA)** evaluates 11 physiologic signs (e.g., pulse, temperature, tremors) to confirm the severity of the addiction in an addict.

◇ The **National Council on Alcoholism Criteria for Diagnosis of Alcoholism (NCA CRIT)** and its **Modified Criteria (MODCRIT)** outline 2 bases on which to make the diagnosis of alcoholism:
  1. physical and clinical parameters,
  2. behavioral, psychological, and attitudinal impact.

◇ The **Addiction Severity Index (ASI)** represents the most comprehensive and lengthy criteria for the diagnosis of chemical dependency. One hundred and eighty items cover 6 areas that are affected by substance use and abuse.

◇ A simple diagnostic aid, the **Michigan Alcoholism Screening Test (MAST)**, uses just 25 questions that are primarily directed at the negative life effects of alcohol on the user (*see Chapter 5*). There is also the **Short Michigan Alcohol Screening Test** with just 13 questions.

◇ The **CAGE Questionnaire** is the simplest assessment tool for problem drinking and consists of just 4 questions.
  1. Have you felt the need to **C**ut down on your drinking?
  2. Do you feel **A**nnoyed by people complaining about your drinking?
  3. Do you ever feel **G**uilty about your drinking?

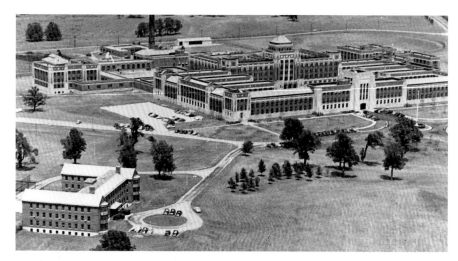

The U.S. government's attitude towards most treatment methods at the end of World War I limited the facilities available for addicts. In 1929 the government allocated funds for two "narcotic farms" to house and rehabilitate addicts who had been convicted of violating federal drug laws or those who wished to commit themselves voluntarily. The Lexington Kentucky Narcotics Farm opened in 1935 and the second facility in Fort Worth, Texas, in November, 1938. The Lexington facility shown in this picture had about 1,000 inmates. Treatment could last up to a year or more. A study of effectiveness showed that 90–96% of addicts returned to active addiction, most within 6 months of discharge (White, 1998).

Courtesy of the U.S. Department of Health and Human Services, Program Support Center

4. Do you ever drink an **Eye-opener** in the morning to relieve the shakes?

Two or more affirmative responses suggest that the client is a problem drinker (Allen, Eckardt, & Wallen, 1988).

TREATMENT OPTIONS

"Let the experiment be fairly tried; let an institution be founded; let the means of cure be provided; let the principles on which it is to be founded be extensively promulgated and, I doubt not, all intelligent people will be satisfied of its feasibility . . . let the principle of total abstinence be rigorously adopted and enforced . . . let appropriate medication be afforded . . . let the mind be soothed . . . let good nutrition be regularly administered—this course, rigorously adopted and pursued, will restore nine out of ten in all cases."

Dr. Samuel Woodward, 1833 (Grinrod, 1840, 1886)

The nineteenth-century expert on mental health Dr. Samuel Woodward

thought that society should support recovery. Addiction is a complex interaction between biological, social, and toxic factors. Given these multiple influences, treatment has evolved along various paths, all of which enjoy some success. However, since each person is unique and the level of addiction different, **no treatment has proven to be universally effective for everyone** who has an addiction. Often, effective treatment requires a variety of techniques in a variety of settings.

"Someone asked me, 'Where would you go to get off drugs? Where would you feel comfortable?' If I had everything I needed, lifetime supplies, and I was shipwrecked on an island, that would be fine."

Recovering 22-year-old methamphetamine abuser

A wide range of options exists for the treatment of alcohol or other chemical addiction. The range is

◇ from "cold turkey" or "white knuckle" dry outs to medically assisted detoxification;

◇ from expensive medical or residential approaches, to free peer groups, 12-step groups, or social model group therapy;

◇ from outpatient treatment, to halfway houses, to residential programs;

◇ from long-term residential treatment (2 years or more) to 7-day hospital detoxification with aftercare;

◇ and from methadone maintenance or other harm reduction techniques to acupuncture, aversion therapies, or a dozen other treatment modalities.

"I believed there were only AA and NA for my 'crank' use and I knew—I just knew these wouldn't work. Then after a particularly nasty run, which I thought I kept from my probation officer, he gave me a choice of getting into treatment or going back to prison. I was startled when he handed me a full-page list of different places I could go. There was a medical program. There was a NA program made up of speed freaks like myself. There was a mental health program near my apartment. There were places I could go to live while kicking. The only problem was waiting for an open slot."

35-year-old recovering "crank" addict

In many of the studies on the effectiveness of different types of programs, what is sometimes forgotten is the process of treatment self-selection. This means that **addicts will often end up in a program that works and drop out of those that feel uncomfortable, are not relevant to their problem, or that they are not ready for** based on the stage of their addiction. So a statistic might read that "this program is only effective for 10% of all addicts" and that's true as far as it goes. However, it could read, "this type of program works for 10% of the addicted population and luckily there are a dozen other programs and if each one is only effective with 10% of the population, then we can offer recovery to most addicts." It also means that we can't put all treatment hopes in just one type of therapy be it drug replacement therapy, a therapeutic community, or 12-step groups. A simile would be that treatment for a heart condition could be diet change, coronary artery bypass, angioplasty, or in the extreme, a heart-replacement operation.

Types of Facilities

Medical model detoxification programs can be hospital inpatient, residential, or outpatient. The treatment in medical model programs is **supervised and managed by medical professionals**. Medications useful for the treatment of the patient can be administered in conjunction with traditional recovery-oriented counseling and educational approaches. These are usually the most expensive types of programs but have the advantage of being able to do a more comprehensive assessment and treatment of the addict's overall physical and mental health. Inpatient medical model programs can cost $3,000 to $25,000 depending on the length of stay (3–28 days) while outpatient medical model programs range from $1,500 to $5,000, again depending on the length of stay (1–6 months). Methadone maintenance is considered a medical model treatment program.

Office-based medical detoxification and maintenance treatment for opiate abusers can now be provided by qualified private medical practitioners. The Food and Drug Administration (FDA) approved the Drug Addiction Treatment Act of 2000 that legalized the prescribing of Schedule III, IV, and V controlled substances to opiate addicts by physicians specially certified with the Drug Enforcement Administration (DEA). Prior to this new law, controlled substances for the treatment of addiction were restricted to registered clinics. This previous restriction threatened the confidentiality of treatment since anyone seen at such a facility could be assumed to be an addict. It also exposed patients to other drug users and often required undue travel by many addicts. Although

physicians have to participate in special training to become certified to treat addicts in their offices, there is some concern that medical treatment detached from immediate, on-site counseling, education, social, and other services for addicts will be ineffective in promoting recovery. This new type of treatment is also known as "office-based opiate addiction treatment" or "O-BOAT."

Social model detoxification programs are nonmedical programs that can be either inpatient or outpatient. These programs are also short term (7–28 days) and aimed at providing a safe and sober environment for addicts to rebalance their body and brain chemistry that was disrupted by abuse of drugs. This then enables them to enter into a full recovery program.

Social model recovery programs (also called "**outpatient drug-free programs**") use a wide variety of approaches to move a client toward recovery. Since social model programs are totally nonmedical, the client usually must be abstinent from drugs for 72 hours before they will be admitted. Approaches include cognitive behavioral therapy, insight-oriented psychotherapy, problem-solving groups, and 12-step programs. Clients may stay in these programs for months or longer (Dodd, 1997).

Therapeutic communities (TC) are generally long-term (1–3 years) self-contained residential programs that provide full rehabilitative and social services under the direction of the facility. These include daily counseling, drug education, vocational and educational rehabilitation, and case management, including referrals to social and health services. Many peer counselors, administrators, and role models in therapeutic communities are ex-addicts. The goals of this type of program are

◇ habilation or rehabilitation of the total individual;

◇ changing negative patterns of behavior, thinking, and feeling that predispose drug use;

◇ and development of a drug-free lifestyle (Institute of Medicine, 1990).

The 3 major stages of treatment in a TC are (1) **induction and early treatment**, usually during the first 30 days, including learning TC policies and procedures, beginning to understand addiction, and committing to the recovery process; (2) **primary treatment**; and (3) **re-entry into the community at large** (National Institute on Drug Abuse [NIDA], 2002b).

Because of funding limitations and availability, variations of the long-term TC concept have developed, e.g., short-term communities (3–6 months), modified therapeutic communities (6–9 months), adolescent therapeutic communities for juveniles that focus on the specific problems of youth, and jail-based TCs (Crowe & Reeves, 1994). There are also day treatment TCs that are less intensive than residential TC treatment but more intensive than the usual outpatient drug treatment program. The keys are maintaining a community approach and the principle of self-help.

Many addicts are often put off by making such a long commitment to being cut off from society. Many programs divide the treatment into 3–6-month phases that permit making commitments to each phase of treatment rather than the full 1–3 years all at one time.

Halfway houses permit addicts to keep their jobs and outside contacts while being involved in a residential treatment program. Addicts receive educational and therapeutic interactions after work hours and live within the facility. Weekends or nonworking days are reserved for more intensive program work that continues for a long duration (1–3 years). Several new religious movements (NRMs) and faith-based treatment initiatives also use the halfway house concept to treat addiction. They are controversial because some critics say that joining a religious movement is exchanging one compulsion for another while the other side says that a spiritual awakening is necessary for true recovery and a NRM halfway house can provide that structure (Muffler, Langrod, Richardson, & Ruiz, 1997).

Sober-living or transitional-

living programs are generally for clients who have completed a long-term residential program. They consist of **apartments or cooperatives for groups of recovering addicts** with strong house rules to maintain a clean and sober living environment that is supportive of each person's recovery effort. Minimal-to-moderate treatment structure is provided for those living arrangements and programs merely monitor compliance to protocols that allow the addicts to reenter the broader society with a drug-free lifestyle.

Partial hospitalization and day hospitals are medical outpatient programs that involve the client in therapeutic activities for 4–6 hours per day while the client still lives at home. These programs provide medical services for detoxification and for medically assisted recovery with medications that either treat withdrawal symptoms, modify craving, or help prevent relapse. Counseling and education are part of these programs. **Intensive outpatient**

programs are a less-intense (6–8 hours per week) modification of this model.

Harm reduction programs, as discussed earlier in this chapter, consist mainly of pharmacotherapy maintenance approaches (also called "agonist maintenance treatment"), particularly methadone maintenance clinics that substitute a long-acting synthetic opioid that is taken orally to prevent opioid withdrawal, block the effects of illicit opioids, and reduce opioid craving. Another harm reduction program that is less successful is controlled drinking or drug use taught through behavioral training programs. There are also education programs that teach how to minimize problems from drug use; **partial detox clinics** that help addicts to lower their drug tolerance to minimize damage to the user; **sobering stations** that provide a safe place for addicts and alcoholics to sleep off their inebriation or hangover, and even **designated driver programs** that seem to sanction heavy drinking by some (Morris, 1995).

Admissions

In 2000 a total of 1.6 million people were treated in various programs and facilities. It is estimated that another 2 million hard-core users also needed treatment and possibly another 3.5 million problematic users needed some kind of care. The totals mean that in 2000 about 7.1 million Americans had serious enough drug and alcohol problems to need treatment.

BEGINNING TREATMENT

It is vital to remember that addiction is a dysfunction of the mind caused by actual biochemical changes in the central nervous system. We are born with most of the brain cells we will ever have (including the reservoir of immature stem cells) unlike tissues such as skin cells that are totally replaced every 8

TABLE 9–1   ADMISSIONS TO DRUG TREATMENT BY PRIMARY SUBSTANCE OF ABUSE, 1992 - 2000

Primary Substance	1992	1994	1996	1998	2000
Alcohol	**898,021**	**858,281**	**804,162**	**764,420**	**724,196**
alcohol only	562,778	504,494	460,366	432,314	413,638
alcohol w/secondary drug	335,243	353,787	343,796	332,106	310,558
Opiates (heroin, OxyContin®, etc.)	**181,876**	**227,757**	**232,934**	**249,426**	**269,362**
Cocaine	**267,292**	**292,649**	**258,033**	**245,010**	**218,311**
smoked cocaine	183,282	216,935	191,124	179,336	158,524
nonsmoked cocaine	84,010	75,714	66,909	65,674	59,787
Marijuana/hashish	**92,414**	**142,707**	**192,614**	**219,059**	**236,638**
Stimulants (amphetamine, methamphetamine, etc.)	**22,117**	**45,159**	**52,937**	**71,181**	**82,883**
Sedative-hypnotics/tranquilizers	**8,350**	**8,046**	**7,459**	**7,740**	**8,411**
Hallucinogens	**3,437**	**2,681**	**2,823**	**2,346**	**2,867**
PCP	**2,833**	**3,433**	**2,501**	**1,833**	**2,589**
Inhalants	**2,918**	**2,675**	**1,971**	**1,592**	**1,251**
Over-the-counter medications	**522**	**583**	**550**	**481**	**739**
Other	**3,007**	**4,056**	**3,704**	**6,468**	**12,333**
None reported	**45,143**	**47,625**	**40,686**	**49,235**	**40,123**
TOTAL ADMISSIONS	**1,527,930**	**1,635,652**	**1,600,374**	**1,618,791**	**1,599,703**

(Substance Abuse and Mental Health Administration, 2003b)

TABLE 9–2   ONE-DAY CENSUS OF CLIENTS IN TREATMENT—BY FACILITY OWNERSHIP & TYPE OF CARE

Year	Private Profit	Private Nonprofit	State/Local Gvmt.	Federal Gvmt.	Tribal Gvmt.	Other	Total	Inpatient Treatment	Outpatient Treatment
1980	17,997	284,483	150,376	25,977	N/C	N/C	**478,793**	N/A	N/A
1984	60,191	395,831	164,232	45,595	N/C	4,430	**670,279**	N/A	N/A
1990	113,522	451,951	172,290	27,025	3,041	N/C	**767,829**	93,888	673,941
1995	179,337	575,002	198,579	46,861	9,348	N/C	**1,009,127**	144,842	864,285
2000	242,184	552,092	153,989	40,549	12,082	N/C	**1,000,896**	109,349	891,547
2002	308,737	646,802	158,384	39,921	9,939	1,046	**1,164,829**	120,755	1,044,074

◇ 72% of all clients were male

◇ 4.9% of female clients were pregnant

◇ close to half of all clients resided in urban areas

◇ one-fourth of all clients were IV drug users at the time of admission

◇ 12% were under 20 years old

◇ 76% were between 21–44 years old

◇ 11% were between the ages of 45 and 64

◇ 1% were over 65 years old

(ONDCP, 2003)

days or so (Snyder et al., 1999). Thus the brain cell disease of addiction is a chronic progressive process that can be treated and arrested but not one that can be reversed to any great extent or cured. The Haight Ashbury Detox Clinic recognizes that **recovery is a lifelong process since the brain cells have been permanently changed**. Addicts (those who have lost control of their drug use) must refrain from ever abusing and, in most cases, even using small amounts of any psychoactive drug if they want to avoid relapsing into addiction.

"Friday I was feeling good. I even went to a meeting. I'd been in this program for 2 years. I thought I could have one

Figure 9-3 •

This is the protocol structure for the Haight Ashbury Detox Clinic (medical model outpatient program). It emphasizes the complexity of treating a compulsive drug user who comes in for treatment, particularly if other problems such as medical complications, mental problems (dual diagnosis), or HIV disease are involved. The limiting factor for many clinics is their budget.

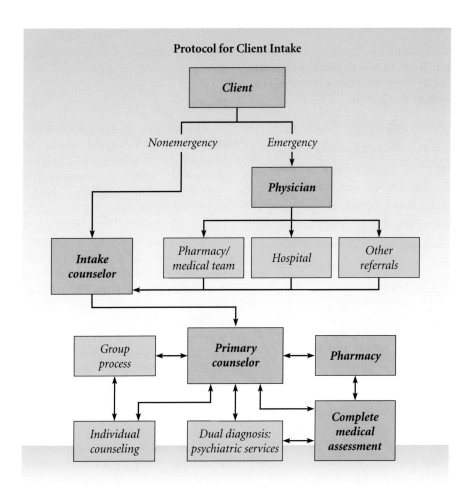

drink to relax with some friends I ran into. I had about five scotches and ended up using coke all night long in a hotel with two prostitutes. I went through about $700 and was broke and then I stole $150 from my room-mate. I was ripped off a couple of times buying stuff and at the end of it, I was tweaked and I still wanted more."

Recovering 24-year-old crack user

RECOGNITION & ACCEPTANCE

Treatment starts with a recognition and acceptance of addiction by the addict. This **self-diagnosis often requires the addict to hit bottom or be the subject of an intervention** with an assessment to support and validate the need for treatment. Only then can an addict be entered into a continuum of lifelong processes to assist her or him in a quest for recovery.

Hitting Bottom

Addiction is a progressive illness that leads to severe life impairment and dysfunction when left to proceed without disruption.

"It really took my soul. I really feel it took my soul. As a human being, it's important to have a soul and I think I was just a hollow shell. It took my family, it took my kids, it took my self-esteem, which is probably the most important facet of all because without that, everything else was just tempo-rary anyway."

Recovering heroin abuser

The earlier addiction is recognized, accepted, and treated, the more likely the addict will have a re-warding life and good health. Hitting bottom doesn't have to be life threatening, it can simply be hopelessness.

"I got up and I looked at my pipe. And then I said, 'No,' and I put it down and I put it in the trash—I didn't break

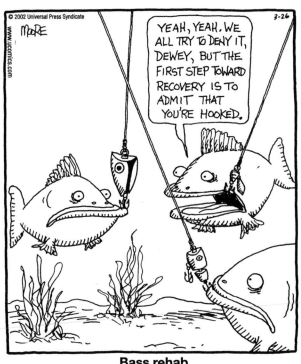

YEAH, YEAH, WE ALL TRY TO DENY IT, DEWEY, BUT THE FIRST STEP TOWARD RECOVERY IS TO ADMIT THAT YOU'RE HOOKED.

Bass rehab.

it—and I rocked myself and I said, 'No dope, no dope, no dope,' and I rocked myself until I could not rock myself any more."

Recovering crack addict

Denial

Overcoming denial, the essential first step in all treatment, is also the most difficult to accomplish. Denial is the universal defense mechanism experienced not only by addicts but also by their families, friends, and associates. Denial prevents or delays the proper recognition and acceptance of a chemical dependency or compulsive behavioral problem. **Denial is a refusal to acknowledge the negative impact that the drug use is having on one's life.** It is also assigning the reason for negative consequences to other causes rather than the drug use or compulsive behavior.

One problem is that many people are unwilling to make the diagnosis or they just don't recognize the signs and symptoms. In particular **the medical profession has a tendency to deny or overlook addiction.** How often or how thoroughly does a physician inquire about a patient's alcohol or other drug

use history? How often is a caffeine in-take assessment done by a physician who is treating anxiety and insomnia in a patient? A study of physician aware-ness in Boston found that about 45% of 1,440 patients with a substance abuse problem said that their physician was unaware of their illness. Uninsured clients, those with a history of medical illness, or those who had been previously treated for substance abuse or mental illness were even more unlikely to be diagnosed correctly by their physician (Saitz, Mulvey, Plough, & Samet, 1998).

"I woke up after passing out in a friend's home, and they had taken my money away from me, and they had posted somebody at the door, and my mother came and said, 'I will not watch your children for you while you go out and party. If you do something about your problem, I'll take care of your kids for a week.' That was the first time anybody had said to me I had a problem and that was the first time anybody said, 'Stop. You can't do this anymore.'"

37-year-old recovering speed user

Breaking Through Denial

Denial plus the toxic effects that psychoactive drugs have on judgment and memory make the addict likely to be the last person to recognize and accept her or his addiction. Usually those closest to the addict, the family or spouse, have the best chance to make the earliest recognition of addiction (not just use) and to help the person break through denial. Besides close relations, others able to recognize addiction include friends, coworkers, employers, ministers, medical professionals, the IRS, and the law. On the other hand, **addiction is the only illness that requires a self-diagnosis for treatment to be effective**. Normally when physicians tell patients that they have high blood pressure, they accept that diagnosis without question and make changes in their lives to improve their health. But when addicts are first confronted with their addiction, they almost always deny any drug problem and continue to abuse drugs.

There are several ways to break through denial.

◇ **Legal Intervention.** The threat of loss of freedom, property, relationships, and professional licensure among others, forces users to accept that they are having a problem with drugs. Legal requirements may mandate treatment while incarceration limits drug use and promotes abstinence in prisons where drug trafficking is supposed to be kept to a minimum. Unfortunately some prison personnel estimate that, if tested, from 10–30% of inmates in many prisons would test positive for an illicit psychoactive drug.

◇ **Workplace Intervention.** Poor performance and the threat of the loss of one's livelihood can break through denial. Strong employee assistance programs work with the at-risk employee.

◇ **Physical Health Problems.** Deteriorating health and doctors' warnings can make the user consider drug problems as a possible cause or complicating factor. The existence of lung cancer, high blood pressure, or heart, liver, kidney, and other diseases caused by drug toxicity can be a powerful tool to confront a patient's denial of addiction.

◇ **Mental Health Problems.** Emotional and mental traumas like depression, anger, and mental confusion that affect day-to-day functioning can also act as a warning signal.

◇ **Financial Difficulties.** Problems such as paying bills, buying food, or covering the rent, which are affected by escalating drug costs, force the user either to deal drugs, turn to other crimes, or cut back on use, thus compelling the user to recognize the financial damage of addiction.

(Miller & Hester, 1989; Heather, 1989)

Table 9-3 shows the sources of referral for people who have entered substance abuse treatment. Some interesting observations: first is that overall, about one-third are self-referred and another one-third are referred by the justice system, usually court-ordered treatment; the percentage of self-referrals for marijuana is only one-half of the number of referrals for other drugs (SAMHSA, 2003b).

"My dad's an alcoholic. I've tried so many things just to get him into treatment but no matter how much I try, he just doesn't listen. So I'm not gonna let him take me down from my recovery. I just told him, you know, 'Forget it. And if you want to be with me, you're going to have to be clean.' And he only loves two things and that's me and my brother. And if we take one of those away, he might want to quit."

Recovering 15-year-old recovering polydrug abuser

Intervention

Special strategies have been developed to attack the denial in drug abusers and addicted people and help them recognize their dependence on drugs. Generally referred to as "interventions," these strategies have been documented since the late 1800s to effectively bring those who are addicted into treatment and hold them there. Further there are now specialists who

TABLE 9–3   ADMISSIONS BY SOURCE OF REFERRAL IN THE UNITED STATES IN 2000

Source of Referral	All Admissions	Alcohol Only	Alcohol w/ Other Drug	Heroin	Crack	Other Cocaine	Marijuana	Methamphetamine
Total # of Admissions	1,599,703	413,638	310,558	243,523	158,524	59,787	236,638	81,764
Individual (self)	33.2%	27.8%	27.4%	64.1%	35.8%	33.4%	56.4%	45.0%
Criminal justice/DUI	36.4%	43.9%	36.3%	12.4%	26.7%	12.0%	6.8%	5.7%
Substance abuse provider	11.7%	10.3%	16.4%	12.7%	6.6%	8.4%	5.3%	5.5%
Other health care provider	7.7%	9.4%	8.5%	5.3%	8.5%	0.3%	3.9%	0.4%
School (educational)	1.1%	0.5%	0.8%	0.1%	0.1%	1.5%	1.3%	0.7%
Employer/EAP	1.0%	1.2%	1.1%	0.3%	0.7%	2.1%	9.6%	15.4%
Other community referral	8.9%	6.9%	9.4%	5.2%	11.6%			

Source: Treatment Episode Data Set: 1992–2000 (SAMHSA/TEDS, 2003b)

help organize and implement interventions (Mersy, 1991). The current style of formal intervention was developed by Dr. Vernon Johnson in the 1960s and refined by a number of treatment professionals.

"Intervention is a process by which the harmful, progressive, and destructive effects of chemical dependency are interrupted and the chemically dependent person is helped to stop using mood-altering chemicals and to develop new healthier ways of coping with his or her needs and problems. It implies that the person need not be an emotional or physical wreck (or hit bottom) before such help can be given."

Vernon E. Johnson, Founder, Johnson Institute (Johnson, 1986)

Generally a formal intervention should be tried after informal interventions have failed or if a professional feels that the wall of denial is too great. Most intervention strategies consist of the following elements:

Love.   An intervention should always start and end with an expression of love and genuine concern for the well-being of the addicted person. Multiple participants should be recruited from various aspects of the addicted person's life—all of whom share a sense of true affection for the user but recognize the progressive impairment of the addiction and are bold enough to commit themselves to participation in the intervention. Generally this intervention team consists of two or more of the following: family members, close friends and coworkers, other recovering addicts, a clergy or community leader, and a lead facilitator.

Facilitator.   A professional intervention specialist or a knowledgeable chemical dependency treatment professional is selected to organize the intervention, educate the participants about addiction and treatment options, train and assist team members in the preparation of their statements, and

support or confirm the diagnosis of addiction. The team meets and prepares its intervention without revealing its activities to the user.

Intervention Statements.   Each team member prepares a statement that he or she will make to the addicted person at the time of the intervention. Each statement consists of 4 parts:

1. a declaration of how much they love, care for, and respect the user;
2. specific incidents they have personally witnessed or experienced related to the addiction and the pain they have personally experienced from the incidents;
3. personal knowledge that the incidents occurred not because of the user's intent but because of the effects that the drug has had on the user's behavior;
4. reassurance of their love, concern, and respect for the user with a strong request that he or she recognize and accept the illness and enter treatment immediately.

Anticipated Defenses & Outcomes.   The facilitator prepares the team to deal with expected defense mechanisms like denial, rationalization, minimization, anger, and accusations. The team also prepares for all logistics (reserving a program or hospital admission, packing clothing and toiletries, covering work and home duties) so that the user will have no excuse or delay entering treatment immediately should a successful intervention ensue. The team also prepares for contingencies and alternative treatments other than the ones they selected should the addict refuse to accept their first recommendation. It is important that the user accepts one of the treatment programs selected by the team and not delay entry by saying they want a different program. In making a program selection, one should be knowledgeable about the addicted person's specific needs, his or her resources to afford treatment, the specific components and deficiencies of available programs, and

the ultimate client goal of these potential programs.

The Intervention.   Timing, location, and surprise are crucial components of the actual intervention. A neutral, nonthreatening, and private location must be secured. It should occur at a time (usually early Sunday morning) when the user is most likely to be sober and not under the influence of a drug. The evidence presented in statements should include current incidents. A reliable plan should be developed to get the addicted person to the location that does not cause her or him to suspect what is about to occur. Finally the facilitator should prepare the order of the statements that have been rehearsed by the team prior to the intervention.

Contingency.   Successful or not, it is important for the intervention team members to continue to meet after the intervention to process their experiences. This also provides the opportunity for team members (especially family members) to explore their own support or treatment needs for issues such as codependency, enabling, or adult children of addicts syndrome.

Despite the inherent risks of anger or rejection that may result from an unsuccessful intervention, the potential benefits from these strategies far outweigh the risks. At a very minimum, the pathological effects of secrecy that pervade an addiction have been brought out to all those who are most affected by it, allowing a chance for successful treatment.

TREATMENT CONTINUUM

"I know it sounds strange but the best thing that ever happened to me was that I became an addict. That's because my addiction forced me into treatment and the recovery process and through recovery I found what was missing in my life."

Nurse with 20 years of recovery time

The chronic, progressive, and relapsing nature of addiction is a depressing and degrading process. Results of a Beck's Depression Inventory (BDI) evaluation of patients entering treatment at the Haight Ashbury Clinic demonstrated that 34–38% tested for maximum depression. Admission interviews also demonstrated that 30–34% had made at least one suicide gesture prior to seeking help for their addiction. Fortunately recovery is a spiritually uplifting and motivating process through which individuals gain a sense of purpose, community, and meaning for their lives. **Recovery is a gradual process and a client passes through several changes, no matter which therapy is used: detoxification, initial abstinence, long-term abstinence (sobriety), and continuous recovery.** It is necessary for the addict to become and remain abstinent through all phases of treatment to be successful, however, slips and relapses are part of the addiction process and often occur during treatment. For this reason they need to be accepted and processed by the client and counselor or therapist. Inclusion of harm reduction education and alternatives should be included during this processing of slips and relapses. The four steps to recovery are the ones used at the Haight Ashbury Detox Clinic.

DETOXIFICATION

The first step is to get the drug out of the body if the client is still using. The user's biochemistry has become so unbalanced that only abstinence will give it time to metabolize the drug and begin to normalize the brain's neurochemical balance. Detoxification will also help normalize clients' thinking processes so they can participate fully in their own recovery. **It takes about a week to completely excrete a drug such as cocaine and perhaps another 4 weeks to 10 months until the body chemistry settles down.** Certain drugs, including marijuana and PCP, take longer to be excreted from the body. Some treatment programs will assist in the detoxification process but most require several days of abstinence prior to

admission to ensure that the patient is no longer at risk to suffer dangerous withdrawal symptoms, such as seizures, particularly when alcohol or sedatives are involved.

"My mother swore off the gin and the Valium® for my wedding. She was too good to her word. She started withdrawing and having convulsions at my reception and almost died in the ambulance. It put somewhat of a damper on the honeymoon."
23-year-old bride

The initial detoxification process is usually through a process called "white knuckling" in which addicts or abusers stop taking the drug on their own and suffer through physical and mental withdrawal symptoms. It can also be done on a normal outpatient basis, an intense outpatient basis, at a residential facility that is medically supervised or a medically managed inpatient facility that can provide treatment in the emergency room of a hospital if the client is in crisis (Chang & Kosten, 1997). **Medically or chemically assisted detoxification is aimed at minimizing the symptoms of withdrawal** that can cause life-endangering effects or an immediate relapse.

For those facilities that assist in detoxification, **assessment of the severity of addiction is important to determine if medical detoxification is necessary** and if so which facility should be used. The level of intoxication, the potential for severe withdrawal symptoms, the presence of other medical or psychological problems, the patient's response to treatment recommendations, the potential for relapse, and the environment for recovery need to be determined.

Severe physical dependence on depressants, major medical or psychiatric complications, and pregnancy are all indications for initiating detoxification in a hospital-based program.

"Something told me I had to stop, so I did. And I stopped by myself for 7 days straight. I didn't know what I was

going through. I was having flashes, I heard people talking to me, and I was sweating. I had the shakes real bad, so I called General Hospital. They gave me poison control and they transferred me to the Haight Ashbury Clinic."
23-year-old recovering cocaine addict

Medication Therapy for Detoxification

A variety of specific medications are used during the detoxification phase to ease the symptoms of withdrawal and minimize the initial drug cravings that occur. (*There is more thorough coverage of potential treatment medications at the end of this chapter.*)

◇ **Clonidine** (Catapres®) dampens the withdrawal symptoms of opioids, alcohol, and even nicotine addiction.

◇ **Phenobarbital** is used to prevent withdrawal seizures and other symptoms associated with alcohol and sedative-hypnotic dependence.

◇ **Methadone**, a long-acting opioid, is one of four federally approved medications for opioid addiction treatment (for detoxification and maintenance). The other three are buprenorphine, levomethadyl acetate (LAAM), and naltrexone.

◇ **Buprenorphine** (Subutex®, Suboxone®) can be used for short-term detoxification or long-term maintenance.

◇ **Naltrexone** (Revia®) blocks the effects of opioids. The addict will have no response to heroin if she or he happens to slip while in treatment. It is also FDA approved for use to prevent craving in recovering alcoholics.

◇ **Antipsychotic medications**, like haloperidol (Haldol®); **antidepressants,** including desipramine and imipramine (Tofranil®); or SSRI antidepressants, like sertraline (Zoloft®) and fluoxetine (Prozac®), have been used in the initial detoxification of cocaine, amphetamine, or other stimulant drug addictions.

◇ **Bromocriptine** (Parlodel®), **amantadine** (Symmetrel®), and **L-Dopa®** have been used to treat the craving associated with cocaine and stimulant drug dependence.

◇ **Acomprosate** is prescribed to decrease alcohol cravings.

◇ **Nicotine patches** (Nicoderm® or Prostep®) are approved to treat the withdrawal symptoms of tobacco whereas nicotine-laced gum (Nicorette®) helps to lessen craving.

◇ **Disulfiram** (Antabuse®) helps to prevent alcoholism relapse by creating unpleasant side effects if alcohol is used.

◇ Finally a number of **amino acids** are used individually or in combination with each other to try to alleviate withdrawal and craving symptoms. The theory is that the brain uses these amino acids to make neurotransmitters that were depleted by the drug addiction. It is believed that the imbalance or depletion of neurotransmitters is the cause of many of the withdrawal symptoms and the intense craving. Common amino acids used for this purpose are tyrosine, taurine, tryptophan, d,1-phenylalanine, lecithin, and glutamine.

Psychosocial Therapy

Medical intervention alone is rarely effective during the detoxification phase. Indeed most programs forego medical treatment if the addict is not in any physiological or psychological danger from drug withdrawal. **Intensive counseling and group work have proven to be the most effective** measures of engaging addicts into a recovery process and should be the main focus of all phases of treatment despite the many medical innovations being developed.

Psychosocial client interactions during detoxification are usually intense (daily encounters in an outpatient program) and highly structured for a 2–6-week duration. **The aim of this treatment phase is to break down residual denial and engage the client**

into the full recovery process. This is accomplished through mandated participation in educational sessions, task-oriented group work, therapy groups, peer recovery groups, 12-step groups, and individual counseling.

Treatment focuses on helping the addict to learn about the disease concept of addiction, the harmful effects of the disease, and the intensity of detoxification symptoms they are experiencing. Clients also receive information about their treatment and any medications used in detoxification. They also develop their recovery or treatment plan with their primary counselor and initiate activities to accomplish their goals during the detoxification phase of treatment. Some programs have also begun to use structured treatment manuals that have a developed curriculum for each phase of treatment with individual daily lesson plans, exercises, and homework assignments.

"I knew I could do it myself. I tried those programs in AA. I stopped using drugs a million times and I never needed one of those programs."
Heroin addict dying from AIDS

INITIAL ABSTINENCE

Once the addict has been detoxified, **body chemistry must be given the opportunity to regain balance**. Continued abstinence during this phase is best promoted by addressing both the continuous craving for drugs and the problems in the addict's life that may present a risk for relapse.

Anticraving medications, such as those used during the detoxification phase, can be continued during the initial abstinence phase when more traditional approaches, like voluntary isolation from environmental triggers or cues (e.g., bars, co-users, drug paraphernalia), counseling, group and 12-step meetings, are ineffective in controlling the episodic drug hunger.

Medical approaches like **Antabus® for alcoholism, naltrexone for opioids and alcohol**, and various amino acids have been used. They continue to suppress or reverse the pleasurable effects

of drugs or decrease the drug craving, all of which helps encourage the addict to stay clean (O'Brien, 1997; Gatch & Lal, 1998).

Research into a cocaine vaccine and a true alcohol antagonist may lead to treatments for these addictions in the same manner that naltrexone is often effective in preventing readdiction to opioids and craving for alcohol.

Environmental Triggers, Relapse Prevention, & Cue Extinction

"When I'm smelling the marijuana here in the building where I live, I smell the 'primos,' which is crack cocaine laced with marijuana, the cravings do come back. And what I do is I call my sponsor. I go to a NA and AA meeting and I mostly talk to my sponsor and I tell her what I'm feeling and I pray to God to give me the strength not to go out to buy me any kind of drugs to use."
38-year-old recovering polydrug abuser

Environmental triggers or cues often precipitate drug cravings. These triggers have been classified into two broad categories: intrapersonal and interpersonal factors (internal states and external influences). Intrapersonal states that have the greatest impact are negative emotional and physical states or internally motivated attempts to regain control and use. External influences include relationship conflicts, social pressures, lack of support systems, negative life events, and so-called slippery people, places, and things (Marlatt, 1995; Carter & Tiffany, 1999). Some other factors that help lead to relapse are exhaustion, dishonesty, impatience, argumentativeness, depression, frustration, self-pity, cockiness, complacency, expecting too much from others, letting up on disciplines, use of any mood-altering drugs, and overconfidence (Pharmacist Rehabilitation Organization, 1999). Addicts have discovered this by themselves and long ago developed handy acronyms like **HALT** (hungry, angry, lonely, tired) and **RID** (restless, irritable, discontent) to remind themselves of the triggers that lead them into relapse.

Relapse prevention has become the focus of almost every treatment program. There are a number of strategies and themes that are used in this process.

◊ Addicts must understand the process of relapse and **learn to recognize their personal triggers** that can be anything from drug odors, seeing friends who use, having money in one's pocket, and even hearing a song about drugs.

◊ They must then **develop behaviors to avoid external cues.** These include avoiding old neighborhoods and dealers, changing one's circle of friends, limiting the amount of money that's carried, and not going into bars or gatherings where drugs are readily available.

◊ They must learn to cope with or **be prepared with an automatic reflex strategy to prevent themselves from using when their craving is activated by internal or external cues.** These include networking with their developed support system, going to a 12-step meeting, using their developed coping skills for negative emotional states and cognitive distortions, doing something that reminds them of their addiction problems or their reasons for wanting to stay clean, remembering their last binge, developing a balanced lifestyle, and possibly using anticraving medications (Daley & Marlatt, 1997).

It is important to note that **drug craving is a true psychological response that is manifested by actual physiological changes** of increased heart rate and blood pressure, sweating, dilation of the pupils, specific electrical changes in the skin, and even an immediate drop of two degrees or more in body temperature.

Deconditioning techniques, stress reduction exercises, expressing one's feelings, and long walks or cold showers are all strategies used by addicts to dissipate the craving response when it arises.

A technique such as **Dr. Anna Rose Childress's Desensitization Program retrains brain cells to not react when confronted by environmental cues.** The procedure involves exposing an addict to progressively stronger environmental cues over 40–50 sessions in a controlled setting. This technique gradually decreases response to the cues until there are no physiologic signs of a craving response even when the addict is exposed to heavy triggers. Every time an addict refrains from using while craving a drug, it lessens the response to the next trigger experience. **Desensitization has also been called "cue extinction"** (Childress, McClellan, Ehrman, & O'Brien, 1988; Childress et al., 1999).

"I did it myself. Every day I would take out my Librium® pills and look at them, touch them, and even smell them. Then I would put them back in the bottle because I knew I couldn't ever use them again. After a while I lost interest in them altogether."
Recovering benzodiazepine addict

Psychosocial Support

Initial abstinence is also the phase during which addicts start to put their lives back in order, working on all the things they neglected while practicing their addiction. A comprehensive analysis of an addict's medical health, psychiatric status, social problems, and environmental needs must be conducted and a plan developed to address all issues presented.

Most importantly **addicts need to build a support system that will give continuing advice, help, and information** when they return to job and home and are subjected to all the pressures and environmental triggers that led to addiction. The support groups and 12-step programs along with involvement in group therapy and continued recovery counseling have been demonstrated to have the most positive treatment outcomes during the initial abstinence phase.

Acupuncture

The use of acupuncture to relieve withdrawal symptoms and reduce craving has been on the increase in the last

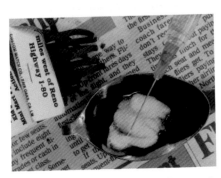
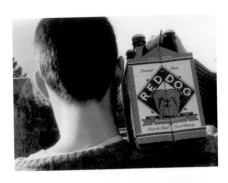
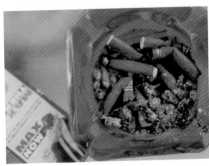

Environmental cues that trigger drug craving can include paraphernalia, drug-using partners, old neighborhoods, and especially money.

30 years since it was first observed to reduce opium withdrawal symptoms (Wen & Cheung, 1973). The hypothesis as to why acupuncture works is that **by stimulating the peripheral nerves, messages are sent to the brain to release natural (endogenous) endorphins that promote a feeling of well-being** (Birch, 2001). Acupuncture has also been shown to alter levels of other neurotransmitters, specifically serotonin and norepinephrine, as well as the hormones prolactin, oxytocin, thyroxin, corticosteroid, and insulin (Boucher, Kiresuk, & Trachtenberg, 1998; Steiner, May, & Davis, 1982). Besides opioid detoxification, acupuncture has been used to reduce craving for alcohol and stimulants with varying results. As with all initial abstinence and detoxification techniques, it is not effective when used as the sole treatment or modality. It can also be used with detox medication (Smith et al., 1997). The problem with acupuncture is that since it is not a replacement therapy for other modalities, it can be expensive, adding an additional therapeutic cost to the treatment process and **its effects last for only a short time often requiring multiple daily treatments to relieve symptoms** during detoxification and initial abstinence.

LONG-TERM ABSTINENCE

The pivotal component of this phase occurs when an addict finally admits and accepts her or his addiction as lifelong and surrenders to the long-term, one-day-at-a-time treatment process. **Continued participation in group, family, and 12-step programs is the key to maintaining long-term abstinence from drugs. The addict must accept that addiction is chronic, progressive, incurable, and potentially fatal and that relapse is always possible.**

"I know that I have another relapse in me. I don't know if I have another recovery in me."
7-year member of Alcoholics Anonymous

It is also vital for recovering addicts to accept that their condition is

chemical dependency or drug compulsivity and not just that of alcoholism, or cocainism, or opioidism. Individuals who manifest addiction to a particular drug, such as cocaine, are well advised to abstain from the use of all psychoactive substances, especially alcohol. A seemingly benign flirtation with marijuana will probably lead to other drug hunger and relapse. It is a common clinical observation that **compulsive drug abusers often switch intoxicants only to find the symptoms of addiction resurfacing through another addictive agent**. Drug switching does not work with recovery-oriented treatment. A study of men and women in treatment found that 80% had a problem with two or more substances during their lifetimes, either concurrently or sequentially (Carrol, 1980). Even abstention from smoking or chewing tobacco can help in the recovery process ("Programs Including Nicotine," 2001).

RECOVERY

"Can we cure addiction? Absolutely not! This is because addiction has caused unrecoverable changes, alterations, and deaths to brain cells. Brain cells can not be regenerated, so the changes caused by drug abuse are permanent. What we can do is arrest the illness, teach new living techniques, rewire the brain to bypass those addicted cells and give the addict in recovery a worthwhile life. It can't be cured but addiction can be effectively prevented and treated."
Darryl Inaba, Pharm.D., CEO, Haight Ashbury Clinics

Treatment and a continued focus on abstinence are not enough to assure recovery and a quality lifestyle. **Recovering addicts also need to restructure their lives and find things they enjoy doing that give them satisfaction and that give them the natural highs instead of the artificial highs they came to seek through drugs.** Without this they may have sobriety but they will not have recovery. This integral phase of

treatment has been validated experimentally by Dr. George Vaillant, Professor of Psychiatry at Harvard University. In studies in 1983 he indicated **4 components necessary to change an ingrained habit of alcohol dependence.** In the following model the generic term "drug" is substituted for Dr. Vaillant's specific reference to alcohol:

1. offering the client or patient a non-chemical substitute dependency for the drug, such as exercise;

2. reminding her or him ritually that even one episode of drug use can lead to pain and relapse;

3. repairing the social, emotional, and medical damage done;

4. restoring self-esteem.

Continued and lifelong participation in the fellowship of 12-step programs along with the concerted effort to seek out natural, healthy, nondrug, rewarding experiences is the formula that most recovering addicts have found to be successful in achieving their treatment goals (Vaillant, 1995).

"I found in sobriety that I love people. I found in sobriety that I have real feelings. I found in sobriety that I have real emotions. I found in sobriety that there's a world of people out there in society that's willing, that's been there all along for me, to assist me. I just never knew it."
56-year-old recovering heroin addict

Natural Highs

"Getting high on life is a skill and just like any other skill—athletic, artistic, musical, or professional—the more you practice it, the more you can improve."
George Obermeier, drug educator

Since psychoactive drugs create sensations or feelings that have a natural counterpart in the body, so **human beings can create virtually all of the sensations and feelings they try to get through drugs** by concentrating on the feelings they experience from natural life situations. Athletic competition releases the same neurotransmitters as cocaine and methamphetamine. Experiencing a second wind or the runner's high from jogging comes from opiate receptor activation by endorphins. Traveling or experiencing new environments activates the same area of the brain that marijuana affects. Being in touch with the natural or drug-free highs available to the brain is what being alive is all about.

OUTCOME & FOLLOW-UP

Primarily promoted by government and other funding sources to justify spending for addiction treatment, **client outcomes and follow-up evaluations have become a major element in treatment program activities**. What is often neglected by this process is an opportunity for treatment programs to utilize the data obtained to modify their treatment protocols and interventions to promote better outcomes for clients. Since addiction by its nature is a chronic, multivaried, and relapsing condition, **there is a need to develop outcome measures that evaluate different phases of the recovery process** including long-term follow up.

Indications most often evaluated to determine successful addiction treatment include:

◇ prevalence of drug slips and relapses (duration of continuous sobriety);

◇ retention in treatment;

◇ completion of a treatment plan and its phases;

◇ family functioning;

◇ social and environmental adjustments;

◇ vocational or educational functioning, including personal finance management;

◇ criminal activity or legal involvement.

It is reassuring to note is that, in general, **all types of addiction treatment have demonstrated positive client outcomes when evaluated by rigorous scientific methods**.

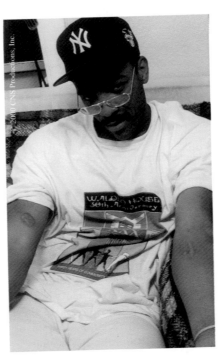

"These abscesses came through my addiction to heroin. Never cleaned my arm, let alone my body. Now I care about myself."
35-year-old recovering addict

INDIVIDUAL VS. GROUP THERAPY

There are two main integrated components of addiction treatment: psychosocial therapy and medical (especially medication) therapy. Recent developments in understanding the neurobiological process of addiction have resulted in an explosive growth of medication treatments and the new medical specialty of addiction medicine also called "addictionology." However, it is important to remember **medical treatments are not effective unless they are integrated with psychosocial therapies**. There are two general types of counseling therapies: individual and group. Most treatment facilities will use a combination of these two methods.

INDIVIDUAL THERAPY

Individual therapy is a process usually conducted by credentialed chemical dependency counselors. **They deal with clients on a one-to-one basis to explore the reasons for their continued use of psychoactive substances and identify all areas of intervention needs.** This may lead to a referral for specialized treatment, such as psychiatry, medical care, and family counseling. The therapist is able to help addicts gain a perspective on their usage and to identify and practice tools that will keep them abstinent from drugs. The most common individual therapies are **cognitive behavioral therapy, reality therapy, aversion therapy, psychodynamic therapy, art therapy, assertiveness training, motivational interviewing, and social skills training** (Stevens-Smith & Smith, 2000).

A treatment plan is developed with the client to guide in this process and individual treatment may continue from one month to several years. Although the majority of treatment is based on group and peer interaction, individual treatment may be more effective for certain types of clients and drugs (e.g., heroin, sedatives).

A drug counselor and a heroin addict in a counseling session at the Haight Ashbury Detox Clinic in San Francisco

Addict: "When I'm going through withdrawal, it's a physical thing, and then after I'm clean, I have the mental problem having to say no every time I get money in my hands: 'Should I or shouldn't I? No, I shouldn't. Go ahead, one more time won't hurt.' After I've passed withdrawal, and I pass by areas where I used to hang out, and I see other people nodding, in my mind, I start feeling like I'm sick again. I want to stay clean."

Counselor: "You can stay clean for a while. Is that what you want? You want to stay clean for a while or for the rest of your life?"

Addict: "I want to stay clean permanently."

Counselor: *"Permanently drug free?"*

Addict: *"But I can do it without attending those [Narcotics Anonymous] meetings."*

Counselor: *"All by yourself?"*

Addict: *"I mean with the medication that I take."*

Counselor: *"But the medications are only going to last you 21 days. They'll help you for a little while with the withdrawal of getting off heroin but what are you going to do when the urges come up?"*

Addict: *"I guess I'll deal with that when the time comes."*

Counselor: *"So you're just going to wait for it? You're going to wait for the urges to come on and start using then?"*

Addict: *"Nah, I can deal with it."*

Counselor: *"You're being highly uncooperative. As a matter of fact, we're going to stop the medications today because we know you're still using heroin and we can't have you using on the program."*

Addict: *"I need those medications."*

Counselor: *"What for? It's just another drug. What you're doing is using it like another drug. I'd like for you to come back to get into that group meeting we have at three o'clock. Also I want you to go to an NA (Narcotics Anonymous) meeting every day. I want you to go to these meetings and participate. Talk every opportunity you can. And also what I want you to do is bring back the signed participation card that you attended. I want you to do that. That's just part of the requirement of being in the program. See, I'm going to assume that you want to stop using drugs."*

Addict: *"Why can't I just get the detoxification drugs?"*

Counselor: *"Because we're not just a medication program. It's a counseling and full recovery program too."*

It is also observed that **individual treatment is less threatening for many individuals** and therefore can be used as a short-term initial basis to introduce addicts to the treatment process.

Motivational Interviewing

One of the most utilized counseling techniques in substance abuse treatment is motivational interviewing coupled with a stages of change model. **The technique uses a nonconfrontational style to involve clients in their own recovery process and help them to change ambivalence about drug use into motivation to make changes that lead to abstinence and recovery.** As in 12-step recovery groups where people look to their own higher power for direction and strength, people make the successful major changes when their motivation is internal not external. The purpose of the counselor is to **guide clients through the stages of change** by helping them reach decisions for themselves rather than forcing them or overdirecting them. This technique helps the clients "release the potential for change that exists in every person."

General principles of motivational interviewing are to

◇ **express empathy**: seeing the world through the clients' eyes and developing empathy is a way to develop rapport with them; reflective listening and acceptance help the counselor to understand the clients;

◇ **roll with resistance**: resistance is not challenged or argued with, rather it is used to help explore the clients' ideas; using that momentum rather than fighting it decreases resistance;

◇ **develop discrepancy**: the counselor needs to help the clients recognize discrepancies between where they are and where they want to be and to see how their current actions will not lead them to their goals;

◇ **support self-efficacy**: by empowering clients to choose their own options, the counselor encourages them to make changes.

(Miller & Rollnick, 2002)

Motivational interviewing techniques are used within the framework of the stages of change model. This requires the counselor to match motivational tasks to the clients' stage of change.

◇ **Precontemplation** is the stage where people do not admit they have a problem and are not thinking about change although others may perceive the problems that need changing. The counselor's task is to raise doubt and increase the clients' perception of risks and problems with current behavior.

◇ **Contemplation** is a stage where clients begin to contemplate if there may be a problem and if they should change. The counselor can tip the balance and evoke reasons to change, show the risks of not changing, and strengthen the clients' self-efficacy for change of current behavior.

◇ **Determination (or preparation)** is a stage where the client decides to do something to change behavior; a conscious decision to do something. The counselor can help the client to determine the best course of action to take in seeking change.

◇ **Action** is the stage of actively doing something; the person chooses a strategy for change and pursues it, taking steps to put that decision into action. The counselor helps the clients take those steps towards change.

◇ **Maintenance** is the stage of actively working on and maintaining change strategies. The counselor helps the clients renew the process of contemplation, determination, and action without becoming stuck or demoralized because of relapse.

(Miller & Rollnick, 2002; Prochaska & Di Clemente, 1994).

GROUP THERAPY

There are several types of group therapies. They are facilitated, peer, 12-step, educational, topic specific, and targeted. Generally **a major focus of group therapy is having clients help each other to break the isolation that chemical dependency induces** so they know they are not alone. Addicts are able to gain experience and understanding from each other about their addiction and learn different ways to combat craving to help prevent further drug impairment or relapse. As peers they are also able to confront one another on issues that may lead to relapse or continued use.

"The group keeps me honest with myself. I get to look at a lot of things and behaviors that are going on with me and I try and keep in the now. I keep thinking about staying clean today and the group keeps me focused on my goal of each day trying to stay clean."
Recovering crack cocaine user

Facilitated Groups

Group therapy usually consists of **six or more clients who meet with one or more therapists on a daily, weekly, or monthly basis.** Therapists facilitate the group by actively leading it, bringing up topics to be discussed, and processing all issues with their clinical insight. The facilitator (counselor) helps to establish a group culture where sharing, trust, and openness become natural to the participants.

Stimulant abuse peer group that uses confrontational techniques and a facilitator

William: "I have two sets of friends. People I use with and people who don't use at all. We've got together and had dinner and so forth."
Facilitator: "That's real safe for you, William. Listen to me, William. They don't know what to look for. They don't know what to expect and
you can manipulate them real easy."
Maria: "The same thing happened to me. You still think you can sit around with alcoholics, with people who drink, like you think you can hang around with dope dealers?"
William: "So the only people I can associate with are people in recovery?"
Maria: "I had to give up my sister."
William: "Okay, admit it. Everybody out there doesn't have a problem."
Maria: "But you do."
William: "That's true."
Facilitator: "Let me ask you a question. Can you see your ears?"
William: "No."
Facilitator: "So that means we can see something you can't see, right? Okay. So far, this group, with your issues, we're batting a thousand. Yes or no?"
William: "Yes."

Peer Groups

Peer group therapy consists of therapists playing a less active role in the dynamics. **They observe interaction and are available to process any conflicts or areas of need but they do not direct or lead the process.**

Drug abuse recovery peer group

John: "I didn't want to come here this morning and then to come here and be faced with, 'Well, you gotta think whether you really want to be here.' It's like I'm ready and I'm scared."
Counselor: "What's scaring you?"
John: "I feel like I'm failing myself."
Bob: "When did you fail before?"
John: "When have I failed before? Oh, I would say the last time was when I got busted buying crack. Just going out there is failing. Knowing I shouldn't be doing that."
Bob: "You gotta put that out there. You gotta deal with that."
John: "The thing is I'm scared of when I'm going to snap again."

Self-Help Groups & Alcoholics Anonymous (12-step group)

The concept of abstinence-based self-help groups goes back hundreds of years in America to fraternal temperance societies and reform clubs where recovering alcoholics could go to maintain their abstinence by discussion, prayer, and social activities. **One of the earliest groups was the Washingtonian Revival started in 1840** by six members of a drinking club in Baltimore, Maryland. They started a weekly temperance meeting and instead of debates, drinking games, and speeches, their main activity was sharing their experiences, starting with confessions of a debasing lifestyle caused by their excessive drinking through their personal recovery. New members, still in the throws of their addiction, were encouraged to tell their own story and sign a pledge of abstinence. This working-class movement spread its message rapidly and chapters formed throughout the country. At the peak of the Washingtonian movement, more than 600,000 pledges were signed. Some meetings had thousands of participants, almost like a revival. The women's auxiliary was called the "Martha Washington Society." The Washingtonian program of recovery was closely mirrored by that of Alcoholics Anonymous created 90 years later.

The Washingtonian Revival program of recovery came to include public confession, public commitment, visits from older members, economic assistance, continued participation in experience sharing, acts of service toward other alcoholics, sober entertainment.

The demise of the movement 7 years after its inception was somewhat of a mystery although everybody had an explanation—that they mostly ignored spirituality in the movement, that they had a weak organizational structure, that they were too sensationalistic, that they didn't have a sustainable recovery program, and that prosperity made them less essential. However, the example of the Washingtonians encouraged other fraternal temperance societies and reform clubs, groups that included the Order of the Good Samaritans, the Order of Good Templars, the Black Templars, the Independent Order of Rechabites, and Osgood's Reformed Drinkers Club. There was continuing debate over whether Prohibition was the real answer to alcoholism. Over the next 50 years, many types of organizations were tried, such as those with a religious basis like rescue missions and the Salvation Army (White, 1998).

It was the evolution and refinement of these groups coupled with the end of Prohibition, the closing down of many drying out institutions and treatment hospitals, and the beginning of the Great Depression that eventually led to **Alcoholics Anonymous (AA) in the 1930s, the most widespread recovery movement in history. It is a peer group concept based on 12 steps of recovery. These groups have no professional therapist present to interact with their members.** Each group is independent and relies on each other's knowledge and successes to help curb alcohol and other drug use. The parent group provides literature, suggestions for meeting format, and general structure. The core book, *Alcoholics Anonymous* (usually referred to as "*The Big Book*"), was written by Bill Wilson (a recovering alcoholic) and Dr. Bob Smith (a physician), the founders of AA, along with 100 recovering alcoholics who tell their stories (Trice, 1995).

"When I went to my first meeting, a 30-year-old beautician was running [telling] her story about how her drinking started, the pain she suffered because of it, and what happened to change her. I was a 49-year-old male with my own business and yet her story was my story. Her reaction to alcohol was the same as mine. Her helplessness after the first drink was mine. Her denial was mine. Her divorce was mine. Her reactions to life's problems were mine. The familiarity

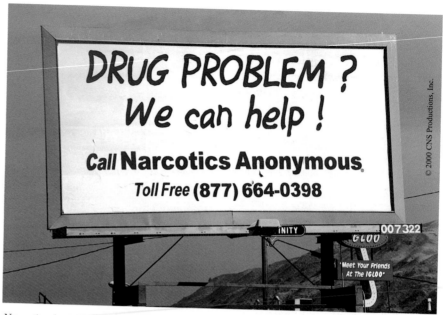

© 2000 CNS Productions, Inc.

Narcotics Anonymous, founded in 1953, has more than 20,000 weekly meetings in 70 countries; 16,000 of the meetings are in the United States. This compares to Alcoholics Anonymous that has more than 100,000 weekly meetings and 2 million current members.

and the sheer power of her running her story have kept me in the group for 5½ years. In AA they say, 'We only have our stories and all we can do is tell what worked for us to stay sober.'
Recovering 54-year-old alcoholic

Some of the other 12-step groups that have formed besides AA are Cocaine Anonymous (CA), Narcotics Anonymous (NA), Marijuana Anonymous (MA), Gamblers Anonymous (GA), Overeaters Anonymous (OA), Sexaholics Anonymous (SA), and Debtors Anonymous (DA).

In addition Al-Anon (for families of alcoholics), Adult Children of Alcoholics (ACoA), and Alateen (for teenagers with alcoholic relatives) use the 12-step process to help those immediately impacted by the behavior of addicts and alcoholics. All 12-step programs are free. They pay their minimal costs through voluntary donations. The only requirement for membership is a desire to stop the addiction.

The 12-step process engages addicts at their level of addiction, breaks the isolation, guilt, and pain, and shows them they are not alone. The process

also fully supports the idea that addiction is a lifelong disease and must be dealt with for the remainder of a person's life. It promotes a program of Honesty, Open-mindedness, and Willingness (HOW) to change. Those are the key elements in sustaining lifelong abstinence from drugs, alcohol, and other addictive behaviors. It breaks down denial and supplies a structure through which people can continue to work on their addiction. **The 12-step programs are based on the concept of solving problems through personal spiritual change**, a concept articulated by the Oxford Group, a popular spiritual movement of the 1920s and 1930s (AA, 1934, 1976; Nace, 1997; Miller, 1998).

"People misunderstand spirituality. They mistake it for religion. Spirituality is people's personal relationship with their higher power as they define him, her, or it. Religion is the way they practice their spirituality. My higher power is God as I learned of Him in my youth. For others their higher power could be an ideal, a philosophy, the goodness within them-

selves, a great person they met in their lives, the stars, or the members of the 12-step group itself. It's something greater than themselves that they can turn to, to get help for their smothering addiction, and to reconstruct their lives. It's only when they give up the need to try to control everything in their lives and give up control to their higher power that they gain the power to overcome their addiction and say no to the first drink."

51-year-old ex-priest who gives talks on spirituality and his recovery from alcoholism

Although most 12-step groups understand and accept spirituality, some users cannot accept the idea of a higher power. For those people *The Big Book* of Alcoholics Anonymous says to take what you want and leave the rest.

The 12 Steps of Alcoholics Anonymous

Step 1: **We admitted we were powerless over alcohol [cocaine, cigarettes, food, gambling, etc.] and that our lives had become unmanageable.**

Step 2: Came to believe that a power greater than ourselves could restore us to sanity.

Step 3: Made a decision to turn our will and our lives over to the care of God as we understood Him.

Step 4: Made a searching and fearless moral inventory of ourselves.

Step 5: Admitted to God, to ourselves, and to another human being the exact nature of our wrongs.

Step 6: Were entirely ready to have God remove all these defects of character.

Step 7: Humbly asked Him to remove our shortcomings.

Step 8: Made a list of all persons we had harmed and became willing to make amends to them all.

Step 9: Made direct amends to such people wherever possible, except when to do so would injure them or others.

Step 10: Continued to take personal inventory and when we were wrong, promptly admitted it.

Step 11: Sought through prayer and meditation to improve our conscious contact with God as we understood Him, praying only for knowledge of His will for us and the power to carry that out.

Step 12: **Having had a spiritual awakening as the result of these steps, we tried to carry this message to alcoholics and to practice these principles in all our affairs.**

In a study of 12-step programs at UCLA by Dr. Robert Fiorentine and his colleagues, it was found that participation in meetings after completing treatment increased the abstinence rate twofold and presumably the recovery rate (Fig. 9-4) (Fiorentine, 1999). The same study found that increasing counseling sessions (four group sessions and one individual session more per month) reduced drug use by 40%.

"I'm not the same person that I was when I entered this fellowship.

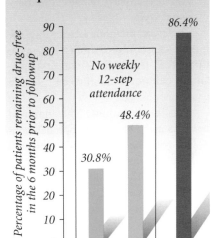

Participation in Drug Abuse Treatment and 12-Step Program Improves Treatment Outcomes

Figure 9-4 •

Weekly attendance at 12-step meetings after treatment almost doubles the abstinence rate of patients (48% vs. 86.4%).

Through my recovery and the 12 steps, I have found meaning and purpose in my life. It feels especially good with my kids because they know that I'm here for them. There's no catch-up anymore. I keep my promises. The challenge of a sober parent is keeping promises."

Recovering heroin addict

The 12 steps work for any addictive behavior. This is because the roots of addiction lie first in the character and lifestyle of the user and second in the use of psychoactive substances.

There are also secular versions of the peer group process used in 12-step groups. These groups do not believe that a higher power is necessary for recovery.

A group like **Rational Recovery (RR)** believes that if you learn to like yourself for who you are, then you will not need to drink or use other drugs. They believe that all addictions come from the same roots. Their approach is based on rational emotive therapy developed by Albert Ellis.

Another group, **Secular Organization for Sobriety (SOS)**, also makes no distinction among the various chemical addictions. Their goal is sobriety, one-day-at-a-time, like AA's and NA's goal.

Women for Sobriety (WFS) does have a spiritual basis but feels that AA principles work better for men. WFS emphasizes the power of positive emotions. **Men for Sobriety (MFS)** has also been formed.

(Horvath, 1997)

Educational Groups

These groups focus primarily on providing information about the addictive process in recovery. **Trained counselors provide the education and often bring in other experts to promote individual lesson plans** to help addicts gain knowledge about their conditions.

Homework assignments are often included to help addicts understand the information. A variety of workbooks and manuals have been written to assist this process. They also teach relapse prevention, coping skills, and even support therapy.

Targeted Groups

These groups can either be part of a formal program or a nonfacilitated peer group and are **directed at specific populations of users**. Such targeted groups include men's groups, women's groups, gay and lesbian groups, physician groups, dual diagnosis groups, bad girls groups (targeted at prostitutes), and priest/minister/rabbi groups (targeted at the clergy). The key element to the success of any group is its ability to develop a group culture that provides relevant, meaningful, acceptable, and insightful knowledge for that selective gathering of participants.

Topic-Specific Groups

Whereas target groups are aimed at certain cultures, topic-specific groups are aimed at certain issues, e.g., AIDS recovery, early recovery, relapse prevention, recovery maintenance, relationships, and codependency. The advantage of these groups is that **they allow the participants to focus on key issues that are a threat to their continued recovery**.

From most studies, **group therapies seem to promote better outcomes and sustain abstinence more than individual therapies**. Specifically, alcohol and cocaine addictions are more responsive to the group process than to individual counseling. From an administrative standpoint, group processes are also much more cost-effective.

Ten Common Errors Made in Group Treatment by Beginning Counselors or Substance Abuse Workers

(Adapted from Geoffrey L. Greif, D.S.W., Associate Dean and Professor, University of Maryland)

1. Failure to have a realistic view of group treatment

Preconceived expectations about the effectiveness of group therapy may cause a new therapist to become impatient with the group's progress when the reality is that each group moves at a different rate of progress from extremely slowly to explosive movement.

Possible solutions: Supervision teaches the therapist to adopt a longer-term perspective. In addition a thorough understanding of the behaviors caused by the specific drug, the way the other groups in the agency function, the cultural backgrounds, and gender-related behaviors of the members make for realistic expectations.

2. Self-disclosure issues and the failure to drop the "mask" of professionalism

New leaders are often challenged by the group members to test the therapist's understanding and/or personal experience with substance abuse.

Possible solutions: A response to any challenge by group members needs to be prepared in advance since too much disclosure by the therapist of personal experience can be as bad as too little disclosure. Leaders needs to accept the humanity of their clients as well as disclosing their own.

3. Agency culture issues and personal style

Different methods of running the groups can confuse clients and make them feel trapped between styles. Group culture vs. facility culture can cause dissonance.

Possible solutions: The therapist needs to make his or her approach consistent with the agency style. Personal styles of treatment that are not contradictory to other counselors' styles should be developed with the help of the supervisor and more experienced therapists.

4. Failure to understand the stages of therapy

Groups pass through specific stages during the recovery process and failure to see the progression can hamper the group process.

Possible solutions: There must be a thorough understanding of the various stages of recovery and how to respond with appropriate and timely exercises and thoughts.

5. Failure to recognize counter-transference issues

Often an inexperienced group leader or therapist will let personal feelings about group members show through or affect their performance, particularly if the age, gender, ethnic background, or lifestyle is different.

Possible solutions: The novice therapist must be aware of and accept such feelings as a normal part of the therapist-client relationship—they should just avoid acting on those feelings in a nontherapeutic manner.

6. Failure to clarify group rules

The largest mistake is failure to clarify group rules (e.g., confidentiality, coming to the group high, arriving late, meeting outside of groups, making personal attacks on other members).

Possible solutions: A written handout that contains clear explanations of the procedures followed by a discussion of the rules will give the group a solid base of understanding.

7. Failure to do group therapy by focusing on individual problem solving

In trying to please individual members of the group by giving insightful and helpful suggestions, the therapist can weaken the group.

Possible solutions: Let the group solve individual problems rather than giving individual help and advice. This gives meaning, purpose, and power to the group.

8. Failure to plan in advance

When the leader decides to wing it and doesn't quite know what the group will be doing, less is accomplished.

Possible solutions: The therapist should have a plan for each session and possibly a backup plan so the group doesn't feel directionless.

9. Failure to integrate new members into the group

If a new member enters the group, integrating them into the established flow can slow the group down. Conversely, if new members are instantly integrated, they don't have time to develop naturally and feel part of the group.

Possible solutions: The therapist can use the opportunity to have the group reevaluate its progress and recommit to the group.

10. Failure to understand interactions in the group as a metaphor for drug-related issues occurring in the group member's family of origin

A new therapist may believe that reactions among group members that are based on a client's familial relationships are true reactions. They might not realize the source of the reactions and so lose an opportunity to use that information to help the client.

Possible solutions: The therapist needs to take the time to establish strong bonds with members of the group so issues and insights raised by group interactions can be used to help the clients.

TREATMENT & THE FAMILY

"I got put into treatment and got out of treatment, you know. I just bullshitted my whole way through treatment. I told them what they wanted to hear and got out and just relapsed again because my dad was like, 'Here, you want to smoke some 'weed'? You want to drink a beer?' It's kinda hard to say no when your dad's sitting there asking you. It makes you feel like it's okay."
15-year-old recovering polydrug abuser

Addiction is a family disease. Abuse of drugs and alcohol greatly impacts all members of an addict's family regardless of whether or not they also abuse psychoactive substances. Analysis of employed addicts and alcoholics demonstrates that their families use the employer's health insurance much more than the families of nonaddicts. This is indicative of the great emotional, physical, and social strain that addicts place on their families.

"Addicts don't have families, they have hostages."
John DeDomenico, family therapist, Haight Ashbury Detox Clinic

Despite this well-established relationship, **the family is often ignored and neglected in the treatment of addictive disease**. This has resulted in family members seeking treatment on their own through traditional family and mental health services or through self-help family treatment systems, like Tough Love, Al-Anon, or Nar-Anon.

More importantly, continued stress from family problems or troubled family members makes it difficult for the recovering addict to remain abstinent.

"A family is ruled by its sickest member."
Moss Hart, dramatist

GOALS OF FAMILY TREATMENT

Treatment of addicts and their families has 4 major goals:

1. **acceptance by all family members that addiction is a treatable disease not a sign of moral weakness**; the addict also needs to accept this point;

2. **establishing and maintaining a drug-free family system** that often includes treatment of the spouse's drug problems or those of the addict's children;

3. **developing a system for family communication and interaction** that continues to reinforce the recovery process of the addict. This is accomplished by integrating family therapy into addiction treatment;

4. **processing the family's readjustment** after cessation of drug and alcohol abuse.

"I burnt every bridge that I've got with pretty much everybody in my whole life. The family sessions here are helping a little bit, you know. My mom comes in—my stepdad doesn't want anything to do with me but my mom

comes in; we're working, we're listening, you know. We're not just fighting anymore. She's not yelling at the top of her lungs. I'm not telling her to f*** off anymore. We're actually working together. It feels good. I might, you know, I might be able to get a life."
18-year-old recovering male polydrug abuser

DIFFERENT FAMILY APPROACHES

Family therapists employ a wide variety of techniques and tools to accomplish these goals once all family members have been motivated to participate. The following are some of the more commonly used models.

Family Systems Approach

This model explores and recognizes how a family regulates its internal and external environment making note of how these interactional patterns change over time. Three major areas of focus of this approach are daily routines, family rituals (e.g., holidays), and short-term problem-solving strategies. **The drug or drinking problem is seen as an integral part of the functioning of all members of the family** not just the person with the problem. Some family systems therapists use 12-step groups as part of their therapy while many feel that correcting family relationships corrects much of the substance abuse problem (Berenson & Schrier, 1998).

Family Behavioral Approach

This approach operates under the concept that interactional behaviors are learned and perpetuated by reinforcements for continuing the behavior. Thus the therapist works with the family to recognize those family behaviors associated with drug use; to categorize the interactions as either negative or positive in reinforcing drug usage; and then to **provide specific interventions to support and reinforce those behaviors that promote a drug-free family system**. Some of the specific strategies used are couples sessions, homework, self-monitoring exercises, communications training, and the development of negotiating and problem-solving skills. A couple might even enter into a behavior change agreement (O'Farrell & Cowles, 1989). Some who use the behavioral approach will focus more on working with the nonabusing spouse.

Family Functioning Approach

This approach first helps the addict or treatment program classify the family system into one of four different types, then uses the classification as a guide for a therapeutic intervention best suited to the functioning of that system.

1. **Functional family systems** are those in which the family of the addict has maintained healthy interactions. Interventions in this system are targeted directly at the addict. Other family members receive limited education and advice to support the recovery of the addict.

2. **Neurotic or enmeshed family systems** usually require intensive family treatment aimed at restructuring the way the family interacts.

3. **Disintegrated family systems** call for a separate yet integrated treatment of addicts and their families. The family may attend Al-Anon while an alcoholic is engaged in an intensive medical detoxification program. Though separated in treatment, this approach needs to be integrated at some point into the common goal of maintaining a drug-free lifestyle by the addict.

4. **Absent family systems** are those in which family members are not available for treatment.

Social Network Approach

This approach focuses mainly on the treatment of the addict but also establishes a concurrent and integrated support network for the family to assist them with the issues caused by the addiction. Through participation in multiple family support or therapy groups, **the family breaks their isolation and develops skills that help them support the recovery effort of its addicted member**.

Tough Love Approach

Though controversial, this movement has grown on the West Coast. The Tough Love approach addresses the major obstacle of denial in both the addict and his or her family. When the addicted family member refuses to accept or deal with dysfunctional drug-using behavior, the family members seek treatment and support from other families experiencing similar problems. **The family learns to establish limits for their interaction with the addict.** This has even included kicking that family member out of the home and severing all contact until the addict agrees to treatment.

OTHER BEHAVIORS

"Even though it was my dad that drank 'til he got sick, doing the intervention was harder for me than for him. I knew he denied his drinking. I didn't realize that I did too even though I didn't drink myself and that I had almost as many problems as he did."
31-year-old adult child of an alcoholic

The stress of living with an alcoholic or drug abuser causes dysfunctional behaviors in the nonusing family members. The most prevalent conditions are codependency, enabling, and manifesting symptoms caused by being children of addicts or adult children of addicts.

Codependency

Just as addicts are dependent upon a substance, **codependents are dependent on the addicts to fulfill some need of their own**. For example, a wife may be dependent on her husband maintaining his addiction in order for her to hold power over the relationship. As long as he's addicted, she has an excuse for her own shortcomings and problems. In this way it creates dysfunction in the addict because it promotes the addiction. Codependency can also be extremely subtle. For example, a person who has been abstinent from alcohol for a week or so has a spouse who offers a drink as a reward for the abstinence. In this kind of household **the chances of recovery are greatly reduced unless the codependents are willing to accept their role in the addictive process and submit to treatment themselves** (Gorski, 1993; Liepman, 1998).

"I was clean for 16 months. My husband had only been clean for 6 weeks. And I tried to show him that being clean and sober does work because my husband, he's not an alcoholic, he basically just smokes crack. And I think he saw what the program was doing for me and that I wasn't going back out or relapsing and buying drugs for him. [In the past] he would sit here and think I would get up and feel sorry for him and go, 'Okay, honey, you're craving, let's get high together.'"
38-year-old recovering polydrug abuser

Enabling

When a family becomes dependent upon the addiction of a family member, **there is a strong tendency to avoid confrontation about the addictive behavior and a subconscious effort to perpetuate the addiction**, often led by a person who benefits greatly from that addiction, the chief enabler. Although enablers may be disgusted with the addict and the addictive behavior, they continue paying off drug debts, paying rent, providing money, or even continuing emotional support for a practicing addict. As with codependents, **the enablers need to accept the role they are playing in this cycle and seek therapy** so they can be more effective in the addict's recovery.

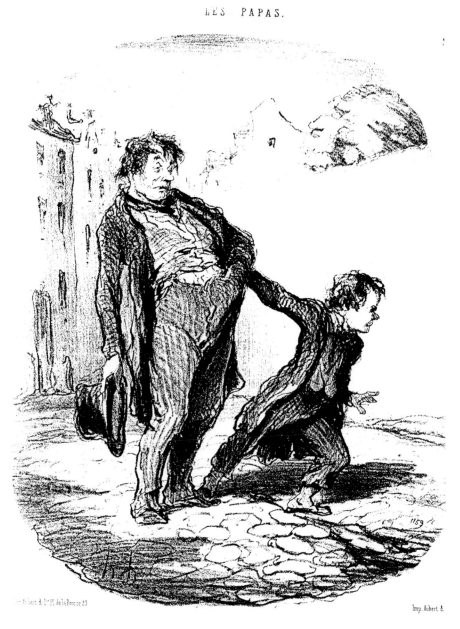

LES PAPAS.

Un fils modèle.

The etching by Henri Daumier is titled "The Fathers" *while the caption reads* "A model son."

● ●

Children of Addicts & Adult Children of Addicts

Many studies have found coping problems in a large percentage of the children of addicts and alcoholics. About 11 million children of alcoholics are under the age of 18 and about 3 million of those will develop alcoholism, other drug problems, and serious coping problems (Windle, 1999). (These statistics also mean that about three-fourths of the children of alcoholics do not develop addiction or serious coping problems.)

Many children of addicts take on predictable behavioral roles within the family that "co" the addiction and often continue on into their adult personalities. In addict families, the roles taken on by the children are usually one or more of the following:

◇ **Model child**: These children are high achievers and are overly responsible. They become chief enablers of addicted parents by taking over their roles and responsibilities.

◇ **Problem child**: These children experience continual multiple personal problems and often manifest early drug or alcohol addiction. They demand and get most of what attention is left from parents and siblings.

◇ **Lost child**: These children are withdrawn, "spaced-out," disconnected from the life and emotions around them. Often avoiding any emotionally confronting issues, they are unable to form close friendships or intimate bonds with others.

◇ **Mascot child or family clown**: These children use another avoidance strategy, which is to make everything trivial by minimizing all serious issues. They are well-liked and easy to befriend but are usually superficial in all relationships, even those with their own family members.

What is important to remember about children of alcoholics/addicts is that **although they may not abuse drugs, their behavior and emotional reactions can be as dysfunctional as those of an addict.** Often they learn very early on that they cannot control the addiction of a loved one, so they often resort to trying to control all other aspects of their life, leading to strained and inappropriate relationships later in life.

Adult children of alcoholics or addicts also

◇ are **isolated and afraid** of people and authority figures;

◇ are **approval seekers** who lose identity in the process;

◇ are **frightened by angry people** and personal criticism;

◇ **become or marry alcoholics** or find another compulsive person to fulfill abandonment needs;

◇ feel guilty when standing up for themselves instead of giving in to others;

◇ become addicted to excitement and stimulation;

◊ confuse love and pity; tend to love people that can be pitied and rescued;

◊ repress feelings from traumatic childhoods and lose the ability to feel or express feelings;

◊ judge themselves harshly and have low self-esteem;

◊ are reactors rather than actors (Sher, 1997; Adger, 1998).

ACoA is a 12-step group to help adult children of alcoholics work through the emotional baggage that followed them into adulthood. ACoA and other similar groups try to help members

◊ understand the disease of addiction and alcoholism because understanding is the beginning of the gift of forgiveness;

◊ put themselves on top of their priority list;

◊ detach with love;

◊ feel, accept, and express feelings and build self-esteem;

◊ learn to love themselves, thus enabling them to love others in healthy ways.

ADJUNCTIVE & COMPLEMENTARY TREATMENT SERVICES

Abuse and addiction to substances have a negative impact on the sufferer's physical, emotional, family, social, and spiritual well-being. Addicts and alcoholics suffer from higher rates of AIDS, viral hepatitis (A, B and C), heart disease, mental illness, emotional disorders, and other physical and psychiatric illnesses as compared to nonaddicts. All of these issues represent serious health and quality of life problems for addicts. The traditional role of addiction treatment has been to help identify these various needs and then case manage addicts towards appropriate treatment or service providers.

Recent concepts believe that treatment that effectively addresses all of these components through a comprehensive, integrated, and "wrap-around" service delivery design within the same program results in increased positive outcomes. Treatment campuses with multimodal and integrated services, merger of county mental health and substance abuse services departments into a single behavioral health department, and the "any door" or "no wrong door" substance abuse treatment access initiatives are all examples of this growing movement towards the direct inclusion of adjunctive and complementary services into a single comprehensive addiction treatment system. The recent interest and growth of faith-based substance abuse treatment initiatives are also part of this development. The U.S. Department of Health and Human Services created the HHS Center for Faith-Based and Community Initiatives to help incorporate nonprofit religious and secular organizations in preventing and treating drug abuse and addiction.

DRUG-SPECIFIC TREATMENT

POLYDRUG ABUSE

Experience at the Haight Ashbury Detox Clinic and treatment centers across the United States shows that although addicts may identify a drug of choice, they are more often than not polysubstance abusers who are using a wide range of substances either concurrently or intermittently. The profile of alcoholics, for example, often includes sedatives, cocaine, and even opioids in addition to their abuse of alcohol. **Treatment programs need to be aggressive about identifying the total drug profile of their clients.** Heroin addicts will often minimize or lie about their use of alcohol even though their drinking may be at a problematic level. **Many substance abusers will also be practicing a behavioral addiction such as gambling, compulsive eating, or even Internet addiction.**

"I have cleaned up off of dope though I've been a drug addict for 23 years. And I have no desire whatsoever to do drugs but alcohol is still there and I do it out of boredom."
42-year-old recovering heroin addict

A recent twin study found high levels of comorbidity for abuse/dependence for 6 different substances (marijuana, cocaine, hallucinogens, sedatives, stimulants, and opiates) and only low levels for single substances. Each twin's environment not heredity was more influential in the specific drug of choice (Kendler, Jacobson, Prescott, & Neale, 2003). **Addiction needs to be addressed as chemical dependency rather than a drug-specific problem.** Treatment is effective in promoting recovery, preventing relapse, and preventing a switch to alternate drug addictions.

"The cravings were just continuous. It was just like—if I was coming off of speed, I wanted heroin. If I was coming off heroin, I wanted to snort cocaine and if I was coming off that, I wanted to stay numb. I wanted to just go from one drug to another."
38-year old recovering polydrug abuser

Given the similarity of the roots of addiction, each drug still has unique effects and problems that should be specifically addressed.

STIMULANTS (cocaine & amphetamines)

The differences between treatment for cocaine and amphetamine abusers indicate that **methamphetamine abusers were more likely to be male, Caucasian, and gay or bisexual.** They were also more likely than cocaine abusers to engage in unsafe sex, share needles, be HIV positive, have a psychiatric diagnosis, and be on psychiatric medications (Copeland & Sorensen, 2001). On the other hand cocaine abusers were similar to methamphetamine abusers in adherence to treatment protocols and recovery rates suggesting that a stimulant abuse program can probably handle both drugs together rather than having separate protocols and groups.

Although admissions for treatment of cocaine abuse decreased more than 25% between 1994 and 2000, there are still 218,000 people that enter treatment each year. This compares to a 90% increase in admissions for methamphetamine and amphetamine abuse in the same period although the total is only 81,764 (SAMHSA, 2003b).

A wide range of drug-induced psychiatric symptoms often accompanies stimulant abuse. Acute paranoia, schizophrenia, major depression, and bipolar disorders are often the initial presentations by a stimulant addict, particularly at the end of a long run. These symptoms require psychiatric intervention to prevent harm and to **assess whether they have been caused by the drug itself or whether the mental illnesses are preexisting** and will continue to be a problem after detoxification and initial abstinence.

Besides psychiatric symptoms, other key effects to watch out for in cocaine or amphetamine abusers who are detoxifying are prolonged craving, anergia (exhaustion), anhedonia (lack of an ability to feel pleasure), and euthymia (a feeling of elation that occurs 3–5 days after stopping use). Euthymia makes users feel that they never were addicted and that they don't need to be in treatment. The anergia and anhedonia start to overtake the euthymia at about 2 weeks after starting detoxification and these feelings, particularly the total lack of ability to feel pleasure, often lead to relapse (Gawin, Khalsa, & Ellinwood, 1994).

Detoxification & Initial Abstinence

After detoxification and treatment for any psychotic symptoms and any life-threatening symptoms, such as extremely high blood pressure and heart rate, **the vast majority of stimulant abusers respond positively to traditional drug counseling approaches**.

However, those stimulant addicts who have not been able to respond to these traditional approaches initially require a more intensive medical approach to bridge the detoxification/ withdrawal period prior to their engagement into recovery. **A variety of drugs are used for medical treatments for stimulant detoxification and initial abstinence.**

◊ **Antidepressant agents**, such as SSRI drugs like fluoxetine (Prozac®) and citalopram (Celexa®) or other newer ones such as mirtzazapine (Remeron®), nefazodone (Serzone®), and venlafaxine (Effexor®), are widely used. These affect serotonin, the neurotransmitter in the brain that deals with both depression and mood.

◊ **Antipsychotic medications** are used to buffer the effects of unbalanced dopamine, e.g., risperidone (Risperadol®), olanzapine (Zyprexa®), ziprasidone (Geodon®), quetiapine (Seroquel®), haloperidol (Haldol®), and others. These are also called "**neuroleptic medications**."

◊ **Sedatives** are prescribed very carefully on a short-term basis to treat anxiety or sleep disturbance problems, e.g., phenobarbital, chloral hydrate, buspirone (BuSpar®) or less often, flurazepam (Dalmane®), chlordiazepoxide (Librium®), or even diazepam (Valium®).

◊ **Nutritional approaches** aimed at enhancing the production of those neurotransmitters that have been depleted by heavy stimulant use help decrease craving and counteract many of the withdrawal symptoms seen in stimulant addiction. Tyrosine, phenylalanine, and tryptophan are proteins used by brain cells to manufacture dopamine, adrenaline, and serotonin that are depleted by stimulant abuse. Their effectiveness has not been proven with conclusive studies, often because it is difficult to isolate the effect of a single substance. Single-substance studies are required for research by the FDA even though these seem to work better in combination.

◊ **Dopamine agonists** like bromocriptine (Parlodel®), amantadine (Symmetrel®), and levodopa (combined with carbidopa in Sinemet®) activate the dopamine receptors in the brain to **suppress withdrawal symptoms and initial craving for stimulants**. Abuse of both cocaine and amphetamines depletes brain dopamine levels that result in craving and other symptoms of withdrawal.

Long-Term Abstinence

A lot of work is currently being put into the treatment of craving and particularly stimulant craving. Two major types of craving have been addressed: endogenous craving and environmentally triggered craving.

Endogenous craving is believed to be caused by the depletion of dopamine in the nucleus accumbens of the limbic system. To treat this situation many medications (as mentioned above) have been used to simulate dopamine in the nucleus cumbers thereby diminishing long-term craving for stimulants. Acupuncture is also used to stimulate dopamine release. Animal research suggests that the dopamine imbalance may last for up to 10 months after cessation of cocaine or amphetamine use (Ricaurte, Seiden, & Schuster, 1984).

Environmentally triggered craving is particularly intense in stimulant addiction. It is more likely to lead to relapse than endogenous craving and has to be treated by intense counseling, group sessions, or desensitization techniques. This type of craving may last throughout one's life but evidence indicates that **continued abstinence weakens the craving response**. This weakening can lead to the extinction of craving caused by environmental triggers.

In an investigation funded by the National Institute on Drug Abuse (NIDA) of 1,600 cocaine-dependent patients with moderate-to-severe problems, researchers found that an absolute minimum of 3 months of treatment was needed to achieve lasting results (8 months maximized effectiveness). About $2^{1}/_{2}$ times more patients relapsed after leaving short-term treatment (38% relapsed) than those leaving long-term residential treatment (15% relapsed) (Simpson, Joe, Fletcher, et al., 1999).

TOBACCO

More and more **treatment centers for drug and alcohol addictions are including treatment for nicotine addiction as part of their program**. Many believe that full recovery from addiction is made more difficult if the recovering client still smokes. The traditional view has been that giving up tobacco might hinder recovery from what they consider more dangerous drugs. In fact recovery rates seem to improve among those who also give up smoking ("Programs Including Nicotine," 2001). More than 80% of alcoholics and drug addicts smoke compared to 25% of the nonaddicted population.

The only guaranteed successful therapy involving tobacco is to never smoke, chew, or use it in any form. Abstinence is necessary because many of the neurological and neurochemical alterations that cause nicotine addiction are permanent. This means that even 10 years after cessation of smoking, a single cigarette can trigger the nicotine craving.

The failure rate for most therapies to stop smoking is extremely high. About 70% of all smokers want to quit and 46% try each year (CDC, 2000). In the past the focus in treatment was the psychological components of the habit of smoking. Unfortunately those approaches didn't fully take into account the lifetime nature of nicotine addiction and therefore recovery. They tried to apply short-term fixes (e.g., 21-day smoking cessation programs) to a long-term problem.

Recently, in recognition of the very real alterations in brain chemistry that trigger nicotine craving during withdrawal, **the treatment community has focused on pharmacological treatments**. The 5-month success rate with the various pharmacological treatments in one study were: nicotine patch,

17.7%; nicotine inhaler, 22.8%; nicotine gum, 23.7%; buproprion SR (Zyban®), 30.5%; nicotine spray, 30.5%; and a combination of two or more, 28.6% (CDC, 2000). The average smoker tries to quit 5–7 times before he or she succeeds.

Nicotine Replacement

Since the main mechanism that causes craving is the drop in blood levels of nicotine that then triggers withdrawal symptoms such as irritability, anxiety, drowsiness, and light-headedness, research has been aimed at nicotine replacement systems. **The purpose of these systems is to slowly reduce the blood plasma nicotine levels to the point where cessation will not trigger withdrawal symptoms** that will cause the smoker to relapse (Thompson & Hunter, 1998). This pharmacological technique of using low controlled dosages of a substance to prevent withdrawal and not reinforce the addiction to it is called "**antipriming**."

The four types of nicotine replacement systems are transdermal nicotine patches, nicotine gum, nicotine sprays, and nicotine nasal inhalers. One of the main advantages of all of these systems is that users are no longer damaging their lungs with some of the 4,000 chemicals found in cigarette smoke. This alone could save almost 200,000 lives per year in the United States. The main problem is that **if relapse prevention, counseling, and self-help groups are not used in conjunction with nicotine replacement therapy, then the chances of smokers returning to their old habits are high** (Rustin, 1998).

Nicotine Patches. Nicotine patches, such as Nicoderm® and Habitrol®, are nicotine-infused adhesive patches that are applied to the skin. Patches can be worn intermittently (daytime only) or continuously. Most of them contain enough nicotine to last for 24–72 hours. **The advantages of patches are the steady rate of release of nicotine, the ease of compliance, and the lack of toxic effects to tissues in the mouth or digestive track.** The

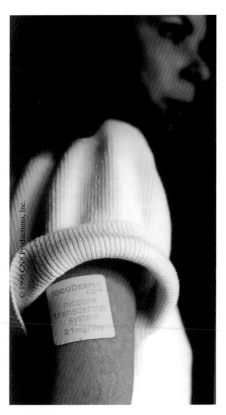

With 47 million Americans addicted to cigarettes, the potential market for devices and drugs, such as a nicotine patch, to help kick the habit is huge.

disadvantages are the cost, the inability to alter the amount being absorbed, and the 4–6 hours it takes for a patch to raise the nicotine level enough to dull nicotine craving. Also, if the user starts smoking while wearing the patch, extremely high and dangerous plasma levels of nicotine can occur.

Nicotine Gum. Nicotine gums, such as Nicorette®, have the advantage of slowing the rise in nicotine levels that smoking brings. **The 10-second rush of an inhaled cigarette gives way to the 15- to 30-minute slow rise that nicotine gum provides when absorbed through the gums** and other mucosal tissues. A slower rise means that craving, which is triggered by the sudden drop in nicotine levels after smoking, doesn't occur. The 15- to 30-minute rise, however, is considerably faster than the 4–6 hours it takes for a transdermal patch to work, so the user

Denial

Denial on the part of the compulsive drinker is the biggest hindrance to beginning treatment. One reason that denial is so common with the use of alcohol is the long time it can take for social or habitual drinking to advance to abuse and addiction (10 years on the average) (Schuckit, 2000). Denial also occurs because alcoholics have no memory of the negative effects they experienced while in an alcoholic blackout. Thus they don't believe that alcohol has really harmed them. Further, alcohol impairs judgment and reason in all users, making them less likely to associate any problem with their drinking.

Detoxification

For a heavy drinker or even an alcoholic, **physical withdrawal is very uncomfortable but usually not dangerous.** Symptoms such as sweating, increased heart rate, increased respiratory rate, and gastrointestinal complaints can often be handled by aspirin, rest, liquids, and any one of hundreds of hangover cures that have been handed down from generation to generation. Symptoms are likely to peak in intensity by 48–72 hours and are greatly diminished by 5 days. On the other hand lesser symptoms including mildly elevated blood pressure, a mild tremor, disturbed sleep, and moodiness can last for weeks to months.

For the small percentage of alcoholics at risk for severe effects, **potentially life-threatening symptoms of withdrawal should be medically managed** with a variety of sedating drugs, such as barbiturates, benzodiazepines (e.g., chlordiazepoxide [Librium®]), paraldehyde, chloral hydrate, and the phenothiazines. Since several of these drugs are addictive, they should be used sparingly and on a very short-term basis. Normally tapering is done on a 5–7 day basis but can be extended to 11–14 days.

Along with emergency medical care, withdrawal and detoxification should also include emotional support and basic physical care such as rest and nutrition (thiamin, folic acid, multi-vitamins, minerals, amino acids, electrolytes, and fructose). Many of the problems will start to abate with detoxification but for the long-term drinker, some damage is irreversible: liver disease, enlarged heart, cancer, and nerve damage among others (Wiehl, Galloway, & Hayner, 1994; Schuckit, 2000).

Initial Abstinence

A common treatment for initial abstinence is the use of Antabuse®, a drug that will make people ill if they drink alcohol. This is used for about 6 months or longer to help get alcoholics through initial abstinence when they're most likely to relapse. A more important part of this process is **encouraging them to go to AA meetings or other support groups** in addition to individual therapy. One procedure is to have the user go to 90 AA meetings within 90 days (called a "90/90 contract").

In 1996 **naltrexone (Revia®) was approved by the FDA for the treatment of alcohol addiction** during the first 3 months of the recovery process; it decreased alcohol relapse by 50–70% when combined with a comprehensive treatment program. Unfortunately naltrexone can be hard on the liver and needs to be used under strict supervision. A number of other drugs are being tried including topiramate (Topamax®) that blocks dopamine so the alcohol doesn't stimulate the reward/reinforcement center (Ross, 2003). Blocking dopamine also seems to help in weight loss and binge-eating disorder (McElroy et al., 2003).

As the alcohol clears from the system, the clinician needs to **evaluate the client for psychiatric problems (especially depression and anxiety) that have developed or were preexisting**. Attempts at suicide should also be considered since the lifetime risk for suicide in alcoholics is 10%.

Long-Term Abstinence & Recovery

In treatment one often encounters someone known as a "dry drunk." This means that the person is not actually drinking alcohol but still has the behavior and mind-set of an alcoholic. Thus the purpose of this stage of treatment, besides avoiding relapse, is to **begin healing the emotional scars, confusion, and immaturity that kept the person drinking for so many years**.

Many treatment centers advertise 30-day drying out programs, implying that detoxification is the key to recovery rather than a small initial step in a long process. As with all addictions, working on recovery throughout one's lifetime is necessary to prevent relapse. Brain cells have been permanently changed by years of drinking, so the recovering alcoholic is always susceptible to relapse.

PSYCHEDELICS

For hallucinogens such as LSD, MDMA, "'shrooms," and ketamine, **the overwhelming majority of users in treatment are male, White, and under the age of 24**. For marijuana smokers, the majority who are in treatment are male and under the age of 24 but more evenly divided ethnically (SAMHSA, 2003b).

Many psychedelics will mimic mental conditions, such as schizophrenia, so the clinician or intake counselor can only make a tentative diagnosis when first seeing the patient until the drug has had time to clear, usually without medications. However, antipsychotic medications, sedatives, and other medications are sometimes used to stabilize the client if they seem a danger to themselves. Although some tissue dependence (physical addiction) is seen with GHB, PCP, ketamine, and marijuana abuse, most all arounders do not result in daily compulsive chronic abuse. **Treatment is therefore most often focused on the psychological, family, and social consequences** that result from their abuse.

Bad Trips (acute anxiety reactions)

The amount of acid or other psychedelic taken, the surroundings, the user's mental state and physical condition all determine the reaction to psychedelics. Because of their effect on the emotional center in the brain, a user is open to the extremes of euphoria and panic. Inexperienced or even experienced users who take too high a dose of LSD or other psychedelic can feel **acute anxiety, paranoia, fear over loss of control, or feelings of grandeur leading to dangerous behaviors**.

"In the 8th grade I started doing acid and drinking a lot and when I was about 15, I took too much acid one night and I tripped out and I cut my arm. Got a big old scar on my arm and took off my clothes and ran down the street naked. Just tripped out. So then I went to rehab after that. I spent 4 days in the hospital."

Ex-LSD user

There are two things to remember when using the ARRRT talk-down technique.

◇ First, if the user seems to be experiencing severe medical, physical, or even emotional reactions that are not responding to the talk-down, medical intervention is needed. Get the person to a hospital or bring in emergency medical personnel experienced in treating that kind of reaction.

◇ Second, although most psychedelic bad trip reactions are responsive to ARRRT, PCP and ketamine may cause unexpected and sudden violent or belligerent behavior. Caution must be exercised in approaching a "bum tripper" suspected of

being under the influence of these drugs.

The best treatment for someone on a bad trip is to talk him or her down in a calm manner without raising one's voice or appearing threatening. Avoid quick movements and let the person move around so there is no feeling of being trapped.

Some of the rave club drugs, like MDMA, ecstasy, GHB, and ketamine, have created addictive behaviors in users who are treated with traditional counseling, education, and self-help groups. GHB also causes true tissue dependence that results in sedative- or alcohol-like withdrawal symptoms requiring medical management.

MARIJUANA

Since the 1980s **there has been a steady increase in the number of people entering treatment for marijuana dependence**. While much of the increase nationally has been because of court-mandated treatment referrals (Fig. 9-6), which account for 56% of admissions, those entering the Haight Ashbury Clinic are, on an increasing basis, predominantly self-referred (SAMHSA, 2003b). Thus through the eyes of marijuana smokers as well as the eyes of the law, there is a growing problem with marijuana dependence. These facts seem to challenge the continued perception that marijuana is a benign drug. Experience at the Haight Ashbury Clinic has shown that marijuana has a true addiction syndrome encompassing both physical and emotional dependence.

"I ain't gonna say I can quit any time. But if I had to stop, I could stop. I ain't gonna say I could quit. I can't go just cold turkey just like that. I could go maybe 3 days without and then I smoke a joint. And then maybe I go like 3 or 4 days without, and then maybe I'll smoke a joint but that'd take some work."

33-year-old chronic marijuana abuser

The physical withdrawal symptoms, though uncomfortable, rarely need medical treatment. They consist of major sleep and appetite disturbances, irritability, anxiety, emotional depression, and even mild muscular discomfort. Craving persists for several months to years upon abstinence. One of the main reasons people deny that these withdrawal symptoms do occur is that **their onset is delayed from 3 weeks to several months after cessation of use**. Marijuana has a wide distribution in body tissues and especially in fat, thus enabling it to persist in the system over a prolonged period of time. Urine tests of chronic marijuana users remain positive sometimes for 3 weeks to several months.

"After I stopped smoking, it took me about 3 or 4 months before I really came out of the fog and really started getting a grasp of what was going on around me . . . and another month or so after that is when I really started to understand that I could do this. And then I started really enjoying it."

28-year-old recovering compulsive marijuana smoker

Treatment for marijuana dependence or addiction is evolving along the same lines as that developed for alcohol dependence and addiction. Psychosocial interventions, education, and peer support have been the most effective in helping people abstain and prevent relapse. **Currently treatment for marijuana addiction is made difficult because much of society still views marijuana as nonproblematic** and therefore views those in treatment

TABLE 9–4   TREATMENT FOR BAD TRIPS

The Haight Ashbury Detox Clinic uses the following ARRRT guidelines in dealing with a person experiencing a bad trip:

A   acceptance: first gain users' trust and confidence;

R   reduction of stimuli: get users to quiet nonthreatening environments;

R   reassurance: educate users that they are experiencing a bad trip and assure them that they are in a safe place, among safe people, and that they will be all right;

R   rest: assist users to relax using stress-reduction techniques that promote a calm state of mind;

T   talk-down: discuss peaceful, nonthreatening subjects with users, avoiding any topic that seems to create more anxiety or a strong reaction.

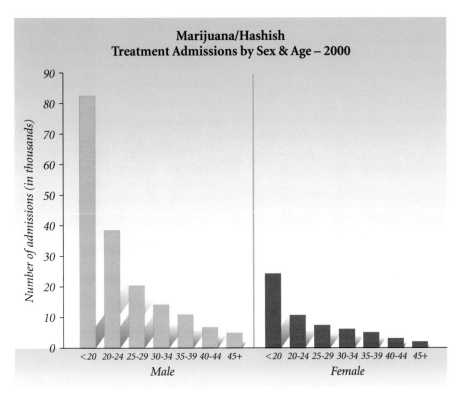

**Marijuana/Hashish
Treatment Admissions by Sex & Age – 2000**

Figure 9-6 •

The vast majority of those entering treatment for marijuana dependence are under the age of 20. The reason is that over half of the referrals for treatment are court mandated while only 17% are self-referred (SAMHSA, 2003b).

as overreacting to their use of the drug. This often undermines the treatment process. Further the 12-step process and other peer-support systems, invaluable in the treatment of other drug dependencies, have not yet evolved fully for marijuana dependence.

Current research on anandamide, the neurotransmitter most affected by marijuana, is giving clues to the nature of marijuana's effects on the body and mind possibly leading to drugs to assist in short- and long-term abstinence. There is already an anandamide antagonist called "SR14176A" that has been used to study the marijuana withdrawal syndrome since the drug will almost instantly block all effects of marijuana, at least temporarily.

INHALANTS

The treatment of those who use inhalants excessively involves **immediate removal from exposure to the substance** to prevent them from aggravating its dangerous effects, such as

lack of oxygen to the brain, damage to the respiratory system, and injuries from accidents. Initial treatment for the delirium that can be caused by inhalants also consists of reassurance and a quiet (nonstimulating) environment. **Patients must then be monitored for potential adverse psychiatric conditions** that may require the use of antipsychotic medications targeted to treat psychoses and suicidal depression. Many inhalants can also produce physical dependence that is similar to the dependence that occurs with sedative-hypnotic drugs. Clients should be monitored for withdrawal seizures and treated with appropriate anticonvulsant medication when warranted.

Each inhalant has its own physical toxic effects and may lead to heart, liver, lung, kidney, and even blood diseases. The symptoms must be evaluated and treated. These substances are reinforcing and can cause psychic dependence and often require long-term psychosocial interventions targeted to prevent relapse into addiction.

Since the majority of these inhalants are easily accessible to adolescents, the majority of abusers are under the age of 20. Almost one-third of inhalant treatment admissions had used inhalants by the age of 12 and another one-third by the age of 13 (SAMHSA, 2003b). What this means in treatment is that there are major developmental problems that must be addressed. Treatment specialists talk about the need to habilitate rather than rehabilitate the "huffer."

About two-thirds of inhalant abusers admitted for treatment reported use of other drugs as well, primarily alcohol and marijuana. These figures emphasize the need to evaluate all "huffers" for possible addiction to other drugs.

TREATMENT FOR BEHAVIORAL ADDICTIONS

It has become increasingly recognized that behavioral addictions that result from a genetic predisposition to addiction, an environment that further predisposes one to compulsive behaviors, and pleasurable reinforcement from the activity itself follow similar brain pathways as drug addiction. **Behavioral addictions require the same intensity of intervention and treatment as substance abuse disorders.** Behavioral addictions include compulsive gambling, sexual addiction, compulsive Internet use, compulsive shopping, and eating disorders (anorexia, bulimia, binge eating).

Since many behavioral addictions have not been studied and treated to the same extent as drug abuse and addiction, there is a scarcity of research data, treatment facilities, and qualified treatment personnel. Besides treatment at mental health facilities, **the front line of treatment has been the evolution of self-help and 12-step support groups for these nonchemical addictions**.

Compulsive Gambling

Americans lost $50 to $60 billion last year in slot and poker machines, at poker, dice, and roulette tables, in sports betting, and on 38 state lotteries. **The**

number of compulsive gamblers has grown dramatically with the increase in games of chance that are found in every state except Utah and Hawaii. The sheer availability of gambling facilities has contributed to the growth of the industry and to multiple relapses during treatment. In one of the few before and after studies, the percentage of Iowans reporting a gambling problem at some time in their lives went from 1.7% in 1989, to 5.4% in 1995 after gambling's introduction, and probably even more today—a three- to fourfold increase (Harden & Swardson, 1996). In a different study the number of pathological gamblers was estimated at 3.6 million in 2002 due to the proliferation of gambling outlets (Califano, 2001). Even the gaming industry estimates that 25–40% of their revenue comes from that 6–8% who are compulsive or problem gamblers. The figures are probably much higher for certain types of gambling, e.g., poker machines in Oregon where it is estimated that 7% of the population spends 60–80% of the money generated by this type of gambling.

"I was at a Gamblers Anonymous meeting in Reno and about 50 people were there. The longest abstinence in that meeting was just 4 months. In meetings I've been to in other states, many people have years of abstinence. The only difference I see is that in Reno, gambling is everywhere and the triggers are everywhere, and the temptation is everywhere."
44-year-old recovering compulsive gambler

With so many compulsive gamblers, there is a **startling lack of facilities to treat this addiction**. Until a few years ago, many states didn't even have a single gambling addiction specialist. Society has been slow to recognize compulsive gambling to be a compulsion as powerful as any drug addiction.

Compulsive gambling has been described as one of the purest addictions since the only substance involved is money. Denial is therefore very powerful in compulsive gamblers and **until a devastating bottom has been reached, most gamblers are reluctant to seek treatment, let alone admit that they have a problem**. Outside interventions, especially those triggered by legal problems (e.g., arrest for embezzlement, declaring bankruptcy), are usually necessary. To most gamblers their trouble is merely a cash flow problem (Brubaker, 1997).

"I figured I was losing $500 here and there, you know, a week. I never thought it was that big a deal because I always thought of myself as going to be successful, going to get a better job down the road where I'll make all this money back, so why quit now?"
21-year-old recovering sports gambler

The Charter Hospital of Las Vegas that treats compulsive gamblers reports **withdrawal symptoms similar to alcoholism, including restlessness, irritability, apprehension about well-being, anger, abdominal pain, headaches, diarrhea, cold sweats, insomnia, tremors, and above all an intense desire to return to gambling**.

"I don't want to sit here and tell anybody anything that's unrealistic. I miss gambling. I miss it still. It brought a sense of—like a power or a satisfaction. I'm learning how to treat it and how to deal with it but that doesn't mean it's over."
42-year-old relapsing compulsive gambler

The standard assessment test for compulsive gambling is the South Oaks Gambling Screen (SOGS) usually accompanied with an in-depth assessment and formal diagnosis. Treatment options developed over the last 30 years include self-help groups such as Gamblers Anonymous (Blume, 1997).

"The problem primarily is that there are no physical gross indicators to a lay person like hangovers, or gross intoxication, or bodily changes, or measurable body fluids that a doctor likes to find. They are mostly psychological and sociological and of course, fiscal or financial. And without that kind of history, we usually don't even get to a diagnosis."
Joel Pursch, M.D., Psychiatrist

The Gamblers Anonymous (GA) program parallels the 12-step process used by Alcoholics Anonymous. It also employs sponsors, group meetings, commitment to complete abstinence, contact numbers, and support to help the gambler particularly through the initial 90-day phase. Additional support groups include Gam-Anon for the families of compulsive gamblers and Gam-A-Teen, a group for children of pathological gamblers.

"Going to GA groups helps me; seeing people who have gone through the same struggles and seeing how every one of them wishes they had quit when they were my age so they didn't have to go through the struggles."
21-year-old recovering compulsive gambler

One of the keys to treating compulsive gamblers is **enabling them to overcome irrational thoughts about chances of winning** since many of them cannot accept the fact that gambling games at casinos, lotteries, race tracks, and in poker machines are meant to take their money. The more they gamble, the more they will lose and if they get ahead, they will compulsively put that money back into the game. Unfortunately almost all pathological gamblers think that they can overcome the computer chips in slot machines and the immutable laws of chance.

"I don't think about those odds. What entices me to stay is I'll see other people winning and I'll think well, my machine hasn't paid out. It's about time that it will."
53-year-old compulsive gambler

The other key in treatment is to get a pathological gambler to recognize that it's the action at a gaming table or the "zoning out" at a machine that is sought, not really the money.

Outpatient along with inpatient or residential treatment programs are available (and scarce) though insurance companies seldom pay for a primary diagnosis of compulsive gambling. It usually takes a diagnosis of a mood disorder or other coexisting condition to get insurance coverage for treatment. Frequently, compulsive gamblers have already lost their jobs and insurance coverage before they seek help for their addiction. In the last few years a few states that have government-controlled lotteries, gambling machines, and various scratch-off games are recognizing their responsibility in providing treatment for the compulsive gamblers. Connecticut spends the most money in treatment. Next is Oregon that passed a bill allotting 1% of its gross gambling revenues, or $2 million a year, towards treatment. California, with 12 times the population, allots much less ($500,000 in 1999).

Even with gambling, several addictions are always involved. **Gambling often coexists with drinking, compulsive spending, and a few other disorders** or the gambling replaced another addiction. Many alcoholics switched to gambling when they quit drinking and it quickly became as compulsive as the alcohol (McElroy, Soutullo, & Goldsmith, 1998). Over 50% of pathological gamblers are also alcohol or substance abusers (Ibanez, Blanco, & Donahue, 2001). All addictions should be treated simultaneously since relapse to one substance or behavior will often trigger another addiction.

Eating Disorders (*also see Chapter 7*)

One of the main elements for effective treatment of all three eating disorders is early intervention. The longer the disorder continues, the more deeply ingrained the behavior and the more physiological and psychological damage. A number of steps are recommended for treating eating disorders:

◇ diagnose and treat any medical complications—hospitalize if necessary;

◇ encourage attendance at Overeaters Anonymous or other 12-step groups to give support to the client;

◇ encourage the client to eat a balanced diet and exercise and educate them as to the components of proper nutrition (Barclay, 2002);

◇ use behavioral and group therapies to encourage weight gain in anorexics and weight loss in bulimics and overeaters;

◇ use cognitive and other therapies to change false attitudes and perceptions of body image and eating;

◇ enhance self-esteem, independence, and development of a stronger identity;

◇ treat and educate the whole family.

In addition to the general guidelines, each of the three eating disorders have their own unique problems to address.

Anorexia. Most severely ill anorexic patients have to be admitted to a hospital because of the extreme weight loss, disturbed heart rhythms, extreme depression, and often suicidal ideation. **It usually takes 10–12 weeks for full nutritional recovery.** Unfortunately most health insurance only covers 15 days. The hospital or home care includes medical treatment and nutritional stabilization requiring weight gain of 1 or 2 lbs. a week even if the patient or family is resistant to gaining weight. Exercise is also recommended. **The complexities of anorexia require a team approach:** physicians for medical complications, dietitians, therapists, counselors, and trained nurses to insure good outcomes.

Bulimia. Clients with bulimia usually have more long-term health problems than those with anorexia such as atherosclerosis and diabetes that rarely need hospitalization but **often need continuing medical care**. Because of the strong link between depression and bulimia and the similarity in serotonin disruption, antidepressants are often used, e.g., selective serotonin reuptake inhibitors (Prozac®, Zoloft®) (Bacaltchuk & Hay, 2003).

Binge-Eating Disorder (includes compulsive overeating). In addition to counseling that focuses on **changing attitudes and ideals**, psychiatric treatment that examines underlying traumas, and **behavioral therapy** to help monitor and control responses to stress and to change eating habits, medications (e.g., Meridia®, serotonin reuptake inhibitors) are used to suppress appetite or treat the depression that can trigger compulsive overeating. However, **support groups including Overeaters Anonymous (OA), TOPS (Take Off Pounds Sensibly), Weight Watchers, and others are crucial in maintaining weight loss and encouraging recovery.** A number of professionals and overeaters believe that abstaining from certain foods, particularly refined carbohydrates (e.g., sugar, refined flour, alcohol, pasta) or fatty substances is needed. These foods are thought to act on the same brain reward systems that reinforce compulsive drug use.

Sexual Addiction

One theory of sexual addiction suggests that predisposed individuals experience an intense form of sexual stimulation when young, identify it with a parent (usually the mother), and come to anticipate that sexual behavior can provide pleasure or relieve pain or tension. The experience is often in conjunction with covert or overt seduction. Because of the relationship between early childhood sexual experiences, the **treatment inevitably has to deal more with childhood development rather than just the mechanics of the addiction**. The treatment often includes behavior modification (e.g., aversion therapy), cognitive behavioral therapy, groups, family or couple therapy, psychodynamic psychotherapy, motivational interviewing, and medications (Goodman, 1997). Again the concurrent use of addictive substances is more prevalent than in the general population because predisposing factors in all addictions are so similar and because psychoactive drugs are often used to affect sexuality, e.g., lower inhibitions or enhance arousal. Recovery from sexual addiction, like recovery from drug addiction, is a lifelong process.

Sexaholics Anonymous.   As with compulsive gambling, sexual addiction is difficult to treat. **The sense of being alone in their addiction or what they consider to be a unique behavior is alleviated when sexaholics realize there are millions of others with the same problems.**

"When we came to SA, we found that in spite of our differences, we shared a common problem—the obsession of lust, usually combined with a compulsive demand for sex in some form. We identified with one another on the inside. Whatever the details of our problem, we were dying spiritually—dying of guilt, fear, and loneliness. As we came to see that we shared a common problem, we also came to see that for us, there is a common solution—the Twelve Steps of Recovery practiced in a fellowship and on a foundation of what we call sexual sobriety."
Sexaholics Anonymous, 1989

One of the main issues that needs to be addressed is the **feelings of shame, guilt, anxiety, and depression that are associated with sexual addiction.** Those issues can be addressed in therapy groups, individual therapy, Sexaholics Anonymous and Sex Addicts Anonymous. Unlike recovery from a drug addiction, complete abstinence from sex is almost impossible, so the goal becomes abstinence from compulsive destructive sexual behaviors. Associated behaviors that need to be addressed are control problems, secrecy, isolation, distorted thinking, and emotional distancing.

Internet Addiction

Internet addiction crosses the line into other computer-related addictions:

cybersexual addiction, cyberrelationship addiction, online gambling and day trading, information overload (compulsive web surfing), computer addiction (game playing), or any combination of the above (Netaddiction, 2000). Along with compulsive gambling, Internet addiction is the fastest-growing addiction exploding from virtually nonexistent 10 years ago. **Because it is so new, treatment personnel and treatment facilities are rare.** Unfortunately the Internet has become so much a part of life and work situations, it is hard to give up use altogether particularly if its use is part of one's job. The usual abstinence model is often impossible to follow. A harm reduction model is often necessary.

Richard Davis from York University, who has studied Internet addiction extensively, has 10 suggestions to help alleviate this condition.

1. Move your computer to a different room in order to change a number of environmental cues that you have become used to.

2. Never go online alone. Always go online with someone else in the room (or at least in the house).

3. Create an Internet usage log. The actual hours of usage are often a surprise to users.

4. Tell people about your problem. It is necessary to break the isolation caused by excessive Internet activity.

5. Do regular exercise. This will overcome sedentary habits of sitting in front of a computer and improve general health.

6. Never use an alias. Be yourself online.

7. Take an Internet holiday, anywhere from one day to several days, even a week.

8. Stop dwelling and obsessing on Internet addiction.

9. Help someone else control their Internet addiction.

10. Get professional help, e.g., a psychotherapist, counselor, or mentor.

(Davis, 2001)

TARGET POPULATIONS

Even though the roots of addiction are similar among all people, treatment works better if it's tailored to specific groups based on gender, sexual orientation, age, ethnic group, job, and even economic status.

MEN VS. WOMEN

Male treatment admissions outnumbered female admissions more than 2 to 1 (1,108,787 male, 484,475 female). Men were more likely to enter treatment through the criminal justice system (SAMHSA, 2003b). In general, **women substance abusers will progress to addiction more rapidly than men**; die at a younger age, and be less likely to ask for and/or receive help.

Research at the Haight Ashbury Detox Clinic has discovered that the process of addiction and especially recovery varies dramatically for men and women. **Men are often external attributers, blaming negative life events like addiction on things outside their control whereas women are more often internal attributers blaming problems on themselves.** When this is extended to their views of addiction, men often blame a wide variety of external forces for their dependence on drugs whereas women often blame themselves for being bad or crazy.

The counseling and intervention used in treatment have focused on early confrontation to break down addicts' denial and make them accept their condition. While appropriate for men, this treatment approach merely reinforces many women's guilt and shame and often prevents them from engaging in treatment or has them leave treatment early. **Treatment approaches that are more supportive and less confrontative result in better outcomes for women.**

Women are usually the primary childcare provider in a family, so for a woman to be able to participate in treatment, childcare must be provided. Further it has been found that women lack transportation more often than their male counterparts. Therefore bus

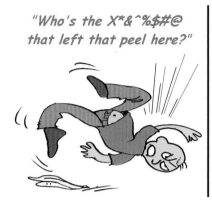

"Who's the X*&^%$#@ that left that peel here?"

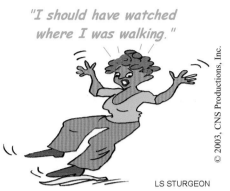

"I should have watched where I was walking."

© 2003, CNS Productions, Inc.

LS STURGEON

tokens, vans, car pooling, or other means of transportation provided to women clients also result in higher success rates. About 60% of treatment facilities offered services such as transportation assistance, transitional employment, family counseling, individual therapy, and relapse prevention to help female clients (SAMHSA, 2002b). A survey of 400 women in recovery attending a conference on recovery, Women Healing: Restoring Connections, said the 3 greatest barriers to their seeking addiction treatment were

1. inability to admit the problem or simply not recognizing their addiction (39%);
2. lack of emotional support for treatment from family members (32%);
3. and adequate childcare while in treatment.

The conference was presented by the Betty Ford Center, Caron Foundation, and the Hazelden Foundation.

YOUTH

Young people often have the perception of invulnerability to drugs and therefore are often in much greater denial about their addiction than adults. Further, studies confirm that **young people are much less willing to accept guidance or intervention from adults but are more willing to listen to their peers** (Hird, Khuri, Dusenbury, & Millman, 1997). Both of these factors call for youth programs targeted around peer interaction and guidance to other youth. **Normal adult programs do not work with young people. Specific**

youth-directed programs have to be provided.

One of the biggest problems with treating teenagers is that they are present-oriented, that is they have problems recognizing consequences that are not immediate. The idea that a 3-month flirtation with cocaine will necessitate a lifetime of recovery is beyond their scope. They also seek instant gratification, much more than even adult addicts, and expect rewards from treatment immediately. Youth programs that include reward incentives for accomplishing different phases of treatment result in better long-term outcomes. Part of the reward structure is that they get included in an acceptable peer group.

OLDER AMERICANS

Because many older Americans view addiction as a character flaw rather than a disease, **they are less likely to seek help for any problematic use of alcohol or other drugs**. Worse, medical professionals often ignore signs of alcoholism or addiction in the elderly out of respect or a mistaken belief that they are less likely to be an addict. Signs of addiction are often misinterpreted as part of the aging process or reaction to prescription medications that are common among the elderly. Also, because of less physical resiliency in those over 55, problematic use of alcohol or other drugs occurs at lower dosages than with younger people. The House Select Committee on Aging has reported that about 70% of hospitalized elderly per-

sons show evidence of alcohol-related problems (although they might be in the hospital for some other condition). It is estimated that about 2.5 million older adults are addicted to alcohol, drugs, or both; this is out of a population of more than 60 million Americans over the age of 55 (U.S. Census Bureau, 2003).

At present **there are few treatment programs aimed specifically at older Americans** but as the percentage of older Americans grows and the baby boomers begin to retire, the need will grow. As with other special groups, older Americans with a substance abuse problem seem to do better in groups with others their own age although mixed groups will work.

Of nine centers set up by NIDA to study addiction, one has been designated specifically to investigate this problem in older Americans. It is located at the University of Florida in Gainesville.

ETHNIC GROUPS

Recognition of cultural variances between groups provides better treatment outcomes. Studies verify that **treatment specifically targeted to different ethnic groups promotes continued abstinence better than general treatment programs** (Perez-Arce, Carr, & Sorensen, 1993). Cultural competency and culturally consistent treatment are now key components of successful programming. It is imperative to note that culture includes a diverse constellation of vital elements: customs, values, rituals, norms, religious beliefs, and ideals. You can't just base a culture upon the color of the skin or general area of the world. The more specific the program is in addressing an identified group's cultural needs, the more effective it will be.

African American

African Americans made up **24% of the admissions to publicly funded substance abuse treatment facilities** although they made up only 12% of the U.S. population. African American female admissions were more likely to

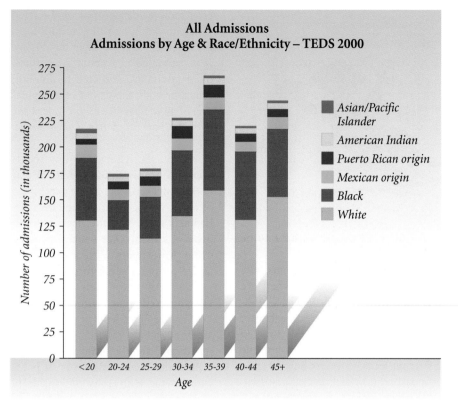

All Admissions
Admissions by Age & Race/Ethnicity – TEDS 2000

Legend:
- Asian/Pacific Islander
- American Indian
- Puerto Rican origin
- Mexican origin
- Black
- White

Y-axis: Number of admissions (in thousands)
X-axis: Age — <20, 20-24, 25-29, 30-34, 35-39, 40-44, 45+

Figure 9-4 •

The racial composition of admissions to drug treatment programs has remained fairly consistent since 1992 and proportionally it is somewhat different than the actual composition of the U.S. population. Whites are 72% of the U.S. population but only 60% of admissions to drug programs while Blacks are 12% of the population but 24% of admissions (SAMHSA, 2003b).

◊ Many neighborhoods with a high African American population have an extremely high infant mortality rate due to drug use by pregnant women who abuse or are addicted.

Drugs as an Economic Resource. Few economic windfalls are available to inner-city African American communities. Reducing drug dealing here means a loss of income to many families. This is in contrast to the European American community where drug/alcohol abuse usually drains the finances of families.

The true economics of the process need to be taught. For example, once the dealer becomes a user, the economic drain starts. Other members of the community are devastated and become dysfunctional; crime is brought to their own backyard.

"Most African Americans come into recovery by way of the criminal justice system, very late in the whole process of addiction, and are compelled to come to programs like Glide or Haight Ashbury by the courts. So you have a whole different attitude from people who have hit rock bottom and decided they've got to seek help. The kids are more concerned about just finishing their term and finishing whatever sentence they have and getting out. They don't want to deal with counselors. They don't want to deal with advice. So what you've got is a chance, at that point, to try to hook them into some kind of system that allows them to get back into the society with a greater chance of success."
Youth drug counselor

involve hard drugs (cocaine, 40% of admissions; alcohol, 27%; opiates, 18%) than were African American male admissions (alcohol 35% of admissions; cocaine, 28%; opiates, 14%) (SAMHSA, 2003b).

The following ideas as to the **differences in the treatment/intervention needs of inner-city African American substance abuser**s are the result of years of experience working with the African American community in San Francisco by members of the Haight Ashbury Detox Clinic and the Black Extended Family Program at Glide Memorial Church (Smith, Buxton, Bilal, & Seymour, 1993).

Higher Pain Threshold. Historically African Americans have developed a high pain threshold to help them survive in a harsh and painful environment. Unfortunately this **greater tolerance for suffering delays a cry for help, leading to more severe addiction and other life problems before entering treatment**. One solution to lowering the pain threshold and getting addicts to treatment sooner is educating the African American community to the true impact of drugs.

◊ In some urban areas, an alarmingly high number of African American babies are born drug affected.

◊ African American teenagers have a greater chance of dying from crack-related crime than they do from being hit by a car.

◊ There are more African American men in their 20s who are in jail from drug-related offenses than are in college.

◊ Since African American women are using crack at a greater rate than any other drug except alcohol, the family structure is dissolving at an alarming rate.

Crime Leads to Chemical Dependency. Most often crime is the first entry into the chemical dependency subculture rather than drug use itself as is true in the White community. Often in the African American community, the pattern is to make sales first and then sample the wares later.

Strong Sense of Boundaries. Intervention is viewed as an inappropriate imposition or violation of one's space. There is resistance from within the community to approaching someone with a chemical dependency problem because that would violate the person's boundaries or turf but not approaching someone also perpetuates denial.

These problems are the most difficult to address. They need a major attitudinal change, i.e., is it better to respect one's turf or to attempt interventions and try to do something about the problem?

Chemical Dependency: Primary or Secondary Problem?   Minority communities often cite underemployment, poor housing, and lack of social/recreational resources as the primary problems instead of chemical dependency. This perpetuates denial and prevents many addicts from getting into treatment early. **Drug users must understand that no other issues can be tackled successfully without tackling recovery first.** The community needs to accept chemical dependency as a primary problem.

"Recovery is a lifetime process. That's a very difficult thing for African Americans to focus on. We're sprinters. We're real good at the 50-yard dash and the 100-yard dash and we have a feeling that, 'Okay, it's a drug problem. Once I stop using and I put it behind me, I can forget it and go about my business.' But no, recovery is a lifetime process and you have to think more in terms of being a marathoner."
Rafiq Bilal, former Director, Black Extended Family Program

Conspiracy Theory.   The belief that the rapid spread of crack (and AIDS) into the African American community is deliberate genocide is very widely held in the African American community. Given the history of slavery, segregation, and defacto segregation, it is understandable. Whether or not the conspiracy theory is true, addiction is still a disease that must be treated in the individual as well as in society as a whole.

Revelations.   In the African American community, organized spirituality has been a key to promoting recovery. Treatment programs based in church settings have been shown to be more effective than more traditional treatment settings.

"The African American community is very spiritually oriented whether from involvement with the church or from historical associations. Most interesting is a recovery pattern of consecutive periods of clean time/relapse, clean time/relapse, until a revelation or 'snapping' occurs that results in a continuous sustained recovery effort. This is different from the more classic expanding periods of sobriety leading towards more sustained long-term recovery."
Rafiq Bilal, former Director, Black Extended Family Program

The Black Extended Family Program under the guidance of Rev. Cecil Williams uses the concept and emotional force of the extended family to help keep people in treatment and give them an alternative to the lonely life of the addict. This concept reestablishes the family, spirituality, and self-worth, qualities that have been weakened by drug use. The Terms of Resistance, a 10-step equivalent of the 12 steps, was developed by Rev. Williams in 1992.

1. I will gain control over my life.
2. I will stop lying.
3. I will be honest with myself.
4. I will accept who I am.
5. I will feel my real feelings.
6. I will feel my pain.
7. I will forgive myself and forgive others.
8. I will rebirth a new life.
9. I will live my spirituality.
10. I will support and love my brothers and sisters (Smith et al., 1993).

Hispanic

The most common primary substances of abuse among Hispanics who presented themselves for treatment were alcohol (36%), opiates (32%), and marijuana (14%). The admissions for opiate abuse were twice that of non-Hispanic groups. Hispanic admissions were 77% male and 23% female compared with 68% male and 31% female among non-Hispanic admissions (SAMHSA, 2003b).

With Hispanics it is important to understand the cultural diversity and the differences between groups as well as the similarities. The most common similarities are: Spanish language, Catholic background, Indian or African traits, Iberian heritage, and strong family structure. The differences are: the number of years or generations they have lived in the United States; the country of origin (the three most prevalent being Mexico, Puerto Rico, and Cuba); their level of education; and their economic status, e.g., are they Mexican migrant workers who immigrate to survive poverty and help their family back home, are they upper-class Mexicans or Costa Ricans looking to protect their wealth, are they middle- and upper-class Cubans who fled Fidel Castro a generation ago and have become a driving force in the Florida economy, or are they lower-, middle-, and upper-class Puerto Ricans (American citizens) who have moved to the East Coast to find a better life for their families?

After addressing any emergency physical or mental health needs, **the first thing a treatment facility has to determine is the level of acculturation of any Hispanic clients coming in for treatment.** For example, how well do they speak English; are they newly arrived immigrants; how integrated are they in the predominantly Anglo society; are they first, second, or third generation Hispanics who have stayed aware of their cultural heritage and kept contact with relatives and friends at home; or are they caught between two cultures without a solid home base?

In New York the rapid influx of Puerto Ricans in the '50s, '60s, and '70s often caused a fragmentation of the extended family system, a polarization between generations, a loss of many aspects of the Puerto Rican culture, and an identity crisis. These stressors, along with language differences, were found responsible (in a New York State survey) for increases in substance abuse. With Cuban Americans, however, the rapid integration into American society has resulted in a level of drug use about half that of the Mexican American and Puerto Rican communities (Ruiz & Langrod, 1997).

What this means in terms of treatment is that **programs have to be flexible, have a diverse staff that has a preponderance of Spanish-speaking and/or bilingual and bicultural counselors and administrators, and be willing to treat the whole family** since the family is so important in Hispanic cultures. Because Hispanic American families have excellent networking systems, these systems can be used extensively in the treatment process. In addition the treatment facility should be aware of the distinct and clear roles that each family member plays in the Hispanic family system. This is in contrast to many Anglo families where the roles of each member can be quite variable.

The core aspects of Hispanic cultures are *dignidad, respeto, y carino—* **dignity, respect, and love.** Even the concept of urine testing can be a touchy subject because the request for a urine test implies a lack of trust. Another aspect is the strong role spirituality plays in Hispanic cultures. In addition to a Catholic heritage, some Hispanic cultures have nonorthodox religious beliefs, such as Spiritualism, Santeria, Brujeria, and Curanderism. Pentecostal and Jehovah's Witness churches are also increasing in Hispanic communities.

"Some of the recent Mexican immigrants I've worked with who have an alcohol problem didn't start drinking heavily until they came to this country at the age of 25 or 30. At home they had to care for their families and had

little money. Here, they are separated from their families and have more money, and so the use of alcohol and other drugs escalates. The other thing I've found is that even if an Hispanic client speaks perfect English, the fact that I'm bilingual and bicultural increases participation in treatment."
Hispanic drug counselor

Asian & Pacific Islander (API)

There are more than 11 million Asian and Pacific Islanders (API) living in the United States and this figure is expected to grow to 41 million by 2050. In California they represent 9.6% of that state's population (about 3.2 million); in New York, 3.9% (693,000); in Hawaii, 61.8% (685,200); in Texas, 1.9% (320,000); and in Illinois, 2.5% of the population (285,000) (U.S. Census Bureau, 2003). As with Hispanic populations, **Asian and Pacific Islanders represent a wide variety of cultures**.

The differences include

◇ a variety of distinct and separate ethnic groups, like Japanese, Filipino, Cambodian, Indian, and Samoan;

◇ a variety of languages, such as Korean, Chinese, Tagalog, and hundreds more;

◇ a variety of religions from Buddhism and Hinduism to Animism, Islam, and Christianity;

◇ a variety of strong cultural characteristics based on thousands of years of history;

◇ a great variety of cultures even within immigrants from the same country, e.g., Cantonese, Shanghaiese, and Taiwanese;

◇ different levels of acculturation depending on the number of generations they have been in the United States. For example, many Chinese Americans and Japanese Americans stretch back four or five generations while the newer immigrants, such as Laotians, Vietnamese, Koreans, and Thai, go back only one or two generations (Westermeyer, 1997).

The similarities are

◇ they live along the Pacific Rim;

◇ they have a strong regard for family;

◇ they generally have a high respect for education;

◇ they are less demonstrative or open in their communication about personal issues;

◇ they are more reserved about expressing accomplishments because they feel this would be a form of arrogant boasting;

◇ they are reluctant to discuss health issues or death because they superstitiously believe that it would make those problems occur.

These and other similarities affect treatment.

Key issues for API populations include immigration, acculturation, and intergenerational conflicts: the difficulties of a new language, the pressures of being a minority, and feelings of loss, grief, separation, and isolation as they adjust to a new country can act as risk factors for drug abuse; the loss of traditional cultural values during the process of assimilation can lead to drinking and other drug use to deal with that stress; finally, the younger generation adapts more quickly to their new culture leading to conflicts with their parents over traditional values (SAMHSA, 2002a).

Asian Americans respond more to credentialed professionals than to peer counselors and prefer individual counseling to group counseling. They rely more on their own responsibility to handle their addiction rather than a higher power or external control. They also feel that if they were to complain about their issues, they would be imposing on others. They feel that saving face and individual honor are important, so they are less responsive and will avoid confrontation. They prefer alternative ways of being able to express their feelings, like creative or expressive arts therapy. They require a strong incorporation of family therapy. Finally, they have strongly developed gender roles, so **separate male and female groups are more effective than mixed groups.**

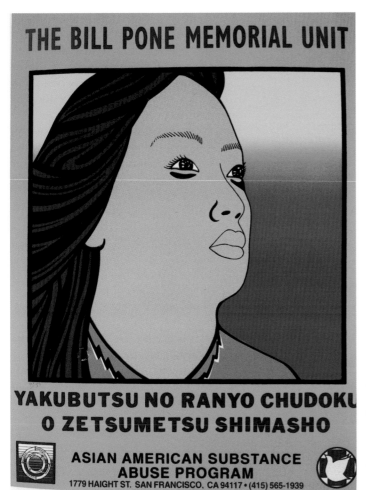

THE BILL PONE MEMORIAL UNIT

YAKUBUTSU NO RANYO CHUDOKU
O ZETSUMETSU SHIMASHO

**ASIAN AMERICAN SUBSTANCE
ABUSE PROGRAM**
1779 HAIGHT ST. SAN FRANCISCO, CA 94117 • (415) 565-1939

Educational material and promotion of a clinic's programs have to be directed at specific communities.

gram incorporating family therapy, treatment of sedative abuse, and personnel who were bicultural and bilingual, it resulted in a dramatic increase of Asian Americans coming into treatment at a level consistent with their overall population in the city.

The most commonly used drugs in API communities vary.

◊ Chinese: tobacco, alcohol

◊ Japanese: alcohol, marijuana, tobacco, crack cocaine, methamphetamine

◊ Koreans: alcohol (whiskey, rice wine), crack cocaine

◊ Filipino: alcohol, marijuana, cocaine

◊ Vietnamese: tobacco, marijuana, alcohol

◊ Cambodian: alcohol, tobacco, crack cocaine, smokable methamphetamine (SAMHSA, 2002a)

Native American

Native American groups have a wide variety of cultural traditions. For example, the five eastern nations (tribes) of Oklahoma, who are literate and successful, have low rates of alcoholism. This is in comparison to some western mountain tribes who, in one study, were found to have a rate of alcoholism 7 times the national average. Overall 65% of Native American/ Alaska Native treatment admissions were for alcohol compared to 45% for the general population (SAMHSA, 2003b). In addition drugs with an historical context, such as tobacco and peyote, are used more often in ceremonies than as recreational drugs, so the introduction of different drugs, particularly alcohol and inhalants, with no cultural tradition of restricted use has caused numerous problems.

Bicultural and bilingual treatment personnel greatly increase the chances of successful treatment. Many nations incorporate cultural traditions in healing, including talking circles, purification ceremonies, sweat lodges, meditative practices, shamanistic ceremonies, and even community "sings."

For Asian Americans, entry into treatment usually occurs late since an admission of addiction is an admission of loss of control. Another problem is that addicts live for the addiction and for themselves rather than for the family and the community, so their addiction and individualism makes them less likely to respond to usual intervention techniques. Finally **the sense of family shame often keeps the family enabling and rescuing the addict again and again rather than insisting they get into treatment**. On the other hand, the strong sense of family makes for greater compliance with protocols once treatment, which incorporates family therapy, has been started. **Programs for Asian Americans must involve the family in any treatment or the chances of success are greatly lowered.**

Available Programs. Because of the wide variety of Asian American

cultures, the historical importance and availability of certain drugs, and the wide geographic distribution in cities and states of various groups, treatment personnel must do surveys of their neighborhoods to make treatment relevant. For example, the utilization of treatment services by Asian Americans in San Francisco was extremely low in the 1980s. This was misinterpreted to mean that Asian Americans had fewer drug problems than other ethnic groups.

Community reports however found as high an incidence of drug abuse in the Asian community as in other ethnic groups, the difference being that the Asian American's drugs of choice were sedatives, particularly street Quaaludes® and Soma® (sedating muscle relaxant), that weren't focused on in most treatment programs. When the Haight Ashbury Detox Clinic developed a specific Asian American pro-

Detoxification centers, halfway houses, outpatient programs, and hospital units have been funded by the Indian Health Service and certain state and county governments. However over 60% of Native Americans live away from traditional communities in multi-ethnic urban areas, so treatment centers in those locales should have the same diversity of bilingual and bicultural personnel for Native Americans as they do for other ethnic and cultural groups.

Talking circles have been used for hundreds of years in various Native American tribes as a way to solve problems and heal members of the tribe. The process is similar to peer groups, though instead of round robin talking with no interruptions, there is cross-talk and questions. The sessions usually last for 2 or 3 hours, though they can last much longer.

"On reservations you get locked into a community where you don't grow and there is a minimum of interaction with other groups. There is virtually no middle class. You have a group who are highly religious who do not drink at all, you have a few who work for the Bureau of Indian Affairs or in limited industry and drink sparingly, and you have another group that lives to drink and drinks to live. There's not enough work, nothing to do, and often nothing to look forward to for many in this group. You're just another Indian and you're not to be trusted. You have to want to be more than just another drunken Indian.

We have to be proud of who we are before we can reach recovery. In the Native American community, the family is very tight. Everyone is your cousin or aunt or uncle. A sense of pride in your people is part of the core of spirituality that helps us survive. As part of this, we've always looked to elders for guidance. The elders would talk to you about your drinking (a form of intervention) to get you to

make changes in your life. The elders have a variety of approaches. They might even do a tough love approach and tell alcoholics to leave the reservation, finish their drinking, and come back when they are sober; or they might tell them to get honest with themselves and make a sobriety pledge to the medicine man or in a pipe ceremony.

We have a variety of tribes that I deal with here in Montana, such as Sioux, Northern Cheyenne, Blackfoot, and Crow. Each one has their own traditions. Unfortunately a number of clinic directors on reservations who are brought in from the outside have trouble understanding the traditions, so they rely more on standard psychosocial therapy, which is not as effective and breeds distrust. Adding to this is the fact that, for many Native Americans, hitting bottom is not as big a trigger for self-referral into treatment as it is in the Anglo community. Often they are not aware of what bottom is. It takes intervention or court mandate to make changes. On the other hand, once they get recovery, they are much less likely to let go. I tell them that alcoholism is like the raven that has stolen your shadow. If your shadow is gone, your spirituality is gone. Be proud of who you are."
Bob Clarkson, Native American drug and alcohol counselor

"Great Spirit, grant me the serenity of a dove to accept the things I cannot change, the courage of an eagle to change the things I can, and the wisdom of an owl to know the difference."
Native American version of the Serenity Prayer used in Alcoholics Anonymous

OTHERS

There are numerous groupings of Americans who require targeted treat-

ment. **Whether they are substance abusers who have physical disabilities, gays or lesbians, homeless, mentally challenged, or a dozen other groups, the key to effective treatment seems to be involvement with peer groups** who have experienced the lifestyle, the problems, the prejudice, the homophobia, the shunning, the joys, the problems with self-esteem or relationships and can speak and help based on personal experience.

The common point that needs to be recognized is that addiction is addiction. To imagine that problems with addictive behavior would disappear if only some other conditions or problems were taken care of is a sure path to continued addictive behavior. On the other hand, the other problems such as racism and mental instability have to be addressed and treated at the same time because **many of the roots of compulsive use lie in a subconscious effort to avoid or cope with the pain experienced in these conditions or lifestyles**.

Physically Disabled

Americans with disabilities represent a much-neglected group of chemically dependent people. Some of the more common disabilities are blindness, deafness, head or brain injury (50,000 a year), and spinal cord injury (10,000–15,000 new cases a year). Despite passage of the Americans with Disabilities Act in 1990, most programs remain inaccessible to many with mobility impairment, visual impairment, and hearing impairment. In addition there is very little interdisciplinary training for working with physically disabled substance abusers. One problem that occurs is that **the counselor can focus too much on the physical disability and miss signs and symptoms of relapse and additional problems or focus too strongly on the addiction and not take into account the extra stress that can be caused by the disability**. Conversely the rehabilitation professional might feel unqualified or leery of handling substance abuse problems or might not even recognize the signs and symptoms. In addition society's attitude towards people with disabilities can promote the concept of learned helplessness and dependency on others and subsequently on drugs. One irony of substance abuse in people with physical disabilities is that substance use is a factor in up to 68% of traumatic disabling injuries (Heinemann, 1997). A thorough medical and drug history is helpful in judging whether the substance abuse predated the disability, was triggered by the disability, or occurred independently of the disability. Because physical disabilities often involve pain, there is an increased use of prescription medications that can be abused.

"I used my disability to the fullest extent of the law. I could go in on the scooter, put on some make-up, and I could coerce them out of anything. I had one doctor going for several months and I remember that I was taking so much Vicodin® at the time that I was throwing up and I would tell him that I had headaches and that caused me to throw up so he would continue to give me the pain medication that would make me throw up. I was down to around 98 pounds at the end of that run. I have been doing that for 17 years, in and out of rehab five times."
58-year-old recovering wheelchair-bound woman

Again it is a preexisting susceptibility to addiction or the increased need for pain relief that usually indicates that the person with a physical disability will have a dependence problem with pain medications (Schnoll, 1993).

In a study of 96 persons with long-term spinal cord injuries, 43% used prescription medications with abuse potential and one-fourth of those, or about 10% of the total, reported misusing the medications. **The group that regularly misused the prescription medications was less accepting of their disability and more depressed.** Another study found that the existence

of a preexisting substance abuse problem made it more likely that the client would not participate fully in rehabilitation thereby slowing recovery and increasing stress (Heinemann, 1993).

Lesbian, Gay, Bisexual, & Transgender (LGBT)

There has been a lack of research on substance abuse in the gay and lesbian communities, so the studies that have been done are not exhaustive, merely suggestive. Even the population of the LGBT community is difficult to determine. One study estimates that in the United States, 9.8% of men and 5% of women report same-gender sexual behavior since puberty while 2.8% of men and 1.4% of women report a homosexual or bisexual identity (Michaels, 1996). The studies that have been done put the incidence of drug and alcohol in the gay community significantly higher than in the general population (SAMHSA, 2001; Bickelhaupt, 1995). A directory of gay and lesbian AA groups listed more than 800 meetings in the United States in the mid-'90s. **Various studies have estimated that 20–25% of gay men and lesbians are heavy alcohol users (compared with 3–10% of heterosexuals** (Hughes & Wilsnack, 1997; Skinner, 1994; Skinner & Otis, 1996). Alcohol was the preferred drug of choice but polydrug use was common. Marijuana was also used at a significantly higher level, almost one-third more than in the general population (Kelly, 1991). A sample of men who have sex with men (MSM) found them 21 times more likely to use nitrite inhalants and 4–7 times more likely to use hallucinogens, stimulants, sedatives, and tranquilizers. Methamphetamine use in particular is nearly epidemic by gay men in certain parts of the United States (Woody et al., 1999; Freese, Obert, Dickow, Cohen, & Lord, 2000).

The high incidence of HIV and AIDS in the gay male community is aggravated by drug or alcohol use for two reasons: the use of drugs lowers inhibitions and leads to unsafe sex and the use of contaminated needles also spreads the HIV virus quickly. This problem is aggravated since **social life often involves bars or other settings that promote drug and alcohol use** (D'Augelli, 1996).

"I'd been using drugs for years and years but when I found out I was positive I said, 'Oh, I'm going to die,' and I just started 'slamming' dope faster and harder, and I did that for 2 years, and when I wasn't dead I said, 'Wait a minute, I'm not dying, I gotta keep going with my life. And I started realizing that I could get clean, and I could stay as healthy as I could, and I could make something out of my life."
Gay recovering substance abuser with AIDS

Though sexual minorities have to suffer through society's hostility, indifference, fear, or misunderstanding and be subject to extra stress, **it is still the roots of addiction that are the greater influence**—genetics tempered by childhood stresses and inflamed by drug use.

"When I first came here, I was so nervous about being gay, one of the minority in the group 'cause there's a lot more straight men, but I really like it now because I can work on my issues about being heterophobic— I get fears around heterosexuals. I stereotype straight guys, 'Oh, they all hate me and they all think I'm less of a man.' And I get to find out that's not true and I get to find out that if someone does have that, then that's theirs. It ain't mine."
Gay recovering polydrug abuser

Societal homophobia, heterosexism, and internalized homophobia (the fear and hatred of one's homosexuality) are often some of the greatest barriers to long-term sobriety and recovery (Kominars, 1995). Fortunately, in recent years there has been a decrease in these feelings mostly due to a decrease in societal homophobia that might lead to better recovery outcomes for sexual minorities (Cabaj, 1997). However in a 1996 Gallup Poll, 50% of Americans said that homosexuality was unacceptable. This can make LGBT clients reluctant to speak about their sexual orientation. This reluctance leaves out pieces of the personality puzzle for treatment personnel (SAMHSA, 2001). For example, **defining the client's family and involving them in treatment can be difficult.** Has the family of origin rejected their son, or daughter, or sibling? What is the structure of the family?

TREATMENT OBSTACLES

Denial and lack of financial or treatment resources have always comprised the biggest obstacles to addiction treatment. But as the treatment of addictive disease continues to evolve, other significant obstacles are being identified that require intervention for successful treatment outcomes.

DEVELOPMENTAL ARREST

The use of psychoactive drugs can delay users' emotional development and keep them from learning how to deal with life's problems. In terms of treatment, the counselors or other professionals have to be aware of the level of development in the individual. They have to be aware of how much of what they or others are teaching is being understood by the client. In addition if a client is not fully detoxified or is not given time to start functioning normally, even the most sophisticated treatment can fall on deaf ears. More extensive assessment is one way to overcome these problems.

FOLLOW-THROUGH (monitoring)

Nothing is more indicative of poor treatment outcome than early program dropout or lack of compliance to the treatment protocol. Ironically client confidentiality that is so vital to the addiction treatment process has contributed to the problem of poor treatment compliance. Clients who have not or will not release information about their treatment progress can be noncompliant to protocols without the awareness of families, employers, or others until more destruction has resulted from their resumed addiction.

Professional licensing boards (medical, nursing, legal) now mandate release of confidentiality as a condition of retaining a license when addicts who are professionals are delivered to treatment after their addiction has been discovered. This practice, though assuring better program compliance, created another obstacle for the treatment professional. How could a therapist engage an addict into deep and sensitive issues about their addiction without being viewed as an extension of the licensing board, the family, or law enforcement? To address this obstacle, some licensing boards and employee assistance programs now employ a program monitor who oversees the progress of an addict in treatment to assure compliance to program protocols.

CONFLICTING GOALS

An individual addict's treatment goal may conflict with a program's goal. Some addicts may enter treatment merely to be able to better manage their abuse of drugs or to qualify for certain social benefits. Most treatment programs insist on an immediate commitment from their clients to a drug-free lifestyle. This difference between goals leads to a poor treatment outcome.

Program goals may conflict with society's goals for treating addicts. Programs naturally focus on the care of their clients using interventions that they hope will lead their clients to the best possible life outcome. Society is more interested in supporting programs that decrease the social costs of addiction (e.g. crime, health costs, accidents, violence).

The problems of **conflicting goals are best managed by development of clear program objectives and goals and better assessment and matching of clients to programs.** Although these concepts seem straightforward and easy to practice, only now is investment in these two areas beginning to occur.

TREATMENT RESOURCES

The biggest obstacle continues to be lack of treatment resources. On a national basis, individuals who apply for treatment are put on a waiting list of 2 weeks to 3 months or longer before they can get into treatment. Studies have shown that for every 100 people put on waiting list, 66% will never make it into treatment. Over the past 30 years, the Haight Ashbury Detox Clinic has found that of those put on their waiting list, 80% never access treatment. What happens to those potential clients is a matter of deep concern. Many die from drugs or from suicide while waiting for treatment (O'Boyle & Brandon, 1998). Most become more heavily involved in drugs and a high proportion end up in the criminal justice system. Since treatment has been shown to be very effective, it is a national tragedy that we continue to have long protracted waiting periods for clients wanting to access treatment.

MEDICAL INTERVENTION DEVELOPMENTS

INTRODUCTION

Drug replacement therapies, medical pharmacotherapy, chemically assisted detoxification, drug-assisted recovery, antipriming medications, drug restoration of homeostasis, and other medical interventions currently in development to treat drug addiction would have been considered to be oxymorons in the field of recovery a few short years ago. Further these terms would have terrified chemical dependency treatment clinicians and recovering addicts as both recognized that the use of psychoactive drugs often resulted in relapse.

Advances in the understanding of the neuropharmacology of addic-

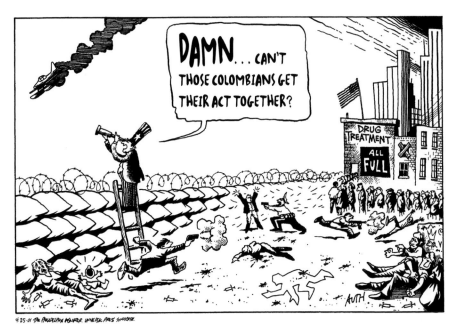

tion during the 1990's Decade of the **Mind led to a virtual flood of medication developments targeted to treat chemical dependencies.** By 2000, the number of new drugs being developed to treat addictions was second only to those in development to treat other mental health disorders and far outnumbered the drugs being developed to treat infections, heart disease, cancer, AIDS, and other illnesses. Chemical dependency treatment specialists now need to broaden their understanding and acceptance of medical therapies as they are certain to be incorporated into addiction treatment in the near future.

TYPES OF MEDICATIONS

The different types of medications being developed to treat addictions can be classified based on the targeted stage of recovery or by their effects on the nervous system and rest of the body (O'Brien, 1997; Vocci, 1999).

Detoxification

Medications that moderate or eliminate the withdrawal syndrome in addicts have been shown to be effective in engaging them into long-term treatment. Some examples of this detoxification development include buprenorphine and lofexidine to treat opioid withdrawal; selegiline, propranolol (a beta blocker), and SSRI antidepressants (paroxetine) for cocaine and stimulant addiction; and phenobarbital or lorazepam for alcohol or sedative-hypnotic dependence (O'Brien, 1997; Vocci, 1999).

Rapid Opioid Detoxification

This technique uses various medications in combination with naloxone or naltrexone and has also been clinically developed to treat opioid addiction. Opioid antagonists like **naloxone and naltrexone are used to precipitate immediate withdrawal and the other medications are used to mitigate the withdrawal symptoms**.

◇ Clonidine is combined with naltrexone to accomplish physical detoxification from opioid tissue dependence within 2–3 days.

◇ The benzodiazepine sedative midazolam is used with naloxone and naltrexone to accomplish opioid detoxification in 24 hours.

◇ A benzodiazepine sedative is combined with clonidine along with naloxone and naltrexone to detoxify an opioid addict within 6–8 hours while they are anesthetized with propofol.

These methods of rapid detoxification are medically dangerous and require intensive medical supervision. Further it is very important to remember that the techniques only accomplish physical detoxification and do not address the long-term behavioral and emotional components of addiction (Lorenzi et al., 1999; Cucchia et al., 1998; Byrne, 1998; Dyer, 1998; Barter et al., 1996; Senft, 1991).

Replacement or Agonist Effects

Controversy over whether this type of therapy is more harm reduction than recovery remains very heated in the addiction treatment community. However, few can deny the effectiveness of methadone replacement therapy in producing positive **benefits for both the addict (reduced morbidity and mortality while increasing overall life functioning) and for society (cost effectiveness and reduction in crime)** (Ball & Ross, 1991). Positive results from methadone maintenance have stimulated the search for other replacement or agonist therapies. LAAM (levomethadyl acetate), methylphenidate, and pemoline for cocaine and stimulant dependence and SSRI antidepressants and GHB (gamma hydroxybutyrate) for alcohol and sedative-hypnotic addiction are examples of replacement therapies in development to treat addictive disorders (O'Brien, 1997; Vocci, 1999). This is in addition to the approval of buprenorphine for treatment of heroin and opiate addiction.

Antagonist (blocking) Medications or Vaccines

Medications or vaccines that block the effects of addictive drugs without inducing their own major psychoactive effects are widely accepted as recovery-oriented treatment approaches. While on these types of agents, addicts will be unable to experience the effects of an abused drug should they have a slip. This destroys the addict's motivation for using and promotes continued abstinence. Significant examples of this treatment approach are the development of depo-naltrexone for opioid addiction and UH-232 for cocaine addiction. A cocaine vaccine that produces antibodies for cocaine, preventing its action for up to 30 days, is also in development (O'Brien, 1997; Vocci, 1999; Carrera et al., 1996; Fox et al., 1996).

Mixed Agonist-Antagonist

A single medication can have an agonist effect at one receptor site and an antagonist effect at another site. Or a combination of drugs are used together that work independently at different receptor sites to accomplish the same overall agonist-antagonist goal. The agonist component of this approach is targeted to prevent withdrawal while the antagonist effects prevent craving by blocking any further drug use. Examples of this approach are the developments of butorphanol and buprenorphine in opioid addiction; cyclazocine in cocaine dependence; and the combination of low-dose nicotine with mecamylamine to treat nicotine addiction. Rapid opioid detoxification described previously also employs this technique of combining agonist with antagonist medication to treat heroin and other opioid addictions (O'Brien, 1997; Rose, Behm, Westman, et al., 1994).

Anticraving & Anticued Craving

Craving or drug hunger is now an established component of addiction. Negative emotional states (e.g., **h**ungry, **a**ngry, **l**onely, **t**ired—HALT; and **r**estless, **i**rritable, **d**iscontent—well as imbalances in brain chemistry due to drug use cause endogenous craving. Environmental cues or triggers (e.g., drug odors, white powders, paraphernalia, crack houses, drug-using acquaintances) also induce a great potential for relapse. **Medications that can mitigate and reduce the craving and the cued-craving responses have witnessed dramatic development in treating addictions** (O'Brien, 1977). Naltrexone has been fully approved as an anticraving treatment for alcoholism and is in development to block cocaine and opioid craving (O'Brien, 1997; Volpicelli, O'Brien, Atterman, & Hayashida, 1992; O'Malley et al., 1992). A concern regarding potential liver toxicity with naltrexone use has limited its use in treating alcohol dependence. Nalmefene, another opioid antagonist, has been shown to reduce alcohol craving without any liver toxicity and is now being developed to treat alcohol addiction (Mason, Ritvo, Morgan, et al., 1994; O'Brien, 1997).

Acamprosate, a nonopioid drug, also exhibits alcohol anticraving effects through modulation of GABA (gamma-aminobutyric acid) and dopamine neurotransmitters (O'Brien, 1997).

Mecamylamine appears to block cocaine-cued craving and is currently in development for this indication, along with its development as a nicotine anticraving medication (Reid, Mickalian, Delucchi, Hall, & Berger, 1999).

The FDA has approved bupropion, an antidepressant medication, for the treatment of nicotine-cued craving. It is also in development as a cocaine anticraving medication. Bupropion research demonstrated that it prevented nicotine craving in patients who did not have symptoms of depression, which indicates that it mitigates craving by another unknown mechanism. Similarly SSRI antidepressants like paroxetine decrease alcohol use in even nondepressed alcoholics (O'Brien, 1997).

The craving response is physiologically similar to a body stress reaction. This has led researchers to study drugs that can antagonize corticotropin releasing factor (CRF) that triggers the stress reaction in the brain. The hypothesis is that craving can be prevented by blocking the body's stress reaction. Ketoconazole and CP154,526 inhibit the release of CRF in the brain and are being developed to treat cocaine craving. Metynapone inhibits the synthesis of body corticoids, which are also involved in the stress reaction. It is also being developed as a drug to treat cocaine craving (Vocci, 1999).

Metabolism Modulation

Medications that can alter the metabolism of an abused drug to render it ineffective or noxious when used are also being developed. Historically disulfiram, used to treat alcoholism, has been the only drug developed in this class. Disulfiram blocks the metabolic processes of alcohol leading to a build-up of acetaldehyde. Acetaldehyde causes nausea, flushing, and negative body reactions. Thus alcoholics suffer immediate adverse consequences from drinking. The effectiveness of disulfiram relies upon the compliance of the alcoholic to take it in support of their stated desire for abstinence. It has therefore had limited success in treating alcoholism in the past. However, the increase of coerced treatments during the past decade has improved disulfiram treatment compliance and increased positive outcomes (O'Brien, 1997; Keane et al., 1984; Keane & Fuller, 1986). This has increased interest in the metabolism modulation approach and some work has begun on the search for medications that can increase the metabolism of cocaine to render it ineffective when abused (Vocci, 1999).

Restoration of Homeostasis

Abuse of addictive drugs imbalances brain chemistry that then reinforces the need to continue using the drug. **Medications and nutrients that restore brain chemical imbalances are theorized to restore homeostasis and mitigate the need for continued drug use.** Drugs that have dopamine-activating effects in the brain (e.g., selegiline, amantadine, pergolide) and antidepressants that increase serotonin in the brain (e.g., desipramine, nefazodone, paroxetine, sertraline, venlafaxine) are all being developed to treat cocaine and alcohol addiction by restoring brain chemical homeostasis (Vocci, 1999).

Amino Acid Precursor Loading

This technique consists of **administering protein supplements** (e.g., tyrosine, taurine, d,l phenylalanine, glutamate, tryptophan) to addicts in an effort to increase the brain's production of its neurochemicals and restore home-ostasis. Though not yet established by rigorous research, many treatment programs report good patient treatment compliance and positive outcomes when amino acid precursor loading is added to the treatment process for cocaine, amphetamine, alcohol, and opioid dependence (Blum et al., 1989).

Modulation of Drug Effects & Antipriming

A fairly recent development is the use of medications that can **modulate or blunt the pleasurable reinforcing effects of addictive drug use**. Calcium channel-blocking medications prevent calcium ions from entering brain cells thus blocking the release of dopamine and therefore the reinforcing effects of cocaine, opioids, and alcohol. Nimodipine, acamprosate, amlodipine, nephedipine, and isadipine are all calcium channel blockers being developed to treat addiction to cocaine, opioids, and alcohol (Vocci, 1999; Shulman, Jagoda, Laycock, & Kelly, 1998).

Sodium Ion Channel Blockers

Medications like riluzole, phenytoin, and lamotrigine **interfere with neuron transmission via this process and result in muting cocaine's reinforcing effects**. Cyclazocine, a mixed opioid agonist-antagonist, also reduces cocaine reinforcement by interfering with cocaine's action on presynaptic neurons' sodium ion channels (Vocci, 1999).

Low Doses of Nicotine

This technique has been shown to **decrease craving without reinforcing the need to increase its dosage** or to continue its use. This effect is known as an "antipriming action" and is the basis for the development of low-dose nicotine delivery systems, like the nicotine patch, to treat nicotine addiction.

Other Drugs

Some medications have clinically been shown to be useful in addiction treatment but by what mechanism they accomplish their positive benefit effect is unknown. Psychedelic drugs like ibogaine and ketamine are said to be effective in treating cocaine and opioid addiction even though the use of ibogaine to treat opioid addiction had resulted in some fatalities. Dextromethorphan (DM), a nonprescription anti-cough medication, is being studied to treat opioid addiction. DM has been shown to be a weak glutamate agonist but its mechanism to decrease opiate withdrawal symptoms, craving, and relapse is unclear. Cycloserine, an antibiotic for the treatment of tuberculosis, is being studied for its ability to decrease opioid use by some unknown mechanism. **Anticonvulsant medications** like valproate and carbamazepine appear to diminish cocaine's craving and "kindling" effects. **Smart drugs**, also known as "nootropic agents," are believed to increase brain activity by unknown mechanisms and are also being tested to treat cocaine and stimulant addiction. Camitine/coenzyme Q10, ginkgo biloba, pentoxifylline, Hydergine®, and piracetam are current nootropics being studied for use in cocaine addiction treatment. Tiagabine and gabapentin are anticonvulsant medications used in the treatment of epilepsy. They are believed to increase brain GABA activity but their ability to decrease cocaine addiction occurs by some yet-to-be-discovered mechanism. These and other clinical observations of drugs that lessen addiction or relapse liability indicate that there is a lot more still to be learned about the addicted brain (Vocci, 1999; O'Brien, 1997).

Some companies, such as Drug Abuse Sciences, Inc., are developing time-release delivery systems for naltrexone (Naltrel®), methadone (Methaliz®), and buprenorphine (Buprel®).

THE NEW DRUG DEVELOPMENT PROCESS

The FDA has established a structured process for the approval of new drugs to treat specific therapeutic indications or the approval of existing drugs to be used for new therapeutic applications. This consists of 3 Steps and 4 Phases.

Step 1: Preclinical Research & Development

This step consists of the initial chemical development of a drug along with animal studies to determine the general effects, toxicity, and projected abuse liability of the substance. If these results indicate that the drug is useful and marketable, the drug's sponsor will apply for an Investigational New Drug (IND) number that will permit human research to be conducted with the substance.

Step 2: Clinical Trials

Step 2 is comprised of 3 Phases that study the efficacy and safety of the drug in humans.

◇ Phase I: Initial Clinical Stage. A small number of human subjects are used to establish drug safety, dosage range for effective treatment, and the occurrence of side effects or adverse reactions.

◇ Phase II: Clinical Pharmacological Evaluation Stage. Double-blind studies (neither the researcher nor the test subject knows if they have received the actual test drug or a placebo) are used to evaluate the effects of the drug, determine side effects, and gauge the effectiveness of its use in treating a specific medical condition.

◇ Phase III: Extended Clinical Evaluation. The new drug is made available to a large number of researchers and patients with the indicated medical condition to further evaluate its safety, effectiveness, recommended dosage, and side effects.

Step 3: Permission to Market

If the drug successfully completes Steps 1 and 2 to demonstrate acceptable efficacy and safety, the FDA can allow the drug to be marketed under its patented name. The process from Step 1 to Step 3 takes up to 12 years to complete. After the drug is marketed, the FDA continues to monitor the drug for adverse or toxic reactions because it can take years for some negative effects to manifest and be discovered. This postmarketing scrutiny is often referred to as "Phase IV" because of the ability of the FDA to remove the drug from the market at any time if negative effects outweigh the positive benefits of using the drug.

OVERVIEW OF MEDICATIONS

A partial list of medications in development for the treatment of addictive disorders was prepared by the authors using information gathered from a large number of references with consultation from the Pharmaceutical Research Center of the Haight Ashbury Free Clinics. It should be noted that the many drugs being developed for cocaine addiction are also being studied to treat amphetamine and other stimulant dependence as well.

TABLE 9–5   MEDICATIONS IN DEVELOPMENT FOR ADDICTIVE DISORDERS

Drug	Brand Name	Current Medical Use	Proposed Use	Theoretical Action	Status
acamprosate or calcium acetyl homotaurine	Campral®	—	alcohol craving	calcium channel blocker, dopamine, GABA & glutamate modulation	Phase III, approved in Europe
amantadine	Symmetrel®	antiviral & Parkinsonism	cocaine addiction	dopamine agonist	Phase II
amlodipine	Lotrel® & Norvasc®	antihypertension	cocaine addiction	calcium channel blocker	clinical observation
baclofen	Lioresal®	muscle relaxant	cocaine addiction	GABA & dopamine agonist	Phase II
BP 897	—	—	cocaine addiction	dopamine d2 & d3 antagonist inhibits cued craving	Step 1
bromocriptine	Parlodel®	antiprolactin	cocaine addiction	dopamine agonist	clinical observation
bupropion	Wellbutrin® & Zyban®	antidepressant	cocaine & nicotine addiction	anticued craving	Phase II, approved for nicotine
butorphanol	Stadol®	analgesia	opioid addiction	opioid agonist-antagonist	Phase II
cabergoline	Dostinex®	antiprolactin	cocaine addiction	dopamine agonist	Phase II
carbamazepine	Tegretol®	anticonvulsant	cocaine addiction	unknown mechanism	clinical observation
carbidopa with levodopa	Atimet® & Sinemet®	Parkinsonism	cocaine addiction	dopamine agonist	clinical observation
carnitine/Co Q (coenzyme Q10)	Ubigold-10®	nootropic (smart drug)	cocaine addiction	mechanism unknown	Phase II
clonidine	Catapres®	antihypertension	opioid withdrawal	alpha 2 agonist	Phase II
cocaine vaccine	ITAC®	—	cocaine addiction	antibodies that prevent cocaine action for 30 days	Phase I
CP-154,526	—	—	cocaine addiction	CRF antagonist	Phase I
cyclazocine	—	—	cocaine addiction	opioid agonist-antagonist, cocaine mechanism unknown	Phase I
cycloserine	Seromycin®	antibiotic	opioid addiction	mechanism unknown	Phase I
depo-naltrexone & depot-naltrexone	— Naltrel®	—	alcohol or opioid addiction opioid	antagonist in depo form blocks opioids for 14–30 days; depo is an injectable pellet and depot is an injectable suspension	Step 1
desipramine	Norpramin®	antidepressant	cocaine withdrawal	serotonin, dopamine, NE & E modulation	Phase II
disulfiram	Antabuse®	alcohol addiction	cocaine addiction	mechanism unknown but decreased alcohol use associated with decreased cocaine relapses	Phase II
dextroampheta-mine	Dexedrine®	narcolepsy & ADD	cocaine & metham-phetamine replacement	CNS stimulant	Phase II
dextrometh-orphan	in various cough meds	anticough	opioid withdrawal & addiction	glutamate antagonist	Phase II
dynorphin 1-13	—	—	opioid addiction	a naturally occurring opioid agonist	Phase II
enadoline	—	—	opioid & cocaine addiction	selective kappa opioid agonist, mechanism in cocaine unknown	Phase I & Phase II

continued

TABLE 9–5 *CONTINUED*

Drug	Brand Name	Current Medical Use	Proposed Use	Theoretical Action	Status
ergot extract	Hydergine®	nootropic	cocaine addiction	dopamine agonist	Phase II
flupenthixol	Fluanxol® Depixol®	antipsychotic	cocaine addiction	dopamine antagonist	Phase II
gabapentin	Neurontin®	anticonvulsant	cocaine addiction	mechanism unknown	Phase II
GBR 12909 or vanoxerine	—	—	cocaine addiction	glutamate agonist	Phase I
gamma hydroxy butyrate (GHB)	Xyrem®	cataplexy of narcolepsy	alcohol & opioid addiction	naturally occurring inhibitory neurotransmitter like GABA	approved for alcoholism in Europe
ginkgo biloba	Bio Ginkgo®	nootropic	cocaine addiction	mechanism unknown	Phase II
isradipine	Dynacirc®	antihypertension	alcohol addiction	calcium channel blocker	clinical observation
ibogaine; also see 18-MC below	Endabuse®	—	opioid & cocaine addiction	mechanism unknown, a toxic psychedelic	Phase I
ketamine	Ketalar®	anesthetic	alcohol addition	mechanism unknown	studied in Russia
ketoconazole	Nizoral®	antifungal	cocaine addiction	CRF antagonist	clinical observation
lamotrigine	Lamictal®	anticonvulsant	cocaine & opioid addiction	sodium channel blocker	Phase II & Phase I
lazabemide	Tempium®	Alzhemier's disease	nicotine addiction	MAO-B inhibitor	Phase III
levo-alpha acetyl methadol or levomethadyl acetate (LAAM)	Orlaam®	opioid addiction	opioid replacement	opioid agonist	approved for use
lobeline	—	—	nicotine and methamphetamine addiction	autonomic ganglia agonist	Phase I
lofexidine	Britlofex®	—	opioid addiction	calcium channel blocker and alpha 2 agonist	Phase II
mazindol	Sanorex, ® & alpha 2 agonist	antiobesity or weight control	cocaine replacement	phenethylamine CNS stimulant	Phase II
mecamylamine	Inversine®	antihypertension	cocaine addiction	blocks nicotine-cued cocaine craving	Step 1
18-methoxycoronaridine (18-MC)	—	—	abolish cravings for cocaine, opiates, nicotine, alcohol & methamphetamine	an ibogaine derivative said to be devoid of hallucinogenic effects, decreases dopamine levels in the habenulo-interpeduncular pathway	research observations in the Caribbean and in Europe
methylphenidate	Ritalin®	ADD & ADHD	cocaine replacement	CNS stimulant	Phase II
metyrapone	Systemic®	hypothalamic-adrenal axis suppression test	cocaine addiction	inhibits corticoid synthesis to inhibit cocaine craving	Phase I
nalmefene	Revex®	opioid overdose and toxic effects	alcohol & opioid addiction	opioid antagonist with no liver toxicity	Phase II for alcohol; approved for opioids
naltrexone	Revia®	alcohol & opioid addiction	cocaine addiction	opioid antagonist inhibits opioid & cocaine craving	Phase II
nefazodone	Serzone®	antidepressant	cocaine addiction	serotonin, dopamine, NE & E modulation	Phase II
nicotine	CigRx®	—	nicotine replacement	low nicotine & carcinogen cigarette	Phase II
nicotine gum	Gumsmoke®	smoking cessation	smokeless tobacco addiction	tobacco-flavored chewing gum alternative to chewing tobacco	Phase II
nicotine with mecamylamine patch	Prostep®	smoking cessation	nicotine addiction	antipriming & anticraving	Phase III
nicotine oral lozenge	Commit Lozenge®	smoking cessation	nicotine addiction	antipriming & anticraving	approved
nifedipine	Adalat® & Procardia®	vasospastic angina	alcohol, opioid, amphetamine, benzodiazepine & marijuana addiction	calcium channel blocker, increased dopamine to mitigate withdrawal and craving	clinical observation
nimodipine	Nimotop®	ischemic stroke	opioid addiction	calcium channel blocker	Phase II

continued

TABLE 9–5 *CONTINUED*

Drug	Brand Name	Current Medical Use	Proposed Use	Theoretical Action	Status
NS 2359	—	—	cocaine addiction	dopamine agonist	Phase II
olanzapine	Zyprexa®	antipsychotic	cocaine addiction	benzodiazepine with antipsychotic effects	Phase II
OT-nicotine	—	—	nicotine addiction	antipriming, anticraving, replacement therapy	Phase II & III
paroxetine	Paxil®	SSRI antidepressant	cocaine & alcohol addiction	serotonin modulation, mechanism in alcoholism unknown	Phase II & clinical observation
pemoline	Cylert®	ADHD	cocaine replacement	CNS stimulant	Phase II
pentoxifylline	Trental®	improve blood flow	cocaine addiction	mechanism unknown	Phase II
pergolide	Permax®	Parkinsonism	cocaine addiction	dopamine d1 & d2 agonist	Phase II
phenytoin	Dilantin®	anticonvulsant	cocaine addiction	sodium channel blocker	Phase II
piracetam	Nootropil®	nootropic	cocaine addiction	mechanism unknown	Phase II
pramipexole	Mirapex®	Parkinsonism	cocaine addiction	dopamine agonist	Phase II
propranolol	Inderal®	antihypertension	cocaine addiction	beta adrenergic blocker but cocaine mechanism unknown	Phase II
reserpine	Reserpoid®	antihypertension	cocaine addiction	dopamine, NE & E modulation	Phase II
riluzole	Rilutek®	ALS disease	cocaine addiction	sodium channel blocker	Phase II
risperidone	Risperdal®	antipsychotic	cocaine addiction	dopamine d2 & serotonin antagonist	Phase II
selegiline (IR & TS)	Eldepryl® & Deprenyl®	Parkinsonism	cocaine addiction	MAO-B inhibitor increased dopamine, NE & E	Phase I & III
sertraline	Zoloft®	SSRI antidepressant	cocaine & alcohol addiction	serotonin modulation, mechanism in alcohol unknown	Phase II & clinical observation
tiagabine	Gabitril®	anticonvulsant	cocaine addiction	GABA modulation	Phase II
topiramate	Topamax®	anticonvulsant	alcohol addiction	dopamine antagonist	being studied in Europe
tramadol	Ultram®	analgesia	opioid replacement	mu opioid receptor agonist	Phase I
tyrosine	—	nutritional supplement	amphetamine & cocaine addiction	increased dopamine synthesis in the brain	Phase I
UH-232	—	—	cocaine addiction	nondysphoric cocaine antagonist	Step 1
valproate	Depacon®	anticonvulsant	cocaine addiction	GABA modulation, Phase II antikindling	
venlafaxine	Effexor®	antidepressant	cocaine addiction	serotonin & NE modulation	Phase II
verapamil	Calan®	angina	alcohol, opiates, amphetamine, benzodiazepine & marijuana addiction	calcium channel blocker	clinical observation

CHAPTER SUMMARY

Introduction

1. The most prevalent disease of the brain is addiction. Annually it causes over $1/2$ million deaths and intense social disruption. The vast majority of deaths are from the legal drugs, tobacco and alcohol.

2. Current issues in treatment include:

◇ the rapidly expanding use of medications to treat detoxification, control craving, and assist relapse prevention; medications include drugs to lessen withdrawal symptoms, anti-craving drugs, antidepressants, substitute medications (e.g., methadone), and nutritional supplements;

◇ the use of imaging techniques and other new diagnostic techniques to visualize the physiological effects of drugs; CAT (computerized axial tomography), MRI (magnetic resonance imaging), PET (positron emission tomography), and SPECT (single photon emission computerized tomography) are four of the methods used;

◊ the lack of resources to provide treatment. Studies have shown that treatment is effective but governments do not allot enough money to provide sufficient treatment;

◊ the use of coerced treatment, such as drug courts, to mandate care for abusers and addicts and thus reduce rearrest rates and cut costs;

◊ the conflict between abstinence-oriented recovery and harm reduction as philosophies of treatment. Most treatment modalities say abstinence is absolutely necessary to recovery while harm reduction advocates say incremental changes are acceptable.

Treatment Effectiveness

3. Treatment is effective. It has a 50% success rate according to the DATOS and CALDATA studies.

4. Each $1 spent on treatment saves at least $4 to $20 in costs related to unchecked addiction.

5. Prison costs $25,000 to $40,000 per inmate a year compared to $1,800 to $3,900 for outpatient treatment or methadone maintenance.

6. Almost two-thirds of arrestees test positive for psychoactive drugs, particularly cocaine and marijuana.

7. There is a shortage of treatment slots for inmates in jails and prisons.

Principles & Goals of Treatment

8. The National Institutes of Health listed 13 principles of effective treatment, e.g., no single treatment is appropriate for all individuals, treatment needs to be readily available, and effective treatment attends to multiple needs of the individual.

9. The two primary treatment goals are motivation towards abstinence and creating a drug-free lifestyle. The secondary goals have to do with creating a better lifestyle by improving job, medical, psychiatric, emotional, and spiritual functioning.

Selection of a Program

10. No single type of treatment is effective for everyone; it must be tailored to the individual.

11. Diagnosis of the type and level of addiction is ascertained through interviews and diagnostic tests, particularly the Addiction Severity Index (ASI).

12. Treatment options include medical model detoxification, social model detoxification, social model recovery, therapeutic communities, halfway houses, sober-living or transitional-living programs, partial hospitalization, and harm reduction programs.

13. About 1.6 million clients are treated each year for drug abuse. About 1,165,000 are in treatment on any given day.

14. Two million more hard-core abusers need treatment.

15. Over 70% of those in treatment are male.

Beginning Treatment

16. Recovery is a lifelong process since brain chemistry is permanently altered by drug abuse.

17. Recognition and acceptance of addiction by the client is crucial to recovery.

18. Breaking through denial is the crucial first step to begin treatment.

19. Denial can be overcome when the addict hits bottom or through a direct intervention (e.g., legal system, family, workplace supervisor, physician).

20. The two major sources of referral are self-referral and legal referrals by the criminal justice system.

21. The elements of a formal intervention are love, a facilitator, intervention statements, anticipated defenses and outcomes, the intervention itself, and contingency plans.

Treatment Continuum

22. Treatment starts with detoxification and escalates through initial abstinence, long-term abstinence, and recovery.

23. It takes about a week for drugs to clear from the body and 4 weeks to 10 months for brain and body chemistry to settle down.

24. Drugs can be cleared from the system through abstinence, medication therapy, and psychosocial therapy.

25. Detoxification medications include clonidine, buprenorphine, naltrexone, phenobarbital, methadone, antipsychotics, and others.

26. Intensive counseling and group therapy are necessary to aid detoxification.

27. Initial abstinence is supported through anticraving medications (e.g., naltrexone, bromocryptine, nicotine replacements), individual counseling, and group therapy.

28. Environmental triggers cause relapse. Cue extinction (desensitization) is one way to avoid relapse. Another is learning automatic responses to cravings.

29. Relapse prevention is the key to initial abstinence.

30. Psychosocial support to help the clients put their lives back in order is crucial: job support, physical and mental health problems support, and housing searches.

31. Acupuncture can help calm withdrawal symptoms and reduce craving to some extent.

32. Addicts must accept that treatment for addiction is a lifelong process and that chemical dependency extends to a variety of substances not just the drug of choice.

33. Long-term abstinence uses individual and group therapy and 12-step groups to prolong abstinence.

34. Recovery entails restructuring one's life, not just staying abstinent.

35. Human beings can naturally experience all the highs they seek through drugs.

36. Follow-up is important not just to satisfy government funding agencies but to know which programs work.

37. Follow-up helps tailor programs to match the client and identify clients who need to be treated again for a relapse.

Individual vs. Group Therapy

38. Individual therapy conducted by a trained counselor helps the recovering client address specific personal issues and identify needs.

39. Some individual therapies include cognitive behavioral therapy, reality therapy, psychodynamic therapy, motivational interviewing, and aversion therapy.

40. Motivational interviewing is a nonconfrontational therapy to resolve a client's ambivalence about wanting recovery and uses the stages of change model to alter their behavior.

41. Group therapy can be used to break the isolation of chemical dependence. The types of groups include facilitated, peer, 12-step, educational, topic-specific, and targeted.

42. Various 12-step groups, such as Alcoholics Anonymous, Narcotics Anonymous, and Overeaters Anonymous, use sponsors, spirituality, and the power of people telling their own stories to teach a clean and sober lifestyle.

43. There are a number of errors that novice counselors make in groups, e.g., unrealistic view of group treatment, self-disclosure confusion, and failure to plan in advance.

Treatment & the Family

44. Addiction affects the whole family, so good treatment should involve the whole family.

45. There are a number of family treatment approaches including the family systems approach, the family behavioral approach, and tough love.

46. Codependency and enabling, whereby family members support the addict in his or her addiction, must be addressed in treatment.

47. In families with adult addicts, the children take on certain roles: model child, problem child, lost child, and family clown.

48. Adults who were raised in addictive households carry many of their problems into adulthood and must face those problems in treatment.

49. Groups such as Al-Anon, Nar-Anon, and ACoA help support and educate the families and friends of alcoholics and addicts.

Adjunctive & Complementary Treatment Services

50. Besides abstinence, treatment needs to provide services to handle physical, emotional, family, social, and spiritual deficits.

Drug-Specific Treatment

51. Most people coming in for treatment are polydrug abusers (including behavioral addictions), even though they have a drug of choice.

52. Stimulant abuse often initially presents treatment professionals with drug-induced symptoms of psychosis and paranoia.

53. Therapy and anticraving medications help overcome anergia, euthymia, and craving during stimulant abstinence.

54. Endogenous (internal) stimulant craving is caused by neurochemical imbalances and bad thinking. Exogenous craving is caused by environmental cues.

55. More and more drug treatment centers include smoking cessation as part of recovery.

56. Because smoking addiction involves nicotine craving, nicotine replacement therapies (e.g., nicotine patches) help taper tobacco craving.

57. Heroin and other opioid treatments usually need medications to alleviate withdrawal during detoxification.

58. Methadone maintenance is a harm reduction therapy that substitutes a controlled opioid for an illicit, problem-causing street opioid. Buprenorphine is also used for detoxification and abstinence maintenance and can be prescribed by certified doctors from their offices.

59. Sedative-hypnotic withdrawal can be life-threatening unless assisted with medical therapy that includes an antiseizure medication like phenobarbital. Withdrawal symptoms can last for weeks even months.

60. Denial is the biggest hindrance to beginning treatment particularly for alcohol abusers. Physical withdrawal is usually not life-threatening.

61. Peer groups and 12-step groups are vital to both long-term abstinence and recovery from alcoholism or any other addiction.

62. Talk-downs with emotional support and time for the drug to leave the body are the usual treatments for bad trips due to LSD or other psychedelics. Antipsychotic or antianxiety medications are also used when needed.

63. There has been a steady increase in people going into treatment for marijuana. The majority of referrals are court ordered.

64. The majority of inhalant abusers are under 20 years old compared to older abusers of other drugs.

65. The treatment for behavioral addictions is similar to the treatment for drug addiction.

66. Sufficient facilities and personnel for treating compulsive gamblers are sorely lacking.

67. Early intervention for eating disorders is very important in treating anorexia, bulimia, and compulsive overeating.

68. Sexual addiction is most often treated by getting at the psychodynamic roots of their compulsion.

69. Internet addiction includes cybersexual addiction, cyberrelationship addiction, information overload, and computer addiction (playing games).

Target Populations

70. Treatment must be tailored to specific groups based on gender, sexual orientation, age, ethnic group, job, and even economic status.

71. Treatment for men should be different than for women. Men often blame external forces while women often blame themselves for their addiction.

72. Youth are less willing to accept guidance, so youth-directed programs that use peer support seem to work best.

73. Older Americans are a fast-growing segment of those with a substance abuse problem and are often reluctant to seek treatment because they view addiction as a character flaw not a disease.

74. Treatment for different ethnic groups works better with culture-specific treatment protocols.

75. African American, Hispanic, Asian American/Pacific Islander, and Native American treatment often requires strong family involvement and accessing the spiritual roots of each community.

76. Little research has been done on treatment for those with physical disabilities. Too much focus is on the handicap and not enough on the addiction.

77. There is also a lack of research for the lesbian, gay, bisexual, and transgender (LGBT) communities. The use of alcohol and drugs lowers inhibitions and abets the spread of disease including HIV. Homophobia and heterophobia complicate substance abuse treatment.

Treatment Obstacles

78. Being aware of the emotional maturity of clients, doing follow-ups to make sure the client is following the program, resolving conflicting goals, and making sure there are enough treatment slots to meet demand are vital to the effectiveness of treatment programs.

Medical Intervention Developments

79. The fastest-growing field in treatment is the development of new medications. Drugs are being developed for: detoxification, replacement therapy (agonist effects), antagonist effects, vaccines, mixed agonist-antagonist effects, anticraving, metabolism modulation, restoration of homeostasis, and modulation of drug effects and antipriming.

80. There are three steps in the new drug development process including preclinical research and development, clinical trials, and permission to market.

REFERENCES

Adger, H. (1998). Children in alcoholic families: Family dynamics and treatment issues. In A. W. Graham & T. K. Schultz (Eds.), *Principles of Addiction Medicine* (2nd ed., pp. 1111–1114). Chevy Chase, MD: American Society of Addiction Medicine, Inc.

Alcoholics Anonymous. (1934, 1976). *Alcoholics Anonymous.* New York: Alcoholics Anonymous World Services, Inc.

Allen, J. P., Eckardt, M. J., & Wallen, J. (1988). Screening for alcoholism: Techniques and issues. *Public Health Reports, 103,* 586–59.

American Association for the Treatment of Opioid Dependence (2002). AMTA. 217 Broadway, New York, NY, 10007. (212) 566–5555.

American Psychiatric Association. (2000). *Diagnostic and Statistical Manual of Mental Disorders* (4th ed., text revisions [DSM-IV-TR]). Washington, DC: Author.

Anglin, M. D., Prendergast, M., & Farabee, D. (1998). The effectiveness of coerced treatment for drug-abusing offenders, ONDCP Conference of Scholars and Policy Makers [Online]. Available: *http://www.ncjrs.org/ondcppubs/treat/consensus/anglin.pdf*

Arrestee Drug Abuse Monitoring Program. (2003). Annual reports on adult and juvenile arrestees. National Institute of Justice [Online]. Available: *http://www.adam-nij.net/files/adam2001.pdf*

Bacaltchuk J., & Hay P. (2003). Antidepressants versus placebo for people with bulimia nervosa. *The Cochrane Library, 2.*

Ball, J. C., & Ross, A. (Eds.). (1991). *The Effectiveness of Methadone Maintenance Treatment.* New York: Springer-Verlag.

Barclay, L. (2002). New treatment achieves 75% remission in eating disorders. *Proceedings of the National Academy of Science, 99*(14), 9486–9491.

Barter, T., et al. (1996). Rapid opiate detoxification. *American Journal of Drug and Alcohol Abuse, 22*(4), 489–495.

Belenko, S. (1998). Research on drug courts: A critical review. *National Drug Court Institute Review, 1*(1) [Online]. Available: *http://www.drugcourt.org/*

Bensen, L. (1879). *Fifteen Years in Hell: An Autobiography.* Indianapolis, IN: Douglas & Carlon.

Berenson, D., & Schrier, E. W. (1998). Current family treatment approaches. In A. W. Graham & T. K. Schultz (Eds.), *Principles of Addiction Medicine* (2nd ed., pp. 1115–1125). Chevy Chase, MD: American Society of Addiction Medicine, Inc.

Bickelhaupt, E. E. (1995). Alcoholism and drug abuse in gay and lesbian persons: A review of incidence studies. In R. J. Kus (Ed.), *Addiction and Recovery in Gay and Lesbian Persons.* New York: Harrington Park Press.

Birch, S. (2001). An overview of acupuncture in the treatment of stroke, addiction, and other health problems. In G. Stux & R. Hammerschlag (Eds.), *Clinical Acupuncture: Scientific Basis*. New York: Springer.

Blum, K., et al. (1989). Cocaine therapy: The reward-cascade link. *Professional Counselor, 27*.

Blume, S. B. (1997). Pathological gambling. In J. H. Lowinson, P. Ruiz, R. B. Millman, & J. G. Langrod (Eds.), *Substance Abuse: A Comprehensive Textbook* (3rd ed., pp. 330–337). Baltimore: Williams & Wilkins.

Boucher, T. A., Kiresuk, T. J., & Trachtenberg, A. I. (1998). Alternative therapies. In A. W. Graham & T. K. Schultz (Eds.), *Principles of Addiction Medicine* (2nd ed., pp. 371–394). Chevy Chase, MD: American Society of Addiction Medicine, Inc.

Brubaker, M. (1997). *Compulsive Gambling & Recovery*. New Orleans, LA: Brubaker Consulting.

Byrne, A. (1998). Rapid opiate detoxification. *British Journal of Psychiatry, 172*, 451, 316(7126), 170.

Cabaj, R. P. (1997). Gays, lesbians, and bisexuals. In J. H. Lowinson, P. Ruiz, R. B. Millman, & J. G. Langrod (Eds.), *Substance Abuse: A Comprehensive Textbook* (3rd ed., pp. 725–732). Baltimore: Williams & Wilkins.

Califano, J. A. (2001). High stakes: Substance abuse and gambling. National Center on Addiction and Substance Abuse [Online]. Available *http://www.casacolumbia.org/newsletter1457/newsletter_show.htm?doc_id=71136*

Carrera, M. R., et al. (1996). *Nature, 378,* 727.

Carrol, J. E. (1980). Uncovering drug abuse by alcoholics and alcohol abuse by addicts. *International Journal of Addiction, 15*, 591–595.

Carter, B. L., & Tiffany, S. T. (1999). Meta-analysis of cue-reactivity in addiction research. *Addiction, 94*(3), 327–340.

Centers for Disease Control. (2000). Treating tobacco use and dependence. U.S. Public Health Service [Online]. Available: *http://www.surgeongeneral.gov/tobacco/smokesum.htm*

Centers for Disease Control. (2001). Cigarette smoking-related mortality. Tobacco Information and Prevention Source (TIPS) [Online]. Available: *http://www.cdc.gov/tobacco/research_data/health_consequences/mortali.htm*

Centers for Disease Control. (2002). MMWR — Annual smoking-attributable mortality, Years of potential life lost, and economic costs — United States, 1995–1999 [Online]. Available: *http://www.cdc.gov/tobacco/research_data/economics/mmwr5114.highlights.htm*

Chang, G., & Kosten, T. R. (1997). Detoxification. In J. H. Lowinson, P. Ruiz, R. B. Millman, & J. G. Langrod (Eds.), *Substance Abuse: A Comprehensive Textbook* (3rd ed., pp. 377–381). Baltimore: Williams & Wilkins.

Cherrington, E. (1920). *The Evolution of Prohibition in the United States*. Westerville, OH: The American Issue Press.

Childress, A. R., McClellan, A. T., Ehrman, R., & O'Brien, C. P. (1988). Classically conditioned responses in opioid and cocaine dependence: A role in relapse? In B. A. Ray (Ed.), *Learning Factors in Substance Abuse*, NIDA Research Monograph 84. Rockville, MD: National Institute on Drug Abuse.

Childress, A. R., McElgin, W., Mozley, P. D., Fitzgerald, J., Reivich, M., & O'Brien, C. P. (1999). Limbic activation during cue-induced cocaine craving. *American Journal of Psychiatry, 156(*1), 11–18.

Copeland, A. L., & Sorensen, J. L. (2001). Differences between methamphetamine users and cocaine users in treatment. *Drug and Alcohol Dependence, 62*, 91–95.

Crowe, A. H., & Reeves, R. (1994). *Treatment for Alcohol and Other Drug Abuse: Opportunities for Coordination.* Technical Assistance Publication Series #11. Rockville, MD: Substance Abuse and Mental Health Services Administration.

Cucchia, A. T., et al. (1998). Ultra-rapid opiate detoxification using deep sedation with oral midazolam: Short and long-term results. *Drug & Alcohol Dependency, 52*(3), 243–250.

D'Augelli, A. R. (1996). Lesbian, gay, and bisexual development during adolescence and young adulthood. In R. P. Cabaj & T. S. Stein (Eds.), *Textbook of Homosexuality and Mental Health* (pp. 267–288). Washington, DC: American Psychiatric Press.

Daley, D. C., & Marlatt, G. A. (1997). Relapse prevention. In J. H. Lowinson, P. Ruiz, R. B. Millman, & J. G. Langrod (Eds.), *Substance Abuse: A Comprehensive Textbook* (3rd ed., pp. 458–467). Baltimore: Williams & Wilkins.

DanceSafe. (2003). Search laboratory pill test results [Online]. Available: *http://www.dancesafe.org/labtesting/*

Dascus, J. (1877). *Battling with the Demon: The Progress of Temperance*. Saint Louis, MO: Scammell & Company.

Davis, R. A. (2001). Freedom from e-slavery: Tips on getting your life back [Online]. Available: *http://www.internetaddiction.ca/internet_addiction_treatment.htm*

Dodd, M. H. (1997). Social model of recovery: Origin, early features, changes, and future. *Journal of Psychoactive Drugs, 29*(2), 133–140.

Dole, V. P., & Nyswander, M. E. (1965). A medical treatment for diacetylmorphine (heroin) addiction: A clinical trial with methadone hydrochloride. *Journal of the American Medical Association, 193*(8), 646–650.

Dorchester, D. (1884). *The Liquor Problem in All Ages*. New York: Phillips & Hunt.

Dyer, C. (1998). Addict died after rapid opiate detoxification. *British Medical Journal, 316*(7126), 170.

Eickelberg, S. J., & Mayo-Smith, M. F. (1998). Management of sedative-hypnotic intoxication and withdrawal. In A. W. Graham & T. K. Schultz (Eds.), *Principles of Addiction Medicine* (2nd ed., pp. 441–454). Chevy Chase, MD: American Society of Addiction Medicine, Inc.

Ethridge, R. M., Craddock, S. G., Dunteman, G. H., & Hubbard, R. L. (1995). Treatment services in two national studies of community-based drug abuse treatment programs. *Journal of Substance Abuse, 7*, 9–26.

Fiorentine, R. (1999). After drug treatment: Are 12-step programs effective in maintaining abstinence? *American Journal of Drug and Alcohol Abuse, 25*(1), 93–116.

Fox, B. S., et al. (1996). Cocaine vaccine. *Nature Medicine, 2*, 1129.

Freese, T. E., Obert, J., Dickow, J., Cohen, R. H., & Lord, R. H. (2000). Methamphetamine abuse: Issues for special populations. *Journal of Psychoactive Drugs, 32*(2), 177–182.

Galanter, M., Keller, D. S., Dermatis, H., & Egelko, S. (2000). The impact of managed care on substance abuse treatment: A report of the American Society of Addiction Medicine. *Journal of Addictive Diseases, 19*(3), 13–34.

Gatch, M. B., & Lal, H. (1998). Pharmacological treatment of alcoholism. *Progress in Neuro-Psychopharmacology and Biological Psychiatry, 22*(6), 917–944.

Gawin, F. H., Khalsa, M. E., & Ellinwood, Jr., E. (1994). Stimulants. In M.

Galanter & H. D. Kleber (Eds.), *Textbook of Substance Abuse Treatment* (pp. 111–139). Washington, DC: American Psychiatric Press.

Geller, A. (1997). Comprehensive treatment programs. In J. H. Lowinson, P. Ruiz, R. B. Millman, & J. G. Langrod (Eds.), *Substance Abuse: A Comprehensive Textbook* (3rd ed., pp. 425–429). Baltimore: Williams & Wilkins.

Gerstein, D. R., et al. (1997). *National Treatment Improvement Evaluation Study (NTIES) Final Report.* Rockville, MD: Center for Substance Abuse Treatment.

Gerstein, D. R., Johnson, R. A., Harwood, H., Fountain, D., Suter, N., & Malloy, K. (1994). *Evaluating Recovery Services: The California Drug and Alcohol Treatment Assessment (CALDATA).* Sacramento, CA: California Department of Alcohol and Drug Programs (Executive Summary: Publication No. ADP94–628). (Copies of study available by calling 916/327–3728.)

Goodman, A. (1997). Sexual addiction. In J. H. Lowinson, P. Ruiz, R. B. Millman, & J. G. Langrod (Eds.), *Substance Abuse: A Comprehensive Textbook* (3rd ed., pp. 340–354). Baltimore: Williams & Wilkins.

Gorski, T. T. (1993). *Addictive Relationships: Why Love Goes Wrong in Recovery.* Independence, MO: Herald House/ Independence Press.

Grinrod, R. (1840, 1886). *Bacchus: An Essay on the Nature, Causes, Effects and Cure of Intemperance.* Columbus, OH: J&H Miller.

Harden, B., & Swardson, A. (1996, March 4). Addiction: Are states preying on the vulnerable? *Washington Post,* p.A1.

Hayner, G., Galloway, G., & Wiehl, W. O. (1993). Haight Ashbury Free Clinics' drug detoxification protocols - Part 3: benzodiazepines and other sedative-hypnotics. *Journal of Psychoactive Drugs, 25*(4), 331–335.

Heather, N. (1989). Brief intervention strategies. In R. K. Hester & W. R. Miller (Eds.), *Handbook of Alcoholism Treatment Approaches* (pp. 93–116). Boston: Allyn and Bacon.

Heinemann, A. W. (1993). An introduction to substance abuse and physical disability. In A. W. Heineman (Ed.), *Substance Abuse & Physical Disability* (pp. 3–9), Binghamton, NY: The Haworth Press, Inc.

Heinemann, A. W. (1997). Persons with disabilities. In J. H. Lowinson, P. Ruiz, R.

B. Millman, & J. G. Langrod (Eds.), *Substance Abuse: A Comprehensive Textbook* (3rd ed., pp. 716–724). Baltimore: Williams & Wilkins.

Hird, S., Khuri, E. T., Dusenbury, L., & Millman, R. B. (1997). Adolescents. In J. H. Lowinson, P. Ruiz, R. B. Millman, & J. G. Langrod (Eds.), *Substance Abuse: A Comprehensive Textbook* (3rd ed., pp. 683–692). Baltimore: Williams & Wilkins.

Horvath, A. T. (1997). Alternative support groups. In J. H. Lowinson, P. Ruiz, R. B. Millman, & J. G. Langrod (Eds.), *Substance Abuse: A Comprehensive Textbook* (3rd ed., pp. 390–395). Baltimore: Williams & Wilkins.

Hubbard, R. L., Craddock, S. G., Flynn, P. M., Anderson, J., & Etheridge, R. M. (1997). Overview of one-year follow-up outcomes in DATOS. *Psychology of Addictive Behavior, 11.*

Hughes, T. L., & Wilsnack, S. C. (1997). Use of alcohol among lesbians. *American Journal of Orthopsychiatry, 678*(1), 20–36.

Ibanez, A., Blanco, C., Donahue, E., et al. (2001). Psychiatric comorbidity in pathological gamblers seeking treatment. *American Journal of Psychiatry, 158,* 1733–1735.

Institute of Medicine. (1990). Treating drug problems (Vol. 1). Washington, DC: The National Academies Press [Online]. Available: *http://books.nap.edu/books/ 0309042852/html/index.html*

Johnson, V. E. (1986). *Intervention.* Minneapolis, MN: Johnson Institute Books.

Keane, T. M., et al. (1984). *Journal of Clinical Psychology, 40,* 340.

Keane, T. M., & Fuller, R. K. (1986). *Journal of the American Medical Association, 256,* 1449.

Kelly, J. (Ed.) (1991). *San Francisco Lesbian, Gay And Bisexual Alcohol And Other Drugs Needs Assessment Study: Vol. I.* Sacramento, CA: EMT Associates, Inc.

Kendler, K. S., Jacobson, K. C., Prescott, C. A., & Neale, M. C. (2003). Specificity of genetic and environmental risk factors for use and abuse/dependence of cannabis, cocaine, hallucinogens, sedatives, stimulants, and opiates in male twins. *American Journal of Psychiatry 160,* 687–695.

Kessler, R. C., McGonagle, K. A., Zhao, S., et al. (1994). Lifetime and 12-month prevalence of DSM-II-R psychiatric disorders in the United States. Results from the National Comorbidity Survey.

Archives of General Psychiatry, 51, 8–19.

Kettler, B. (2003, February 5). Methadone cuts will spur crime. *Medford Mail Tribune,* p.1A.

Kominars, S. B. (1995). Homophobia: The heart of the darkness. In R. J. Kus (Ed.), *Addiction and Recovery in Gay and Lesbian Persons.* New York: Harrington Park Press.

Lewis, J. A., Dana, R. Q., & Blevins, G. A. (1994). *Substance Abuse Counseling.* (2nd ed.). Pacific Grove, CA: Brooks/ Cole Publishing Company.

Liepman, M. R. (1998). The family in addiction. In A. W. Graham & T. K. Schultz (Eds.), *Principles of Addiction Medicine* (2nd ed., pp. 1093–1110). Chevy Chase, MD: American Society of Addiction Medicine, Inc.

Lorenzi, P., et al. (1999). Searching for a general anaesthesia protocol for rapid detoxification from opioids. *European Journal of Anaesthesiology, 10,* 719–727.

Lowinson, J. H., Payte, J. T., Salsitz, E. A., Joseph, H., Marlon, I. J., & Dole, V. P. (1997). Methadone maintenance. In J. H. Lowinson, P. Ruiz, R. B. Millman, & J. G. Langrod (Eds.), *Substance Abuse: A Comprehensive Textbook* (3rd ed., pp. 405–414). Baltimore: Williams & Wilkins.

Mahon, N. (1997). Treatment in prisons and jails. In J. H. Lowinson, P. Ruiz, R. B. Millman, & J. G. Langrod (Eds.), *Substance Abuse: A Comprehensive Textbook* (3rd ed., pp. 455–457). Baltimore: Williams & Wilkins.

Marlatt, G. A. (1995). Relapse prevention: Theoretical rational and overview of the model. In G. A. Marlatt & J. Gorden (Eds.), *Relapse Prevention: A Self-Control Strategy in the Maintenance of Behavior Change.* New York: Guilford Publications.

Marlatt, G. A., & Tapert, S. F. (1993). Harm reduction: Reducing the risks of addictive behaviors. In J. S. Baer, G. A. Marlatt, & R. J. McMahon (Eds.), *Addictive Behaviors Across the Lifespan* (pp. 243–271). Newbury Park, CA: Sage Publications.

Mason, B. J., Ritvo, E. C., Morgan, R. O., et al. (1994). A double-blind, placebo-controlled pilot study to evaluate the efficacy and safety of oral nalmefene HCL for alcohol dependence. *Alcoholism, 18,* 1162–1167.

Mathias, R. (1999). The basics of brain imaging. *NIDA Notes, 11*(5).

McClellan, A. T., Grissom, G. R., Zanis, D., Randall, M., Brill, P., & O'Brien, C. P. (1997). Problem-service "matching" in addiction treatment: A prospective study in four programs. *Archives of General Psychiatry, 54*, 730–735.

McElroy, S. L., et al. (2003). Topiramate in the treatment of binge eating disorder associated with obesity: A randomized, placebo-controlled trial. *American Journal of Psychiatry, 160*, 255–261.

McElroy, S. L., Soutullo, C. A., & Goldsmith, R. J. (1998). Other impulse control disorders. In A. W. Graham & T. K. Schultz (Eds.), *Principles of Addiction Medicine* (2nd ed.). Chevy Chase, MD: American Society of Addiction Medicine, Inc.

Mecca, A. M. (1997). Blending policy and research: The California outcomes study. *Journal of Psychoactive Drugs, 29*(2), 161–164.

Mersy, D. J. (1991). Interventions for recovery in drug and alcohol addiction. In N. S. Miller (Ed.), *Comprehensive Handbook of Drug and Alcohol Addiction* (pp. 1063–1077). New York: Marcel Dekker, Inc.

Meuller, M. D. (1999). NIDA-supported researchers use brain imaging to deepen understanding of addiction. *NIDA Notes, 11*(5).

Meuller, M. D., & Wyman, J. R. (1997). Study sheds new light on the state of drug abuse treatment nationwide (DATOS). *NIDA Notes, 12*(5).

Michaels, S. (1996). The prevalence of homosexuality in the United States. In R. P. Cabaj & T. S. Stein (Eds.), *Textbook of Homosexuality and Mental Health* (pp. 43–63). Washington, DC: American Psychiatric Press.

Miller, W. R. (1998). Researching the spiritual dimensions of alcohol and other drug problems. *Addiction, 93*(7), 979–990.

Miller, W. R., & Hester, R. K. (1989). Treating alcohol problems: Toward an informed eclecticism. In R. K. Hester & W. R. Miller (Eds.), *Handbook of Alcoholism Treatment Approaches* (pp. 3–13). Boston: Allyn and Bacon.

Miller, W., & Rollnick, S. (2002). *Motivational Interviewing* (2nd ed.). New York: Guilford Publications.

Morris, S. (1995). *Harm reduction vs. disease model: Challenge for educators.* Presented at the conference of the International Coalition of Addiction Studies Educators (INCASE), Boston, MA.

Muffler, J., Langrod, J. G., Richardson, J. T., & Ruiz, P. (1997). Religion. In J. H. Lowinson, P. Ruiz, R. B. Millman, & J. G. Langrod (Eds.), *Substance Abuse: A Comprehensive Textbook* (3rd ed., pp. 492–295). Baltimore: Williams & Wilkins.

Nace, E. P. (1997). Alcoholics anonymous. In J. H. Lowinson, P. Ruiz, R. B. Millman, & J. G. Langrod (Eds.), *Substance Abuse: A Comprehensive Textbook* (3rd ed. pp. 383–389). Baltimore: Williams & Wilkins.

National Center on Addiction and Substance Abuse. (2001). Shoveling up: The impact of substance abuse on state budgets [Online]. Available: *http://www.casacolumbia.org/publications1456/publications_show.htm?doc_id=47299*

National Center on Addiction and Substance Abuse. (2003). Crossing the bridge: An evaluation of the drug treatment alternative-to-prison (DTAP) program [Online]. Available: *http://www.casacolumbia.org/usr_doc/Crossing_the_bridge_March2003.pdf*

National Criminal Justice Reference System. (2003). Drug court resources: Facts and figures [Online]. Available: *http://www.ncjrs.org/drug_courts/facts.html*

National Institute on Alcohol Abuse and Alcoholism. (2000). 10th special report to the U.S. Congress on alcohol and health. Bethesda, MD: U.S. Department of Health and Human Services, REP 023. [Online]. Available: *http://www.niaaa.nih.gov/publications/10report/intro.pdf*

National Institute on Drug Abuse. (1999). Principles of drug addiction treatment. NIH Publication No. 99-4180 [Online]. Available: *http://www.nida.nih.gov/PODAT/PODATindex.html*

National Institute on Drug Abuse. (2002a). Buprenorphine approval expands options for addiction treatment. *NIDA Notes, 17*(4).

National Institute on Drug Abuse. (2002b). Research report series – Therapeutic community. [Online]. Available: *http://www.drugabuse.gov/ResearchReports/Therapeutic/Therapeutic3.html*

National Institutes of Health. (1997). *Effective Medical Treatment of Heroin Addiction. NIH Consensus Statement.* Bethesda, MD: National Institutes of Health.

Netaddiction. (2000). What is Internet addiction? Center for online addiction [Online]. Available: *http://www.netaddiction.com/faqsindex.htm*

Nielsen, B., Nielsen, A. S., & Wrae, O. (1998). Patient-treatment matching improves compliance of alcoholics in outpatient treatment. *Journal of Nervous and Mental Disease, 186*(12), 752–760.

O'Boyle, M., & Brandon, E. A. (1998). Suicide attempts, substance abuse, and personality. *Journal of Substance Abuse Treatment, 15*(4), 353–356.

O'Brien, C. P. (1997). A range of research-based pharmacotherapies for addiction. *Science, 278*(5335), 66–70.

O'Farrell, T. J., & Cowles, K. S. (1989). Marital and family therapy. In R. K. Hester & W. R. Miller (Eds.), *Handbook of Alcoholism Treatment Approaches* (pp. 183–205). Boston: Allyn and Bacon.

O'Malley, S. S., Jaffe, A. J., Chang, G., Schottenfeld, R. S., Meyer, R. E., & Rounsaville, B. (1992). Naltrexone and coping skills therapy for alcohol dependence. *Archives of General Psychiatry, 49*, 881–887.

Office of National Drug Control Policy. (2001). Drug treatment in the criminal justice system [Online]. Available: *http://www.whitehousedrugpolicy.gov/publications/factsht/treatment/index.html*

Office of National Drug Control Policy. (2003). National drug control strategy: 2003 [Online]. Available: *http://www.whitehousedrugpolicy.gov/publications/policy/ndcs03/drug_related_data.pdf*

Payte, J. T. (1997) Methadone maintenance treatment: The first thirty years. *Journal of Psychoactive Drugs, 29*(2), 149–154.

Payte, J. T., & Zweben, J. E. (1998). Opioid maintenance therapies. In A. W. Graham & T. K. Schultz (Eds.), *Principles of Addiction Medicine* (2nd ed., pp. 557–570). Chevy Chase, MD: American Society of Addiction Medicine, Inc.

Peele, S. (1995). Controlled drinking versus abstinence. *Encyclopedia of Drugs and Alcohol* (Vol. 1, pp. 92–97). New York: Simon & Schuster Macmillan.

Perez-Arce, P., Carr, K. D., & Sorensen, J. L. (1993). Cultural issues in an outpatient program for stimulant abusers. *Journal of Psychoactive Drugs, 25*(1), 35–44.

Pharmacist Rehabilitation Organization. (1999). A checklist of symptoms leading to relapse. *Pharmacists Rehabilitation Organization Newsletter, 3*(1).

Prochaska, D. R., & Di Clemente, C. C. (1994). *Transtheoretical Approach: Crossing Traditional Boundaries of Therapy.* Melbourne, FL: Krieger Publishing Company.

Programs including nicotine addiction as part of treatment. (2001). *Alcoholism & Drug Abuse Weekly, 13*(38), 1–3.

Raine, A., Phil, D., Lencz, T., Bihrle, S., LaCasse, L., & Colletti, P. (2000). Reduced prefrontal gray matter volume and reduced autonomic activity in antisocial personality disorder. *Archives of General Psychiatry, 57*, 119–127.

Reid, M. S., Mickalian, J. D., Delucchi, K. L., Hall, S. M., & Berger, S. P. (1999). An acute dose of nicotine enhances cue-induced cocaine craving. *Drug and Alcohol Dependence, 49*, 95–104.

Reiger, D. A., Narrow, W. E., & Rae, D. S. (1999). *Unpublished National Institute of Mental Health (NIMH) analyses.*

Ricaurte, G. A., Seiden, L. S., & Schuster, C. R. (1984). Further evidence that amphetamines produce long-lasting dopamine neurochemical deficits by destroying dopamine nerve fibers. *Brain Research, 303*, 359–364.

Rose, J. E., Behm, F. M., Westman, E. C., et al. (1994). Mecamylamine combined with nicotine skin patch facilitates smoking cessation beyond nicotine patch treatment alone. *Clinical Trials Therapy, 56*, 86–99.

Ross, E. (2003, May 16). Epilepsy drug helps alcoholics quit drinking. *Medford Mail Tribune*, p. 1A.

Ruiz, P., & Langrod, J. G. (1997). Hispanic Americans. In J. H. Lowinson, P. Ruiz, R. B. Millman, & J. G. Langrod (Eds.), *Substance Abuse: A Comprehensive Textbook* (3rd ed., pp. 705–712). Baltimore: Williams & Wilkins.

Rustin, T. A. (1998). Management of nicotine withdrawal. In A. W. Graham & T. K. Schultz (Eds.), *Principles of Addiction Medicine* (2nd ed., pp. 571–582). Chevy Chase, MD: American Society of Addiction Medicine, Inc.

Saitz, R., Mulvey, K. P., Plough, A., & Samet, J. H. (1998). Physician unawareness of serious substance abuse. *American Journal of Drug and Alcohol Abuse, 23*(3), 343–354.

Schnoll, S. (1993). Prescription medication in rehabilitation. In A. W. Heineman (Ed.), *Substance Abuse & Physical Disability* (pp. 79–91). Binghamton, NY: The Haworth Press, Inc.

Schuckit, M. A. (1994). Goals of treatment. In M. Galanter & H. D. Kleber (Eds.), *Textbook of Substance Abuse Treatment*, (pp. 3–10). Washington, DC: American Psychiatric Press.

Schuckit, M. A. (2000). *Drug and Alcohol Abuse* (5th ed.). New York: Kluwer Academic/Plenum Publishers.

Schwetz, B. (2001). Labeling changes for Orlaam. *Journal of the American Medical Association, 285*(21).

Senft, R. A. (1991). Experience with clonidine-naltrexone for rapid opiate detoxification. *Journal of Substance Abuse Treatment, 8*(4), 257–259.

Sher, K. J. (1997). Psychological characteristics of children of alcoholics. *Alcohol Health & Research World, Children of Alcoholics, 21*(3), 247–254.

Shulman, A., Jagoda, J., Laycock, G., & Kelly, H. (1998). Calcium channel-blocking drugs in the management of drug dependence, withdrawal and craving. A clinical pilot study with niphedipine and verapamil. *Australian Family Physician, Supplement 1:S*, 19–24.

Simpson, D. D., Joe, G. W., Fletcher, B. W., et al. (1999). A national evaluation of treatment outcomes for cocaine dependence. *Archives of General Psychiatry, 57*(6), 507–514.

Skinner, W. F. (1994). Prevalence and demographic predictors of illicit drug use among lesbians and gay men. *American Journal of Public Health, 84*, 1307–1310.

Skinner, W. F., & Otis, M. D. (1996). Drug and alcohol use among lesbian and gay people in a Southern U. S. Sample. *Journal of Homosexuality, 30*(3), 59–62.

Smith, D. E., Buxton, M. E., Bilal, R., & Seymour, R. B. (1993). Cultural points of resistance to the 12-step recovery process. *Journal of Psychoactive Drugs, 25*(1), 97–108.

Smith, M. O., Brewington, V., Culliton, P., Lorenz, K., Ng, Y., Wen, H. I., & Lowinson, J. H. (1997). Acupuncture. In J. H. Lowinson, P. Ruiz, R. B. Millman, & J. G. Langrod (Eds.), *Substance Abuse: A Comprehensive Textbook* (3rd ed., pp. 484–492). Baltimore: Williams & Wilkins.

Snyder, E., et al. (1999). Human neural stem cells advance distant prospect of reseeding damaged brain. *Nature Biotechnology, 17*(1).

Steiner, R. P., May, D. L., & Davis, A. W. (1982). Acupuncture therapy for the treatment of tobacco smoking addiction. *American Journal of Chinese Medicine, 10*(1–4), 107–121.

Stevens-Smith, P., & Smith, R. L. (2000). *Substance Abuse Counseling: Theory & Practice* (2nd ed). Upper Saddle River, NJ: Prentice-Hall College Division.

Strain, E. C., Bigelow, G. E., Liebson, I. A., & Stitzer, M. L. (1999). Moderate vs. high-dose methadone in the treatment of opioid dependence. *Journal of the American Medical Association, 281*, 1000–1005.

Substance Abuse and Mental Health Services Administration. (2000). *Substance Abuse Treatment in Adult and Juvenile Correctional Facilities*. (DHHS Publication No. SMA DO-3380). Rockville, MD: Author.

Substance Abuse and Mental Health Services Administration. (2001). *A Provider's Introduction to Substance Abuse Treatment for Lesbian, Gay, Bisexual, and Transgender Individuals*. DHHS Publication No. (SMA) 01-3498). Rockville, MD: Center for Substance Abuse Treatment.

Substance Abuse and Mental Health Services Administration. (2002a). Communicating appropriately with Asian and Pacific Islander audiences [Online]. Available: *http://ncadi.samhsa.gov/govpubs/MS701/*

Substance Abuse and Mental Health Services Administration (2002b). National survey of substance abuse treatment services: N-SSATS: 2000 [Online]. Available: *http://wwwdasis.samhsa.gov/00nssats/nssats2000report.pdf*

Substance Abuse and Mental Health Services Administration. (2003a). 2001 National survey on drug abuse. Office of Applied Studies [Online]. Available: *http://www.samhsa.gov/oas/nhsda/2k1nhsda/vol1/toc.htm*

Substance Abuse and Mental Health Services Administration. (2003b). Treatment episode data sets 1992–2000. Office of Applied Studies [Online]. Available: *http://wwwdasis.samhsa.gov/teds00/2.1a.htm*

Thompson, G. H., & Hunter, D. A. (1998). Nicotine replacement therapy. *Annals of Pharmacotherapy, 32*(10), 1067–1075.

Trice, H. M. (1995). Alcoholics Anonymous. In D. B. Heath (Ed.), *Encyclopedia of Drugs and Alcohol* (Vol. 1, pp. 85–92). New York: Simon & Schuster Macmillan.

U.S. Census Bureau. (2003). Projections of the resident population by age, sex, race, and Hispanic origin [Online]. Available: *http://www.census.gov/population/projections/nation/detail/d2001_10.pdf*

U.S. Department of Justice. (2003a). Bureau of Justice statistics special report: Substance abuse and treatment, state and federal prisoners, 1998 [Online]. Available: *http://www.ojp.usdoj.gov/bjs/crimoff.htm#recidivism*

U.S. Department of Justice. (2003b). Prison statistics [Online]. Available: *http://www.ojp.usdoj.gov/bjs/prisons.htm*

U.S. Public Health Service. (1999). Mental health: A report of the Surgeon General [Online]. Available: *http://www.surgeongeneral.gov/library/mentalhealth/home.html*

Vaillant, G. E. (1995). *The Natural History of Alcoholism Revisited*. Cambridge, MA: Harvard University Press.

Vocci, F. (1999, October). *Medications in the pipeline*. Paper presented at the CSAM Conference, Addiction Medicine: State of the Art, Marina Del Rey, CA.

Volkow, N. D., Fowler, J. S., & Wang, G. (2003). The addicted brain: Insights from imaging studies. *The Journal of Clinical Investigation, 111*(10), 1444–1451.

Volpicelli, J. R., O'Brien , C., Alterman, A., & Hayashida, M. (1992). Naltrexone in the treatment of alcohol dependence. *Archives of General Psychiatry, 49*, 876.

Wen, H. L., & Cheung, S. Y. C. (1973). Treatment of drug addiction by acupuncture and electrical stimulation. *Asian Journal of Medicine, 9*, 23–24.

Westermeyer, J. (1997). Native Americans, Asians, and new immigrants. In J. H. Lowinson, P. Ruiz, R. B. Millman, & J. G. Langrod (Eds.), *Substance Abuse: A Comprehensive Textbook* (3rd ed., pp. 712–715). Baltimore: Williams & Wilkins.

White, W. L. (1998). *Slaying the Dragon: The History of Addiction Treatment and Recovery in America*. Bloomington, IL: Chestnut Health Systems/Lighthouse Institute.

Wiehl, W. O., Galloway, G., & Hayner, G. (1994). Haight Ashbury Free Clinics' drug detoxification protocols, Part 4: Alcohol. *Journal of Psychoactive Drugs, 26*(1), 57–59.

Windle, M. T. (1999). *Alcohol Use Among Adolescents*. Thousand Oaks, CA: Sage Publications.

Woody, G. E., Donnell, G. R., Seage, D., Metzger, M., Marmor, B. A., & Koblin, B. A. (1999). Non-injection substance use correlates with risky sex among men having sex with men. *Drug and Alcohol Dependence, 53*(3).

Mental Health & Drugs

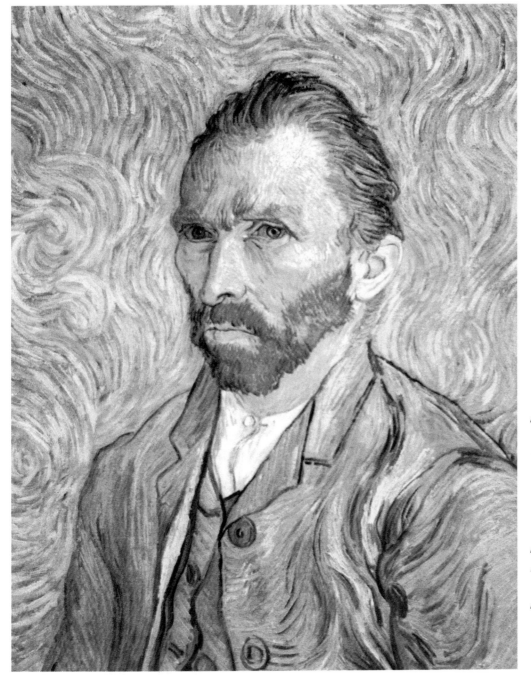

T he image of Vincent van Gogh was that of a person with mental illness and alcoholism who cut off his ear. Recently researchers at the University of California in Berkeley discovered that the liqueur absinthe, which contains the potent toxin alpha-thujone found in wormwood that can cause delirium, was partially responsible for his madness.

Musee D'Orsay, Paris.

MENTAL HEALTH & DRUGS

- **Introduction:** About one-third of adults with any mental disorder, such as depression, schizophrenia, bipolar disorder, or anxiety disorder, also have a co-occurring substance use disorder. Conversely between 50% and 70% of substance abusers also have a co-occurring mental disorder.
  - ◇ The neurotransmitters, receptor sites, and other brain mechanisms involved in mental and emotional problems and illnesses are the same ones affected by psychoactive drugs.
  - ◇ Substance-related disorders are divided into substance use disorders and substance-induced disorders.
- **Determining Factors:** Heredity, environment, and the use of psychoactive drugs affect mental health in much the same way as they affect drug use and addiction.

DUAL DIAGNOSIS (CO-OCCURRING DISORDERS)

- **Definition:** Dual diagnosis is the co-occurrence of an interrelated mental disorder and substance use disorder. The number of individuals suffering from both a substance abuse problem and a mental illness is growing. The decrease of inpatient mental facilities has magnified this problem.

- **Epidemiology:** There is a high incidence of mental imbalances among drug users and conversely many people with mental/emotional problems use drugs, often to self-medicate.

- **Patterns of Dual Diagnosis:** A mental illness can be preexisting or substance induced (temporary or permanent). Drug use can aggravate a mental illness or mask it.

- **Making the Diagnosis:** Because the direct effects as well as the withdrawal effects of drugs can mimic mental illnesses, initial diagnoses need to be "rule-out" diagnoses.

- **Mental Health vs. Substance Abuse:** The previous distrust between these two treatment communities has partly given way to cooperation and recognition of the duality of drug abuse and mental illness.

- **Psychiatric Disorders:** Thought (psychotic), affective, anxiety, and personality disorders are the most common psychiatric problems. These include schizophrenia, major depression, bipolar disorder, post-traumatic stress disorder, panic disorder, and borderline personality disorder.

- **Treatment:** Mental illness and substance-related disorders have to be treated simultaneously or treatment will not be effective. Treatment can include individual therapy, group therapy, self-help groups, and psychiatric medications. Treatment takes place in a variety of facilities from outpatient to residential.

- **Psychopharmacology:** Antidepressants, antipsychotics, mood stabilizers, and antianxiety drugs are the principal medications used to control mental illnesses.

The authors are indebted to Pablo Stewart, M.D., Chief of Psychiatry, Haight Ashbury Free Clinics, Associate Clinical Professor of Psychiatry, University of California, San Francisco, School of Medicine for his invaluable guidance and contributions in cowriting this chapter.

Surge in anti-psychotic drugs given to kids draws concern

By Karen Thomas
USA TODAY

An estimated half-million schoolki
now taking powerful anti-psychotic
— more than 10 times the number a
ade ago — and some experts worr
too many children are getting these
inappropriately to control aggressiv
havior.

About 532,000 children ages 6-1
taking these drugs

scribe them to children "off-label."
Driven by these new drugs, more than
33.5 million prescriptions were written for

■ **Tobacco**: Special programs
may be needed to

Strong medicine
Number of kids 6 to 18 who

about 500 children for one year.
A spokesman for Janssen Pharmaceu-

contained classrooms.
The report

Mentally Ill Twice as Likely to Be Smokers, Study Finds

previous research. And because people
with

morbidity Survey, was com-
early 1990s but is still appli-
se patterns of smoking and
tal illness have not changed

articipants answered ques-

said there appears to be a genetic tendency in some addicts that makes them
more likely to abuse an array of different
drugs. The link between other mental illnesses and cigarette smoking is also well-
known

pulse control and the ability to
personalize risk—all that much harder to
do when one's thinking is impaired by
mental illness.

However, the authors found that a siz-
able number of people with a history of
psychiatric disorders had been able to
quit smoking, though at a lower rate than
those who weren't mentally ill.

"This was

Inmates: Prison boom occurs as states abandon mental hospitals

Continued from Page One

when new antipsychotic drugs
made medicating patients in the
a humane alter

victed of murder, compared with
11.4 percent of other prisoners,
and 12.4 percent of mentally ill inmates had been convicted of sexual assault, compared with 7.9 per-

ed rates of mental illness varie
race and sex, with white an
male inmates reporting h
rates than African American
male inmates.

'P' Is for Preschoole and Proza

■ **Health**: The overprescri
of mood-altering drugs for
has gotten out of hand.

By ARIANNA HUFFINGTON

At a White House meeting on
with health and education c
Hillary Rodham Clinton tapped
growing national concern and
proposals for warning labels and
ranging study on the use of
"Some of these young people," s

Mentally ill could be forced into care

Davis signs bill to allow
involuntary treatment

By Robert Salladay
CHRONICLE SACRAMENTO BUREAU

Drug, alcohol abusers likelier to suffer mental ills, study says

By Alison Bass
BOSTON GLOBE

BOSTON — Researchers said
Wednesday that people who abuse
alcohol or drugs are much more
likely than nonabusers to suffer
from pre-existing mental disorders,
such as manic-depression, anxiety
and schizophrenia.

American Medical Association.
"If you get drug abusers detoxed
and sober but fail to recognize their
underlying depression, they are
much more likely to resume drugs,"
Goodwin said. "Conversely, if you
try to treat a manic-depressive person while that person is still actively using drugs, you can forget about
it. It won't work."

an underlying psychiatric disorder.
For example, teen-agers who
have a depressive or anxiety disorder are twice as likely to develop a
drug or alcohol problem later on,
suggesting that they may be drinking or taking drugs to ease their
psychological pain, Goodwin said.
While the connection between
mental illness and substance abuse

MENTAL HEALTH & DRUGS

INTRODUCTION

"I didn't think that I was a mentally ill person. I thought, 'Well, I'm a drug addict and I'm an alcoholic and if I don't drink and I don't use, then it should just be a simple matter of just changing my entire life; and I felt a little bit overwhelmed by the thought."
35-year-old man with major depression

Mental Health: A Report to the Surgeon General, released in December of 1999, states that **of the 40 million Americans who experience any mental disorder such as schizophrenia, major depression, bipolar disorder, an anxiety disorder, or a personality disorder in the course of a year, about 7–10 million also experience a substance-related disorder** (National Institute of Mental Health [NIMH], 1999; Regier et al., 1990).

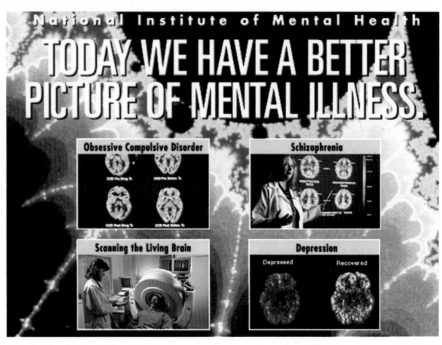

Diagnosis of mental illness has been as much an art as a science. With the advent of sophisticated imaging devices and measuring techniques, art and science have developed a more supportive partnership. This web site from the National Institute of Mental Health offers pictures of schizophrenia and other mental illnesses.
Courtesy of the National Institute of Mental Health

BRAIN CHEMISTRY

The interconnection between mental/emotional health and drug use is so pervasive that understanding this link gives a valuable insight into the functioning of the human mind at all levels. The reason for the link is that **the neurotransmitters affected by psychoactive drugs are the same ones involved in mental illness. Many people with mental problems are drawn to psychoactive drugs in an effort to rebalance their brain chemistry and control their agitation, depression, or other mental problems.** The opposite is also true. For some people who abuse drugs, their chemistry becomes unbalanced enough to aggravate a preexisting mental illness or mimic the symptoms of one (Barondes, 1993; Zimberg, 1999).

"I wound up preferring the heroin because I felt relaxed when I would snort it. I felt like I didn't have any troubles. I felt like I had some peace of mind and the drugs that were up, like speed and cocaine, made me feel really anxious."
Recovering drug abuser with major depression

This connection between mental health and drug use can be seen in the **similarity between the symptoms of psychiatric disorders and the direct effects of psychoactive drugs or their withdrawal effects**. For example,

◇ cocaine or amphetamine intoxication mimics mania, anxiety, or psychosis;

◇ cocaine or amphetamine withdrawal looks like major depressive disorder or generalized anxiety disorder;

◇ the manic effects of cocaine or amphetamine, followed by the exhaustion of withdrawal, mimic a bipolar illness that includes manic delusions and then depression;

◇ excessive use of alcohol causes a depressed mood, lack of interest in surroundings, and a disruptive sleep pattern characteristic of a major depressive disorder;

◇ psychedelic drugs, e.g., mescaline and LSD, mimic the delusional hallucinations associated with a psychotic disorder (Goldsmith & Ries, 1998).

CLASSIFICATION OF SUBSTANCE-RELATED DISORDERS

Substance-related disorders are classified in the *Diagnostic and Statistical Manual of Mental Disorders* (*DSM-IV-TR*) as mental disorders (American Psychiatric Association [APA], 2000). They are divided into 2 general categories:

1. **Substance use disorders** involve patterns of drug use and are divided into substance dependence and substance abuse. (Note that the word "addiction" is not used.)

   ◇ **Substance dependence** is defined in the *DSM-IV-TR* as "**a maladaptive pattern of substance use leading to clinically significant impairment or distress** as manifested by three or more of the following: tolerance, withdrawal, the need for larger amounts, unsuccessful efforts to cut down use, an expenditure of large amounts of time to get, use, and think about the drug, important social, employment, or recreational activities are limited or curtailed, and there is continued use despite adverse consequences."

   ◇ **Substance abuse** is defined as "recurrent substance use that results in disruption of work, school, or home obligations, recurrent use in physically hazardous situations, recurrent legal problems, and there is **continued use despite adverse consequences**."

2. **Substance-induced disorders** include **conditions that are caused by use of the specific substances**. These conditions usually disappear after a period of abstinence, however, some of the damage can last weeks, months, years, and even a lifetime. Substance-induced **disorders include intoxication, withdrawal, and certain mental disorders**, e.g., delirium, dementia, amnestic disorder, psychotic disorder, mood disorder, anxiety disorder, sexual dysfunction, and sleep disorder. The substances specifically defined in the *DSM-IV-TR* include alcohol, amphetamines, *Cannabis*, cocaine, hallucinogens, inhalants, opioids, PCP, and sedative-hypnotics.

DETERMINING FACTORS

The three main factors that affect the central nervous system's balance and therefore a human being's susceptibility to mental illness as well as addiction are heredity, environment, and the use of psychoactive drugs (Brady, Myrick, & Sonne, 1998; Brehm & Khantzian, 1997). For example, nearly every neurochemical system involved in depression is also found to be abnormal in substance use and substance-induced disorders (McDowell, 1999).

HEREDITY & MENTAL BALANCE

How does heredity affect our mental health? Research has already shown a **close link between heredity and schizophrenia, bipolar disorder, depression, and even anxiety**. The risk of a child developing schizophrenia is somewhere between 0.5% and 1% if the child has no close-order relatives with schizophrenia. On the other hand if the child has a close relative who has schizophrenia, the risk jumps 15–30-fold (Gottesman, 1991).

"My great uncle's got schizophrenia and my nephew's got schizophrenia. He's got it really bad because he can't control his fits. I didn't think about that growing up, only when I started hearing the voices. Then I thought, 'Hmm, just like my nephew.'"
28-year-old man with schizophrenia

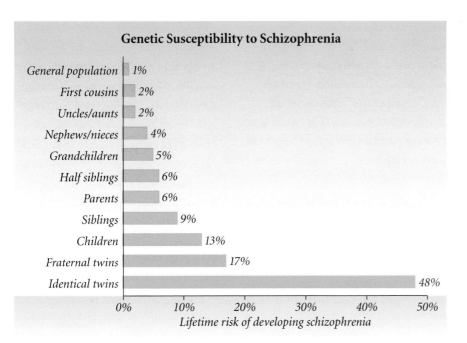

Figure 10-1 •

The risk of developing schizophrenia if a genetic relation has the disease varies with the number of shared genes. Second-degree relatives, such as nieces, only share 25% of one's genes, a parent shares 50%, and an identical twin shares 100% (Gottesman, 1991).

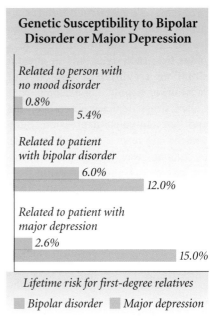

Figure 10-2 •

The risk of developing depression or bipolar disorder is greatly increased if a first-degree relative (parent, sibling, child) has the disease (Goodwin, 1990).

Some individuals are born with a brain chemistry that gives them a susceptibility to certain mental illnesses. **If the genetically susceptible brain chemistry is then stressed by a hostile environment or psychoactive drug use, then that person has an increased likelihood of developing mental illness.** If there is a very heavy genetic susceptibility, it may not take as severe an environmental stress. If there's a low genetic susceptibility, it will take a much stronger environmental or chemical stress to trigger the illness. Even if there is a high susceptibility with strong environmental stresses, mental illness may still not develop. The statistics show that even if there is a close relative with major depression, 5 out of 6 children or siblings will not develop that illness (Goodwin, 1990; Kendler & Diehl, 1993).

"In my family, my mom, my aunt, and my grandmother were diagnosed as manic-depressive [bipolar disorder]. It runs in the family. It didn't have

anything to do with drugs. It was just a lack of something in the brain."
16-year-old boy in treatment for bipolar illness

Genetic links for behavioral disorders, such as binge-eating disorder, compulsive gambling, and even attention-deficit disorder, have been found in twin surveys. Identical twins raised by two different sets of foster parents often exhibit the same character traits and behaviors regardless of their different environments (Zickler, 1999).

It is important to remember that heredity affects susceptibility to drug or behavioral addiction in much the same pattern that heredity affects susceptibility to mental illness. **A high genetic susceptibility does not mean that that mental illness or addiction will occur, only that there is a greater chance that it will occur.**

"Both my parents were alcoholics. My brother's an addict and alcoholic. I basically followed in my father's

footsteps—the drinking, the running around, losing wives, kids, all that."
38-year-old recovering alcoholic with major depression

The relationship between heredity, mental illness, and psychoactive drugs can be seen by examining the connections between the neurotransmitter dopamine, the drug cocaine, and schizophrenia. Heredity can affect the formation of dopamine receptor sites and the ability of the brain to produce dopamine. Schizophrenia seems to be caused in part by the brain having too much dopamine. Cocaine stimulates the release of dopamine, so long-term or high-dose use can induce a schizophrenic-like psychosis. With both the real psychosis and the drug-induced psychosis, excess dopamine seems to be a key element (Blum et al., 2000).

ENVIRONMENT & MENTAL BALANCE

The same environmental factors that can induce a susceptibility to drug abuse can induce mental/emotional problems. **The neurochemistry of people subject to extreme stress can be disrupted and unbalanced to a point that their reactions to normal situations are different than those of most other people.** For example, continued stress depletes norepinephrine and that can cause depression. Such persons may react to stressful situations by running away, falling apart, becoming extremely angry, or using psychoactive drugs. The stressors they respond to don't even have to be dramatic. They can merely be normal family expectations. For such individuals, mother saying, "It's eleven o'clock, I wish you'd get out of bed," can result in extreme anger that further disrupts the child's balance, thought processes, and, therefore, behavior (Barondes, 1993).

"My parents had a troubled marriage and they'd fight and argue and my mother would be beaten. I think maybe some of the rage and some of the anger manifested itself into the schizophrenia or just triggered it. After my schizophrenia became really prominent, I noticed that little things, like on-the-job stress, would get to me and I'd move on because it would trigger all sorts of problems."
28-year-old dually diagnosed client

Abuse and sexual molestation can be major negative environmental factors. Well over 50% of the young adults who are psychotic and have a problem with drugs experienced at least one form of abuse when they were children and the rate is much greater for women than for men. In addition over 75% of female addicts have suffered incest, molestation, or physical abuse as a child or adult (Zweben, 1996; Substance Abuse and Mental Health Services Administration [SAMHSA], 2002a).

"My dad beat my mom when he was under the influence of alcohol. He was an alcoholic. He also beat my older sister and me. When he came home, I was always running and hiding. A few years after he left the family, I was molested. I was screwed up but when I went into the service, I found that the marijuana and the heroin I abused in 'Nam kept my emotions under control."
Vietnam veteran with posttraumatic stress disorder

PSYCHOACTIVE DRUGS & MENTAL BALANCE

Along with heredity and environment, the use of psychoactive drugs can deplete, increase, mimic, or otherwise disrupt the neurochemistry of the brain. This disruption of brain chemistry can lead to mental illness, drug addiction, or both.

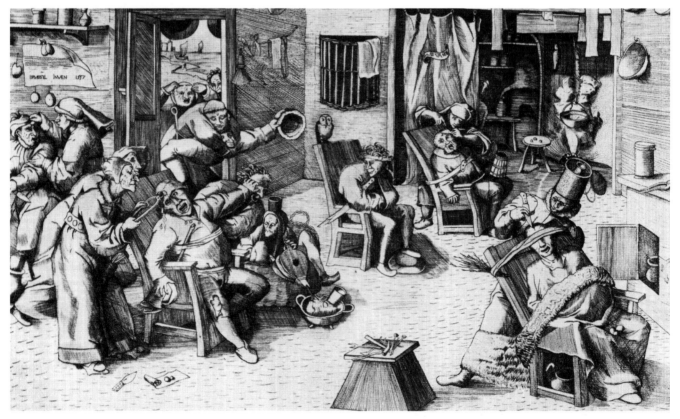

This illustration, The Extraction of the Stone of Madness *by Pieter Bruegal, the Elder, is a satire of ways to treat mental illness. It shows that even 300 years ago people thought that mental illness was caused by something physical inside the brain. Compare this to the modern view of many clinicians that mental illness can be treated by changing the neurochemistry inside the brain through psychotropic medications.*
Courtesy of the National Library of Medicine, Bethesda, MD

If a nervous system is impacted by enough psychoactive drugs, any individual may develop mental/emotional problems but it is the predisposed brain that is more likely to have prolonged or permanent difficulties. There is no set time for this to happen. The process may take years or, as in the case of psychedelic drugs, just one use can release an underlying psychopathology (Smith & Seymour, 2001). The brain that is not predisposed is the one most likely to return to its predrug functioning during abstinence.

"Apparently, through three generations of my family and our alcohol drinking or opium smoking, I inherited a tendency to manic depression that wouldn't awaken under just alcohol abuse. It took a more exotic drug, one that was a little bit beyond the range of a northern European family, to bring out my illness and that was marijuana."

45-year-old client with bipolar disorder

The type of drug has a great impact on symptoms of co-occurring disorders. For example, women with a dual diagnosis of cocaine abuse and post traumatic stress disorder (cocaine/PTSD) had greater occupational impairment, less monthly income, more legal problems (e.g. greater number of arrests for prostitution) and greater social impairment (e.g., fewer friends, unmarried) than those who had a PTSD/alcohol dual diagnosis. On the other hand, those with PTSD/alcohol dual diagnosis were more likely to have serious accidents and extraordinarily stressful life events. Rates of major depression and social phobia were also higher among this group than the cocaine/PTSD group (Back et al., 2003).

Every time a psychoactive substance enters the brain, it changes the equilibrium and the neurochemistry has to adjust. When exposure to that drug has ended, the brain does not always return to its original balance. For example, **a brain predisposed to major depression can aggravate that mental problem by heavy abuse of alcohol and sedative-hypnotics or withdrawal from stimulant drugs** (Drake & Mueser, 1996, 2002). **A brain predisposed toward schizophrenia can be activated and a psychotic episode triggered by psychedelic abuse.** One mental disorder, hallucinogen persisting perception disorder (HPPD), is marked by the transient recurrence of disturbances of perception (flashbacks) similar to those experienced while actually using a hallucinogen. The symptoms are disturbing and can cause impairment in everyday functioning. They may disappear in a few months or may last for years.

DUAL DIAGNOSIS (CO-OCCURRING DISORDERS)

DEFINITION

A growing number of chemically dependent individuals are under treatment for dual diagnosis. In this book, this is defined as "**the co-occurrence of an interrelated mental disorder and a substance use disorder**." What this means is that a cocaine user might also have a psychosis even when not using drugs. An alcoholic might have severe depression that persists even when clean and sober. A further example is the person with a preexisting attention-deficit/hyperactivity disorder (ADHD) who continually self-medicates his condition with methamphetamine.

Although the term "dual diagnosis" has been widely used in the substance abuse and mental health fields, other terms like "comorbidity," "double trouble," "substance abusing mentally ill" (SAMI), and "mentally ill chemical abuser" (MICA) have also been used. In the last few years the term "co-occurring disorders" has come into wide use (Evans & Sullivan, 1990; SAMHSA, 2002b). In this chapter we will use dual diagnosis and co-occurring disorders interchangeably.

"After more than 30 years of use, when I gave up the codeine and the Valium® in treatment, I started to remember the pain. You know the first thing that flashed through my mind was my uncle's face when he was hurting me real bad when I was 10. I hadn't remembered it for 32 years."

45-year-old woman with major depression

"The previous patient is a case where the diagnosis becomes clearer the longer she is clean and sober. She appears to have suffered from a major depressive disorder but there's also evidence of a posttraumatic stress disorder. The symptoms for the PTSD did not emerge until she was able to remain clean and sober for a period of time. Her treatment would necessarily include the simultaneous addressing of her substance abuse and mental health problems."

Pablo Stewart, M.D., Chief of Psychiatry, Haight Ashbury Free Clinics

The mental health conditions most often diagnosed as part of dual diagnosis fall into two categories: preexisting and substance induced. Examples of **preexisting mental disorders** are

◇ thought disorders (psychotic disorders), e.g., schizophrenia;

◇ mood disorders (affective disorders), e.g., major depressive disorder and bipolar disorder;

◇ anxiety disorders, e.g., panic disorders, obsessive-compulsive disorders, posttraumatic stress disorder, and ADHD.

(APA, 2000; Levin & Donovan, 1998; Lilenfield & Kaye, 1996; McElroy, Soutullo, & Goldsmith, 1998; O'Conner & Ziedonis, 1998; Salloum & Daley, 1994; Schuckit, 2000)

Examples of **substance-induced mental disorders** are

◇ stimulant-induced psychotic disorders;

◇ alcohol-induced mood disorders;

◇ marijuana-induced delirium.

"I have this illness, mental illness, with manic depression and when I take the alcohol, my functioning isn't as clear cut, not as sharp as say the average person who isn't suffering any mental problems."

52-year-old client with dual diagnosis

It is important to distinguish between having symptoms of mental illness and actually having a major psychiatric disorder. Everyone feels blue and sad sometimes. Everyone has the capacity for grief and loneliness but this does not mean that a person is medically depressed, requiring medication or psychiatric treatment. It's really a question of severity and persistence of these symptoms (Woody, 1996; Zimberg, 1999). The connection between substance abuse and mental disorders is real. One study found the chance of major depression combined with alcoholism in women was substantially higher and probably was mainly the result of genetic factors but environment still had an influence (Kendler, Heath, Neale, & Eaves, 1993).

It is common for people who are abusing substances to present with symptoms of a personality disorder particularly borderline or antisocial personality disorders. However as a person achieves and maintains sobriety, **the majority of the symptoms of the personality disorder will often dissipate** unless the person has a preexisting condition. There is much debate as to

the actual prevalence of personality disorders.

EPIDEMIOLOGY

In an earlier study published in *Journal of the American Medical Association (JAMA)*, **44% of alcohol abusers and 64.4% of other substance abusers actually admitted for treatment had, in addition to their drug problem, at least one serious mental illness** (Regier et al., 1990). Certain drugs increase the likelihood of mental illness. For example, three-fourths of cocaine abusers had a diagnosable mental disorder as did one-half of all compulsive marijuana users. The majority of the mental illnesses were caused by substances; however some were self-medicating their preexisting psychiatric disorders with street drugs (Kessler et al., 1994).

"I believe I had depression all along, even before I started using, and so through alcohol, marijuana, and even heroin, I was treating that depression."

24-year-old dual diagnosis client

Conversely 29–34% of all mentally ill people had a problem with either alcohol or other drugs (Regier et al., 1990; Merikangas, Stevens, & Fenton, 1996). The overlap is even greater with certain mental disorders. Sixty-one percent of people with manic-depressive illness and 47% of people with schizophrenia also had a problem with substance abuse. Finally, in prisons the prevalence of a psychiatric illness when the prisoner had an addictive disorder was a remarkable 81% (Beeder & Millman, 1997).

Unfortunately **of the 7–13 million people that do have co-occurring disorders**, about 23% received mental health care only, 9% received substance abuse treatment only, leaving just 8% that received both and 60% that received none (Watkins, Audrey, Kung, & Paddock, 2001).

PATTERNS OF DUAL DIAGNOSIS

Which substance is used and how it is used help determine the two general patterns of dual diagnosis.

PREEXISTING MENTAL ILLNESS

One kind of dual diagnosis involves **the person who has a clearly defined mental illness and then gets involved in drugs**, e.g., the teen with major depression who discovers amphetamines. Here the drugs are often used to self-medicate symptoms of the mental illness.

"My mom asked my little brother if he thought I'd been depressed a lot in my life and he said I'd been depressed ever since he could remember. The speed got me out of it except when I was coming down."

16-year-old boy

The presence of a preexisting mental illness does not prevent the user from developing a substance abuse condition. Therefore mentally ill people often have a concurrent substance abuse problem that does not involve self-medication. An example of this would be a schizophrenic who also suffers from alcoholism.

SUBSTANCE-INDUCED MENTAL ILLNESS

This type of dual diagnosis happens when there isn't a preexisting problem. However as a result of substance abuse and/or withdrawal, the user develops psychiatric problems because the toxic effects of the drug disrupt the brain chemistry (Ziedonis & Wyatt, 1998; Drake & Mueser, 1996). The imbalance in the brain chemistry in this type of diagnosis is usually temporary and with abstinence the mental illness will disappear within a few weeks to a year (Smith & Seymour, 2001). However, a significant number of these problems manifest as unresolved and chronic mental illnesses. This is more likely to occur in those with a preexisting susceptibility to mental illness.

"My initial flip out was in 1986 after snorting 'crank' for 6 weeks straight, about a half gram a day. I started hearing voices and thinking that my phones were tapped. Friends brought me to the psychiatric hospital where I was treated with antipsychotic medication. My diagnosis was methamphetamine-induced psychotic disorder."

28-year-old client

Substance-induced mental disorders include delirium, dementia, persisting amnestic disorder, psychotic disorder, mood disorder, anxiety disorder, sexual dysfunction, sleep disorder, and hallucinogen persisting perception disorder.

"This speed run's only been 13 days but I get these sores and I get paranoid and real crazy. After I come down it'll be weird. It will take weeks to get back into shape. And all that other crap will disappear."

43-year-old heavy IV methamphetamine addict

MAKING THE DIAGNOSIS

ASSESSMENT

When people see a relative or friend acting oddly and having trouble coping with everyday life over a prolonged period, they don't know whether they should ascribe that difficulty to relationship problems, trouble at home, drug use, or mental illness. Substance abuse and mental health professionals have the same problem, as is evident from the variations in diagnoses of the many mental health disorders cited above. Thus when assessing mental illness in a substance abuser, a general rule used by

treatment professionals is that **the initial diagnosis should be a "rule-out diagnosis." This means that several possible diagnoses will be considered during the period of assessment.**

"The doctor told me that a person who drank 25 years like me would probably take a year to clear. That was one reason that I never figured out that I was manic-depressive. I didn't notice it. I figured I was depressed because I was drunk all the time."

35-year-old man

Since many psychiatric symptoms can be the result of drug toxicity and or withdrawal, it is incorrect to immediately assume that all of these symptoms are due to a preexisting mental illness. **The prudent clinician addresses all symptoms but avoids making a specific psychiatric diagnosis until the drug abuser has had time to get sober** and beyond drug withdrawal (Senay, 1997; Shivani, Goldsmith, & Anthenelli, 2002).

"I was on opiates and antidepressants and I would have very severe respiratory problems at night, got no sleep, wanted to crawl out of my skin. I was paranoid. I thought that everybody was against me and it probably took me a good 2 weeks of being in treatment to be completely through withdrawals. The nice thing about coming into treatment is they do taper you. They help you through those first few days of withdrawal when you feel like you want to die."

38-year-old pharmaceutical opiate abuser

Factors that may influence the diagnosis include

◇ the particular pattern of substance use;
◇ the presence of a preexisting mental illness;
◇ the evidence of any self-medication;
◇ the age of onset of any psychiatric symptoms;

◇ the relationship of the psychiatric symptoms to the substance use.

Reasons for Increased Diagnoses

There are several possible reasons why the number of dually diagnosed clients on the streets seems dramatically higher in the 1990s and 2000s than during the '60s and '70s. These include

◇ the **diminishing number of inpatient mental health facilities** (Fig. 10-3) due to decreasing mental health budgets, decreasing mental health coverage by HMOs and other insurance programs, and occasionally misguided governmental policies on mental health support;

◇ the **proliferation of substances of abuse** particularly stimulants. Since strong stimulants are more toxic to brain chemistry than most substances, except inhalants and alcohol, those with fragile brain chemistry are more likely to be pushed over the edge into chronic neurochemical imbalance and mental illness (Keller & Dermatis, 1999);

◇ the **increasing number and greater expertise of licensed professionals** working in the field of chemical dependency treatment have resulted in a greater recognition and documentation of dual diagnosis;

◇ the **increasing awareness of substance abuse and its effects by mental health workers** has resulted in their increased recognition of it as an important co-occurring condition;

◇ finally, managed care and diagnosis-related group (DRG) payments for treatment services usually provide more financial incentives for the treatment of multiple medical and psychiatric problems than for just addiction treatment (Guydish & Muck, 1999). These **payment structures can pressure some clinicians to overdiagnose mental illness in the substance abuser**.

(Smith, Lawlor, & Seymour, 1996; Soderstrom et al., 1997)

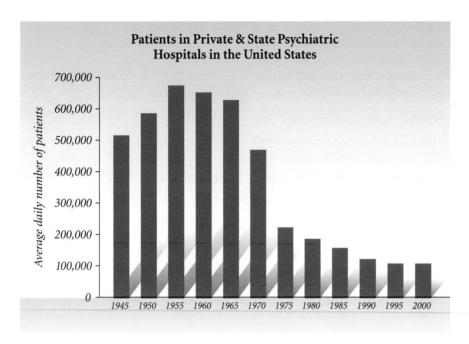

Patients in Private & State Psychiatric Hospitals in the United States

Average daily number of patients

Figure 10-3 •

The psychiatric hospital census has gone down while the number of people diagnosed with mental illnesses has gone up.

For these reasons an increasing number of people with psychiatric disorders have been forced to deal with their problems on an outpatient basis or on their own. Being detached from hospital supervision, clients are more likely to exhibit poor control of their prescribed medication thus aggravating their mental problems and making them more likely to turn to street drugs for help. All of these factors have also led to increases in mentally ill homeless people whose problems are exacerbated by the lack of a support system. The number of homeless in the United States in any given week is estimated at 500,000 to 600,000 (Rahav, Rivera, Nuttbrock, et al., 1995). Approximately one-half to two-thirds of this homeless population meet diagnostic criteria for substance dependence. Also **at least 25% of the total homeless population also suffer from preexisting mental illness. Of the mentally ill homeless, over 70% suffer from substance dependence** (Crome, 1999).

"I had used heroin to control my depression sort of as a mood stabilizer, so withdrawing from it caused an even worse depression. When I came out of the sort of fog from the first 5 days of not having it, I felt better but the pink cloud feeling vanished quite quickly and was replaced with the depression that I was used to."
Patient with major depression

UNDERSTANDING THE DUALLY DIAGNOSED PATIENT

Understanding and adapting to the treatment complexities of the client with a mental health problem and a substance abuse problem is a challenge for treatment professionals.

"When I went into the hospital, I would tell them I had a problem, that I was on Valium® and codeine. The first thing they would then give me was a shot of Valium®. I told them that Valium® addiction was one of my problems. They still gave it to me."
40-year-old dually diagnosed woman

In the past, inability to treat a person who manifested both substance abuse and mental problems, combined with an outright refusal to develop treatment strategies for the dually diag-

nosed client, resulted in inappropriate and potentially dangerous interactions with clients. **They were often shuffled aimlessly back and forth between the mental health care system and the substance abuse treatment system without receiving adequate treatment from either.** Even though there's been an increase in facilities that address the dually diagnosed client, inappropriate care is all too often still the rule rather than the exception. Budget considerations and lack of expertise have much to do with this problem.

Substance abuse treatment facilities do not usually want these patients because they see them as too disorganized and too disruptive or, in many cases, too inattentive to participate in group therapy, which is frequently the core element of treatment. **Psychiatric treatment centers also avoid these patients because they're perceived as substance abusers, disruptive, and manipulative.** They also frequently relapse into active substance abuse that interferes with medications used to treat mental illnesses (Wu, Kouzis, & Leaf, 1999).

MENTAL HEALTH VS. SUBSTANCE ABUSE

The following list contains 11 differences that have existed between the mental health (MH) treatment community and the substance abuse (SA) treatment community. While certain differences continue, these two communities are moving toward a closer working relationship. An increasing number of facilities employ both mental health and substance abuse treatment staff utilizing a team approach to treatment. They offer on-site treatment for the dually diagnosed client or at least provide a cross-referral team approach to a separate mental health treatment provider.

1. **MH used to say, "Control the underlying psychiatric problem and then the drug abuse will disappear." Substance abuse treat-**

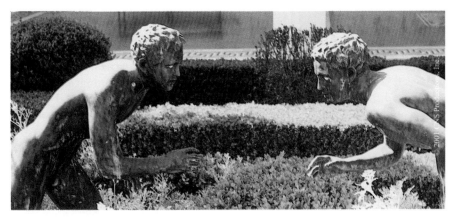

Courtesy of the Getty Museum.

● ●

ment providers used to say, "Get the patient clean and sober and the mental health problems will resolve themselves." While these statements have some validity, both disciplines are coming to recognize that perhaps one-third to three-fourths of their clients are legitimately dually diagnosed and require concurrent treatment of both the substance abuse and the mental health problems.

2. **In the MH system, partial recovery from one's problems is more readily acceptable** than in SA programs where most professionals believe that lifelong abstinence from all abused drugs is necessary, including alcohol and marijuana. This abstinence and a supporting program of recovery coupled with a rigorous SA treatment are necessary for ongoing recovery in a dual diagnosis client.

3. **Clients are more reluctant to seek help from the MH system than from SA treatment programs.** This is probably because of the stigma of mental illness. Clients and their families hope that the problem is only addiction from which they believe they can recover more fully than they can from mental illness.

"I tell members of my family that I'm in a halfway house for drug addiction as opposed to mental health because it seems with drug addiction, I can get

better but with mental health, people see it as a chronic long-term problem."
19-year-old dually diagnosed male with major depression

4. **MH relies more on medication to treat the client whereas SA programs tend to be divided between promoting a drug-free philosophy and substituting a less-damaging drug such as methadone in a harm reduction maintenance program.** Medically oriented SA programs, as opposed to social model SA programs, utilize medications to help clients detoxify before getting them into a long-term drug-free philosophy.

"I refused to take any psychiatric medication for a long time. I thought you had to be really crazy to take it and I thought that this was a big conflict that would limit my recovery. If I take medication, I'm a drug addict. But I'm glad I'm taking it now. I'm able to sleep and think better."
35-year-old client with major depression

5. **MH uses case management, shepherding clients from one service to another, whereas SA programs have traditionally emphasized self-reliance** because they neither want to enable clients nor make clients transfer their dependence to the program. In spite of that, case management is being

used in many SA treatment programs. Traditional SA treatment staff now utilize outside resources to provide a more holistic treatment approach. SA programs that do not have in-house mental health treatment capacity should refer their dually diagnosed clients to outside agencies to receive appropriate mental health care at the same time that they are in SA treatment.

6. **MH has traditionally utilized a supportive psychotherapeutic approach whereas many SA programs continue to use confrontation techniques** that many MH professionals think are inappropriate. A major conflict often occurs when a patient is not responding to traditional SA treatment because he also suffers from a psychiatric disorder. **One can't use the same behavioral threshold to terminate a dual diagnosis patient from treatment as one would with someone who only suffers from substance abuse.** In programs that provide dual diagnosis services, the staff needs to learn to recognize psychiatric symptoms that can often interfere with SA treatment. It is inappropriate to discharge patients from treatment who are psychiatrically unstable.

7. Both the MH system and the SA system have problems with sharing information because of confidentiality laws and regulations. In general however MH shares information with allied fields more readily than does SA.

8. In **MH the treatment team is composed of professionally prepared individuals**: social workers, nurses, psychiatrists, psychologists, and licensed counselors. **In some SA programs recovering substance abusers often make up the bulk of the treatment staff.** Personal recovery does not professionally prepare someone to treat substance abusers and most states now require special training and credentialing to be able to work

with addicts. All staff working with mentally ill substance abusers also require specialized professional preparation to adequately treat these difficult patients.

9. **MH relies on scientifically based treatment approaches. SA programs often rely on the philosophy "what works for me will work for you."** No longer can traditional SA treatment programs rely solely on self-experience and tradition. MH staff however can learn much from traditional SA treatment especially as it applies to spirituality in recovery.

"All I can tell someone is, 'I have a problem. I don't know which way you're going to deal with it or tackle it but I have a problem, and I can't function, and I need help.'"
Dual diagnosis patient with major depression

10. **MH pays a lot of attention to the idea of preventing the client from getting worse. In the past, SA programs, taking their cue from early 12-step fellowship beliefs, had a tendency to allow people to hit bottom in order to break through the denial of addiction.** Most SA programs now see that approach as outmoded and dangerous. They rely more on motivational interviewing to engage people in treatment. Motivational interviewing, a way to help people recognize and do something about their problems, is particularly useful with people who are reluctant to change or are ambivalent about changing (Miller & Rollnick, 2000; Swanson & Arthur, 2003). The dually diagnosed client needs support throughout the change process, much more so than the singly diagnosed client (Finnell, 2003).

11. **In MH, treatment is individualized. Many traditional SA programs tend to be one size fits all.** Best practices dictate that appropriate techniques from both disciplines be utilized with the dually

diagnosed patient since both conditions require simultaneous treatment. Traditional education approaches used in SA treatment need to be integrated into individualized mental health treatment plans.

While the situation may be improving from the perspective of the MH treatment community, dual diagnosis has represented an almost insurmountable challenge to the clinical expertise of the staff of SA programs. Their assessment skills and even their underlying concept of recovery or sobriety have been challenged by patients with a dual diagnosis. It can be difficult to differentiate preexisting mental illness from a substance-induced mental illness. **Patients are often misdiagnosed with mental illness early in the treatment or assessment processes resulting in patients being referred to MH programs that, all too often, then reject these individuals because of their concurrent SA problems.**

Substance abuse programs often resist developing the expertise needed to diagnose and treat MH problems. Fiscal and other limited resource problems prevent the expansion of their services to meet the needs of dually diagnosed clients, creating a tendency to establish MH problems as an exclusionary criteria for treatment admission or continued treatment in many SA programs. Even SA programs with expertise in this area often mistake psychoactive substance-induced mental illness for proof that there is an existing psychiatric diagnosis.

RECOMMENDATIONS

"Our consumers do not have the opportunity to separate their addiction from their mental illness, so why should we do so administratively and programmatically?"
(Osher, 2001)

Research over the past decade confirms that **the dually diagnosed patient must be treated for both disorders simultaneously**. They are best

treated **in a single program when appropriate resources are available** (Kosten & Ziedonis, 1997). Where programs equipped to handle dual diagnosis cases are not available, **SA programs need to establish linkages with MH service providers and vice versa** so that they can work together in providing the client with their combined treatment expertise. This is particularly important because when patients are admitted for treatment for psychiatric problems, they are more willing to acknowledge coexisting SA problems and more receptive to facing the need for additional treatment (RachBeisel, Dixon, & Gearon, 1999).

Each discipline needs to recognize that MH and SA treatment are both long-term propositions and therefore **they need to establish both short-term and long-range services to address the problems of dual diagnosis** (Minkoff & Regner, 1999). Recent research also suggests that incorporating behavioral (motivational) approaches to substance abuse treatment is more effective for the dually diagnosed client because the structure is better suited to overcoming cognitive difficulties that accompany schizophrenia and certain other mental illnesses (Drake, Mercer-McFadden, Mueser, McHugo, & Bond, 1998). Most importantly, some research has found that **intensive case management was associated with the greatest improvement in dually diagnosed clients**. A smaller but measurable improvement was also shown with standard aftercare and outpatient psychoeducational groups (Dumaine, 2003).

MULTIPLE DIAGNOSES

As the substance abuse treatment community becomes more aware of other simultaneous disorders that complicate the treatment of addiction, it must be must willing to accept new challenges such as

◇ multiple drug (polydrug) abuse;
◇ other medical disorders such as chronic pain syndrome, hepatitis, epilepsy, cancer, heart and kidney disease, diabetes, sickle cell anemia, and even sexual dysfunction;

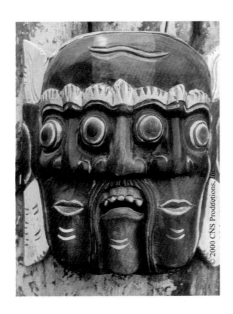

© 2000 CNS Productions, Inc.

◇ and triple diagnosis (dual diagnosis complicated by the presence of HIV disease).

"One of the biggest things that caused me the most anxiety is, you know, I'm HIV positive and I really started having problems with sleep. I found that out and I was really torn between cleaning up and staying clean or just going out and using. I felt like, 'Well, I'm going to die anyway, a nasty horrible death,' and I had nightmares and then my feelings surfaced to a point where a lot of other feelings came up about old stuff."
Recovering HIV-positive alcohol abuser with a general anxiety disorder

The literature is very clear that **a person must achieve sobriety from all drugs of abuse not just their drug of choice particularly when they are dually diagnosed**. This means that recovering heroin addicts, for example, need to refrain from alcohol and marijuana use even though they have never had a stated problem with these substances.

Research using the Addiction Severity Index links successful substance abuse treatment with addressing a person's medical problems. **Substance abuse treatment therefore must be linked to appropriate medical care in order for clients to achieve**

any degree of long-term sobriety. This includes the treatment of legitimate pain syndromes that may require treatment with narcotic analgesics. Substance abuse treatment programs need to creatively incorporate the treatment of legitimate pain syndromes into their overall treatment approaches.

Of special significance is the **epidemic growth of hepatitis C and other severe liver diseases in chemically dependent patients**. The prevalence of hepatitis C in IV drug users is now much greater than that of HIV emphasizing the need to avoid hepatotoxic drugs, especially alcohol.

In addition a variety of medical disabilities such as hearing or mobility impairment, social concerns including cultural attitudes toward chemical dependency and mental health treatment, and language barriers may also provide impediments to successful treatment of those with multiple diagnoses.

Although not a disability issue, women, particularly those who are pregnant and/or parenting, have special treatment needs. For example, women process psychiatric medications differently than men and will have higher plasma levels for a given dose of a prescribed drug and therefore need lower doses (Zweben, 1996). In addition programs that treat the pregnant woman's addiction or her mental illness are usually organized separately thus the pregnant addict with a mental illness can receive conflicting information (Grella, 1996). Finally the health risks to the fetus or newborn are greatly increased since both drug use and mental illness interfere with the normal nurturing qualities of the mother (Mallouh, 1996). **These problems require the development of future drug programs that are holistic, use several modalities, and are multidisciplinary** in order to meet the challenge of the evolving complicated clinical needs of the chemically dependent patient (Selwyn & Merino, 1997).

Triple diagnosis is defined as "the presence of an HIV infection in the dually diagnosed client." Persons with AIDS, an AIDS-related condition, an HIV-positive blood test who are a partner of someone with AIDS require

additional treatment expertise and specific services to effectively address their chemical dependency.

As the AIDS epidemic has progressed out of strictly gay and intravenous drug-using populations and into the cocaine- and other drug-using heterosexual populations, **triple diagnosis is straining health department resources and further complicating treatment** (Wechsberg et al., 1999).

"When we looked at the first 49 consecutive HIV-infected patients who came into our substance abuse services at San Francisco General Hospital, the bottom line was that 84% had some Axis I psychiatric diagnosis. A third had depressive disorders and another third had anxiety disorders. And 18% had organic brain syndromes, mild-to-moderate dementia, or organic psychosis."
Steven L. Batki, M.D., psychiatrist, Medical Director, SF General Hospital Substance Abuse Services

According to the National Treatment Improvement Evaluation Study (NTIES), **dually diagnosed patients were more likely to share a needle, have sex for money, have sex with an intravenous drug user, and report being raped** than someone with no psychiatric co-occurring disorder. Dually diagnosed clients should be targeted for more intense HIV interventions to avoid adding AIDS to their difficulties (Dausey & Desai, 2003).

NOTE: The following sections will examine the different kinds of psychiatric disorders; discuss the relationship between heredity, environment, and psychoactive drugs as related to mental illness and drug addiction; then examine the various treatments available for the mentally ill substance-abusing patient, particularly the use of psychotropic medications in therapy.

PSYCHIATRIC DISORDERS

"A neurotic is the person who builds a castle in the air. A psychotic is the

TABLE 10–1   BRAIN DISORDERS IN AMERICANS (1-YEAR PREVALENCE)

Diagnosis	Percent of Adults 18-54	Percent of Adults 55 & Up	Percent of Children & Adolescents
Schizophrenia	1.3%	0.6%	1.2%
Mood disorders	**7.1%**	**4.4%**	**6.2%**
bipolar I disorder	1.1%	0.2%	
major depressive episode	5.3%	3.8%	
unipolar major depression	5.3%	3.7%	
Anxiety disorders	**16.4%**	**11.4%**	**13.0%**
obsessive-compulsive disorder (OCD)	2.4%	1.5%	
panic disorder	1.6%	0.5%	
simple phobia	8.3%	7.3%	
posttraumatic stress disorder (PTSD)	3.6%	—	
agoraphobia	4.9%	4.1%	
Any brain disorder (one person might have multiple disorders)	**21.0%**	**19.8%**	**20.9%**

(NIMH, 1999; Shaffer, Fisher, Dulcan, et al., 1996)

person who lives in it. And a psychiatrist is the person who collects the rent."

Anonymous

Overall about 21% of the U.S. population is affected by mental disorders during a given year (Table 10-1). Anxiety disorders are the most prevalent followed by mood disorders (especially depression). Schizophrenia is extremely debilitating but occurs much less frequently than anxiety or mood disorders (NIMH, 1999).

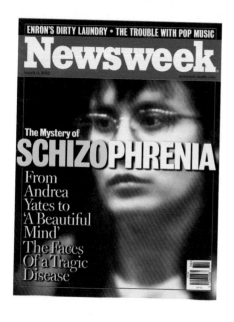

PREEXISTING MENTAL DISORDERS

Although there are hundreds of mental illnesses as classified by the mental health community, the following are the principal ones that are most often associated with dual diagnosis.

Thought Disorder (schizophrenia)

Schizophrenia is a chronic psychotic illness that affects approximately 1% of the population. There are many psychiatric illnesses that have psychotic symptoms as part of their presentation. These include but are not limited to schizoaffective disorder, bipolar disorder with psychotic features, major depressive disorder with psychotic features, delusional disorder, and substance-induced psychotic disorder.

A thought disorder such as schizophrenia is believed to be mostly inherited. It is characterized by

◇ **hallucinations** (false visual, auditory, or tactile sensations and perceptions);

◇ **delusions** (false beliefs);

◇ an **inappropriate affect** (an illogical emotional response to any situation);

◇ **ambivalence** (difficulty in making even the simplest decisions);

◇ **poor association** (difficulty in connecting thoughts and ideas);

◇ an **impaired ability to care for oneself**;

◇ autistic symptoms (a pronounced detachment from reality);

◇ poor job performance;

◇ strained social relations.

The signs have to be present for at least 6 months for the diagnosis to be made (APA, 2000).

"I was hearing voices, and the voices wouldn't go away, and they followed me wherever I went. I got into creating scenarios as to who they were and what they were doing."

28-year-old man with schizophrenia

Schizophrenia usually strikes individuals in their late teens to early adulthood and can be with them for life although occasionally there is spontaneous remission. Schizophrenia is extremely destructive to those with the illness as well as to their friends and families.

When diagnosing schizophrenia, clinicians try to determine which psychoactive drugs are being used by the patient. When these are not taken into consideration, clinicians may end up with a false or incomplete diagnosis. Clinicians can accomplish this assessment by taking a thorough medical history, interviewing close friends and family, or by using urinalysis or hair analysis. Unfortunately a large percentage of drug and alcohol problems are still missed.

Several abused drugs mimic schizophrenia and psychosis, producing symptoms that can be easily misdiagnosed.

◇ **Cocaine and amphetamines can cause a toxic psychosis** (especially when used to excess) that is almost indistinguishable from a true paranoid psychosis.

◇ **Steroids can also cause a psychosis.** Drug-induced paranoia can be indistinguishable from true paranoia.

◇ **Uppers**, such as MDMA (ecstasy) and related stimulant/hallucinogens, **and even marijuana can cause paranoia**.

◇ The **psychedelics**, such as LSD, peyote, psilocybin, and PCP, **disassociate users from their surroundings**, so hallucinogenic abuse can also be mistaken for a thought disorder.

◇ Also **withdrawal from downers can be mistaken for a thought disorder because of extreme agitation**.

Many of the drug-induced psychiatric symptoms should disappear as the body's drug levels subside upon detoxification and treatment (Senay, 1997, 1998; Delgado & Mereno, 1998).

Major Depressive Disorder

Mood disorders (affective disorders) include major depressive disorder, bipolar affective disorder, and dysthymia (mild depression). They are the second most prevalent psychiatric disorders after anxiety disorders. **Almost 15% of Americans will experience a major depressive disorder in their lifetime; 8.6% in any 1 yr. period** (Kessler et al., 2003). It has been estimated that depression costs employers $44 billion a year. Depressed people may make it to work but their performance is substandard. And although more Americans are seeking help for their depression, only one-fourth of the total are receiving adequate help (Stewart, Ricci, Chee, Hahn, & Morganstein, 2003).

Major depression is characterized by depressed mood, diminished interest and diminished pleasure in most activities, disturbances of sleep patterns and appetite, decreased ability to concentrate, feelings of worthlessness, and suicidal thoughts (APA, 2000). All of these symptoms may persist without any life situation to provoke them. For example, a patient with major depression may win a lot of money in a lottery and respond to it by staying depressed. For the diagnosis of major depression, **these feelings have to occur every day, most of the day, for at least 1 week running**. Causes such as medical illness or drug abuse would probably rule out a diagnosis of major depression as would natural reactions to the death of a loved one, a strained relationship, or divorce. These conditions however can cause the susceptible individual to develop major depression.

"The depression just came when it wanted to come. I just sat there and thought about something and I got depressed. The anger came because every male that has ever been in my life has beaten me or used me, you know, mentally and physically—not sexually thank goodness."
17-year-old boy with major depression

Excessive alcohol use, stimulant withdrawal (cocaine or amphetamine), and the comedown or resolution phase of a psychedelic (LSD, ecstasy) result in temporary drug-induced depression that is almost indistinguishable from that of major depression but will clear in time with the completion of withdrawal or comedown. Depression and/or anxiety found in substance abusers are, in about 80% of the cases, due to the drugs and not to a preexisting mental disorder (Nunes, Donovan, Brady, & Guitkin, 1994).

Bipolar Affective Disorder

Bipolar affective disorder (formerly called "manic depression") is **characterized by alternating periods of depression, normalcy, and mania**. The depression phase is described above. The depression is as severe as

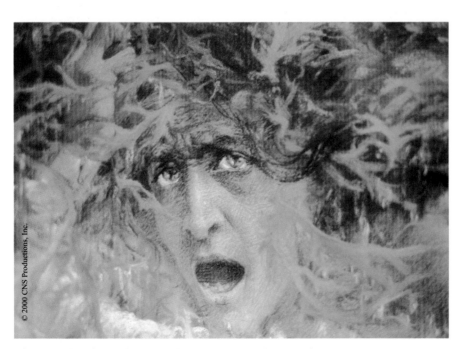

The Angry Wave by Lucien-Lévy Dhurmer. Musee D'Orsay, Paris.

that which occurs in major depression. If untreated, **many bipolar patients have frequent suicide attempts**.

The mania, on the other hand, is characterized by

◇ **a persistently elevated, expansive, and irritated mood;**

◇ **inflated self-esteem or grandiosity;**

◇ **decreased need for sleep;**

◇ **the pressure to keep talking** and being more talkative than usual;

◇ flight of ideas;

◇ distractibility;

◇ an increase in goal-directed activity or psychomotor agitation;

◇ **excessive involvement in pleasurable activities** that have a high potential for painful consequences (e.g., drug abuse, gambling, inappropriate sexual advances often leading to unsafe sex) (APA, 2000).

These symptoms can be severe enough to cause marked impairment in job, social activities, and relationships.

"The manic feeling is a real feeling of elation and euphoria. There's that grinding angry sort of—I don't really get angry and violent, well I did in jail, but I don't really want to hurt anybody or anything. And as far as being depressed goes, I can really say I've only been depressed about three times, once to the point of being suicidal."

30-year-old man with a bipolar disorder

Bipolar affective disorder usually begins in a person's 20s and affects men and women equally. Many researchers believe this disease is genetic in origin. **Toxic effects of stimulant or psychedelic abuse will often resemble a bipolar disorder.** Users experience swings from mania to depression depending upon the phase of the drug's action, the surroundings, and their own subconscious feelings and beliefs. More than half of those with a bipolar diagnosis (56%) had an alcohol use disorder (Regier et al., 1990; Sonne & Brady, 2002).

OTHER PSYCHIATRIC DISORDERS

Anxiety Disorders

Anxiety disorders are the most common psychiatric disturbances seen in medical offices. About 16% of adults (18–54 years old) will experience an anxiety disorder in a given year (NIMH, 1999). There are a number of anxiety disorders.

Posttraumatic stress disorder (PTSD). PTSD is a persistent reexperiencing of a traumatic event that involved actual or threatened death or serious injury (e.g., combat, sexual assault, motor vehicle accident). Associated symptoms include persistent avoidance of stimuli associated with the trauma and persistent symptoms of increased arousal, e.g., sleep problems, irritability, anger, and hypervigilance. This disorder can be chronic in nature and very disabling (Reilly, Clark, Shopshire, Lewis, & Sorensen, 1994). One study estimated that **20–25% of those in treatment for substance use disorders may have PTSD** (Brady, 1999). At Veteran's Administration (VA) hospitals, treatment centers, and domiciliaries, the incidence of PTSD among substance abusers is even higher (Ruzek, 2003). PTSD is twice as common in women as in men often due to physical and sexual abuse.

"I broke down after about 6 months over in Vietnam and I was in charge of a gun crew. And when I broke down from seeing the deaths and all the abuse over there, some people's lives were lost. I'm responsible and it hurts. When I was medically evacuated back to the States, I immediately jumped into alcohol and heroin."

50-year-old Vietnam veteran with PTSD

Panic disorder with and without agoraphobia (fear of open spaces). This is another common anxiety disorder. It consists of recurrent unexpected panic attacks. The person also has a persistent concern about having additional attacks, worries about the implications of having an attack, and changes behavior due to the attacks. **A panic attack is a discreet period of intense fear or discomfort in the absence of real danger** that is accompanied by at least 4 of 13 somatic or cognitive symptoms. These symptoms include palpitations, sweating, trembling or shaking, sensations of shortness of breath or smothering, feeling of choking, chest pain or discomfort, nausea or abdominal distress, dizziness or lightheadedness, derealization or depersonalization, fear of losing control or going crazy, fear of dying, paresthesias (numbness), and chills or hot flushes. The attack has a sudden onset and builds to a peak rapidly (usually in 10 minutes or less) and is often accompanied by a sense of imminent danger or impending doom and an urge to escape (APA, 2000).

"I'd be waiting for my prescription at a drugstore and someone would just look at me and all of a sudden, my whole body just went inside itself and I started shaking. My heart was racing. I couldn't say anything. I was just in total panic. I couldn't move. My mind kept saying there's nothing to be scared of but I couldn't control it. I had no idea what really triggered it. My husband would come up and hold me and sit there and say, "Breathe." And after a couple of minutes I would be all right and I would use one of my pills for anxiety, Lorazepam®, a benzodiazepine. I think that my use of cocaine over a period of several years messed up my neurochemistry, particularly my adrenaline system."

50-year-old woman with a panic disorder

Panic attacks can occur in someone who has a panic disorder, major depressive disorder, and a cardiac patient experiencing tachycardia. Panic attacks can also be induced by stimulants and marijuana.

Others anxiety disorders include

◇ **agoraphobia** without history of panic disorder (a generalized fear of open spaces);

◇ **social phobia** (fear of being seen by others acting in a humiliating or embarrassing way, e.g., fear of eating in public);

◇ **simple phobia** (irrational fear of a specific thing or place);

◇ **obsessive-compulsive disorder** (uncontrollable intrusive thoughts and irresistible often distressing actions, such as cutting one's hair or repeated hand washing).

"I had a number of obsessions. The obvious one right now is my hair. I cut my hair obsessively in a crew cut, constantly, by my own hand. The thought would just come into my mind. It was something I didn't really have control over. I would smoke marijuana almost as compulsively as I cut my hair."
Client with an obsessive-compulsive disorder

Generalized anxiety disorder (GAD). GAD is defined by unrealistic worry about several life situations that lasts for 6 months or longer. It is another common anxiety disorder along with several miscellaneous disorders such as acute stress disorder (APA, 2000).

Sometimes it is extremely difficult to differentiate the anxiety disorders. Many are defined more by symptoms than specific names. Some of the more common symptoms in anxiety disorders are shortness of breath, muscle tension, restlessness, stomach irritation, sweating, palpitations, hypervigilance, difficulty concentrating, and excessive worry. **Often anxiety and depression are mixed together.** Some physicians think that many anxiety disorders are really an outgrowth of depression (Gastfriend & Lillard, 1998).

Toxic effects of stimulant drugs and withdrawal from opioids, sedatives, and alcohol (downers) also cause symptoms similar to those described in anxiety disorders and can be easily misdiagnosed as such (Nunes et al., 1994). In one study of college students, the odds of having an anxiety disorder were much greater if alcohol abuse and dependence were present and the odds of having alcohol dependence were also greater if an anxiety disorder was present (Kushner, Sher, & Erickson, 1999).

Dementias

These are **problems of brain dysfunction brought on by physical changes in the brain** caused by aging, miscellaneous diseases, injury to the brain, or psychoactive drug toxicities. Alzheimer's disease in which older people suffer the unusually rapid death of brain cells, resulting in memory loss, confusion, loss of emotions, and gradually the ability to care for themselves is one example of this mental disorder. Mental confusion from heavy marijuana use and various prescription drugs may mimic symptoms of this disorder.

Developmental Disorders

These disorders, usually first diagnosed in infancy, childhood, or adolescence, include **mental retardation, autism, communication disorders, and attention-deficit/hyperactivity disorders.** (*See Chapter 3 for more information on ADHD.*) Heavy and frequent use of psychedelics like LSD or PCP can be mistaken for developmental disorders.

Somatoform Disorders

These disorders have **physical symptoms without a known or discoverable physical cause and are likely to be psychologically caused,** e.g., hypochondria (abnormal anxiety over one's health accompanied by imaginary symptoms). Cocaine, amphetamine, and other stimulant psychosis create a delusion that the user's skin is infested with bugs when no infestation exists.

Personality Disorders

These disorders, such as borderline personality disorder, are characterized by **inflexible behavioral patterns that lead to substantial distress or functional impairment.** Most of these patients with personality disorders act out, that is, exhibit behavioral patterns that have an angry hostile tone, that violate social conventions, and that result in negative consequences. **Anger is intrinsic to personality disorders as are chronic feelings of unhappiness and alienation from others, conflicts with authority, and family discord. These disorders frequently coexist with substance abuse** and are particularly hard to treat because of the acting out, which may include relapsing to drug use or creating a major disruption in their treatment setting (Smith & Seymour, 2001; Dimeoff, Comtois, & Linehan, 1998; Schuckit, 1986). In children and adolescents, conduct disorder and oppositional defiant disorder are predictors of alcohol and drug use problems (Clark, Vanyukov, & Cornelius, 2002).

Eating Disorders

Eating disorders (bulimia, anorexia, and binge-eating) often co-occur with substance use disorders and other psychiatric and personality disorders. A **weak impulse control is often found in eating disorders and substance use disorders,** a possible common etiology along with genetic factors for both conditions (Grillo, Sinha, & O'Malley, 2002). Eating disorders are often found in conjunction with major depression and PTSD (Dansky, Brewerton, & Kilpatrick, 2000).

Pathological Gambling

Pathological gambling, an impulse control disorder, is more common in clients who abuse or are dependent on alcohol. Gamblers will often drink in conjunction with their gambling trips to casinos or bars. Methamphetamine abuse is also found in many compulsive gamblers since it gives them the ability to remain in the casino or at a poker machine for long hours. Often though, a recovering alcoholic or addict will switch addictions and become just as pathological about gambling as he or she was about drinking or using other drugs (Grant, Kushner, & Kim, 2002).

Other Disorders

There are dozens of other mental disorders including adjustment disorders, sleep disorders, sexual and gender identity disorders, and factitious disorders that can exist independently or in combination with other mental disorders and drug use disorders.

SUBSTANCE-INDUCED MENTAL DISORDERS

Among patients who suffer from a dual diagnosis **the majority of the mental health problems encountered are caused by substance use rather than it being a preexisting mental disorder**. As mentioned, a clinically sound approach in dealing with these patients is to first assume their mental illness is substance induced until proven otherwise (Shivani et al., 2002).

Alcohol-Induced Mental Illness

Impulse Control Problems. People who abuse alcohol often demonstrate impulse control problems. These problems include but are not limited to **violence, suicide, unsafe sex, and other high-risk behaviors**. These behaviors are not due to an independent impulse control disorder if they only occur in the context of alcohol use.

Sleep Disorders. Sleep problems are a common symptom that clinicians use to establish the presence of a mental disorder. Alcohol, however, significantly contributes to a person's sleep problems. These include difficulty staying asleep as well as early morning awakening. Alcohol causes sleep problems due to its powerful suppression of REM sleep. **Sleep problems induced by alcohol can last for months after a person attains stabile sobriety.** If a person's sleep problems occur in the context of alcohol use, they may not indicate the presence of an independent mental disorder.

Anxiety. Alcohol is a minor tranquilizer that has antianxiety properties. However when a person's alcohol intake exceeds their body's ability to metabolize it, the person will then experience alcohol withdrawal upon cessation. **Symptoms of alcohol withdrawal include increased pulse rate, body temperature, and blood pressure as well as a variety of anxiety-like symptoms.** These alcohol-induced anxiety symptoms will dissipate over a period of 2–3 days. The clinician needs to take into consideration the patient's alcohol use prior to diagnosing an independent anxiety disorder.

Depression. **Studies indicate that up to 45% of alcoholics present with concurrent symptoms of major depressive disorder. However after a period of 4 weeks of sobriety, only 6% of alcoholics will persist with these depressive symptoms** (Brown & Schuckit, 1988). Therefore a clinician cannot make the diagnosis of major depressive disorder in a person who is drinking alcohol until they've had a period of at least 4 weeks of sobriety. There's conflicting data in the literature regarding the association between major depressive disorder and a history of alcoholism. Some authors suggest that recovering alcoholics are at 4-fold risk of developing major depressive disorder (Hasin & Grant, 2002). However, the mechanism of this association has not been identified. **Treatment with antidepressant medication is contraindicated in people who are drinking alcohol.**

"It's an egg and chicken situation because when I sober up I could say I was like a depressed personality. I have a problem of depression. Then I found that alcohol totally matched my needs. Then I drank a long time, so I start seeking stimulants. Then I found cocaine, it totally matched my needs. I think my problem comes first before my drug use but at first when I drank it was total self-medication for my depression.
34-year-old female with major depression

Psychosis. This clinical syndrome is marked by the **development of psychotic symptoms after many decades of heavy drinking**. These symptoms exist in the absence of intoxication and withdrawal. This syndrome has gone by a variety of names in the past with the most current one being **"alcohol-induced psychotic disorder."** Any and all psychotic symptoms can be seen with this disorder. These include but are not limited to auditory and visual hallucinations, delusional thought content, and ideas of reference. Of note, alcohol-induced psychotic disorder is extremely sensitive to treatment with antipsychotic medication. The actual mechanism is unclear. Clinicians should be cautioned to avoid the use of antipsychotic medication during periods of acute alcohol withdrawal. Conversely, alcohol use disorder is the most common co-occurring disorder found in clients with schizophrenia (Drake & Mueser, 2002).

Dementia. The neurotoxic effects of alcohol are well-established. Alcohol abuse is capable of causing a dementia-like syndrome with prominent cognitive deficits. Alcohol-induced dementia can mimic other similar conditions such as Alzheimer's disease. Even in its most severe form **the patient with alcohol-induced dementia can regain some cognitive functioning in sobriety**. This process may take up to a year to occur. The clinician should be mindful that patients in early recovery from alcoholism will often present with severe memory problems that can interfere with their treatment. Thoughtful clinicians need to be aware of this fact and modify their treatment approaches accordingly.

Stimulant-Induced Mental Illness

Impulse Control Problems. As is seen with alcohol abuse, stimulant abusers also demonstrate impulse control problems. These behaviors are not due to an independent impulse control disorder if they only occur in the context of stimulant use.

Mania. The person who is acutely intoxicated with stimulants can present in an identical fashion as someone who is in the acute manic phase of a bipolar disorder. The clinician should be cautioned to not assume that this manic-like behavior is solely attributable to a bipolar disorder if it only occurs in the context of stimulant abuse. **If the manic-like symptoms are solely due to stimulant intoxication, they will completely resolve upon cessation of the period of intoxication.** Antimanic medications such as depakote or lithium are not indicated for stimulant-induced manic disorder; rather this syndrome is best treated by helping the patient achieve stable abstinence.

Panic Disorder. The use of **stimulants can induce a panic attack**. This panic focus in the brain increases in size each time a person has a stimulant-induced panic attack. (Panic focus is that part of your brain from which panic attacks originate. Excess drug use turns neighboring cells into more panic cells. It is very similar to what is called a "seizure focus.") At a certain point, which is unique to the individual, this panic focus can take on a life of its own—**a person can go on to have a chronic panic disorder even if they never use stimulants again.**

Depression. Depression is caused by an imbalance of neurotransmitters, like serotonin, in the brain. Stimulant drugs, such as methamphetamine, cause a temporary imbalance of these neurochemicals. **This imbalance can last up to 10 weeks after a person stops using stimulants.** During this period the person will present with depressed mood, anhedonia (lack of ability to feel pleasure), suicidality, anxiety, and sleep disturbance, symptoms that are identical to those of someone suffering from a major depressive disorder. **If the symptoms of depression are caused by stimulant abuse alone, antidepressants may help with the symptoms only during the initial detoxification phase** of treatment and probably should not be continued on a long-term basis as in the treatment of

major depression. The proper treatment approach for those people who are suffering from stimulant-induced mood disorder is monitoring their suicidality while engaging them in substance abuse treatment.

In the early days of the crack cocaine epidemic in the mid-1980s, there was great enthusiasm for the use of antidepressants to treat stimulant abuse. The initial reports were very promising. However when this treatment approach was studied in a double-blind manner, the initial benefits were not replicated.

Anxiety. As with alcohol-induced anxiety, this can also be induced by stimulant abuse. These **stimulant-induced anxiety disorders occur both in the context of acute intoxication and withdrawal**. Again, the proper treatment of stimulant-induced anxiety includes engaging people in substance abuse treatment.

Psychosis. It is a well-known medical fact that stimulants are capable of causing both short-term and long-term psychotic symptoms. Not everyone who abuses stimulants will experience psychotic symptoms. **Those individuals who do experience psychotic symptoms will almost surely reexperience those same symptoms each time they use and as abuse continues, the duration of the effects will increase.** Medical literature (especially from Japan that has had many stimulant epidemics) reports that psychotic symptoms can last up to 5 years after cessation of use. Although this 5-year figure represents one end of the spectrum, it is certainly **common for people to experience psychotic symptoms for many months after cessation of stimulant abuse**. Proper treatment includes the use of antipsychotic medications in these individuals. The exact dosing and duration of treatment with antipsychotic medications depends on the severity of the stimulant-induced psychotic disorder.

Cognitive Impairment. With the advent of high-tech neuroimaging, in-

vestigators have been able to demonstrate that **stimulant abuse causes both transient and permanent damage to the brain**. This brain damage is thought to be responsible for the cognitive impairment often seen in stimulant abusers.

Marijuana-Induced Mental Illness

In many circles marijuana is felt to be a benign substance. Upon closer scrutiny, however, marijuana has been shown to be a potent psychoactive substance. This is especially problematic given the fact of the easy availability of higher-potency marijuana. **The higher concentration of the active ingredient THC is thought to be responsible for the psychiatric syndromes noted in marijuana users.**

Delirium. The use of the term "delirium" is often connected to a person who is ranting and raving; however, the essential feature of a marijuana-induced delirium is a **disturbance of consciousness that is accompanied by a change in cognition** that cannot be better accounted for by a preexisting or evolving dementia. Most people who are suffering from a delirium are not readily recognizable by the general public or by the clinician who's not adept at diagnosing subtle neurocognitive problems. This is also true of the person who's experiencing the delirium. Marijuana is thought to be responsible for causing delirium in chronic users. This delirium looks like the typical "stoner" (people who use marijuana on a regular basis) who is spaced out, detached, and oblivious to the world around them. These individuals often have **difficulty with memory, multistep tasking and other simple cognitive processes.** The current thinking is that it **may take up to 3 months or even longer for this delirium to clear after a person stops using marijuana.**

Psychosis. Again, due in part to the high concentrations of THC currently available, it is not uncommon for people to experience psychotic symptoms while intoxicated on marijuana. These include but are not limited to **paranoia and auditory and visual hallucinations.** Fortunately these **symptoms tend to be transient and only occur while a person is intoxicated on marijuana.** However there are increased reports of hallucinogen persisting perceptual disorder (HPPD) occurring in marijuana abusers with symptoms lasting for several months even though there is no further exposure to the substance. If the psychotic symptoms persist after a person has stopped using marijuana, then the clinician should be alerted to consider alternate explanations for the psychotic symptoms.

Panic. As with stimulant abuse, **marijuana is capable of inducing a panic attack while intoxicated.** However the role of marijuana in causing a chronic panic disorder, as is seen in stimulant abuse, has not been studied. It would follow that people who continue to experience marijuana-induced panic attacks would increase the size of the panic focus.

Amotivational Syndrome. As stated in Chapter 6 the traditional notion is that marijuana makes you unmotivated. The reality of this is still unclear. **Does marijuana make you amotivational or do amotivational people tend to smoke marijuana?** To date there have not been any good scientific studies explaining the relationship between marijuana and amotivational syndrome.

Other Drug-Induced Mental Illnesses

Most psychoactive substances are capable of inducing transitory or more enduring psychiatric syndromes. But remember, the incidence of substance-induced psychiatric symptoms is much greater than the incidence of preexisting psychiatric problems (and symptoms). Of particular concern lately is the emergence of psychiatric syndromes secondary to the psycho-stimulant MDMA (ecstasy). Although this has not been rigorously studied to date, it appears that ecstasy can cause both mood and psychotic problems in susceptible individuals. Symptoms of serotonin syndrome should be considered.

TREATMENT

The close association of unbalanced brain chemistry in mental illness with the distorting brain effects of heredity, environment, and psychoactive drug use suggests that **treatment of mental illness and/or addiction should be directed towards rebalancing brain chemistry.**

REBALANCING BRAIN CHEMISTRY

Heredity & Treatment

As of yet, we cannot alter a person's genetic code. As of yet, we can't change a person with alcoholic marker genes that signal a susceptibility to alcoholism, drug addiction, or other addictive behavior. As of yet, we can't decrease the genetic vulnerability of a teenager with a mother and grandmother who have schizophrenia. **We can however alert some people that they are more at risk for a certain mental illness, drug addiction, or other compulsive behavior due to their heredity** (Blum et al., 2000). Hopefully current research in gene therapy that is aimed towards altering genetic factors will be a giant step in controlling inherited mental illnesses. We are getting closer and closer to being able to manipulate individual genes (gene therapy).

Environment & Treatment

Since we currently aren't able to correct heredity, **we can attempt to improve the environment thereby influencing brain chemistry.** If people change where and how they live, they can avoid those stressors and environmental cues that keep them in a state of turmoil, continually unbalance their neurochemistry, and make them more likely to abuse drugs thereby intensifying their mental illness. People can leave an abusive relationship, avoid their drug-using associates, get enough sleep, avoid situations that make them angry, seek out new friends in self-help groups to avoid isolation, and make sure they get good nutrition.

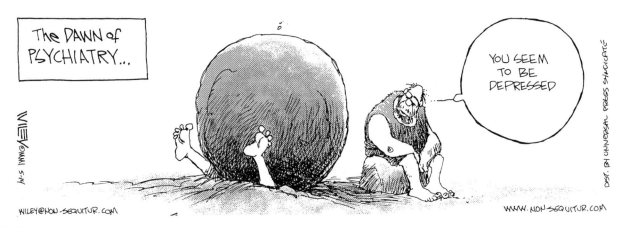

Psychoactive Drugs & Treatment

We are currently **in the midst of a psychopharmacologic revolution**. Outstanding new treatments are available to patients to alleviate their suffering. It is imperative that all **substance abuse treatment providers familiarize themselves with the basics of psychopharmacology as it is the cornerstone for mental health treatment**. This notion may be contrary to the beliefs of many people who have been in the field for a while; however the success of many of these therapies may help people let go of some of their prejudices regarding psychopharmacology.

Oftentimes patients will use self-prescribed substances to treat their mental illness.

"I took both alcohol and lithium for my manic depression. The difference is that one is faster working. The alcohol works quickly, the lithium takes time to get there. But the alcohol caused other problems in my life in addition to my depression. I think I'll stick to the lithium."

52-year-old woman

There is an **ever-expanding group of drugs called "psychotropic" or "psychiatric" medications (e.g., antidepressants, antipsychotics or neuroleptics, antianxiety drugs)** that are prescribed by physicians to try to counteract neurochemical imbalance caused by mental illness or addiction and that help the dually diagnosed client lead a less-destructive life. (The various psychotropic medications will be examined in detail later.)

Starting Treatment

With many dually diagnosed clients, it is hard to know where to start treatment. Do you start treating the mental illness or the addiction or do you treat them simultaneously right from the beginning? Best practice currently is to address both problems simultaneously; that is to **stabilize both the substance and mental health**

problems in an attempt to make the most accurate assessment possible. This means acute stabilization of the homicidal or suicidal patient as well as detoxification from drug dependence. It should be noted however that formal treatment can only proceed after a thorough diagnostic assessment.

"It is often difficult to know where to start with a dually diagnosed patient. Upon initial evaluation it is almost impossible to know which came first, the substance abuse or mental illness. My approach to these very difficult patients is to assume that all psychiatric symptoms are substance induced until proven otherwise."

Pablo Stewart, M.D., Chief of Psychiatry, Haight Ashbury Free Clinics

Impaired Cognition

A very common but underappreciated condition of dually diagnosed clients is significant cognitive impairment. Unfortunately many clinicians involved in treatment believe that once dually diagnosed individuals put down the booze or drugs, they should be able to engage in treatment but that's not always the case. A study of a number of dually diagnosed clients at a public hospital found that the majority were mildly-to-severely cognitively impaired and that they had difficulty participating in treatment. Reviewing screening exams on neurocognitive function at a VA hospital, researchers found that approximately 50% of the patients were mildly-to-severely impaired (Blume, Davis, & Schmaling, 1999).

For the treatment provider, what this means is the patient often appears normal but is suffering from significant cognitive impairment. For example they can repeat what they hear but the information and therapy don't sink in. **It may take weeks or months after detoxification for reasoning, memory, and thinking to come back to a point where the dually diagnosed individual can begin to fully engage in treatment.** As the patient remains in treatment, treatment techniques have to

be tailored to the person's ability to process the information that the doctor and staff are providing.

Developmental Arrest

Drug abuse and mental illness often result in the arresting of emotional development. Take the case of a young man in his late teens or early 20s who's fully grown and intelligent but has been using drugs since the age of 12 and has also had emotional and mental problems. This type of patient comes to treatment with all kinds of difficulties. One of the worst problems is that he's suffered developmental arrest at age 12, the point where most people begin to work through issues and stresses in their lives. Most people mature through all the struggles and go on to become adults but those who use drugs, who have avoided difficult emotions, and have not gone through that process of maturation will still experience all the emotions that they avoided 5 or 6 years ago.

"It's all those issues as a child that I seemed to take into my adulthood and they come out. I'd get my buttons pressed. Someone gets me a little pissed off. You know, I really thought when I came into recovery I wouldn't be angry anymore. Well it took me almost 3 years in treatment to realize that anger is a legitimate feeling. It's how I deal with it today and how I used to deal with it. That's what I'm learning about."

30-year-old dually diagnosed client

What happens is that **many dually diagnosed clients have the character traits that are normal in children but abnormal in adults thus making treatment extremely difficult.** Dr. Burt Pepper, a psychiatrist who treats young dually diagnosed clients, lists 11 of these characteristics.

1. They have a **low frustration tolerance**.

2. They **can't work persistently for a goal** without constant encourage-

ment and guidance, partially because of their low tolerance for frustration.

3. They **lie to avoid punishment**.

4. They have mixed feelings about independence and dependence and then, feeling hostile about dependency, they test limits.

5. **They test limits constantly** because they haven't learned them yet or have rejected them.

6. **Their feelings are expressed as behaviors.** They cry, run away, and hit rather than talk, reason, explain, or apologize.

7. **They have a shallow labile affect that means a shallowness of mood.** Give a kid a toy, they laugh; take it away, they cry.

8. They have a **fear of being rejected**. Extreme rejection sensitivity can even be expressed as paranoid schizophrenia.

9. Some live in the present only but most of the older teens or young adults live in the past. **Most dually diagnosed clients have no hope for the future** possibly because they remember the past too well or have trouble thinking.

10. **Denial is a common characteristic in young children.** One form is a refusal to deal with unpleasant but necessary duties. Another form is an unwillingness to stop something that's pleasurable, like kids playing roughhouse until one gets hurt badly.

11. **They have the feeling, "Either you're for me or against me,"** a black and white approach to every judgment in life, with no modulation or moderation.

These characteristics are also very common in people being treated solely for chemical dependency. What this situation suggests is that developmental assessment must be performed on clients; that is **treatment providers need to appreciate where a person is in their developmental process and address treatment accordingly**. An example might be that a person was un-able to establish basic trust, a developmental step that is usually accomplished in early childhood. Treatment would have to be directed to help this person establish basic trust before addressing more-advanced developmental issues.

The above difficulties are all chronic or even lifelong problems that cannot be treated with short-term therapy. **These are problems of living, of living sober, and of living with the symptoms of the mental illness.** The best treatment consists of addressing all of those issues that the individual client brings into the treatment setting. These issues are unique to any given client and must be addressed in an individualized manner.

Psychotherapy, Individual Counseling, & Group Therapy

"Look into the depths of your own soul and learn first to know yourself, then you will understand why this illness was bound to come upon you and perhaps you will thenceforth avoid falling ill."
Sigmund Freud, 1924

Psychotherapy is a very effective way of treating both a person's mental illness and substance abuse illness. Psychotherapy can be applied in either an individual or a group manner. **Group therapy has become the standard for substance abuse and mental illness treatments** (Zweben, 1998). The exact strategies for employing psychotherapy for mental illness is not the focus of this chapter.

The therapist should be cautioned however that **the primary treatment of severe mental illness is psychopharmacology and not psychotherapy**. Patients are often allowed to suffer needlessly during the course of psychotherapy when they actually need medication. This is not to imply that the clinician doesn't talk to the patient while they're being stabilized on medication.

In the recent past the psychotherapeutic approach for substance abuse disorders focused on working through the substance abuser's denial. It was strongly believed that a person could not get clean and sober if they did not deal with the denial about their illness. Although this psychotherapeutic strategy was very appealing to clinicians, it did little for the substance abuser. Current thinking regarding the proper use of psychotherapy in substance use disorders includes a **phase model**.

The first phase of a psychotherapeutic approach for a dually diagnosed client is achieving abstinence. This is at least a 6-month period where the therapist would emphasize supportive psychotherapeutic techniques. These techniques would include relapse prevention work, education on stress reduction and mental illness, and abstinence psychotherapy. The wise therapist would avoid confronting the patient with their denial during this phase.

The next phase is called "maintaining abstinence." This period occurs after the patient has between 6 and 24 months of sobriety. It is during this phase that the therapist would begin to introduce notions of denial and other maladaptive defense mechanisms.

At the end of this period the psychotherapy for **the substance abuser would be indistinguishable from any other psychodynamically oriented treatment** except for the increased emphasis on education and abstinence from addictive drugs. (Davis, Klar, & Coyle, 1991; Zimberg, 1994).

PSYCHOPHAR-MACOLOGY

The field of medicine that addresses the use of medications to help correct or help control mental illnesses and drug addiction is called "psychopharmacology." The scope of this branch of medicine has grown rapidly in the last 15 years producing hundreds of new medications and greatly expanding this approach to mental illness.

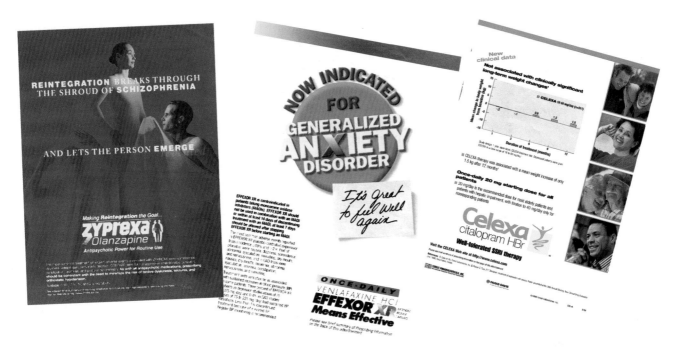

Zyprexa®, an antipsychotic; Effexor®, an antianxiety drug; and Celexa®, an antidepressant are widely used, often due to an abundance of advertising.

Quite often the dual diagnosis patient does need medication for psychiatric disorders, such as **antidepressants and mood stabilizers for mood disorders, antipsychotic (neuroleptic) medications for thought disorders, and antianxiety medications for anxiety disorders.** These medications should only be prescribed after a thorough assessment has been accomplished. Care should also be taken in the use of these medications given the individual's difficulty in dealing with drugs. The clinician has to make sure the medication used for the psychiatric problem does not aggravate or complicate the substance abuse problem.

Medications are used on a short-term, medium-term, or even lifetime basis to try to rebalance the brain chemistry that has become unbalanced either through hereditary anomalies, environmental stress, and/or the use of psychoactive drugs and compulsive behaviors. These medications are used in conjunction with individual or group therapy and with lifestyle changes.

Previously one of the biggest debates in treatment centers was about the reliance upon psychiatric medications. Some clinicians looked at medications only as a last resort. Others felt that they should be the first step in treatment. Due to recent advances in the mental and substance abuse fields, psychiatric medications are much more acceptable to treatment providers.

The various **psychiatric medications currently in use affect the manner in which neurotransmitters work** in different ways.

◇ They can increase the presynaptic release of neurotransmitters (methylphenidate).

◇ They can block the neurotransmitter from connecting with a given receptor site (antipsychotics).

◇ They can inhibit the reuptake of neurotransmitters by the presynaptic neuron thus increasing the amount of neurotransmitter available in the synapse (SSRIs such as Prozac® and Zoloft® work this way on serotonin).

◇ They can inhibit the metabolism of neurotransmitters (Nardil® and MAO inhibitors) thereby enhancing the action of norepinephrine or dopamine.

◇ They can enhance the effect of existing neurotransmitters (benzodi-

azepines such as Valium® increase the effects of GABA).

Besides manipulating brain chemistry, **some drugs act directly to control symptoms**. For example, beta blockers (Inderal®) calm the sympathetic nervous system that controls heart rate, blood pressure, and other functions that can go out of control in a panic attack or drug withdrawal state.

One problem with psychiatric medications is that it's **very hard to design a drug that will only work on a certain neurotransmitter in a particular way**. Advances have occurred in this regard. For example, the new atypical antipsychotics are designed to work on the specific dopamine receptors involved in psychotic symptoms. However even with these advance medications, there is some overlap to dopamine receptors in other parts of the central nervous system not involved in the psychotic process. Therefore there will always be side effects even to these newer medications. **It is imperative to constantly monitor each patient's reactions to the drug and adjust the dose accordingly.** A careful explanation of the drug along with possible side effects and a specific plan of use should be fully explained to each patient.

"The medication that we are talking about giving you in this treatment program is really designed to correct some of the damage that you did to your body and to your mind with the drugs or damage that had been happening as a result of some emotional or psychological problem. It does not mean you're sick, it does not mean you're defective, and it does not mean you're weak. It just means that your biochemistry somehow got out of balance and the medications that we're recommending, especially the antidepressant medications, are to rebalance those chemicals and bring you to a point where you can fully and effectively function and then begin to work on your other problems."

Stanley Yantis, M.D., psychiatrist – consulting with a dual-diagnosed client

PSYCHIATRIC MEDICATIONS VS. STREET DRUGS

One of the advantages of physician-prescribed medications over street drugs is that generally, except for the benzodiazepines and stimulants, they are not addicting. In fact **the treatment of anxiety, depression, and other mental problems through psychiatric medications can relieve many of the reasons and triggers for drug abuse**. A study of the risk of substance use disorders in boys who were treated with methylphenidate and other ADHD treatment drugs found a significant decrease in the risk of having drug use problems as adults compared to patients who were not treated (Biederman, Wilens, Mick, Spencer, & Farone, 1999).

Sometimes prescribing psychiatric medications can cause problems for dually diagnosed clients because they are often taught to stay away from all drugs during recovery. The treatment profession has developed and distributed pamphlets to the various recovery fellowships explaining the need for psychiatric medications by many dual diagnosis patients in recovery. Nevertheless there are well-meaning members of these fellowships who insist that no one taking these medications is really recovering. The patient may be talked into flushing his or her medicine down the toilet with potentially adverse psychiatric results. Consequently it is essential that those responsible for treating dual diagnosis clients who are in recovery understand and support those clients through the potential problems of early recovery (Buxton, Smith, & Seymour, 1987; Center for Substance Abuse Treatment, 1995; Alcoholics Anonymous, 1995).

When using street drugs, patients feel a false sense of control over which drugs they ingest, inject, or otherwise self-administer. The same patients, when receiving medication from a doctor, often express the feeling that they are not in control of their lives. Thus they are more apt to rely on street drugs rather than on psychiatric medications for relief of their emotional problems. It is up to the physician to work with the patient regarding any and all issues raised by the use of prescription medications.

"Before I came to the clinic, I thought that using antidepressants was taboo. I wanted to use street drugs but not any of these clinical ones. There's a stigma to it. I used marijuana to deal with my depression and I could take it when I felt I needed it, not a pill that I had to take every so often as prescribed by my psychiatrist."

35-year-old client with depression and a problem with marijuana

The following Table 10-2 is a compilation of many of the ideas that have been covered in these pages regarding the relationship between brain chemistry, drug addiction, and mental illness. When studying the table, notice how many different neurotransmitters are affected by a single street drug especially cocaine or alcohol. Also notice the physical and mental traits that are affected by a neurotransmitter and how a street drug affects those functions (Lavine, 1999; Physician's Desk Reference [PDR], 2003).

We will discuss the drugs under the heading of the mental illness that they are generally used to treat (Table 10-2). There is some overlap, for example, when a drug used for depression, such as Prozac®, is also used to treat obsessive-compulsive disorder or when an antidepressant is also used for bipolar disorder.

DRUGS USED TO TREAT DEPRESSION

Many in the psychiatric field feel that **depression is caused by an abnormality in the production of the neurotransmitters serotonin, norepinephrine (noradrenaline)**, plus a few others. Antidepressants are usually meant to increase the amount of serotonin or norepinephrine available to the brain to correct this imbalance. The number of people receiving outpatient treatment for depression has more than tripled since 1987. During that same period, the number of clients receiving psychotherapy dropped about 15%, so the primary treatment for those suffering from depression is medication rather than psychotherapy.

The newer antidepressants such as Prozac®, Paxil®, Zoloft®, Welbutrin®, Remeron®, Serzone®, Celexa®, and Effexor® work through a variety of mechanisms mostly by increasing the levels of certain neurotransmitters including serotonin, dopamine, and norepinephrine.

Selective Serotonin Reuptake Inhibitors (SSRIs)

Fuoxetine (Prozac®) was the first and most popular of the newer antidepressants and has received a large amount of publicity both pro and con since its release in 1988. It seems quite effective in the treatment of depression with fewer side effects than tricyclic antidepressants or the MAO inhibitors. It is also used to treat obsessive-compulsive disorder, panic disorder, and eating disorders.

Fluoxetine along with sertraline

TABLE 10–2   THE RELATIONSHIP BETWEEN NEUROTRANSMITTERS, THEIR FUNCTIONS, STREET DRUGS, MENTAL ILLNESS, & PSYCHIATRIC MEDICATIONS

COLUMN 1	COLUMN 2	COLUMN 3	COLUMN 4	COLUMN 5
Neurotransmitter	Normal Functions	Street Drugs That Disrupt the Neurotransmitter	Associated Mental Illnesses	Some Examples of Medications to Rebalance Neurotransmitters
Serotonin	Mood stability, appetite, sleep control, sexual activity aggression, self-esteem	Alcohol, nicotine, amphetamine, cocaine, PCP, LSD, MDMA (ecstasy)	Anxiety disorders e.g. PTSD, panic disorder, obsessive-compulsive disorder, generalized anxiety disorder; mood disorders, e.g., bipolar disorder, major depressive disorder, depression	Selective serotonin reuptake inhibitors (e.g. Prozac® Zoloft®, Paxil®, Celexa®), BuSpar®, Elavil®, Desyrel®
Dopamine	Muscle tone/control, motor behavior, energy, reward mech., attention span, pleasure, mental stability, hunger/ thirst/sexual satiation	Cocaine, nicotine, PCP, amphetamine, caffeine, LSD, marijuana, alcohol, opioid	Psychotic disorders, e.g., schizophrenia, schizoaffective disorder, Parkinson's disease	Antipsychotics, e.g. Risperdol®, L-dopa, amantadine , bromocryptine
Norepinephrine, epinephrine	Energy, motivation, eating, attention span, pleasure, heart rate, blood pressure, dilation of bronchi, assertiveness, alertness, confidence	Cocaine, nicotine, amphetamine, caffeine, marijuana, MDMA, 2CB, CBR	Anxiety disorders, mood disorders, narcolepsy	Bupropion, desipramine, methylphenidate, clonidine, beta blockers
Endorphin, enkephalin	Pain control, reward mechanism, stress control (physical and emotional)	Heroin, other opioids, PCP, alcohol, marijuana	Psychotic disorders, mood disorders	Methadone, LAAM, naltrexone, buprenorphine
GABA (gamma aminobutyric acid)	Inhibitor of many neurotransmitters, muscle relaxant, control of aggression, arousal	Alcohol, marijuana, barbiturates, PCP, benzodiazepines	Anxiety, sleep disorders, narcolepsy	Benzodiazepines, glutamine, THC
Acetylcholine	Memory, learning, muscular reflexes, aggression, attention, blood pressure, heart rate, sexual behavior, mental acuity, sleep, muscle control	Marijuana, nicotine, alcohol, PCP, cocaine, amphetamine, LSD	Alzheimer's disease, schizophrenia, tremors	Vistaril®, Artane®, Cogentin®, Benadryl®, tacrine (Cognes®), donepezil (Aricept®), rivastigmine (Exelon®), galantamine (Reminyl®)
Cortisone, corticotrophin	Immune system, healing, stress	Heroin, cocaine	Schizophrenia, depression, insomnia, anxiety	Corticosteroids (Prednisone®, cortisone), ACTH, cortisol
Histamine	Sleep, inflammation of tissues, stomach acid, secretion, allergic response	Antihistamines, opioids	Depressive illness	Antihistamines
Anandimide	Natural function is still unknown but several receptors still discovered	Marijuana	Not known	Marijuana antagonist (SR14176A)

(Zoloft®), citalopram (Celexa®), paroxetine (Paxil®), and fluvoxamine (Luvox®) are classified as selective serotonin reuptake inhibitors (SSRIs) that **increase the amount of serotonin available to the nervous system**. The amount needed to be effective varies widely from patient to patient and has to be adjusted. It generally takes 2–4 weeks for the full effect to be felt. The most common side effects are insomnia, nausea, diarrhea, headache, and nervousness. Most of the side effects are mild and will go away in a few weeks. Recently the Food and Drug Administration warned against the use of paroxetine (Paxil®) for those under age 18 due to increased risk of suicide. The drug is not approved for pediatric use but some physicians had been prescribing it anyway. However they did approve another SSRI, fluoxene (Prozac®), for pediatric use (U.S. Food and Drug Administration, 2003).

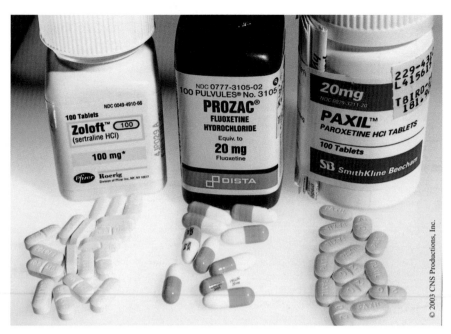

Three of the most widely used SSRI antidepressants are sertraline (Zoloft®), fluoxetine (Prozac®), and paroxetine (Paxil®).

One potential problem with SSRIs is that when used in conjunction with street drugs that stimulate the release of serotonin (e.g., methamphetamine), they can lead to what is called "**serotonin syndrome**." Caused by excess serotonin, the symptoms include elevated body temperature, shivering and tremors, mental changes, rigidity, autonomic nervous system instability, and occasionally death. The use of SSRIs by people who abuse stimulants (e.g. cocaine and amphetamine) can result in severe stimulant toxicity. By this we mean that people are much more susceptible to the medical and psychiatric side effects of the stimulants (e.g., convulsions, psychosis, severe manic-like behavior).

Tricyclic Antidepressants

Tricyclic antidepressants used to be the main drugs used to treat depression but over the last 15 years the newer antidepressants have proved to have fewer toxic effects and side effects resulting in their becoming the preferred medication.

Tricyclic antidepressants, such as imipramine (Tofranil®) and desipramine (Norpramine®), are thought to **block reabsorption of serotonin and norepinephrine by the sending neuron** thereby increasing the activity of those biochemicals at the receiving neuron. This blocking effect in turn **forces the synthesis of more receptor sites for these neurochemicals**. The delay in the creation of new receptor sites may account for the lag time in effecting a change in the patient's mood. It usually takes 2–6 weeks for a patient to respond to the drug therapy.

The tricyclics are very effective in treating patients with chronic symptoms of depression. People without depression do not get a lift from tricyclic antidepressants as they do with a stimulant. In fact most of these medications actually cause drowsiness.

"The antidepressants did not get me high as far as what I could feel. It wasn't like feeling drunk or stoned. You don't get that sensation. The high I got is more like a lift, a mood lift. It's the difference between being lethargic and sad or active and happy."

41-year-old man with depression

The tricyclic antidepressants, available mainly as pills, can be dangerous if taken in overdose. Careful monitoring of not only compliance by the patient with prescribed dosage but also **constant feedback from the patient as to the effects and side effects is also necessary**. Major side effects are dry mouth, blurred vision, inhibited urination, hypotension, and sleepiness (Zwillich, 1999).

"I went off antidepressants. And after a month, 6 weeks, I began getting depressed again but I had to be convinced that I was depressed again. And they said, 'You really should go back on medication' and I didn't want to admit that I didn't want to be on medication. I wanted to exist without it."

35-year-old patient with major depression

These drugs are also dangerous to the heart when mixed with street drugs or alcohol. Of note, tricyclics are rarely prescribed for depressive disorders due to the overwhelming superiority of the newer antidepressant medications.

Monamine Oxidase (MAO) Inhibitors

Monamine oxidase (MAO) inhibitors such as phenelzine (Nardil®), tranylcypromine (Parnate®), and isocarboxazid (Marplan®) are also used to treat depression. These very strong drugs **work by blocking an enzyme (monoamine oxidase) that metabolizes the neurotransmitters norepinephrine and serotonin. This in essence raises the level of these neurotransmitters.** Unfortunately MAO inhibitors have several potentially dangerous side effects, so care and close monitoring are necessary. They do give fairly quick relief from a major depression or panic disorder but the user has to be on a special diet and remain aware of the possibility of high blood pressure, headaches, and several other side effects. Combined use of MAO inhibitors with stimulants, depressants, and alcohol can be fatal. There are also a number of over-the-counter drugs that should not be taken with MAO inhibitors (PDR, 2003). As with the tricyclic antidepressants, the MAO inhibitors are rarely used due to the severity of their side effect profile.

Stimulants

In the past, amphetamine or amphetamine congeners including Dexedrine®, Biphetamine®, Desoxyn®, Ritalin®, and Cylert® were used to treat depression. They work by increasing the amount of norepinephrine and epinephrine in the central nervous system. They are mood elevators when used in moderation but the problem was that **since tolerance develops rapidly and the mood lift proved to be too alluring, misuse and addiction developed fairly rapidly**. The overuse led to various physical and mental problems such as agitation, aggression, paranoia, and psychosis. Stimulants are no longer indicated for the treatment of depression. Ritalin® is prescribed for patients with attention-deficit/hyperactivity disorder. In the recovering dually diagnosed client suffering from ADHD and a substance-abuse problem, stimulants are also contraindicated. Psychiatrists are now prescribing nonstimulant medication such as buproprion and atomoxetine (Strattera®) to treat ADHD.

DRUGS USED TO TREAT BIPOLAR DISORDER

The main drug used for the treatment of bipolar disorder over the last 30 years has been lithium. Other medications have been developed during this time that include carbamazapine (Tegretol®), valproic acid (Depakene®), divalpoex sodium (Depakote®), oxcarbozepine (Trileptal®), gabapentin (Neurontin®), and topirmate (Topamax®). Each of these medications is well-tolerated by patients and very effective in the treatment of bipolar disorder. However each of these medicines has a very distinct side effect profile and requires a thorough medical evaluation prior to initiation.

Lithium

Lithium is a naturally occurring mineral that helps stabilize both the highs and lows of bipolar disorder. It is more effective, however, in stabilizing the highs. Although it is generally safe, it carries with it some potentially serious medical side effects such as hypothyroidism and requires close medical monitoring. A patient can expect to see clinical improvement in as soon as 2 weeks after initiation of the medication. As with the other psychiatric medications, the use of street drugs and alcohol is contraindicated in patients being prescribed lithium.

"The way manic depression works, at least for me, is the medicine can control about 20% of it. The other 80% is me. I have to learn how to control my moods with my mind because the medication is only a small part."
40-year-old with bipolar disorder

The remaining drugs currently used to treat bipolar disorder are also antiseizure medications. As in seizure disorders, these medications help the bipolar patient by stabilizing their misfiring neurons. Each one of these medications has its own unique set of medical side effects, requires close monitoring, and like lithium should not be taken with street drugs or alcohol.

DRUGS USED TO TREAT PSYCHOSES (antipsychotics or neuroleptics)

In the early 1950s a new class of drugs, **phenothiazines, was found to be effective in controlling the symptoms of schizophrenia**. Some of the drugs such as Thorazine®, Mellaril®, Proloxin®, and Compazine® were initially referred to as major tranquilizers to differentiate them from barbiturates and benzodiazepines that were called "minor tranquilizers." More recently nonphenothiazines like Haldol®, Risperdal®, Zyprexa®, Clozaril®, Loxitane®, and Moban® have been developed and have become widely used. They act like phenothiazines and have similar side effects. Even newer antipsychotics are being developed. In 2002 aripiprazole (Abilify®), a dopa-

mine system stabilizer, was approved (Stahl, 2002).

Researchers found that **one of the major causes of psychotic symptoms in schizophrenia is an excess of dopamine**. Most of the **antipsychotic medications work by blocking the dopamine receptors in the brain** thereby inhibiting the effects of the excess dopamine. Generally antipsychotic drugs work to alleviate the psychotic symptoms but do not cure the illness itself. This is true for all of the mental illnesses that have psychoses associated with them. The antipsychotic drugs are not without potentially serious side effects. The main difference between many of the antipsychotic drugs is their side effects profile.

The main side effects of antipsychotics have to do with the blockage of dopamine. From Table 10-2 you can see that dopamine controls muscle tone and motor behavior. **By blocking the dopamine, symptoms such as involuntary movement and the inability to sit still are common.** Parkinsonian syndrome (mainly a tremor but also loss of facial expression and slowed movements), akathisia (agitation, jumpiness exhibited by 75% of patients), akinesia (temporary loss of movement and apathy), and even the more serious tardive dyskinesia (involuntary movements of the jaws, head, neck, trunk, and extremities) are the most common complications when using these medications. Often anticholinergic medications, such as Cogentin®, Artane®, or even an antihistamine like Benadryl® are given to block side effects.

Please note however that there are other potentially serious side effects associated with antipsychotics. Although these medicines are relatively safe, extreme care should be taken before they are prescribed.

Another commonly encountered side effect of antipsychotic medications is sedation; **patients on antipsychotics may seem drugged**. Sedation is an unwanted side effect and is not the primary purpose of prescribing antipsychotic medications. There are times however that the astute clinician will take advantage of this side effect of sedation when treating the agitated psychotic patient. These drugs are dangerous when used as sleeping pills by patients who are not psychotic. They should never be used only to help control an agitated patient or as a sleep aid.

There is a trend toward using atypical antipsychotics such as risperidone (Risperdol®) in the acutely psychotic patient. As the antipsychotic drugs do not have an immediate effect on the patient's psychotic symptom, it may take several weeks to achieve full antipsychotic effect. During this time the patient should be treated with the lowest dose possible that is still exerting a clinical effect. After several weeks at this low dose, the amount may be slowly increased if the person remains with intractable psychotic symptoms. If after 4–6 weeks at this higher dose, the patient's symptoms remain unchanged then the clinician usually switches to a different type of antipsychotic. The patient's dose of antipsychotic medication can usually be safely lowered after the symptoms are under better control. This approach is particularly important in treating elderly patients.

Newer atypical antipsychotic drugs have recently been tested. Clozapine (Clozaril®) is usually effective in the 30% of patients who do not respond to standard antipsychotic drug therapy. Unfortunately weekly blood tests are necessary to monitor the side effects of clozapine, which make its use very expensive. Even newer atypical antipsychotics, like risperidone (Risperdal®) and olanzapine (Zyprexa®), do not have this problem but are still more expensive than the older antipsychotics. However, current best practice promotes the use of atypical antipsychotics over their less-expensive predecessors.

More than 33.5 million prescriptions were written for antipsychotic medications in the United States in 2001, up 34% from the previous 2 years. Even more dramatic is a 10-fold increase in the number of children who are using antipsychotics over the past decade (from 50,000 to 532,000) (Thomas, 2002).

Patients with a preexisting psychotic illness such as schizophrenia or schizoaffective disorder often self medicate with street drugs in an attempt to control their symptoms. The street drugs commonly used include heroin as well as other opiates, alcohol, marijuana, or sedative-hypnotics. Since all of these street drugs have dangerous toxic effects when combined with antipsychotic drugs, patients are exhorted to cease using them while under psychiatric treatment (Brier et al., 1997).

"I would drink alcohol with some of these pills that I was taking and I would really blackout, and I would loose consciousness pass out, and it was pretty bad, and I would have different types of side effects like blotchy skin, and it was bad, really, really, bad."

28-year-old addict with schizophrenia and bipolar disorder

DRUGS USED TO TREAT ANXIETY DISORDERS

For generalized anxiety disorder as well as some of the other anxiety disorders, the **benzodiazepines are widely used**. The most commonly prescribed are alprazolam (Xanax®), diazepam (Valium®), chlordiazepoxide (Librium®), and clorazepate (Tranxene®). Developed in the early 1960s, the benzodiazepines were considered safe substitutes for barbiturates and meprobamate (e.g., Miltown®). They act very quickly, particularly Valium®. **The calming effects are apparent within 30 minutes.** Some of the benzodiazepines are long acting (diazepam, chlordiazepoxide, clorazepate, clonazepam, prazepam, halazepam) and some are short acting (triazolam, lorazepam, temazepam). These drugs work because they facilitate inhibition by GABA, the major inhibitory neurotransmitter.

The main problem with benzodiazepines is that they are habit forming, even at clinical doses, and do have dangerous withdrawal symptoms. They should be avoided in treating the dually

diagnosed patient for whom they can retrigger drug abuse. There are many other medications that can be safely used with the dually diagnosed patient. These include BuSpar® and the beta blockers. Recently SSRI antidepressants such as Paxil®, have been approved for use in anxiety disorder (Ikeda, 1994; PDR, 2003).

With SSRIs and for almost all psychiatric medications, care should be taken when stopping the medication.

"I went off the Paxil®. I stopped immediately instead of tapering off of them and I had headaches; and again I was just really angry. My anxiety level, that is why I was taking it for, just shot up to the roof. I thought a couple of times I was having a heart attack. I went to my doctor and he told me flat out that you can not just stop taking the Paxil®, that you will have huge withdrawal symptoms."

38-year-old dual diagnosis patient

Buspirone (BuSpar®) is one of the only other drugs labeled for generalized anxiety disorder. It is a serotonin modulator and **will block the transmission of excess serotonin, one of the causes of the symptoms of many forms of anxiety**. It also mimics serotonin, so it can substitute for low levels of serotonin, a feature used by some doctors to treat depression. It takes 1–2 weeks to work and is not nearly as dramatic, initially, as the benzodiazepines. Consequently many patients are reluctant to use it. Its advantage however is that side effects are minimal and have not been shown to be habit forming.

As stated, the SSRIs such as Paxil® and Zoloft® are currently indicated for use in anxiety disorders. These drugs have a direct antianxiety effect and are not just used with depressed patients who also have anxious symptoms.

Drugs for Obsessive-Compulsive Disorder (OCD)

For the obsessive-compulsive disorder (OCD), almost every type of psychotropic medication has been tried in the past, usually with relatively poor results. Anafranil® (clomipramine) has recently been used with reasonable results. SSRIs like paroxetine, sertraline, and fluoxetine have also been used.

Drugs for Panic Disorder

Several drugs are used to control panic attacks and panic disorder. Previously benzodiazepines were the primary drug of choice for the treatment of panic disorders. As noted above, benzodiazepine-type medication should be avoided in the patient with dual diagnosis. **Current treatment recommendations include the use of SSRI antidepressant medications.** These are very effective in the treatment of panic and generally have a favorable side effect profile. These medications need to be taken daily and are not designed to treat a person with an acute panic attack.

Other frequently used medications in the treatment of panic are the beta blockers. They help to control both the physical and psychological symptoms associated with panic. Care should be taken when using beta blockers as they can have serious cardiac side effects in certain patients.

COMPLIANCE & FEEDBACK

The biggest problem with psychiatric medications (and with any prescription medication) is compliance with the physician's instructions. If patients aren't getting the desired effects, they will often alter the dosage on their own, simply stop taking the medication, or combine it with other medications causing dangerous interactions.

"I stopped taking it and got so depressed I took the remnants of both prescriptions, which was 1,000 mg of Seroquel® and 1,500 mg of Zoloft®. I took all at one time because I became so depressed. My fiancée and I had a fight and I wanted to kill myself."
38-year-old dually diagnosed male

Since the insurance coverage for office visits can be limited and because publicly funded treatment slots are limited, a patient might only see the physician once a month or less even at the beginning of use of a psychiatric medication when feedback is necessary to select the right drug and adjust the dose. The physician and client must both work in tandem for the greatest success. At the Haight Ashbury Detox Clinic, the clients have to come in almost every day.

"This clinic has been a lifesaver for me. I'm able to come in every day and talk to a therapist about how I'm feeling but also I'm able to talk to doctors and a pharmacist about how the medications are working, so they're able to make adjustments, modifications, changes on a daily basis, which has really helped me stabilize my moods and thoughts."
35-year-old patient at the Haight Ashbury Detox Clinic with schizoaffective diosorder

---

TABLE 10–3   MEDICATIONS USED TO HANDLE PSYCHIATRIC PROBLEMS

MAJOR DEPRESSION (antidepressants)

Selective serotonin reuptake inhibitors (SSRIs): citalopram (Celexa®), fluoxetine (Prozac®, Sarafem®), fluvoxamine (Luvox®), paroxetine (Paxil®), sertraline (Zoloft®), escitalopram (Lexapro®)

Tricyclic antidepressants: *tertiary amine tricyclics:* amitriptyline, (Elavil®, Endep®), clomipramine (Anafranil®), doxepin (Sinequan®, Adapin®), imipramine (Tofranil®, Janimine®), trimipramine (Surmontil®); *secondary amine tricyclics:* desipramine (Norpramin®, Pertofrane®), nortriptyline (Aventyl®, Pamelor®), protriptyline (Vivactil®); *tetracyclics:* amoxapine (Asendin®), maprotiline (Ludiomil®)

Dopamine-norepinephrine reuptake inhibitors: bupropion (Welbutrin®), bupropion SR (Wellbutrin SR®, Zyban®)

Serotonin-norepinephrine reuptake inhibitors: venlafaxine (Effexor®), venlafaxine XR (Effexor XR®), duloxetine

Serotonin modulators: nefazodone (Serzone®), trazodone (Desyrel®)

Norepinephrine-serotonin modulators: mirtazapine (Remeron®)

Monoamine oxidase (MAO) inhibitors: phenelzine (Nardil®), tranylcypromine (Parnate®), selegiline (Eldepryl®)

Stimulants used as antidepressants: amphetamine/methamphetamine (Adderall®, Dexadrine®, Biphetamine®, Desoxyn®), methylphenidate (Ritalin®), pemoline (Cylert®)

BIPOLAR AFFECTIVE DISORDER (mood stabilizers)

Lithium: Eskalith®, Lithobid®, carbamazepine (Tegretol®), valproic acid (Depakene®), divalproex sodium (Depakote®), olanzapine (Zyprexa®), oxcarbazepine (Trileptal®), gabapentin (Neurontin®), and topiramate (Topamax®)

THOUGHT DISORDERS (antipsychotics)

Butyrophenones: haloperidol (Haldol®)

Dibenzoxazepines: loxapine (Loxitane®), molindone (Moban®, Lidone®)

Heterocyclics: chlorprothixene (Taractan®), triflupromazine (Vesprin®)

Phenothiazines: chlorpromazine (Thorazine®), prochlorperazine (Compazine®)

Piperazines: acetophenazine (Tindal®), fluphenazine (Prolixin®, Permitil®), perphenazine (Trilafon®, Etrafon®), trifluoperazine (Stelazine®)

(continued)

TABLE 10–3   MEDICATIONS USED TO HANDLE PSYCHIATRIC PROBLEMS (*continued*)

Piperidines: mesoridazine (Serentil®), pimozide (Orap®), piperacetazine (Quide®), thioridazine (Mellaril®)
Thioxanthenes: thiothixene (Navane®)
Atypical antipsychotics: aripiprazole (Abilify®), clozapine (Clozaril®), olanzapine (Zyprexa®), quetiapine (Seroquel®), risperidone (Risperdal®), ziprasidone (Geodon®)
Drugs used to treat extrapyramidal side effects of antipsychotics: amantadine (Symmetrel®), benztropine (Cogentin®), diphenhydramine (Benadryl®), propranolol (Inderal®), trihexyphenidyl (Artane®)

GENERALIZED ANXIETY DISORDER (anxiolytics)

Benzodiazepines: *short-acting* (2–4-hour duration of action): alprazolam (Xanax®), lorazepam (Ativan®), oxazepam (Serax®), temazepam (Restoril®), triazolam (Halcion®); *long-acting* (6–24-hour duration of action): chlordiazepoxide (Librium®), clonazepam (Klonopin®), clorazepate (Tranxene®), diazepam (Valium®), halazepam (Paxipam®), prazepam (Centrax®)
Nonbenzodazepines: buspirone (BuSpar®), citalopram (Celexa®), paroxetine (Paxil®), venlafaxine (Effexor®)

OBSESSIVE-COMPULSIVE DISORDER (OCD)

Clomipramine (Anafranil®), fluoxetine (Prozac®), fluvoxamine maleate (Luvox®), sertraline (Zoloft®)

PANIC DISORDER

First-line drugs (medications that should be tried first to control panic): SSRIs (Zoloft®, Prozac®, Paxil®), alprazolam (Xanax®), clonazepam (Klonopin®), desipramine (Norpramin®, Pertofrane®), imipramine (Tofranil®)
Beta blockers: atenolol (Tenormin®), propranolol (Inderal®)
Others: MAO inhibitors, e.g., phenelzine (Nardil®) and tranycypromine (Parnate®)

SOCIAL PHOBIA

Beta blockers: atenolol (Tenormin®), propranolol (Inderal®)

POSTTRAUMATIC STRESS DISORDER

First-line drugs: SSRIs (Zoloft®, Paxil®)
Second-line drugs: beta-blockers (atenolol, pindolol [Visken®], propranolol [Prolixin®])

SLEEPING DISORDER

Benzodiazepines: clonazepam (Klonopin®), clorazepate (Tranxene®), extazolam (ProSom®), flurazepam (Dalmane®), oxazepam (Serax®), quazepam (Doral®), temazepam (Restoril®), triazolam (Halcion®), zaleplon (Sonata®), zolpidem (Ambien®)
Nonbenzodazepines: amitriptyline (Elavil®), chloral hydrate, diphenhydramine (Benadryl®), doxepin (Sinequan®), trazodone (Desyrel®)

ATTENTION-DEFICIT/HYPERACTIVITY DISORDER (ADHD)

Stimulants: amphetamine (Adderall®, Adderall XR®), pemoline (Cylert®), dextroamphetamine (Dexedrine®, DextroStat®, Dexedrine Spansule®), dexmethylphenidate (Focalin®), methylphenidate (Ritalin®, Methylin®, Metadate®, Concerta®)
Nonstimulant: atomoxetine (Strattera®)

(Keltner & Folks, 1997; PDR, 2003; Marangell, Silver, Martinez, & Yudofsky, 2002)

CHAPTER SUMMARY

MENTAL HEALTH & DRUGS

Introduction

1. Of the 40 million Americans with a mental illness, 7–10 million also have a substance-related disorder.

2. The neurotransmitters that are involved in mental illness are the same ones involved in drug abuse and addiction.

3. The direct effects of many psychoactive drugs as well as the withdrawal effects mimic many mental illnesses.

4. Substance-related disorders include substance use disorders (substance dependence and substance abuse) and substance-induced disorders (e.g., amphetamine psychosis, alcohol depression).

Determining Factors

5. Heredity, environment, and psychoactive drugs affect one's susceptibility to mental illness in much the same way they affect susceptibility to drug abuse and dependence.

6. The risk of developing a mental illness depends on heredity. The risk of a person developing schizophrenia if they have a close relative with schizophrenia jumps from 1% to 15%; for major depression it jumps from 5% to 15%; for a bipolar illness it jumps from 1% to 12%.

7. Environmental influences, such as extreme stress, can increase susceptibility to mental illness. Physical abuse in childhood is very common (50–75%) in those who are psychotic.

8. Psychoactive drugs can alter neurochemistry and aggravate preexisting mental illnesses, mimicking the symptoms of mental illness.

DUAL DIAGNOSIS (CO-OCCURRING DISORDERS)

Definition

9. Dual diagnosis is defined as "the co-occurrence of an interrelated mental disorder and a substance use disorder."

10. Preexisting mental disorders used to define dual diagnosis include thought or psychotic disorders (schizophrenia), mood or affective disorders (major depression, bipolar affective disorder), and anxiety disorders (panic disorder, posttraumatic stress disorder [PTSD]).

11. Substance-induced mental disorders include stimulant-induced psychotic disorders and alcohol-induced mood disorders. The symptoms usually disappear with abstinence.

12. It is common for drug abusers to present with symptoms of a personality disorder, e.g. antisocial personality disorder or borderline personality disorder. The symptoms can usually be minimized with abstinence.

Epidemiology

13. About 44% of alcohol abusers and 64.4% of substance abusers admitted for treatment also have a serious mental illness. Conversely 29–34% of mentally ill people have a problem with either alcohol or other drugs.

14. Up to 81% of those in prison with a drug problem also have a mental illness.

Patterns of Dual Diagnosis

15. One type of dual diagnosis is the person who has a clearly defined mental illness and then gets involved in drugs.

16. The second type of dual diagnosis is the direct result of substance abuse where the abuser develops psychiatric problems that are usually temporary but occasionally persist and evolve into a chronic mental health problem.

Making the Diagnosis

17. A psychiatric diagnosis should be a "rule-out diagnosis" where several possible diagnoses are considered. The clinician should avoid a specific diagnosis until the client has had time to get sober.

18. The number of dually diagnosed patients has increased due to the diminishing number of mental health care facilities, the proliferation of substances of abuse, the increasing numbers and greater expertise of licensed professionals in the field, and the pressures from managed care to diagnose a reimbursable illness.

19. Patients were often shuffled back and forth between the mental health care system and the substance abuse treatment system.

Mental Health vs. Substance Abuse

20. Five of the 11 main differences between the mental health (MH) treatment community and the substance abuse (SA) treatment community are

◇ MH says, "Control the psychiatric problem and the drug abuse will disappear." SA says, "Get the patient clean and sober and the mental health problem will disappear." Simultaneous treatment is necessary for one-third to three-fourths of the clients depending on the survey;

◇ in MH partial recovery is more acceptable whereas in SA most believe that lifetime abstinence is possible;

◇ MH often uses psychiatric drugs to treat the dual diagnosis patient whereas SA promotes a drug-free philosophy or occasionally a drug substitution (e.g., methadone) method;

◇ MH has a supportive psychotherapeutic approach philosophy whereas SA often uses a confrontative philosophy;

◇ MH keeps the client from getting worse while SA has a tendency to let people hit bottom to break through denial.

21. Health professionals need to reconcile the two philosophies of treatment to develop programs that treat both illnesses (mental illness and addiction).

22. Multiple diagnoses can include polydrug abuse, medical diseases, and hepatitis C in addition to a dually diagnosed client.

23. A triple diagnosis is defined as "HIV, drug abuse, and a mental illness." The explosive growth of triple diagnoses is straining health department resources. Comprehensive drug treatment programs that use multiple treatment modalities are necessary.

Psychiatric Disorders

24. Overall about 21% of the U.S. population is affected by mental disorders during a given year with anxiety disorders as the most prevalent.

25. A thought disorder, such as schizophrenia, is characterized by hallucinations, delusions, an inappropriate affect, poor association, and an impaired ability to care for oneself. It usually strikes individuals in their late teens and early adulthood. Several abused drugs can mimic schizophrenia particularly stimulants and psychedelics.

26. Major depressive disorder is characterized by a depressed mood, diminished interest and pleasure in most activities, sleep and appetite disturbances, feelings of worthlessness, and suicidal thoughts. Excessive alcohol use and stimulant drug withdrawal can cause temporary drug-induced depression.

27. A bipolar affective disorder involves manic phases alternating with depressive phases. Excess

stimulant or psychedelic abuse will often resemble a bipolar disorder.

28. Anxiety disorders include post-traumatic stress disorder (PTSD), panic disorder, agoraphobia, social phobia, simple phobia, obsessive-compulsive disorder, and a generalized anxiety disorder. Often anxiety and depression are mixed together.

29. Other mental illnesses include dementias (e.g., Alzheimer's disease), developmental disorders (e.g., ADHD), somatoform disorders (e.g., hypochondria), personality disorders, eating disorders, and compulsive gambling.

30. Substance-induced mental disorders are much more prevalent in substance abusers than psychiatric disorders.

31. Alcohol-induced mental illnesses include impulse control problems, sleep disturbance, anxiety, depression, psychosis, and dementia.

32. Stimulant-induced mental illnesses include impulse control problems, mania, panic disorder, depression, anxiety, psychosis, and cognitive impairment.

33. Marijuana-induced mental illnesses include delirium, psychosis, panic, and amotivational syndrome.

Treatment

34. Treatment for dual diagnosis can be done through psychotherapy, counseling, the group process, and especially with psychiatric medications.

35. Clients can be alerted to any genetic predisposition to addiction. Environment can be changed reducing stressors and drug-using cues. Psychiatric medications can be used to rebalance the neurochemistry of mental illness.

36. The drug dependence or abuse and the mental health problem need to be stabilized and then treated simultaneously.

37. Impaired cognition and developmental arrest make treatment of dual diagnosis difficult. Many people coming in for treatment are much younger emotionally than they are physically.

38. Group therapy has become the standard for substance abuse and mental illness treatments. For mental illness, psychopharmacology is the primary form of clinical treatment.

39. The three phases of psychotherapy are achieving abstinence, maintaining abstinence, and continuing psychotherapy along with psychiatric medication.

Psychopharmacology

40. The major classes of psychiatric drugs are antidepressants and mood stabilizers for mood disorders, antipsychotics (neuroleptics) for thought disorders (psychoses), and antianxiety medications for anxiety disorders. They can be used on a short-term, medium-term, and even lifetime basis.

41. Psychiatric medications manipulate brain chemistry in a variety of ways and relieve symptoms of mental illness. They can also cause undesirable and severe side effects and so should be closely monitored.

42. Many with mental illnesses try to self-medicate with street drugs or alcohol in order to feel in control of their lives.

43. Drugs used to treat depression are selective serotonin reuptake inhibitors (SSRIs) such as Prozac®, Zoloft®, Paxil®; tricyclic antidepressants; monoamine oxidase (MAO) inhibitors; and stimulants (e.g., amphetamines, methylphenidate).

44. The main drug used to treat a bipolar disorder is lithium. Carbamazepine (Tegretol®), valproic acid (Depakene®), and divalproex sodium (Depakote®) are also used.

45. Some of the drugs used to treat psychoses, such as schizophrenia, are halperidol (Haldol®), clozapine (Clozaril®), risperidine (Risperdal®), olanzapine (Zyprexa®), and the phenothiazines, e.g., chlorpromazine (Thorazine®). Mostly they control dopamine levels in the brain.

46. The principal drugs used to treat anxiety are the benzodiazepines, such as Valium® and Xanax®, and the nonbenzodiazepine buspirone (BuSpar®). Normally the benzodiazepines begin acting within 30 minutes while buspirone requires 1–2 weeks before its full effects are realized.

REFERENCES

Alcoholics Anonymous. (1995). *The AA Member—Medications and Other Drugs.* New York: Alcoholics Anonymous World Services, Inc.

American Psychiatric Association. (2000). *Diagnostic and Statistical Manual of Mental Disorders* (4th ed., text revision [DSM-IV-TR]). Washington, DC: Author.

Back, S. E., Sonne, S. C., Therese, K., Killeen, T., Dansky, B. S., & Brady, D. T. (2003). Comparative profiles of women with PTSD and comorbid cocaine or alcohol dependence. *American Journal of Drug & Alcohol Abuse, 29*(1), 169–189.

Barondes, S. H. (1993). *Molecules and Mental Illness.* New York: Scientific American Library.

Beeder, A. B., & Millman, R. B. (1997). Patients with psychopathology. In J. H. Lowenson, P. Ruiz, R. B. Millman, & J. G. Langrod (Eds.), *Substance Abuse, A Comprehensive Textbook* (3rd ed., pp. 551–562). Baltimore: Williams & Wilkins.

Biederman, J., Wilens, T., Mick, E., Spencer, T., & Faraone, S. V. (1999). Pharmacotherapy of attention deficit/hyperactivity disorder reduces risk for substance use disorder. *Pediatrics, 5.*

Blum, K., Braverman, E. R., Cull, J. G., Holder, J. M., Luck, R., Lubar, J., Miller, D., & Comings, D. E. (2000). "Reward deficiency syndrome" (RDS): A biogenetic model for the diagnosis and treatment of impulsive, addictive, and compulsive behaviors. *Journal of Psychoactive Drugs, 32*(supplement).

Blume, A. W., Davis, J. M., & Schmaling, K. B. (1999). Neurocognitive dysfunction in dually diagnosed patients: A potential roadblock to motivating behavior change. *Journal of Psychoactive Drugs, 31*(2), 111–115.

Brady, K. T. (1999). *Treatment of PTSD and substance use disorders.* Paper presented at the 152nd annual meeting of the American Psychiatric Association, Washington, DC.

Brady, K. T., Myrick, H., & Sonne, S. (1998). Comorbid addiction and affective disorders. In A. W. Graham & T. K. Schultz (Eds.), *Principles of Addiction Medicine* (2nd ed., pp. 983–992). Chevy Chase, MD: American Society of Addiction Medicine, Inc.

Brehm, N. M., & Khantzian, E. J. (1997). Psychodynamics. In J. H. Lowenson, P. Ruiz, R. B. Millman, & J. G. Langrod (Eds.), *Substance Abuse, A Comprehensive Textbook* (3rd ed., pp. 90–100). Baltimore: Williams & Wilkins.

Brier, A., Su, T. P., Saunders, R., Carson, R. E., Kolachana, B. S., De Bartolomeis, A., Weinberger, D. R., Weisenfeld, N., Malhotra, A. K., Eckelman, W. C., & Pickar, D. (1997). Schizophrenia is associated with elevated amphetamine-induced synaptic dopamine concentrations: Evidence from a novel positron emission tomography method. *Proceedings of the National Academy of Science, 94*, 2569–2574.

Brown, S. A., & Schuckit, M. A. (1988). Changes in depression among abstinent alcoholics. *Journal of Studies on Alcohol, 49*(5), 412–417.

Buxton, M. E., Smith, D. E., & Seymour, R. B. (1987). Spirituality and other points of resistance to the 12-step process. *Journal of Psychoactive Drugs, 19*(3), 275–286.

Clark, D. B., Vanyukov, M., & Cornelius, J. (2002). Childhood antisocial behavior and adolescent alcohol use disorders. *Alcohol Research & Health, 26*(2), 109–115.

Crome, I. B. (1999). Substance misuse and psychiatric comorbidity: Towards improved service provision. *Drugs: Education, Prevention and Policy, Source Id: 6*(2), 151–174.

Center for Substance Abuse Treatment. (1995). *Assessment and Treatment of Patients with Coexisting Mental Illness and Alcohol and Other Drug Abuse* (DHHS Publication No. (SMA) 95-3061). Rockville, MD: U.S. Department of Health and Human Services.

Dansky, B. S., Brewerton, T. D., & Kilpatrick, D. G. (2000). Comorbidity of bulimia nervosa and alcohol use disorders: Results from the National Women's Study. *International Journal of Eating Disorders, 27*, 180–190.

Dausey, D. J., & Desai, R. A. (2003). Psychiatric comorbidity and the prevalence of HIV infection in a sample of patients in treatment for substance abuse. *Journal of Nervous & Mental Disease, 191*(1), 10–17).

Davis, K., Klar, H., & Coyle, J. T. (1991). *Foundations of Psychiatry.* Philadelphia: Harcourt Brace Jovanovich, Inc.

Delgado, P. L., & Mereno, F. A. (1998). Hallucinogens, serotonin, and obsessive-compulsive disorder. *Journal of Psychoactive Drugs, 30*(4), 359–366.

Dimeoff, L. A., Comtois, K. A., & Linehan, M. M. (1998). Personality disorders. In A. W. Graham & T. K. Schultz (Eds.), *Principles of Addiction Medicine* (2nd ed., pp. 1062–1081). Chevy Chase, MD: American Society of Addiction Medicine, Inc.

Drake, R. E., Mercer-McFadden, C., Mueser, K. T., McHugo, G. J., & Bond, G. R. (1998). Review of integrated mental health and substance abuse treatment for patients with dual disorders. *Schizophrenia Bulletin, 24*, 589–608.

Drake, R. E., & Mueser, K. T. (1996). Alcohol-use disorder and severe mental illness. *Alcohol Health & Research World, 20*(2), 87–93.

Drake, R. E., & Mueser, K. T. (2002). Co-occurring alcohol use disorder and schizophrenia. *Alcohol Research & Health, 26*(2), 99–102.

Dumaine, M. L. (2003). Meta-analysis of interventions with co-occurring disorders of severe mental illness and substance abuse: Implications for social work practice. *Research on Social Work Practice, 13*(2), 142–165.

Evans, K., & Sullivan, J. M. (1990). *Dual Diagnosis: Counseling the Mentally Ill Substance Abuser.* New York: Guilford Publications.

Finnell, D. S. (2003). Use of the transtheoretical model for individuals with co-occurring disorders. *Community Mental Health Journal, 39*(1), 3–15.

Gastfriend, D. R., & Lillard, P. (1998). Anxiety disorders. In A. W. Graham & T. K. Schultz (Eds.), *Principles of Addiction Medicine* (2nd ed., pp. 983–1006). Chevy Chase, MD: American Society of Addiction Medicine, Inc.

Goldsmith, R. J., & Ries, R. K. (1998). Substance-induced mental disorders. In A. W. Graham & T. K. Schultz (Eds.), *Principles of Addiction Medicine* (2nd ed., pp. 969–982). Chevy Chase, MD: American Society of Addiction Medicine, Inc.

Goodwin, M.D. (1990). *Manic-Depressive Illness.* London: Oxford University Press.

Gottesman, I. I. (1991). *Schizophrenia Genetics: The Origins of Madness.* New York: W. H. Freeman and Co.

Grant, J. E., Kushner, M. G., & Kim, S. W. (2002). Pathological gambling and alcohol use disorder. *Alcohol Research & Health, 26*(2), 143–150.

Grella, C. (1996). Background and overview of mental health and substance abuse treatment systems: Meeting the needs of women who are pregnant and parenting. *Journal of Psychoactive Drugs, 28*(4), 319–344.

Grillo, C. M., Sinha, R., & O'Malley, S. S. (2002). Eating disorders and alcohol use disorders. *Alcohol Research & Health, 26*(2), 151–160.

Guydish, J., & Muck, R. (1999). The challenge of managed care in drug abuse treatment. *Journal of Psychoactive Drugs, 31*(3), 193–195.

Hasin, D. S., & Grant, B. F. (2002). Major depression in 6,050 former drinkers. *Archives of General Psychiatry, 59*(9), 794–800.

Ikeda, R. (1994). Prescribing for chronic anxiety disorders. *Journal of Psychoactive Drugs, 26*(1), 75–76.

Keller, D. S., & Dermatis, H. (1999). Current status of professional training in the addictions. *Substance Abuses: Journal of the Association for Medical Education and Research in Substance Abuse, 20*(3), 123–140.

Keltner, N. L., & Folks, D. G. (1997). *Psychotropic Drugs.* St. Louis: Mosby-Year Book, Inc.

Kendler, K. S., & Diehl, S. R. (1993). The genetics of schizophrenia: A current genetic-epidemiological perspective. *Schizophrenia Bulletin, 19*, 261–295.

Kendler, K. S., Heath, A. C., Neale, M. C., & Eaves, L. J. (1993). Alcoholism and major depression in women. A twin study of the causes of comorbidity.

Archives of General Psychiatry, 50(9), 690–698.

Kessler, R. C., Berglund, P., Demler, O., Jin, R., Koretz, D., Merikangas, K. R., Rush, J., Walters, E. E., & Wang, P. W. (2003). The epidemiology of major depressive disorder. *Journal of the American Medical Association, 289*, 3095–3105.

Kessler, R. C., McGonagle, K. A., Zhao, S., Nelson, C. B., Hughes, M., Eshleman, S., Wittchen, H. U., & Kendler, K. S. (1994). Lifetime and 12-month prevalence of DSM-III-R psychiatric disorders in the United States. Results from the National Comorbidity Survey. *Archives of General Psychiatry, 51*, 8–19.

Kosten, T. R., & Ziedonis, D. M. (1997). Substance abuse and schizophrenia: Editors' introduction. *Schizophrenia Bulletin, 23*, 181–186.

Kushner, M. G., Sher, K. J., & Erickson, D. J. (1999). Prospective analysis of the relation between DSM-III anxiety disorders and alcohol use disorders. *American Journal of Psychiatry, 156*(5), 723–732.

Lavine, R. (1999). Roles of the psychiatrist and the addiction medicine specialist in the treatment of addiction. *San Francisco Medicine, 72*(4), 20–22.

Levin, F. R., & Donovan, S. J. (1998). Attention deficit/hyperactivity disorder, intermittent explosive disorder, and eating disorders. In A. W. Graham & T. K. Schultz (Eds.), *Principles of Addiction Medicine* (2nd ed., pp. 1029–1046). Chevy Chase, MD: American Society of Addiction Medicine, Inc.

Lilenfeld, L. R., & Kaye, W. H. (1996). The link between alcoholism and eating disorders. *Alcohol Health & Research World, 20*(2), 94–99.

Mallouh, C. (1996). The effects of dual diagnosis on pregnancy and parenting. *Journal of Psychoactive Drugs, 26*(4), 367–380.

Marangell, L. B., Silver, J. M., Martinez, J. M., & Yudofsky, S. C. (2002). *Psychopharmacology*. Washington, DC: American Psychiatric Publishing, Inc.

McDowell, D. M. (1999). *Evaluation of depression in substance abuse*. Paper presented at the 152nd annual meeting of the American Psychiatric Association, Washington, DC.

McElroy, S. L., Soutullo, C. A., & Goldsmith, R. J. (1998). Other impulse control disorders. In A. W. Graham & T. K. Schultz (Eds.), *Principles of Addiction Medicine* (2nd ed., pp. 1047–1062).

Chevy Chase, MD: American Society of Addiction Medicine, Inc.

Merikangas, K. R., Stevens, D., & Fenton, B. (1996). Comorbidity of alcoholism and anxiety disorders: The role of family studies. *Alcohol Health & Research World, 20*(2), 100–106.

Miller, W., & Rollnick, S. (2000). *Motivational Interviewing*. New York: Guilford Publications.

Minkoff, K., & Regner, J. (1999). Innovations in integrated dual diagnosis treatment in public managed care: The Choate Dual Diagnosis Case Rate Program. *Journal of Psychoactive Drugs, 31*(1), 3–12.

National Institute of Mental Health. (1999). *Mental Health: A Report of the Surgeon General*. Rockville, MD: National Institute of Mental Health. Also [Online]. Available: *http://www.samhsa.gov/reports/congress2002/execsummary.htm*

Nunes, E. V., Donovan, S. J., Brady, R., & Guitkin, F. M. (1994). Evaluation and treatment of mood and anxiety disorders in opioid-dependent patients. *Journal of Psychoactive Drugs, 26*(2), 147–154.

O'Conner, P. G., & Ziedonis, D. M. (1998). Linkages of substance abuse with primary care and mental health treatment. In A. W. Graham & T. K. Schultz (Eds.), *Principles of Addiction Medicine* (2nd ed., pp. 353–362). Chevy Chase, MD: American Society of Addiction Medicine, Inc.

Osher, F. C. (2001). Co-occurring addictive and mental disorders. In R. W. Manderscheid & M. J. Henderson (Eds.), *Mental Health, United States, 2000*. DHHS Publication No. (SMA) o1-3537. Rockville, MD: Center for Mental Health Services.

Physician's Desk Reference. (2003). *Physicians Desk Reference (*57th ed.). Montvale, NJ: Medical Economics Company, Inc.

RachBeisel, J. Dixon, L., & Gearon, J. (1999). Awareness of substance abuse problems among dually diagnosed psychiatric inpatients. *Journal of Psychoactive Drugs, 31*(1), 53–7.

Rahav, M., Rivera, J. J., Nuttbrock, L., et al. (1995). Characteristics and treatment of homeless, mentally ill chemical-abusing men. *Journal of Psychoactive Drugs, 27*(1), 93–104.

Regier, D. A., Farmer, M. E., Rae, D. S., Locke, B. Z., Keith, S. J., Judd, L. L., & Goodwin, F. K. (1990). Comorbidity of mental disorders with alcohol and other drug abuse. Results from the Epidemi-

ological Catchment Area (ECA). *Journal of the American Medical Association, 264*(19), 2511–2518.

Reilly, P. M., Clark, H. W., Shopshire, M. S., Lewis, E. W., & Sorensen, D. J. (1994). Anger management and temper control: Critical components of posttraumatic stress disorder and substance abuse treatment. *Journal of Psychoactive Drugs, 26*(4), 401–408.

Ruzek, J. I. (2003). Concurrent posttraumatic stress disorder and substance use disorder among veterans. In P. Ouimette & P. J. Brown, (Eds.), *Trauma and Substance Abuse*. Washington, DC: American Psychological Association.

Salloum, I. M., & Daley, D. C. (1994). *Understanding Major Anxiety Disorders and Addiction*. Center City, MN: Hazelden Foundation.

Schuckit, M. A. (1986). Alcoholism and affective disorders: Genetic and clinical implications. *American Journal of Psychiatry, 143*, 140–147.

Schuckit, M. A. (2000). *Drug and Alcohol Abuse*. New York: Kluwer Academic/Plenum Publishers.

Selwyn, P. A., & Merino, F. L. (1997). Medical complications and treatment. In J. H. Lowenson, P. Ruiz, R. B. Millman, & J. G. Langrod (Eds.), *Substance Abuse, A Comprehensive Textbook* (3rd ed., pp. 597–682). Baltimore: Williams & Wilkins.

Senay, E. C. (1997). Diagnostic interview and mental status examination. In J. H. Lowenson, P. Ruiz, R. B. Millman, & J. G. Langrod (Eds.), *Substance Abuse, A Comprehensive Textbook* (3rd ed., pp. 364–368). Baltimore: Williams & Wilkins.

Senay, E. C. (1998). *Substance Abuse Disorders in Clinical Practice*. New York: W. W. Norton & Company.

Shaffer, D., Fisher, P., Dulcan, M. K., et al. (1996). The NIMH Diagnostic Interview Schedule for Children, Version 2.3. *Journal of the American Academy of Child and Adolescent Psychiatry, 35*, 865–877.

Shivani, R., Goldsmith, J., & Anthenelli, R. M. (2002). Alcoholsm and psychiatric disorders: Diagnostic challenges. *Alcohol Research & Health, 26*(2), 90–98.

Smith, D. E., Lawlor, B., & Seymour, R. B. (1996). Healthcare at the Crossroads. *San Francisco Medicine, 69*(6).

Smith, D. E., & Seymour, R. B. (2001). *The Clinician's Guide to Substance Abuse*. Center City, MN: Hazelden/McGraw Hill.

Soderstrom, C. A., Smith, G. S., Dischinger, P. C., McDuff, D. R., Hebel, J. R., Gorelick, D. A., Kerns, T. J, Ho, S. M., & Read, K. M. (1997). Psychoactive substance use disorders among seriously injured trauma center patients. *Journal of the American Medical Association, 277*(22), 1769–1775.

Sonne, S. C., & Brady, M. D. (2002). Bipolar disorder and alcoholism. *Alcohol Research & Health, 26*(2), 103–108.

Stahl, S. M. (2002). Dopamine system stabilizers, aripiprazole, and the next generation of antipsychotics. *Journal of Clinical Psychiatry, 62*(11–12).

Stewart, W. F., Ricci, J. A., Chee, E., Hahn, S., & Morganstein, D. (2003). Cost of lost productive work time among U.S. workers with depression. *Journal of the American Medical Association, 289*, 3135–3144.

Substance Abuse and Mental Health Services Administration. (2002a). Report to Congress on the prevention and treatment of co-occurring substance abuse disorders and mental disorders [Online]. Available: *http://www.samhsa. gov/reports/congress2002/foreword. htm*

Substance Abuse and Mental Health Services Administration. (2002b). Women, Co-Occurring Disorders and Violence Study [Online]. Available: *http://www.wcdvs.com/publications/default.asp*

Swanson, M. V., & Arthur, J. (2003). Use of the University of Rhode Island change assessment to measure motivational readiness to change in psychiatric and dually diagnosed individuals. *Psychology of Addictive Behaviors, 17*(2), 91–97.

Thomas, K. (2002, July 23). Surge in antipsychotic drugs given to kids draws concern. *USA Today*, p. D8.

U.S. Food and Drug Administration. (2003). FDA approves Prozac for pediatric use used to treat depression and OCD [Online]. Available: *http://www.fda.gov/ bbs/topics/ANSWERS/2003/ANS01187. html*

Watkins, K. E., Audrey, B., Kung, F. Y., & Paddock, S.(2001). A national survey of care for persons with co-occurring mental and substance abuse disorders. *Psychiatric Services, 52*(8), 1062–1068.

Wechsberg, W. M., Desmond, D., Inciardi, J. A., Leukefeld, C. G., Cottler, L. B., & Hoffman, J. (1999). HIV prevention protocols: Adaptation to evolving trends in drug use. *Journal of Psychoactive Drugs, 30*(3), 291–298.

Woody, G. E. (1996). The challenge of dual diagnosis. *Alcohol Health & Research World*, 20(2), 76–80.

Wu, L., Kouzis, A. C., & Leaf, P. J. (1999). Influence of comorbid alcohol and psychiatric disorders on utilization of mental health services in the National Comorbidity Survey. *American Journal of Psychiatry, 156*(8), 1230–1243.

Zickler, P. (1999). Twin studies help define the role of genes in vulnerability to drug abuse. *NIDA Notes, 14*(4).

Ziedonis, D., & Wyatt, S. (1998). Psychotic disorders. In A. W. Graham & T. K. Schultz (Eds.), *Principles of Addiction Medicine* (2nd ed., pp. 353–362). Chevy Chase, MD: American Society of Addiction Medicine, Inc.

Zimberg, S. (1994). Individual psychotherapy: Alcohol. In M. Galanter & H. D. Kleber (Eds.), *The American Psychiatric Press Textbook of Substance Abuse Treatment* (pp. 263–273). Washington, DC: American Psychiatric Press, Inc.

Zimberg, S. (1999). A dual diagnosis typology to improve diagnosis and treatment of dual disorder patients. *Journal of Psychoactive Drugs. 31*(1), 47–51.

Zweben, J. E. (1996). Psychiatric problems among alcohol and other drug-dependent women. *Journal of Psychoactive Drugs, 28*(4), 345–366.

Zweben, J. E. (1998). Integrating psychotherapy and pharmacotherapies in addiction treatment. In A. W. Graham & T. K. Schultz (Eds.), *Principles of Addiction Medicine* (2nd ed., pp. 1081–1089). Chevy Chase, MD: American Society of Addiction Medicine, Inc.

Zwillich, T. (1999). Beware of long-term effects of antidepressants. *Clinical Psychiatry News, 27*(9), 16.

INDEX